The Essence of Analgesia and Analgesics

The Essence of Analgesia and Analgesics

Edited by

Raymond S. Sinatra

Jonathan S. Jahr

J. Michael Watkins-Pitchford

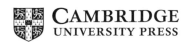
CAMBRIDGE
UNIVERSITY PRESS

CAMBRIDGE UNIVERSITY PRESS
Cambridge, New York, Melbourne, Madrid, Cape Town,
Singapore, São Paulo, Delhi, Dubai, Tokyo, Mexico City

Cambridge University Press
The Edinburgh Building, Cambridge CB2 8RU, UK

Published in the United States of America by Cambridge
University Press, New York

www.cambridge.org
Information on this title:
www.cambridge.org/9780521144506

First published 2011

Printed in the United Kingdom at the University Press,
Cambridge

*A catalog record for this publication is available from the
British Library*

Library of Congress Cataloging in Publication data

The essence of analgesia and analgesics / edited by Raymond
S. Sinatra, Jonathan S. Jahr, J. Michael Watkins-Pitchford.
    p. cm.
ISBN 978-0-521-14450-6 (pbk.)
1. Analgesics. 2. Analgesia. I. Sinatra, Raymond S. II. Jahr,
Jonathan S. III. Watkins-Pitchford, J. Michael.

RM319.E87 2010
615'.783–dc22   2010034377

ISBN 978-0-521-14450-6 Paperback

Contents

Section 3. Neuraxial Opioid Analgesics

Section 4. NSAIDs

Contributors

Shamsuddin Akhtar MD
Assistant Professor of Anesthesiology, Yale University School of Medicine, New Haven, CT, USA

Greg Albert MD
Resident in Anesthesiology, Yale University School of Medicine, New Haven, CT, USA

Sidney Allison
University at Buffalo, School of Medicine and Biomedical Sciences, Roswell Park Cancer Institute, Buffalo, NY, USA

Muhammad Anwar MD
Clinical Assistant Professor, Department of Anesthesiology, Yale University, School of Medicine, New Haven, CT, USA

Haruo Arita MD
Assistant Clinical Professor of Anesthesiology, Department of Anesthesiology, David Geffen School of Medicine at UCLA, Ronald Reagan UCLA Medical Center, Los Angeles, CA, USA

Amanda Barker
Pain Fellow, Department of Anesthesiology and Perioperative Care, UC Irvine School of Medicine, Irvine, CA, USA

Mary Hanna Bekhit MD
Assistant Clinical Professor of Anesthesiology, Department of Anesthesiology, David Geffen School of Medicine at UCLA, Ronald Reagan UCLA Medical Center, Los Angeles, CA, USA

Jeanna Blitz
NYU School of Medicine, New York City, NY, USA

Tyson Bolinske MD
Medical Student, University of North Dakota, and Research Associate in Anesthesiology, Department of Anesthesiology, Yale University School of Medicine, New Haven, CT, USA

David Burbulys MD
Assistant Clinical Professor of Anesthesiology, David Geffen School of Medicine at UCLA, Department of Anesthesiology, Harbor-UCLA Medical Center, Torrance, CA, USA

Asokumar Buvanendran MD
Associate Professor of Anesthesiology, Rush Presbyterian Medical Center, Chicago, IL, USA

Gregory Cain MSN, CRNA
Department of Anesthesiology, Yale University School of Medicine, New Haven, CT, USA

Keith A. Candiotti MD
Professor of Pain Medicine, and Vice-Chair University of Miami School of Medicine, Miami, FL, USA

Daniel B. Carr MD
Saltonstall Professor of Pain Research, Tufts Medical Center, Boston, MA, and Chief Medical Officer, Javelin Pharmaceuticals, Inc., Cambridge, MA, USA

Derek Chalmers PhD, DSc
President & CEO, Cara Therapeutics, Inc., Shelton, CT, USA

John Charney MD
Assistant Clinical Professor of Anesthesiology, David Geffen School of Medicine at UCLA, Department of Anesthesiology Harbor-UCLA Medical Center, Torrance, CA, USA

Rex Cheng MD
Assistant Clinical Professor of Anesthesiology, David Geffen School of Medicine at UCLA, Department of Anesthesiology, Harbor-UCLA Medical Center, Torrance, CA, USA

Roger Chou MD
Associate Professor of Medicine, Department of Medicine and Department of Medical Informatics and Clinical Epidemiology, Oregon Health & Science University, Portland, OR, USA

Keun Sam Chung MD
Assistant Professor of Anesthesiology, Yale University School of Medicine, New Haven, CT, USA

Anna Clebone MD
Resident in Anesthesiology, Yale University School of Medicine, New Haven, CT, USA

Frederick Conlin MD
Resident in Anesthesiology, Yale University School of Medicine, New Haven, CT, USA

Susan Dabu-Bondoc MD
Assistant Professor of Anesthesiology, Yale University School of Medicine, New Haven, CT, USA

Tiffany Denepitiya-Balicki MD
Resident in Anesthesiology, Yale University School of Medicine, Cedar Street, New Haven, CT, USA

Jeanette Derdemezi MD
Assistant Clinical Professor of Anesthesiology, David Geffen School of Medicine at UCLA, Department of Anesthesiology, Harbor-UCLA Medical Center, Torrance, CA, USA

Anahat Kaur Dhillon MD
Assistant Clinical Professor of Anesthesiology, Department of Anesthesiology, David Geffen School of Medicine at UCLA, Ronald Reagan UCLA Medical Center, Los Angeles, CA, USA

Ho Dzung MD
Pain Fellow, Department of Anesthesiology, University at Buffalo, Buffalo, NY, USA

Juan Jose Egas MD
Resident in Anesthesiology, Yale University School of Medicine, New Haven, CT, USA

Stephen M. Eskaros MD
Assistant Clinical Professor of Anesthesiology, Department of Anesthesiology, David Geffen School of Medicine at UCLA, Ronald Reagan UCLA Medical Center, Los Angeles, CA, USA

Zhuang T. Fang MD
Assistant Clinical Professor of Anesthesiology, Department of Anesthesiology, David Geffen School of Medicine at UCLA, Ronald Reagan UCLA Medical Center, Los Angeles, CA, USA

Claudia R. Fernandez Robles MD
Assistant Professor of Pain Medicine, University of Miami School of Medicine, Miami, FL, USA

Victor A. Filadora II
University at Buffalo, School of Medicine and Biomedical Sciences, Roswell Park Cancer Institute, Buffalo, NY, USA

Ellen Flanagan
Assistant Professor of Anesthesiology, Duke University Medical Center, Durham, NC, USA

Dan Froicu MD
Resident in Anesthesiology, Yale University School of Medicine, New Haven, CT, USA

Allison Gandey BJ, MJ
Senior Journalist, Medscape Neurology, WebMD Professional News, New York, NY, USA

Nehal Gatha MD
Resident in Anesthesiology, Yale University School of Medicine, New Haven, CT, USA

Boris Gelman MD
Assistant Professor of Anesthesiology, Department of Anesthesiology, David Geffen School of Medicine at UCLA, Ronald Reagan UCLA Medical Center, Los Angeles, CA, USA

Christopher Gharibo MD
Pain Management Clinic, NYU Department of Anesthesiology, New York, NY, USA

Muhammad K. Ghori MD
Assistant Professor of Anesthesiology, Yale University School of Medicine, and Attending Anesthesiologist, West Haven VA Medical Center, New Haven, CT, USA

Brian Ginsberg MB BCh, FFA
Associate Professor, Medical Director, Acute Pain Service, Duke University Medical Center, Durham, NC, USA

Michael E. Goldberg MD
Professor and Chief, Department of Anesthesiology,
Cooper University Hospital, The Robert Wood
Johnson Medical School – UMDNJ, Camden, NJ,
USA

Jeff Gudin MD
Director, Pain Management, Englewood Hospital,
Englewood, NJ, USA

Thomas Halaszynski DMD, MD, MBA
Associate Professor of Anesthesiology, Yale
University School of Medicine, New Haven, CT, USA

Martin Hale MD
Medical Director, Gold Coast Research LLC, Weston,
FL, USA

Dorothea Hall MD
Clinical Assistant Professor of Anesthesiology,
Department of Anesthesiology, David Geffen School
of Medicine at UCLA, Ronald Reagan UCLA Medical
Center, Los Angeles, CA, USA

Craig T. Hartrick MD
Director, Academic Affairs, Beaumont Hospital,
Royal Oak, MI, USA

Justin Hata MD
Assistant Clinical Professor, Departments of Anesthesio-
logy & Perioperative Care, PM&R Acting Director,
Division of Pain Medicine, and Co-director, UC Irvine
Comprehensive Spine Program, UCI Medical Center, USA

Lars E. Helgeson MD
Assistant Professor of Anesthesiology, Yale University
School of Medicine, New Haven, CT, USA

Joe C. Hong MD
Assistant Clinical Professor of Anesthesiology,
Department of Anesthesiology, David Geffen School
of Medicine at UCLA, Ronald Reagan UCLA Medical
Center, Los Angeles, CA, USA

Richard W. Hong MD
Assistant Clinical Professor of Anesthesiology,
Department of Anesthesiology, David Geffen School
of Medicine at UCLA, Ronald Reagan UCLA Medical
Center, Los Angeles, CA, USA

Balazs Horvath MD
Assistant Professor of Anesthesiology, Yale University
School of Medicine, New Haven, CT, USA

Eric S. Hsu MD
Clinical Professor of Anesthesiology and Director Pain
Fellowship Program, Department of Anesthesiology,
David Geffen School of Medicine at UCLA, Ronald
Reagan UCLA Medical Center, Los Angeles, CA, USA

Gabriel Jacobs
Resident in Anesthesiology, Yale University School of
Medicine, New Haven, CT, USA

Jonathan S. Jahr MD
Professor of Clinical Anesthesiology, David Geffen
School of Medicine at UCLA, Ronald Reagan UCLA
Medical Center, Los Angeles, CA, USA

Rongjie Jaing MD
Resident in Anesthesiology, Yale University School of
Medicine, New Haven, CT, USA

Inderjeet Singh Julka MD
Assistant Clinical Professor of Anesthesiology, David
Geffen School of Medicine at UCLA, Department
of Anesthesiology, Harbor-UCLA Medical Center,
Torrance, CA, USA

Zeev N. Kain MD, MBA
Professor of Anesthesiology and Pediatrics and
Psychiatry, Chair Department of Anesthesiology
and Perioperative Care, Associate Dean of Clinical
Research, School of Medicine, University of
California, Irvine, Orange, CA, USA

Clinton Kakazu MD
Assistant Clinical Professor of Anesthesiology, David
Geffen School of Medicine at UCLA, Department
of Anesthesiology, Harbor-UCLA Medical Center,
Torrance, CA, USA

Kianusch Kiai MD
Associate Clinical Professor of Anesthesiology,
Department of Anesthesiology, David Geffen School
of Medicine at UCLA, Ronald Reagan UCLA Medical
Center, Los Angeles, CA, USA

Mary Keyes MD
Clinical Professor of Anesthesiology, Department of
Anesthesiology, David Geffen School of Medicine at
UCLA, Ronald Reagan UCLA Medical Center, Los
Angeles, CA, USA

Michael M. Kim MD
Director, Resident Education in Pain Medicine,
Department of Anesthesiology & Perioperative Care,

University of California, Irvine Medical Center, Orange, CA, USA

Peter G. Lacouture MS, PhD
Executive Director, Scientific & Medical Affairs, Magidom Discovery, Lithia, FL, USA, and Adjust Assistant Professor of Medicine, Brown University School of Medicine, Providence, RI, USA

Ryan Lanier
Senior scientist, Rock Creek Pharmaceuticals, Gloucester, MA, USA

Vivian K. Lee MD
Resident Physician, Department of Anesthesiology, David Geffen School of Medicine at UCLA, Ronald Reagan UCLA Medical Center, Los Angeles, CA, USA

Mark J. Lema MD
Professor and Chair, Department of Anesthesiology, University at Buffalo – SUNY, Roswell Park Cancer Institute, Buffalo, NY, USA

Oscar A. de Leon-Casasola MD
Director, Pain Management, Department of Anesthesiology, Roswell-Park Cancer Center, Buffalo, NY, USA

Imanuel Lerman MD
Internal Medicine Doctor, Department of Neurology, Yale University School of Medicine New Haven, CT, USA

Philip Levin MD
Associate Clinical Professor of Anesthesiology, Department of Anesthesiology, David Geffen School of Medicine at UCLA, Santa Monica/UCLA and Orthopaedics Hospital and Medical Center, Los Angeles, CA, USA

Steven Levin MD
Advanced Diagnostic Pain Treatment Centers, Yale New Haven Medical at Long Wharf, New Haven, CT, USA

JinLei Li MD
Resident in Anesthesiology, Yale University School of Medicine, New Haven, CT, USA

Eric C. Lin
Yale University School of Medicine, New Haven, CT, USA

Sharon Lin MD
Assistant Clinical Professor, University of California, Irvine, Department of Anesthesiology and Perioperative Care, Orange, CA, USA

David A. Lindley DO
Anesthesiology and Pain Management, University of Miami, Miami, FL, USA

Ana M. Lobo MD
Assistant Professor of Anesthesiology, Yale University School of Medicine, Department of Anesthesiology, New Haven CT, USA

Marisa Lomanto MD
Pain Fellow, Yale-New Haven Hospital, Yale University School of Medicine, Department of Anesthesiology, New Haven, CT, USA

Mirjana Lovrincevic MD
Associate Professor of Anesthesiology and Oncology, University at Buffalo-SUNY, School of Medicine and Biomedical Sciences, Buffalo, NY, USA

Brenda C. McClain MD
Associate Professor of Anesthesiology, Yale University School of Medicine, New Haven, CT, USA

Tariq Malik MD
Assistant Professor of Anesthesiology, University of Chicago School of Medicine, Department of Anesthesia and Critical Care, Chicago, IL, USA

Jure Marijic MD
Associate Clinical Professor of Anesthesiology, Department of Anesthesiology, David Geffen School of Medicine at UCLA, Ronald Reagan UCLA Medical Center, Los Angeles, CA, USA

Joseph Marino MD
Attending Anesthesiologist and Director, Acute Pain Management Service, Huntington Hospital, Huntington, NY, USA

Laura Mechtler
Medical Student, Hungary

Alan Miller MD
Section of Interventional Pain Management, Jefferson Medical College, Philadelphia, PA, USA

Carly Miller MD
Section of Interventional Pain Management, Jefferson Medical College, Philadelphia, PA, USA

Amit Mirchandani MD
Resident in Anesthesiology, Yale University School of Medicine, New Haven, CT, USA

Sukanya Mitra MD
Associate Professor, Department of Anaesthesia and Intensive Care, Government Medical College and Hospital, Chandigarh, India

Fleurise Montecillo
Resident in Anesthesiology, NYU Department of Anesthesiology, New York, NY, USA

James M. Moore MD
Associate Clinical Professor of Anesthesiology, Department of Anesthesiology, David Geffen School of Medicine at UCLA, Ronald Reagan UCLA Medical Center, Los Angeles, CA, USA

Debra E. Morrison MD
Director, Pediatric & Neonatal Anesthesia Services, School of Medicine, University of California, Irvine, Orange, CA, USA

Philip F. Morway MD
Assistant Clinical Professor of Anesthesiology, Department of Anesthesiology, David Geffen School of Medicine at UCLA, Santa Monica/UCLA and Orthopaedics Hospital and Medical Center, Los Angeles, CA, USA

Carsten Nadjat-Haiem MD
Assistant Clinical Professor of Anesthesiology, Department of Anesthesiology, David Geffen School of Medicine at UCLA, Ronald Reagan UCLA Medical Center, Los Angeles, CA, USA

Hamid Nourmand MD
Associate Clinical Professor of Anesthesiology, Department of Anesthesiology, David Geffen School of Medicine at UCLA, Ronald Reagan UCLA Medical Center, Los Angeles, CA, USA

Dana Oprea MD
Fellow in Anesthesiology, Yale University School of Medicine, New Haven, CT, USA

Sunil J. Panchal MD
Director, National Institute of Pain, Lutz, FL, USA

Edward J. Park MD
Assistant Clinical Professor of Anesthesiology, Department of Anesthesiology, David Geffen School of Medicine at UCLA, Ronald Reagan UCLA Medical Center, Los Angeles, CA, USA

Kathleen Ji Park
University at Buffalo, School of Medicine and Biomedical Sciences, Roswell Park Cancer Institute, Buffalo, NY, USA

Kellie Park MD
Resident in Anesthesiology, Yale University School of Medicine, New Haven, CT, USA

Parisa Partownavid MD
Assistant Clinical Professor of Anesthesiology, Department of Anesthesiology, David Geffen School of Medicine at UCLA, Ronald Reagan UCLA Medical Center, Los Angeles, CA, USA

Akta Patel
Thomas Jefferson University, Philadelphia, PA, USA

Bijal Patel
Resident in Anesthesiology, Yale University School of Medicine, New Haven, CT, USA

Komal D. Patel MD
Assistant Clinical Professor of Anesthesiology, Department of Anesthesiology, David Geffen School of Medicine at UCLA, Ronald Reagan UCLA Medical Center, Los Angeles, CA, USA

Neesa Patel MD
Assistant Clinical Professor of Anesthesiology, Department of Anesthesiology, David Geffen School of Medicine at UCLA, Ronald Reagan UCLA Medical Center, Los Angeles, CA, USA

Swati Patel MD
Associate Clinical Professor of Anesthesiology, Department of Anesthesiology, David Geffen School of Medicine at UCLA, Ronald Reagen UCLA Medical Center, Los Angeles, CA, USA

Paul M. Peloso MD, MSc
Merck & Co., Inc., NJ, USA

Danielle Perret MD
Director, Fellowship Training Program in Pain Medicine, Department of Anesthesiology & Perioperative Care, and Department of Physical Medicine and Rehabilitation, University of California, Irvine Medical Center, Orange, CA, USA

Anthony DePlato
University at Buffalo, School of Medicine and Biomedical Sciences, Roswell Park Cancer Institute, Buffalo, NY, USA

Marjorie Podraza Stiegler MD
Assistant Clinical Professor of Anesthesiology, Department of Anesthesiology, David Geffen School of Medicine at UCLA, Ronald Reagan UCLA Medical Center, Los Angeles, CA, USA

Despina Psillides MD
Department of Anesthesiology, Yale University School of Medicine, New Haven, CT, USA

Mamatha Punjala MD
Assistant Professor of Anesthesiology, Yale University School of Medicine, New Haven, CT, USA

Johan Raeder MD, PhD
Professor in Anaesthesiology and Chairman of Clinical Ambulatory Anaesthesia, Oslo University Hospital, Ullevaal, Oslo, Norway

Siamak Rahman MD
Assistant Clinical Professor of Anesthesiology, Department of Anesthesiology, David Geffen School of Medicine at UCLA, Ronald Reagan UCLA Medical Center, Los Angeles, CA, USA

Aziz M. Razzuk MD
Research Associate, Occupational Health Services, Kaiser Permanente, Honolulu, Hawaii

Maggy G. Riad MD
Assistant Clinical Professor of Anesthesiology, Department of Anesthesiology, David Geffen School of Medicine at UCLA, Ronald Reagan UCLA Medical Center, Los Angeles, CA, USA

Kristin L. Richards MD
Resident in Anesthesiology, Yale University School of Medicine, New Haven, CT, USA

R. Todd Rinnier DO
Chief Resident, Department of Anesthesiology, Cooper University Hospital, The Robert Wood Johnson Medical School – UMDNJ, Camden, NJ, USA

Ian W. Rodger BSc, PhD, MRPharmS, FRCP
Vice President, Research & Academic, St Joseph's Healthcare Hamilton, and Professor, Department of Medicine, McMaster University, Hamilton, Ontario, Canada

Joseph Rosa MD
Clinical Professor of Anesthesiology, Department of Anesthesiology, David Geffen School of Medicine at UCLA, Ronald Reagan UCLA Medical Center, Los Angeles, CA, USA

Abraham Rosenbaum MD
Assistant Professor of Clinical Anesthesia, Section of Pediatric Anesthesia, University of California Irvine Medical Center, Orange, CA, USA

Alireza Sadoughi MD
Associate Clinical Professor of Anesthesiology, Department of Anesthesiology, David Geffen School of Medicine at UCLA, Ronald Reagan UCLA Medical Center, Los Angeles, CA, USA

Veena Salgar MD
Assistant Professor of Anesthesiology, Yale University School of Medicine, New Haven, CT, USA

Leslie Schechter
Department of Pharmacy, Thomas Jefferson University Hospital, Philadelphia, PA, USA

Michael Seneca MSN, CRNA
Department of Anesthesiology, Yale University School of Medicine, New Haven, CT, USA

Yasser F. Shaheen MD
Assistant Clinical Professor, Division Director, NORA, Department of Anesthesia, Yale University School of Medicine , New Haven, CT, USA

James H. Shull MD
Resident in Anesthesiology, Yale University School of Medicine, New Haven, CT, USA

Elizabeth Sinatra BS
Research Associate in Anesthesiology, Yale University School of Medicine, New Haven, CT, USA

Raymond S. Sinatra MD
Professor of Anesthesiology, Yale University School of Medicine, New Haven, CT, USA

Neil Singla MD
Director of Clinical Research, Department of Anesthesia, Lotus Clinical Research, Huntington Hospital, Pasadena, CA, USA

Neil Sinha MD
Resident in Anesthesiology, Yale University School of Medicine, New Haven, CT, USA

Denis V. Snegovskikh MD
Assistant Professor of Anesthesiology, Department of Anesthesiology, Yale University School of Medicine, New Haven, CT, USA

Dmitri Souzdalnitski MD
Resident in Anesthesiology, Yale University School of Medicine, New Haven, CT, USA

Julie Sramcik MD
Assistant Professor of Anesthesiology, Yale University School of Medicine, New Haven, CT, USA

Zoreh Steffens MD
Assistant Clinical Professor of Anesthesiology, Department of Anesthesiology, David Geffen School of Medicine at UCLA, Harbor-UCLA Medical Center, Torrance, CA, USA

Alexander Timchenko MD
Resident in Anesthesiology, Yale University School of Medicine, New Haven, CT, USA

Vadim Tokhner MD
Assistant Clinical Professor of Anesthesiology, Department of Anesthesiology, David Geffen School of Medicine at UCLA, Harbor-UCLA Medical Center, Torrance, CA, USA

Marc C. Torjman PhD
Professor and Director of Research, Department of Anesthesiology, Cooper University Hospital, The Robert Wood Johnson Medical School – UMDNJ, Camden, New Jersey, USA

Co T. Truong MD
University of California Irvine Medical Center, Los Angeles, CA, USA

Nalini Vadivelu MD
Associate Professor of Anesthesiology, Yale University School of Medicine, New Haven, CT, USA

Ashley Vaughn MSN, CRNA
Department of Anesthesiology, Yale University School of Medicine, New Haven, CT, USA

Anjali Vira MD
Resident in Anesthesiology, Yale University School of Medicine, New Haven, CT, USA

Eugene R. Viscusi MD
Associate Professor of Anesthesiology, Jefferson Medical College, Philadelphia, PA, USA

Dajie Wang MD
Jefferson Medical College, Philadelphia, PA, USA

Shu-ming Wang MD
Associate Professor of Anesthesiology, Yale University School of Medicine, New Haven, CT, USA

J. Michael Watkins-Pitchford MD
Assistant Professor of Anesthesiology, Yale University School of Medicine, New Haven, CT, USA

Steven J. Weisman MD
Jane B. Pettit Chair in Pain Management, Children's Hospital of Wisconsin, and Professor of Anesthesiology and Pediatrics, Medical College of Wisconsin, Milwaukee, WI, USA

Ira Whitten MD
Resident in Anesthesiology, Yale University School of Medicine, New Haven, CT, USA

Bryan S. Williams MD MPH
Assistant Professor of Anesthesiology, Division of Pain Medicine, Rush Presbyterian Medical Center, Chicago, IL, USA

Jeremy M. Wong MD
Assistant Professor of Anesthesiology, Department of Anesthesiology, David Geffen School of Medicine at UCLA, Ronald Reagan UCLA Medical Center, Los Angeles, CA, USA

Thomas Wong MD
Instructor of Anesthesiology, Yale University School of Medicine, New Haven, CT, USA

Christopher Wray MD
Assistant Clinical Professor of Anesthesiology,
Department of Anesthesiology, David Geffen School
of Medicine at UCLA, Ronald Reagan UCLA Medical
Center, Los Angeles, CA, USA

Yaw Wu MD
Assistant Clinical Professor of Anesthesiology,
Department of Anesthesiology, David Geffen School
of Medicine at UCLA, Harbor-UCLA Medical
Center, Torrance, CA, USA

Anthony T. Yarussi MD
Assistant Professor of Anesthesiology, University
at Buffalo, School of Medicine and Biomedical
Sciences, Roswell Park Cancer Institute, Buffalo, NY,
USA

Laurie Yonemoto MD
Resident in Anesthesiology, Yale University School of
Medicine, New Haven, CT, USA

Bita H. Zadeh MD
Assistant Clinical Professor of Anesthesiology,
Department of Anesthesiology, David Geffen
School of Medicine at UCLA, Ronald Reagan
UCLA Medical Center, Los Angeles, CA, USA

Jill Zafar MD
Assistant Professor of Anesthesiology, University at
Buffalo, School of Medicine and Biomedical Sciences,
Roswell Park Cancer Institute, Buffalo, NY, USA

Martha Zegarra MD
Resident in Anesthesiology, Yale University School of
Medicine, New Haven, CT, USA

Keren Ziv MD
Assistant Clinical Professor of Anesthesiology,
Department of Anesthesiology, David Geffen
School of Medicine at UCLA, Ronald Reagan
UCLA Medical Center, Los Angeles, CA,
USA

Introduction

Ian W. Rodger

Pain is a wholly tormenting, disagreeable, multi-factorial sensory experience. It is defined by the International Association for the Study of Pain (IASP) as *"An unpleasant sensory and emotional experience associated with actual or potential tissue damage, or described in terms of such damage"*. Pain intensity can vary from mild to severe. Its duration can be transient, acute, intermittent or persistent. Several distinct, but frequently overlapping, types of pain are recognized: nociceptive/physiological, inflammatory and neuropathic. All pain is initially detected by a highly specialized sensory apparatus, the nociceptor, located on sensory nerve terminals. Once activated by a noxious stimulus the nociceptor transduces the signal into an electrical impulse (action potential) that travels up the primary sensory neuron *en route* to the brain. Given the extensive neural and neurochemical processes that are involved in pain signaling it is apparent that there are abundant points at which chemical/drug interference with these processes can occur. The vast array of analgesics and analgesic adjuncts that we have available today all have one thing in common; they interfere with the pain signaling cascade in delivering their analgesic effect(s).

Today healthcare providers are faced with a bewildering number of analgesics and adjunct agents in addressing different pain conditions in their patients. Indeed, the variety of analgesic agents available is also frequently mystifying to experts in the field. Furthermore, the intensity of pain research has accelerated dramatically in recent years given the recognition that there is an enormous unmet medical need for improved pain therapies, especially for those difficult to treat, intractable pain states. Thus, under the glare of this spotlight the complex molecular, genetic and pathophysiological mechanisms underlying different types of pain are steadily being unraveled. With this understanding has come the consequent realization that improved pain control is entirely feasible not only with the analgesics available today but also with those that are on the horizon for tomorrow. That said, however, today we work with analgesics that have unique sites of action. They work peripherally and/or centrally, frequently have several sites of action, come in a variety of dose strengths and formulations and have a wide variety of durations of action. It is no surprise, therefore, that many analgesics also come burdened with a far less than desirable side-effect profile and significant potential for interactions and toxicity.

In this textbook the editors have chosen to divide the subject literature available into twelve sections, each with a particular focus. Section 1 concentrates on setting the stage for an understanding of analgesic action. Thus, it describes the definitions and characteristics of different types of pain, the various pain pathways including mechanisms underlying both peripheral and central sensitization (aspects of wind-up) and other elements of analgesic theory. Sections 2 through 11 describe the essence of commonly prescribed acute and chronic pain medications. As a deliberate policy, and for both convenience and continuity, the editors have opted to list each analgesic according to its drug class. The final section (12) deals with new and emerging therapies. This section provides details of how existing therapies are being re-engineered and reformulated to provide superior analgesic control. It also provides a glimpse of the future by identifying new molecular targets that hold promise for the discovery and development of novel analgesics with completely new mechanisms of action.

In the final analysis this textbook provides a host of welcome information, tightly packaged, that provides a much needed reference source on analgesia and analgesics. It will benefit all healthcare professionals tasked with the responsibility of optimizing the control, and ideally the elimination, of pain and suffering.

The Essence of Analgesia and Analgesics, ed. Raymond S. Sinatra, Jonathan S. Jahr and J. Michael Watkins-Pitchford. Published by Cambridge University Press. © Cambridge University Press 2011.

Pain definitions and assessment

Raymond S. Sinatra

Introduction

Pain is among the most common of patient complaints encountered by health professionals and it remains the number one cause of absenteeism and disability. Each year, more than 60 million trauma-related pain episodes occur in the USA, as well as acute pain related to over 40 million surgical procedures [1]. Pain has been defined by the International Association for the Study of Pain as "an unpleasant sensory and emotional experience associated with actual or potential tissue damage" [2]. In clinical settings, it has been suggested that presence of pain and the intensity of discomfort are whatever the patient says they are unless proven otherwise by poor adherence to an agreed treatment plan [3–5]. We now recognize that in addition to the ethical and humanitarian reasons for minimizing discomfort and suffering, pain-related anxiety, sleeplessness and release of stress hormones or catecholamines may have deleterious effects upon post-surgical outcome, and may lead to the development of chronic pain [6–8].

Classification of pain

Pain is a complex physiological process that can be classified in terms of its intensity (mild, moderate, severe) its duration (acute, convalescent, chronic), its mechanism (physiological, nociceptive, neuropathic), and its clinical context, (post-surgical, malignancy-related, neuropathic, degenerative, etc.) [2]. Pain detection, or nociception, requires the activation of specialized transducers called nociceptors, which are the peripheral endings of A-delta (Aδ) and (C) sensory fibers. Nociceptors are activated following thermal, mechanical or chemical tissue injuries, and initiate afferent transmission of action potentials to the dorsal horn of the spinal cord. Pain perception follows activation of second-order sensory neurons which relay noxious signals to higher thalamic and cortical centers (Figure 2.1).

The mechanistic classification of pain is as follows [2,4,5]. (1) Physiological pain is defined as brief, rapidly perceived, non-traumatic discomfort that identifies a potentially dangerous stimulus. This adaptive alerting response involves cortical perception and localization and a reflex withdrawal that prevent and/or minimize tissue injury. Physiological pain is also associated with learned avoidance and adaptation that can modify future behavior. (2) Nociceptive pain results from the activation of physiologically normal nerve fibers in response to tissue injury. In addition to cellular damage and neural irritation, humoral mediators and peripheral inflammatory responses play a major role in its initiation and progression. Nociceptive pain can be further divided into somatic and visceral pain subtypes. Somatic nociceptive pain is well localized, sharp, crushing, or tearing pain that follows traumatic injury to dermatomally inervated structures. It includes cutaneous, muscular and ligamentous pain, but also includes headache and osteogenic pain. In contrast, visceral nociceptive pain is poorly localized non-dermatomal specific discomfort that is usually described as dull, cramping, or colicky. Visceral pain includes discomfort related to bowel obstruction, first-stage labor, dilatation of hollow viscus, early appendicitis and peritoneal irritation. Visceral pain is mediated by free nerve endings in gastro intestinal organs and peritoneum that respond to irritation or distention. Referred pain is a special form of visceral pain that radiates in a somatic dermatomal pattern. Referred pain may be explained by convergence of spinal input theory, or reflex response theory [2].(3) Neuropathic pain results from irritation, infection, degeneration, transaction or compression injury to nervous tissue. It is usually characterized as burning, electrical and/or shooting in nature. Pain following injury to sensory nerves is termed causalgia or chronic regional pain syndrome II. Pain associated with injury or abnormal activity

The Essence of Analgesia and Analgesics, ed. Raymond S. Sinatra, Jonathan S. Jahr and J. Michael Watkins-Pitchford. Published by Cambridge University Press. © Cambridge University Press 2011.

PAIN PERCEPTION

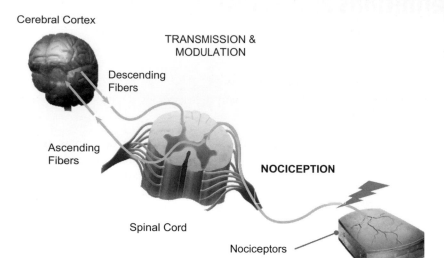

Figure 2.1. A mechanistic representation of nociception and pain perception.

Table 2.1.

Category	Cause	Symptom	Examples
Physiological	Brief exposure to a noxious stimulus	Rapid, yet brief pain perception	Touching a pin or hot object
Nociceptive/inflammatory	Somatic or visceral tissue injury with mediators impacting on intact nervous tissue	Moderate to severe pain, described as crushing or stabbing; usually worsens after the first 24 hours	Surgical pain, traumatic pain, sickle cell crisis
Neuropathic	Damage or dysfunction of peripheral nerves or CNS	Severe lancinating, burning or electrical shock-like pain	Neuropathy, chronic regional pain syndrome, postherpetic neuralgia
Mixed	Combined somatic and nervous tissue injury	Combinations of symptoms; soft tissue pain plus radicular pain	Low back pain, back surgery pain

of sympathetic fibers is termed reflex sympathetic dystrophy or chronic regional pain syndrome I. Neuropathic pain is often associated with peripheral and central sensitization, secondary hyperalgesia and alterations in sympathetic tone and regional perfusion. A common characteristic of neuropathic pain is the coexistence of sensory deficits or sensory abnormalities in the setting of increased pain sensation. These abnormalities include hyperpathia, or increased or exaggerated pain intensity with minor stimulation; allodynia, in which non-noxious sensory stimulation is perceived as painful; dysesthesia/paresthesia, which are unpleasant sensations at rest

or following touch and movement. Differences between physiological, nociceptive and neuropathic pain are described in Table 2.1.

Hyperalgesia

Hyperalgesia describes a state of increased pain sensitivity and enhanced perception following acute injury which is related to peripheral release of intracellular or humoral noxious mediators [7,9–11]. Primary hyperalgesia (peripheral sensitization) describes an altered state of sensibility in which the intensity of painful sensation induced by noxious and non-noxious stimulation is greatly increased. Hyperalgesia results in dynamic or "effort-dependent" pain, in which discomfort during ambulation, coughing and physical therapy is significantly increased [10]. Continued activation of nociceptors secondary to neural compression, stretch, infection, hematoma, and edema can result in prolonged disability and impaired rehabilitation. Secondary hyperalgesia (central sensitization) is related to ongoing noxious transmission and "sensitization" of second-order neurons in the dorsal horn [11]. Clinical alterations associated with secondary hyperalgesia include allodynia, multi-segmental flexion reflexes (splinting, muscle spasm) and alterations in sympathetic tone and regional perfusion. As a result, discomfort may be perceived at dermatomes above and below the site of trauma. The duration of central sensitization generally outlasts the initial barrage of high-threshold input and may become independent of further depolarization [6,7].

Pain temporality and duration

Acute pain

Acute pain is an adaptive physiological response that follows traumatic injuries and surgery. It has two primary components. (1) The sensory discriminative component describes the location and quality of the stimulus. It is characterized by rapid response, short latency to peak response, and short duration of action. Noxious information is conveyed by rapidly conducting A-delta fibers, and monosynaptic transmission to the sensory cortex [10,12]. This component rapidly identifies the site of injury or potential injury, and initiates reflexive/cognitive withdrawal responses. (2) The affective-motivational component underlies suffering and the emotional components of pain and is responsible for learned avoidance and other adaptive and non-adaptive behavioral responses.

The affective motivational component is mediated by slowly conducting c-fibers, and polysynaptic transmission to the limbic cortex [10,12]. It is responsible for continued pain perception, suffering, pain-related behaviors, hyperalgesia, reflex spasm (splinting behavior). It is also responsible for immobilization, and protection of the injury site.

In general, acute pain is limited in duration (1–14 days) and is associated with temporal reductions in intensity. Optimally controlled acute pain may be mild–moderate at rest but generally worsens during movement (effort-dependent or incident pain). Poorly controlled acute pain is associated with peripheral sensitization, spinal facilitation, hypothalamic/adrenal responses, and emotional/behavioral changes [7,9,12].

Rehabilitative/convalescent pain

A subacute pain state associated with convalescence and rehabilitation may persist for 1–2 months after surgery or traumatic injury. Patients may experience moderate to severe incident pain and require opioid analgesics for sleep and mobilization. Severe rehabilitative pain has a negative impact on physical therapy, return to normal functionality and quality of life.

Chronic pain

Chronic pain refers to persistent or progressively increasing discomfort beyond the normal time frame of healing [2,10]. An alternative definition is moderate to severe discomfort persisting 3 months or more following tissue injury (post-operative pain syndromes) or initial symptoms of cellular degeneration (osteoarthritic disease). The etiological classification of chronic pain refers to the clinical context in which pain perception takes place, and can be categorized as benign, malignancy-related, post-surgical, neuropathic, degenerative, or mixed.

Chronic pain is often associated with sensitization and plasticity changes in the peripheral and central nervous system that facilitate pain transmission and impair intrinsic noxious modulatory mechanisms [7,9,13]. Transition from acute pain to chronic pain involves ongoing peripheral and central sensitization, persistent hyperalgesia, the development of neuropathic symptoms and maladaptive emotional responses (pain behavior) [10]. Patients with chronic pain may be troubled by a persistent pain state that remains constant or gradually increases in frequency and intensity (malignancy-associated pain, osteoarthritis), or an intermittent pain state that has peaks (flare) and troughs in intensity (vasculopathic pain, gout, low back pain). Others may present with a combination of persistent pain plus intermittent flare, and complain of pain that is constant or gradually increasing, with episodes of increased intensity or flare (rheumatoid arthritis, neuropathic pain).

Chronic pain may also be characterized by its localization. Peripheral pain is is associated with

Table 2.2.

Acute pain	Chronic pain
1. Usually obvious tissue damage	1. Multiple causes (malignancy, benign)
2. Distinct onset	2. Gradual or distinct onset
3. Short, well-characterized duration	3. Persists after 3–6 months of healing
4. Resolves with healing	4. Can be a symptom or diagnosis
5. Serves a protective function	5. Serves no adaptive purpose
6. Effective therapy is available	6. May be refractory to treatment

Table 2.3.

Temporal	Onset, duration, periodicity
Variability	Constant, effort-dependent, waxing and waning, episodic "flare"
Intensity	Average pain, worst pain, least pain, pain with activity of living
Topography	Focal, dermatomal, diffuse, referred, superficial, deep
Character	Sharp, aching, cramping, stabbing, burning, shooting
Exacerbating/relieving	Worse at rest, with movement or no difference
Quality of life	Interferes with movement, ambulation, daily life tasks or work

ongoing nociceptor sensitization, neuropathic injury and stimulation of sympathetic efferents. Myelopathic pain is associated with spinal injuries and includes localized irritative and compression-related pain, radicular pain and skeletal muscular irritability. Central pain describes pain syndromes that follow CNS injury (post-stroke, CNS tumor) that are generally ill defined or poorly localized and difficult to treat. While some forms of chronic pain have an unclear etiology and unpredictable course, most begin as acute inflammatory or neuropathic pain. An increasing body of evidence suggests that severe acute pain, analgesic undermedication, nerve injury and genetic variabilities are responsible for the development of chronic pain [13,14].

Although acute and chronic pain have distinguishing characteristics, there is often overlap, making the diagnosis and management of pain challenging. Differences between acute and chronic pain are outlined in Table 2.2.

Qualitative aspects of pain perception

Appreciating the clinical features of the different types of pain not only helps properly classify pain and its etiology, but also helps guide the often complex multimodal medical management that accompanies pain management [10,13,14]. The healthcare provider must be detailed in attaining the qualitative factors and history associated with a patient's pain. The McGill Pain Questionnaire may be used to measure the quality, character, and intensity of acute and chronic pain. The qualitative aspects of pain perception are outlined in Table 2.3.

Finally, it is well recognized that certain acute traumatic and chronic pain conditions are associated with a mixture of noiciceptive inflammatory and neuropathic pain. For example, tissue injury and a marked inflammatory response following laparotomy or thoracotomy initiates a somatic nociceptive component responsible for incisional and muscular pain, while peritoneal or pleuritic irritation is responsible for a visceral nociceptive component. Neural injury related to retraction or transection initiates a neuropathic component. Clinical pain complaint, intensity of symptoms, pain characteristics and choice of analgesic are related to the extent of inflammation, visceral versus somatic nociception, and neural tissue injuries.

References

1. Warfield CA, Kahn CH. *Anesthesiology* 1995;**83**: 1090–1094.

2. Bonica JJ. Definitions and taxonomy of pain. In Bonica JJ, ed. *Management of Pain*. Philadelphia: Lea & Febiger, 1990.

3. Fishman SM, et al. *J Pain Sympt Manag* 2000;20.

4. Bonica JJ. The need of a taxonomy. IASP Subcommittee on the Taxonomy of Pain 1979;6(3):247–252.

5. Melzack R, Wall PD. *Science* 1965;**150**:971.

6. Woolf CJ. *Pulm Pharmacol* 1995;**8**:161–167.

7. Woolf and Salter. *Science* 2000;**288**: 1765.

8. Urban and Gebhart. *Med Clin North Am* 1999;**83**: 585.

9. Samad et al. *Nature* 2001;**410**:471.

10. Bonica JJ. Anatomic and physiologic basis of nociception and pain. In Bonica JJ, ed. *Management of Pain*. Philadelphia: Lea & Febiger, 1990, pp. 28–94.

11. LaMotte RH, Thalhammer JG, Robinson CJ. Peripheral neural correlates of magnitude of cutaneous pain and hyperalgesia. *J Neurophysiol* 1983;**50**:1–26.

12. Sinatra RS, Bigham M. The anatomy and pathophysiology of acute pain. In Grass JA, ed. *Problems in Anesthesiology*. Philadelphia: Lippincott-Raven, 1997.

13. Fields HL, Martin JB. Pain: pathophysiology and management. In Braunwald E, Fauci AS, Isselbacher KJ, et al., eds. *Harrison's Principles of Internal Medicine*, 15th ed. New York: McGraw-Hill, 2001.

14. Mannion RJ, Woolf CJ. *Clin J Pain* 2000;**16**(suppl):S144–S156.

15. Kehlet H. *Br J Anaesth* 1989;**63**:189–195.

Section 1
Chapter

3

Pain Definitions

Pain pathways and pain processing

Amit Mirchandani and Shamsuddin Akhtar

Introduction

Understanding the anatomical pathways and key neurochemical mediators involved in noxious transmission and pain perception is fundamental to optimizing the management of patients with acute and chronic pain. In this chapter we will outline the basic anatomy of the pain pathway and identify key neurochemical mediators involved in pain modulation.

Nociception

The conduction of pain does not simply involve conduction of impulses from the periphery to the cortical centers in the brain. Transmission of pain or nociception is a complex phenomenon and involves multiple stages that can be grouped broadly into three processes: (1) activation of specialized peripheral nerve endings; (2) conduction of noxious impulses to the spinal cord; and (3) transmission of impulses from the spinal cord to the supra-spinal and cortical centers. The culmination of these processes results in the localization and perception of pain. At each of these stages, nociceptive impulses can be suppressed by local interneurons or by descending inhibitory fibers and modulated by a variety of neurotransmitters and neuromodulators. Any abnormality of peripheral and central pain pathways including pathological activation, or the imbalance of activation and inhibitory pathways, may increase the severity of acute pain and contribute to the development of persistent pain [1].

7

Activation of sensory end organs and/or nerve endings

The nociception begins with the activation of peripheral sensory afferent receptors, also known as nociceptors, which are widely distributed throughout the body. Nociceptors are the peripheral endings of pseudo-unipolar neurons, whose cell bodies are located in the dorsal root ganglia (DRG). The nociceptor central ending terminates in the spinal cord and transmits noxious impulses to the dorsal horn [1,2].

Nociceptors convey noxious sensation, either externally (i.e. skin, mucosa) or internally (i.e. joints, intestines). They can be activated by any noxious insult, most of which can be categorized as either mechanical, chemical, or thermal in nature. Nociceptor activation is associated with a depolarizing Ca^{2+} current or a "generator potential". Once a certain threshold is met, the distal axonal segment depolarizes via an inward Na^+ current, and an action potential is conducted centrally.

Noxious stimuli are conducted from peripheral nociceptors to the dorsal horn via both unmyelinated and myelinated fibers. Nociceptive nerve fibers are classified according to their degree of myelination, diameter, and conduction velocity. For instance, A-delta axons are myelinated and allow action potentials to travel at a very fast rate of approximately 6–30 meters/second towards the central nervous system. They are responsible for "first pain" or "fast pain", a rapid (1 second) well-localized, discriminative sensation (sharp, stinging) of short duration [1,2]. Perception of first pain alerts the individual of actual or potential tissue injury and initiates the reflex withdrawal mechanism. The more slowly conducting non-myelinated C fiber axons conduct at speeds of about 2 meters/second. These unmyelinated C-fibers (termed polymodal-nociceptive fibers) respond to mechanical, thermal, and chemical injuries. C-fibers mediate the sensation of "second pain", which has a delayed latency (seconds to minutes) and is described as a diffuse burning or stabbing sensation that persists for a prolonged period of time. Larger A-beta axons, which respond to maximally light touch and/or movement stimuli, typically do not produce pain, except in pathological conditions [1,2].

Multiple receptors located on the primary afferent nerves are involved in specific transduction of particular noxious stimuli. Vanilloid receptors (VRI) and vanilloid receptor like-1 are excited by heat. VRI and acid-sensing ion channels are also stimulated by mechanical stimuli. Inotropic purinergic (P2X) receptors are excited by stretch and modulated by low pH [1,3]. Temperature is sensed by receptors called transient receptor potential (TRP) channels. An important TRP channel termed the TRPV-1 receptor has been widely studied. Capsacian and other TRPV-1 blockers initially activate and then deactivate nociceptors for prolonged periods of time. These compounds may provide long-term blockade of nociceptor function and prolonged suppression of acute pain.

A number of inflammatory and noxious mediators are involved in peripheral pain transduction [1] (Figure 3.1).

1. Substance P is a neuropeptide released from the unmyelinated primary afferent fibers, and its role in nociception is well established. Its effects can be blocked by treatment with the neurotoxin capsaicin, which destroys afferent nerve terminals. The pro-inflammatory effects of substance P include: vasodilatation and plasma extravasation, degranulation of mast cells, resulting in histamine release, chemo-attraction and proliferation of leukocytes, and cytokine release.

2. Bradykinin is a markedly algesic (pain-producing) substance that has direct activating effects on peripheral nociceptors.

3. Histamine is stored in mast-cell granules and is released by substance P and other noxious mediators. The effects of histamine are mediated by its interaction with specific receptors, resulting in vasodilatation and edema and swelling resulting from the enhanced permeability of postcapillary venules.

4. Serotonin or (5-hydroxytryptamine; 5-HT) is stored in the dense-body granules of platelets. 5-HT enhances microvascular permeability.

5. Prostaglandins (PGs) play a substantial role in the initial activation of nociceptors and exacerbate inflammation and tissue swelling at the site of injury. Up-regulation of cyclooxygenase-2 leads to rapid conversion of arachidonic acid from injured cell membranes into a variety of prostanoids (PGs and thromboxane A2).

6. Cytokines and interleukins released as part of the peripheral inflammatory response can circulate to and increase production of PGs in the brain. The accumulation of noxious mediators at the site of injury results in ongoing nociceptor stimulation, nociceptor recruitment and development of primary hyperalgesia.

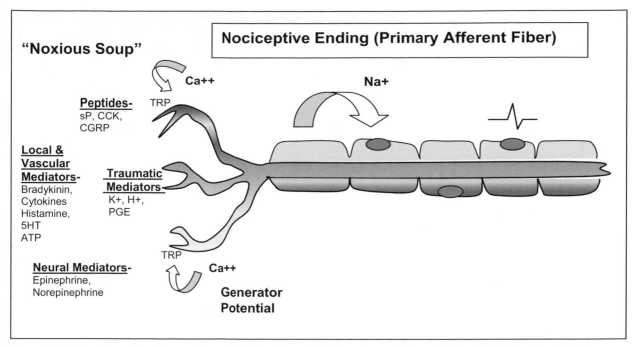

Figure 3.1. Nociceptive ending (primary afferent fiber). From: Sinatra RS. Pain pathways. In Sinatra RS, Viscusi G, de Leon-Casasola O, Ginsberg B, eds. *Acute Pain Management*. Cambridge University Press, 2009.

Conduction of pain to the spinal cord (and medulla)

Nearly all sensory afferents, regardless of peripheral origin, terminate in the dorsal horns of the spinal cord and medulla. Unmyelinated C fiber nociceptors terminate principally in lamina II (substantia gelatinosa). Small myelinated A-delta nociceptors terminate lamina I of the dorsal horn. The terminal endings of the primary afferent neurons in the spinal cord transmit pain signals to second-order neurons via several neurotransmitters, including glutamate and substance P. The second-order neurons involved in the pain pathway are principally of two types; (1) nociceptor-specific neurons that respond exclusively to inputs from A-delta and C fibers, and (2) wide-dynamic-range (WDR) neurons that respond to both noxious and non-noxious stimuli [1,4,5]. Higher-frequency stimulation leads to NMDA receptor activation, gradual increases in WDR neuronal discharge and a sustained burst of activity termed "wind-up". In this situation, WDR neurons become sensitized and hyperresponsive and transmit normal tactile responses as painful stimuli [1,5]. These central sensitizing changes are responsible for secondary hyperalgesia which increases the intensity of acute pain (refer to Chapter 5: hyperalgesia).

Reflexive intraspinal pathways connect primary nociceptor afferents to motor neurons and the autonomic efferents. Activation of these pathways leads to reflex skeletal muscular responses (muscle splinting/spasm) and autonomic responses (increased vascular tone hypertension, tachycardia, adrenal activation) [3].

A number of neurotransmitters, neuromodulators and their respective receptors are involved in the neurotransmission at the dorsal horn. They can be broadly classified into two groups.

1. Excitatory transmitters that are released from the primary afferent nociceptors or interneurons within the spinal cord.
2. Inhibitory transmitters that are released by interneurons within the spinal cord or supraspinal sources.

Most often more than one neurotransmitter is released at the same time. Aspartate and glutamate are excitatory amino-acids (EAAs) involved in pain transmission [4,5]. Glutamate is the main excitatory CNS neurotransmitter and mediates rapid, short-duration depolarization of second-order neurons. Peptides such as substance P and neurokinin are responsible for delayed long-lasting depolarization. EAAs act on various receptors, which principally include alpha-amino-3-hydroxy-5-methyl-4-isoxazolepropionic

9

acid (AMPA) receptors, *N*-demethyl-D-asprtate (NMDA) receptors, kaniate receptors (KA) and metabotropic glutamate receptors [3, 4]. EAAs activate AMPA receptors, which mediate sodium influx, cell depolarization and rapid priming of NMDA receptors. Substance P and other peptides bind to neurokinin receptors, leading to the activation of second messengers, culminating in changes in protein synthesis, genomic activation and slow activation of NMDA receptors (Figure 3.2). Activation of the NMDA receptor is associated with Ca^{2+} mobilization, and causes large and prolonged depolarization in the already partially depolarized neurons. Increase in intracellular calcium leads to the activation of multiple downstream pathways triggering

second messengers including PG, inositol triphosphate (IP_3), cGMP, eicosanoids, nitric oxide and protein kinase C [4,5] (Figure 3.3). Persistent pathological activation of these pathways leads to central sensitization and potential chronic pain conditions. Metabotropic glutamate receptors are a family of receptors that are coupled to G-protein. Though they do not appear to be involved in acute pain, there is compelling evidence that they play a modulatory role in nociceptive processing, central sensitization and pain behavior.

Afferent impulses arriving in the dorsal horn are tempered and modulated by inhibitory mechanisms. Inhibition occurs through local inhibitory interneurons and descending pathways from the brain.

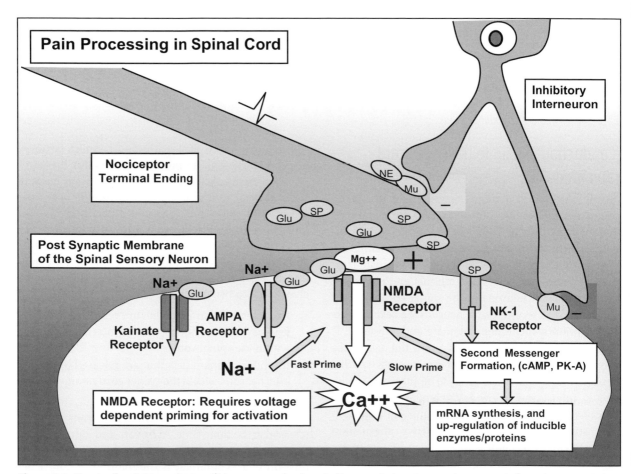

Figure 3.2. Targets of excitatory noxious mediators on second-order cells. Glutamate is the primary excitatory agonist for noxious transmission. Glutamate activates specific binding sites located on AMPA, kainate, and NMDA receptors. Ion channels on activated AMPA and kainate receptors allow Na^+ to enter and depolarize the cell. Changes in intracellular voltage rapidly prime the NMDA receptor and allow an Mg^{2+} plug to be dislodged. Following dislodgement an inward flux of Ca^{2+} is initiated. Glutamate binding to NMDARs maintains the inward Ca^{2+} flux. Substance P binds and activates NK-1 receptors. This receptor up-regulates second messengers including cAMP and PKA which slowly prime and maintain excitability of NMDARs. Activation of second messengers in turn up-regulates inducible enzymes, initiates transcription of mRNA, and mediates synthesis of acute reaction proteins. These changes increase neuronal excitability and underlie subsequent plasticity. From: Sinatra RS. Pain pathways. In Sinatra RS, Viscusi G, de Leon-Casasola O, Ginsberg B, eds. *Acute Pain Management.* Cambridge University Press, 2009.

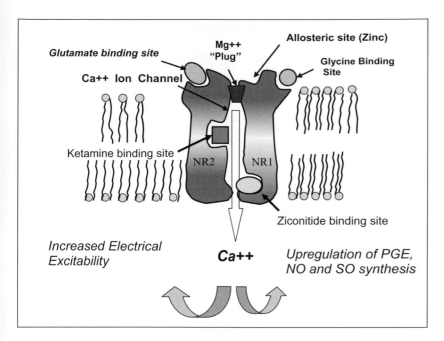

Figure 3.3. The NMDA receptor is a four-subunit, voltage-gated ligand-specific ion channel. The four subunits include two NR-2 units which contain glutamate binding sites and two NR-1 units which contain glycine binding sites and an allosteric site that is sensitive to zinc ions. Glutamate is the primary agonist of NMDR while glycine functions as a modulator. The central ion channel is normally blocked by a magnesium ion. Once dislodged, Ca^{2+} ions can pass through the channel and induce neuronal excitability. From: Sinatra RS. Pain pathways. In Sinatra RS, Viscusi G, de Leon-Casasola O, Ginsberg B, eds. *Acute Pain Management*. Cambridge University Press, 2009.

GABAergic and glycinergic interneurons are involved in tonic inhibition of nociceptive input and loss of these neurons is implicated in the development of chronic and neuropathic pain [5]. Endogenous opioids and noradrenergic pathways are also involved in inhibitory pain modulation.

Transmission of impulses from the spinal cord to the supraspinal structures

Several ascending tracts are responsible for transmitting nociceptive impulses from the dorsal horn to supraspinal targets. These include spinothalamic, spinoreticular, spinomesencephalic and spinolimbic tracts. The spinocervicothalamic and post-synaptic dorsal column are also involved in nociception. Of these, the spinothalamic tract is considered the primary perception pathway [1]. Axons traveling in the spinothalamic tract (STT) travel to several regions of the thalamus where pain signals diverge to broad areas of the cerebral cortex. The STT is divided into two tracts: the lateral neo-spinothalamic tract (nSTT) and the more medial paleo-spinothalamic tract (pSTT). The nSTT projects directly to the neothalamus. The neothalamus is a highly somatotopically organized region with cells conveying nociceptive impulses directly to the somatosensory cortex for rapid perception (localization) and prompt withdrawal from the noxious stimulus [1,5]. The lateral tracts are also discriminative and account for sensory qualities, such as throbbing or burning. The pSTT is a slow multisynaptic pathway that projects to the reticular activating system (RAS), periaqueductal gray (PAG), and medial thalamus. The medial thalamus is not somatotopically organized, and its cells project to the frontal and limbic cortex. The pSTT is associated with prolonged acute pain and chronic pain, and is responsible for diffuse, unpleasant feelings, and suffering long after an injury has occurred. Nociceptive impulses transmitted by the pSTT lead to persistent supraspinal responses affecting circulatory, respiratory, and endocrine function and underlie emotional and behavioral responses such as fear, anxiety, helplessness, and learned avoidance [1,5].

Descending control of pain

Descending neural pathways inhibit pain perception and efferent responses to pain. The cerebral cortex, hypothalamus, thalamus and brainstem centers (periaqueductal gray [PAG], nucleus rhaphe magnus [NRM] and locus coeruleus [LC]) send descending axons to the brainstem and spinal cord that modulate pain transmission in the dorsal horn. These axonal terminals either inhibit release of noxious neurotransmitters from primary afferents, or diminish the response of second-order neurons to the noxious input. Several neurotransmitters play critical roles in

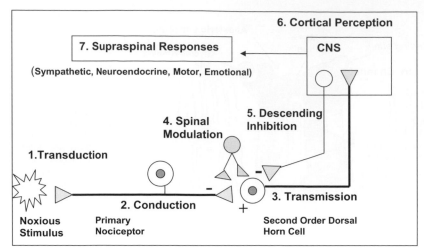

Figure 3.4. (1) Peripheral noxious mediators activate nociceptor endings via a process termed transduction. (2) Noxious impulses are delivered to the spinal cord dorsal horn via the process of conduction in afferent fibers. (3) The process of transmission describes synaptic transfer of noxious impulses from primary afferents to second-order cells in dorsal horn. (4) Modulation describes inhibitory and facilitatory effects of spinal interneurons on noxious transmission. (5) Descending inhibition refers to descending brainstem, midbrain, and cortical inhibitor nerve endings which supress pain transmission. (6) Cortical perception includes neocortical sites of pain localization and limbic centers responsible for emotional and suffering components of pain. (7) Supraspinal responses include sympathetic, neuromuscular, and neuroendocrine responses to pain. From: Sinatra RS. Pain pathways. In Sinatra RS, Viscusi G, de Leon-Casasola O, Ginsberg B, eds. *Acute Pain Management*. Cambridge University Press, 2009.

modulating pain transmission, including the endogenous opioids (enkephalin, dynorphin), gamma-aminobutyric acid (GABA), and norepinephrine. The PAG is an enkephalinergic brainstem nucleus responsible for both morphine- and stimulation-produced analgesia. Descending axons from the PAG project to nuclei in the reticular formation of the medulla, including NRM, and then descend to the dorsal horn where they synapse with and inhibit WDR and other neurons [1,5]. Axon terminals from the NRM project to the dorsal horn, where they release serotonin and norepinephrine. Axons descending from the LC modulate nociceptive transmission in the dorsal horn primarily via release of norepinephrine and activation of postsynaptic alpha-2-adrenergic receptors. GABAergic and enkephalinergic interneurons in the dorsal horn also provide local suppression of pain transmission [5].

From the preceding discussion it is very clear that generation of acute pain is a complex process involving many neural structures, neurotransmitters and neuromodulators. Key aspects of afferent pain signaling, cortical perception and efferent responses are outlined in Figure 3.4.

Conclusion

Transmission of pain impulses from specialized sensory end-organs or nerve endings to the cortical centers is a complex phenomenon and involves multiple stages, neurotransmitters, neuromodulators, inflammatory mediators, and excitatory and inhibitory pathways. Transition from acute to chronic pain is an even more complex and less understood process. However, it is clear that peripheral and central sensitization processes play an important role in the pathological development of chronic pain.

References

1. Sinatra RS, Bigham M. The anatomy and pathophysiology of acute pain. In Grass JA, ed. *Problems in Anesthesiology*. Philadelphia: Lippincott-Raven, 1997.

2. Hudspith MJ, Siddall PJ, Munglani R. Physiology of pain. In Hemmings HC, Hopkins P, eds. *Foundations of Anesthesia*, 2nd ed. Elsevier, 2000, pp. 267–286.

3. Benzon H. *Essentials of Pain Medicine and Regional Anesthesia*, 2nd ed. Churchill Livingstone, 2005, pp. 3–12.

4. Barash PG, Cullen BF, Stoelting RK, eds. *Clinical Anesthesia*, 5th ed. Lippincott, Williams & Wilkins, 2006, pp. 1442–1449.

5. Sinatra R. Pain pathways and pain processing. In Sinatra RS, deLeon-Cassasola O, Ginsberg B, Viscusi G. *Acute Pain Management*. Cambridge University Press, 2009, pp. 3–21.

4 Pain characteristics

Alireza Sadoughi

Introduction

A variety of approaches for classifying pain have been developed; the two most frequently used are based on pain duration (i.e. acute vs. chronic pain) and underlying pathophysiology (i.e. nociceptive vs. neuropathic pain). During the past several decades medicine has focused on the mechanism of pain, its management, and the possible prevention of complications, including neuropathic pain. There has been extensive research on neuropathic pain and the neurotransmitters that are involved. Pain has several different pathophysiological mechanisms, most commonly described as nociceptive, inflammatory, and neuropathic. With an acute noxious stimulus (an actual or potentially damaging event), the peripheral nervous system transmits noxious information to the central nervous system. However, with ongoing and intense stimulation, acute pain can become persistent and lead to the development of chronic pain.

This chapter will highlight the mechanisms that are particularly important for a rational, rather than an empirical, approach to pain management. It takes into account the concept that pain is an experience, and it cannot be separated from the patient's mental state, including their environmental and cultural background. These factors hold great importance because they can cause the brain to trigger or abolish the experience of pain, independent of what is occurring elsewhere in the body. Therefore, when assessing a complaint of pain, it is critical to also investigate the appropriate mental and environmental factors. In the clinical setting, a physician must infer the pathophysiological aspect of a pain syndrome from the patient's clinical evaluation.

Temporal classifications

Acute pain is temporally associated with a noxious stimulus secondary to an identifiable tissue injury, disease process, or abnormal function of a muscle or viscera, and is the normal physiological survival response to potential harm. The function of acute pain is to protect tissues from actual or potential injury by muscular reflex responses, alerting processes, and autonomic responses in vascular, visceral, and endocrine tissues. The global response to pain is produced by a complex interaction of cognitive interpretations and emotional responses, which are influenced by the individual's general physical state, past experiences, psychological state, social environment, and expectations. The source of acute pain is usually identifiable and localizable. The pain intensity is usually proportional to the severity of tissue injury, and it subsides as it heals. Acute pain is associated with an autonomic nervous system response, which causes tachycardia, increased blood pressure, anxiety, and stereotypic behaviors of withdrawal, splinting, rubbing, grimacing, or a combination of these responses.

In contrast, patients with sustained or chronic pain do not have autonomic over-activity, but have varying degrees of physical dysfunction, anxiety, depression, social isolation, and personality changes that cause a decrease in their quality of life. The term chronic pain is imprecise, but refers to pain lasting longer than 3 to 6 months. In some patients, the pain is chronic because the underlying pathological condition is chronic. Chronic neurogenic pain may be central pain resulting from pathology in the spinal cord, brainstem, thalamus, or cortex. Neuropathic pain may also be pain arising from damage to primary afferent neurons. Examples of chronic nociceptive pain include rheumatoid arthritis, osteoarthritis, degenerative disk and joint disease, osteoporosis fractures, chronic gout, and ankylosing spondylitis. Chronic pain associated with musculoskeletal disease is a combination of chronic persistent pain with intermittent acute exacerbations. The pain that is associated with movement, pressure, and light touch is neuropathic pain. Hyperalgesia and allodynia are expressions of sensitization of peripheral nociceptors and plasticity-induced central mechanisms in the spinal cord or brain. Hyperalgesia is a higher pain intensity felt upon noxious heat stimulation (thermal hyperalgesia) or noxious mechanical stimulation (mechanical hyperalgesia). Allodynia is the occurrence of pain that is elicited by stimuli that are normally below the pain threshold. Some authors include this lowering of the threshold in the term hyperalgesia in non-neuropathic pain [1].

Nociception and pain

The International Association for the Study of Pain (IASP) has defined pain as an unpleasant sensory and emotional experience that is evoked by actual or potential noxious (i.e. tissue-damaging) stimuli or by tissue injury. Normally, pain is the subjective result of nociception. Nociception is the encoding and processing of noxious stimuli in the nervous system. It can be objectively measured with various techniques, i.e. with electrophysiological recordings. By contrast, pain as a subjective experience can be verbally or visually described by humans, and it cannot be measured objectively. However, animals (as well as humans) show reflex responses to acute noxious stimuli, which can be assessed for the relationship between nociception and pain.

Nociceptive (tissue) pain

Nociceptive receptors are in skin, muscles, bone, joints, and viscera. Nociceptors refer to specialized pain receptors that are equipped in the periphery with receptors that are sensitive to noxious or potentially noxious mechanical and chemical stimuli [1,2]. In normal, non-damaged tissue, nociceptors or protective nociceptors (PN) are activated. High-threshold mechanoreceptor skin afferents come in two forms; lightly myelinated fast-conducting A-delta fibers and smaller unmyelinated slow-conducting C fibers. C fibers comprise around 70% of all nociceptors. C fibers contain a variety of neuropeptides, including substance P (SP) and calcitonin gene-related peptide (CGRP), as well as a high-affinity receptor for nerve growth factor (NGF). The tissue innervated as well as the rate of stimulation determine the quality of pain sensation. Furthermore, as a potent vasodilator, SP increases the nitric oxide (NO) release and causes axon reflex-mediated wheal and flare reaction. Then nociceptors project to the outermost region of the

spinal dorsal horn (lamina I and outer lamina II) and terminate largely on spinal neurons, which project to higher-order pain centers in the brain.

Nociceptive pain is further subdivided into somatic and visceral pain. Somatic pain, usually from muscles, fascia, joints, bones, and tissue trauma, can be well localized and described as dull, aching, throbbing, or gnawing pain. This type of pain is associated with bone metastases, soft tissue inflammation, and postoperative pain. Visceral pain usually comes from injury by infiltration, compression, distention, or dilatation to the sympathetic nervous system innervated organs, and is described as deep, squeezing, dragging, or pressure-like. Visceral pain is usually poorly localized and often referred to distant locations. Primary or metastatic tumors tend to distend, infiltrate, compress, or stretch the thoracic and abdominal viscera causing visceral pain. Visceral pain is typically referred to somatic structures and is often associated with greater autonomic, motor, and emotional responses compared to somatic pain [1].

All viscera receive dual innervation. Thus, in contrast to somatic input to the central nervous system, which has a single, usually spinal, destination, input to the central nervous system from organs in the thoracic cavity arrives at two locations: (1) the brainstem nucleus tractus solitarii (vagal afferent input) and (2) the thoracic spinal cord. Furthermore, visceral afferent fibers are disproportionately fewer than somatic afferent fibers. Consequently, the low number of visceral afferents and greater intraspinal distribution lead to a loss of spatial discrimination, consistent with the diffuse, difficult-to-localize nature of visceral pain [1].

In the peripheral and central nervous system, there are several inhibitory mechanisms such as A-beta neurons and enkephalins. Repetitive stimulation of nerve fibers called A-beta mechanoreceptives, for example, initially excites and then inhibits dorsal horn spinothalamic tract (STT) neurons via interposed interneurons releasing γ-aminobutyric acid (GABA) or enkephalin, which decreases the stimulation of C fibers.

The purpose of PN is to act as an early warning system, with a sharp initial pain from the A-delta fibers followed by a dull pain from the slower C fibers. This mechanism prevents tissue damage by alerting the body to the presence of an intense, potentially damaging stimulus in the environment. The resulting pain protects tissue from being further damaged because withdrawal reflexes are usually elicited. In patients who lack the capacity to feel nociceptive pain, there is enormous damage. For instance, patients who have congenital analgesia have deformities of the tips of their fingers, lips, and tongues, and their life expectancy is reduced. Generally, nociceptive pain is responsive to nonsteroidal anti-inflammatory drugs (NSAIDs) and opioids. Conditions associated with inflammation, bone pain, and joint disease are particularly responsive to NSAIDs, which will be addressed.

Inflammatory pain

Inflammatory pain is often caused by direct injury to tissue such as by a surgical scalpel or trauma. There are several processes that contribute to this type of pain. For example, silent nociceptors (SN), which are completely insensitive to mechanical or thermal stimuli in normal tissue, start to respond to stimuli and are sensitized. These SN are important in mediating neurogenic inflammation. Cyclooxygenase-2 (COX-2) is a protein that acts as an enzyme and catalyzes the production of prostaglandins. Hours after peripheral inflammation, there is a massive increase in COX-2. COX-2 leads to the production of prostaglandins that bind to specific receptors and initiate a cascade of kinases causing sensitization of the nociceptors [1,2]. The cascade leads to both hyperexcitability and hypersensitivity through the activation of two kinases, specifically protein kinase A and protein kinase C. These kinases serve to transduce proteins that are responsive. For instance, they heat stimuli, reducing the threshold of activation as well as the phosphorylate sodium channels, which are expressed in the membrane causing a hyperexcitable state. These two mechanisms allow peripheral sensitization of the peripheral nociceptors and are responsible for reduction of the pain threshold at the site of tissue damage.

As mentioned earlier, SP is released by nociceptors, causing vasodilatation, plasma extravasation and other effects, i.e. attraction of macrophages or degranulation of mast cells. These events cause signs of inflammation such as heat, redness, and swelling. In spite of the complexity of the cytokines and neurotransmitters involved in inflammation, researchers have identified interleukin-1 (IL-1) and tumor necrosis factor alpha (TNF-a) [2].These chemicals cause release of other mediators, which can produce further sensitization or activation of primary afferent fibers and nearby primary afferent nociceptors [1,2]. This process is the basis of the neurogenic inflammation associated with these changes that can be observed following an injury.

Neuropathic (nerve) pain

Neuropathic pain is a state of complex, chronic pain that is usually accompanied by neural and non-neural tissue injury. It can be caused by trigeminal neuralgia, HIV infection, herpes zoster, and diabetes. Among intact nerves and tissue, a stimulus that is noxious will usually induce a subjective pain response; however, under clinically relevant conditions, e.g. surgical incisions, this association is not predictable. With constant activity from nociceptive afferents, sensitization of the nociceptors occurs. Central and peripheral pain-processing neurons or nerve fibers may be dysfunctional or injured. Damaged nerve fibers send incorrect signals to the central nervous system and cause a change in nerve function both at the site of injury and in the surrounding areas (primary and secondary hyperalgesia respectively). The pain may persist for months or years beyond the apparent healing of damaged tissues [1,3]. Plasticity is a term used to refer to these changes that occur in the established nervous system. Changes in neuronal structure, connections between neurons, and alterations in the quantities and properties of neurotransmitters, receptors, and ion channels ultimately result in increased functional activity of neurons in the pain pathway. Conversely, plasticity can decrease the body's own pain inhibitory systems, resulting ultimately in increased pain. Plasticity can result in short-term changes, which last from minutes to hours, or long-term changes, which may become permanent. Both peripheral and central nervous systems have a role in neuronal plasticity [1–3].

In injury, commonly, the inhibiting A-beta fibers begin to express SP and CGRP; low-threshold stimuli can lead to SP release in the dorsal horn. These transmitters cause hyperexcitability by decreasing the stimuli threshold of the nociceptors. Moreover, Schwann cells in damaged nerves start to produce increased mRNA for NGF, leading to regenerative events. Often, damaged axons also express adrenoreceptors, causing discharges in response to circulating epinephrine and norepinephrine. These neurotrophins may cause aberrant regeneration, such as the ingrowths of sympathetic postganglionic axons or large myelinated afferents, forming abnormal connections in the nociceptive processing circuits within the dorsal horn. These sprouts develop active sodium channels that become sites of tonic impulse generations (in the absence of noxious stimuli), known as ectopic foci. Regenerative sprouts "rewire" the afferent sensory system and cause alllodynia (i.e. pain resulting from a nonpainful stimulus) [3]. Persistent allodynia is a common characteristic of neuropathic pain. A light stroke of the patient's face may feel like a shock or lightning bolt and result in the sudden pain of trigeminal neuralgia. In contrast, patients with diabetic neuropathy suffer from dysesthesia; an unpleasantly strange or tingly sensation, rather than a painful feeling.

In the central nervous system (CNS), low- and high-frequency synaptic activation and the release of neuromodulators and glutamate cause an increase in the number of discharged action potentials with each stimulus. These reversible changes in the excitability of neurons via post-translational means are called modulation. As a result of repeated exposure to sensitizing stimuli, such as inflammatory mediators, modulation of peripheral neurons leads to "heterosensitization", an increase in the excitability of the nociceptor terminal membrane [2,3]. Centrally, there is a loss of inhibitory interneurons and the stimulus-response system is greatly distorted. The result is persistent, pathological pain. At the level of transcriptional change, inflammation produces up-regulation of genes and increased expression of TRPV1 and sensory nerve-specific sodium channels in response to injury and inflammatory mediators [3]. Consequently, the nerve growth factor decreases the threshold to noxious stimulation, resulting in hyperalgesia. Clustering of sodium channels in the axon membrane produces foci of irritability and ectopic discharges, which is a major contributor to spontaneous neuropathic pain. These sodium channels can be blocked by lidocaine, mexiletine, and anticonvulsants. The number of opioid mu receptors decreases, and the number of $\alpha2\gamma$ calcium channel subunits increases, producing diminished effectiveness of morphine and enhanced effectiveness of gabapentin for neuropathic pain [3].

Mixed-category pain

In some conditions, the pain appears to be caused by a complex mixture of nociceptive and neuropathic factors. An initial nervous system dysfunction or injury may trigger the neural release of inflammatory mediators and subsequent neurogenic inflammation. For example, migraine headaches probably represent a mixture of neuropathic and nociceptive pain. Myofascial pain is probably secondary to nociceptive input from the muscles, but the abnormal muscle activity may be the result of neuropathic conditions.

Pharmacological management

Generally, neuropathic problems are not completely reversible, but improvement is often possible with appropriate treatment. Examples of conditions amenable to treatment include post-herpetic neuralgia, reflex sympathetic dystrophy/causalgia (nerve trauma), components of cancer pain, phantom limb pain, entrapment neuropathy (e.g., carpal tunnel syndrome), and peripheral neuropathy (widespread nerve damage). Diabetes is the most common cause of peripheral neuropathy, but other causes include chronic alcohol use, exposure to other toxins (e.g. chemotherapies), vitamin deficiencies, and a variety of other medical conditions. When considering pharmacological options to treat chronic pain, options in order of use include non-opioids (e.g. acetaminophen, NSAIDs), opioids, and co-analgesics. Generally, the non-opioids are unlikely to provide any significant degree of pain relief in patients with neuropathic pain. Given the complicated nature of neuropathic pain, it is not surprising to find that, at best, an opioid or co-analgesic agent will decrease the pain to half. In fact, careful analgesic selection and dosage titration are required, since many patients with neuropathic pain are elderly, taking multiple medications, and carrying numerous comorbid conditions.

NSAIDs' mechanism of action relays inhibition of production of prostanoids to prevent the inflammatory pain. Two cyclooxygenase enzymes contribute to the conversion of arachidonic acid to prostaglandin H2; cyclooxygenase-1 (COX-1) is a constitutive form of cyclooxygenase but COX-2 tends to be induced primarily by inflammation in most tissues. Many recent medications and investigations are directed at inhibiting COX-2 to relieve pain, such as celecoxib.

Clustering of sodium channels in the axon membrane produces foci of irritability and ectopic discharges, which are a major contributor to spontaneous neuropathic pain. Treatments that reduce peripheral sensitization are drugs that affect the sodium channels (e.g. carbamazepine, oxcarbazepine, phenytoin, topiramate, lamotrigine, lidocaine, and mexiletine). Co-analgesics that address central sensitization by affecting calcium channels include gabapentin, pregabalin, levetiracetam, oxcarbazepine, lamotrigine, topiramate, and ziconotide. Tricyclic antidepressants (TCAs), serotonin-norepinephrine reuptake inhibitor (SNRIs), tramadol, and opioids will enhance the descending inhibitory pathway.

Currently, there are a few agents that are US Food and Drug Administration (FDA)-approved for neuropathic pain. These are carbamazepine (Tegretol) for trigeminal neuralgia, duloxetine (Cymbalta) for diabetic neuropathy, gabapentin (Neurontin) and transdermal lidocaine (LidoDerm) for post-herpetic neuralgia, and pregabalin (Lyrica) for both diabetic neuropathy and post-herpetic neuralgia. However, there are a significant number of studies demonstrating the effectiveness of these and other co-analgesics in treating a wide variety of neuropathic pain states. Gabapentin and pregabalin are alpha2-delta ligands that were introduced to the market as anti-epileptic drugs. However, they have been effective in treating post-herpetic neuralgia, painful diabetic neuropathy, mixed neuropathic pain syndromes, phantom limb pain, Guillain-Barré syndrome, and spinal cord injury pain.

Opioids have proven less effective in management of neuropathic pain. Nevertheless, the synergic effect of opioids and co-analgesics such as gabapentin has been proven to be very successful. Tramadol (Ultram) is a norepinephrine and serotonin reuptake inhibitor that has a weak mu opioid agonist as one of its metabolites. Tramadol is effective in treating painful diabetic neuropathy and polyneuropathy of various causes. Several studies have also demonstrated the effectiveness of neutralizing antibodies to IL-1 and TNF receptors to reduce pain-associated behaviors.

The recent decades have brought a greater focus on pain management and the medical community has had more success in understanding pain and its management. With time, it is certain that more pathways and neurotransmitters will be discovered, which will bring about better medications and methods of treating acute as well as chronic neuropathic pain.

References

1. *Bonica's Management of Pain*, 3rd ed. Philadelphia: Lippincott Williams & Wilkins, 2001.

2. Firestein G. *Kelley's Textbook of Rheumatology*, 8th ed. Philadelphia: W.B. Saunders, 2008.

3. Stucky C. Mechanisms of pain. *PNAS* 2001;**98**:11845–11846.

Section 1
Chapter

5

Pain Definitions

Primary and secondary hyperalgesia

Brenda C. McClain

Introduction

Hyperalgesia is defined by the International Association for the Study of Pain (IASP) as "an increased response to a stimulus which is normally painful". Primary hyperalgesia or peripheral sensitization reflects the activation and sensitization of nociceptive A delta and polymodal C-fiber terminal endings within the injured area. Secondary hyperalgesia, or central sensitization, involves spinal neuroplasticity and facilitation of supraspinal noxious transmission. The stimulus response associated with primary hyperalgesia is shifted to the left, such that reduction in noxious stimulation intensity is associated with increased intensity of pain perception (Figure 5.1).

Primary hyperalgesia

Primary hyperalgesia follows primary nociceptor activation (or transduction) in response to mechanical,

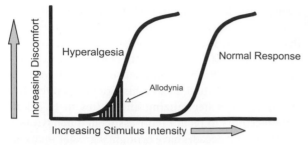

Figure 5.1. Physiological alterations associated with hyperalgesia.

thermal, and chemical noxious stimulation [1]. Peripheral mediators of mechanical and thermal injury include K^+ and H^+ ions, prostaglandins (PGE-2), cytokines (IL-6, IL-10, TNFα), and autacoids (substance P, angiotensin II, bradykinin, histamine, and serotonin). Following exposure to this "noxious soup" of algesic, inflammatory, and pro-inflammatory mediators, nociceptors become sensitized (peripheral sensitization) and depolarize either spontaneously or at lower stimulating thresholds. Several membrane receptors and ion channels are specifically expressed in terminal nociceptor endings. These include certain vanilloid receptors (TRPV-1), purinergic receptors, and tetrodotoxin- resistant sodium channels. TRPV-1 receptors initiate generator potentials within terminal endings and are primarily responsible for encoding noxious stimuli into a barrage of action potentials [2] (Figure 5.2).

Up-regulation of cyclooxygenase-2 (COX-2) converts arachidonic acid released from damaged cell membranes into prostaglandin E_2 (PGE_2), a primary noxious mediator and transduction initiator. Bradykinin and kallidin bind to constitutive G-protein coupled receptors termed B_2 receptors, which in turn activate phospholipases A_2 and C, as well as protein kinase C. Bradykinin also activates voltage-gated ion channels by altering K^+ and Na^+ ion flux, resulting in enhanced excitability of mechano-heat-sensitive C nociceptors [3]. The co-localization of bradykinin with the vanilloid receptor TRPV1 has been recently shown to play a major role in bradykinin-induced hyperalgesia. TRPV1 receptors are activated at lower temperatures when sensitized by bradykinin [3,4]. Although the earliest phases of primary hyperalgesia are mediated by the inflammatory soup of noxious substances, later phases involve pathophysiological alterations including neural injury, effects of efferent sympathetic potentiation, and the effects of neutrophils and lymphocytic infiltration. This later phase is associated with ectopic discharges and stimulus-independent activity (Figure 5.3).

The process of neural sensitization and the clinical term "hyperalgesia" also relate to discomfort in response to sensations that normally would not be perceived as painful. The term hyperpathia describes exaggerated perception resulting from minor amounts of peripheral noxious stimulation. Allodynia defines a state in which non-noxious stimulation is perceived as being painful. Allodynia is commonly observed following severe or extensive injuries, and in patients developing persistent and neuropathic pain. Clinical characteristics associated with hyperalgesia are presented in Table 5.1.

Secondary hyperalgesia

Secondary hyperalgesia is a form of central sensitization that follows ongoing tissue injury and inflammation. Its clinical manifestations include an exaggerated response to noxious and innocuous stimuli applied to undamaged tissue surrounding the site of injury. An important role of secondary hyperalgesia and central sensitization is to increase effort-dependent pain, thereby limiting movement and further tissue damage following acute injuries; however, an increasing body of evidence suggests that these physiological adaptations are also responsible for pain persistence, symptoms of neuropathic pain, and the development of chronic pain states [5,6].

Neurophysiology

Secondary hyperalgesia refers to the activation and progressive sensitization of second-order nociceptive specific (NS) and wide-dynamic-range (WDR) neurons in the dorsal horn as well as activation of other nociceptive neurons in brainstem and thalamus [6]. These cells are activated by barrages of noxious afferent input from the injury site. WDR sensitization is primarily limited to afferent mechanoreceptor input and exaggerated responses to temperature input are less obvious. Two forms of secondary hyperalgesia have been described: hyperalgesia to light touch, which is also referred to as allodynia, and hyperalgesia to punctate stimuli. Hyperalgesia in response to heat and light-touch stimuli is more difficult to induce, less pronounced, of shorter duration and encompasses a smaller receptive field than secondary hyperalgesia to punctate stimuli.

The mechanisms leading to stimulation and sensitization of dorsal horn neurons include enhanced

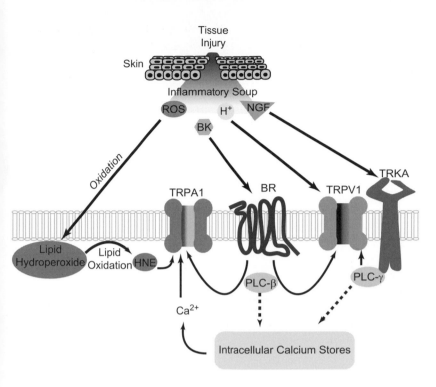

Figure 5.2. Inflammatory agents regulate TRPV1 through direct and indirect mechanisms. Tissue injury, ischemia, or cellular stress generates an array of pro-algesic and pro-inflammatory agents, collectively referred to as the "inflammatory soup". This includes extracellular protons (H^+), prostaglandin (PGE), bradykinin (BK), and nerve growth factor (NGF). Some factors, such as H^+ and K^+, activate TRPA1 or TRPV1 directly, whereas others, such as BK and NGF, modulate channel gating indirectly. TRPA1 and TRPV1 function as polymodal signal integrators capable of detecting products of cell and tissue injury. These channels promote pain hypersensitivity by depolarizing the primary afferent nerve fiber and/or lowering thermal or mechanical activation thresholds. (Adapted from Trevisani et al. *PNAS* 2007; 104(33):13519–13524.)

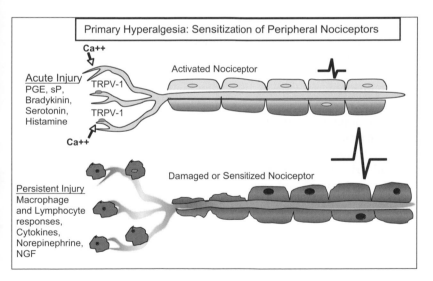

Figure 5.3. Following acute injury, primary noxious mediators including PGE, sP. and bradykinin activate TRPV-1 receptors, which initiates intracellular Ca^{2+} flux and depolarization of peripheral terminal endings. This Ca^{2+} generator potential in turn initiates Na^+-mediated axon potentials. With ongoing inflammation, terminal endings become sensitized and depolarize independently. With persistent injury, macrophages and lymphocytes infiltrate the terminal endings and release cytokines, interleukins and nerve growth factor, which further sensitizes the nociceptor. Courtesy of Sinatra RS: Lecture presented at NYS PGA 2009.

afferent signaling, wind-up and long-term potentiation. (Refer to Chapter 2: Pain pathways). A study by Zeigler et al. [7] has shown that intradermal injection of capsaicin into the dorsum of the hand elicits a stable state of secondary hyperalgesia for at least 2 h that is characterized by a leftward shift of the stimulus-response function for punctate mechanical stimuli. They also demonstrated that conduction blockade in both small-diameter A-fiber subtypes where C fibers were unaffected showed that intradermal injection of capsaicin produced pain that was equal in magnitude to the pain produced without a nerve block; however, no hyperalgesia to punctate stimuli could be detected. After the block had been released, punctate hyperalgesia was present. These findings indicate that C-fiber discharges induce central sensitization and that

Table 5.1. Characteristics of hyperalgesia

Hyperalgesia

- Defines a state of increased pain sensitivity and enhanced perception following acute injury which may persist chronically
- The hyperalgesic region may extend dermatomes above and below the area of injury and is associated with ipsilateral (and occasionally contralateral) muscular spasm/immobility
- Hyperalgesia may be observed following incision, crush, amputation, and blunt trauma

Primary hyperalgesia

- Describes increased pain sensitivity at the injury site
- Related to peripheral release of intracellular or humoral noxious mediators

Secondary hyperalgesia

- Describes increased pain sensitivity at adjacent, uninjured sites
- Related to changes in excitability of spinal and supraspinal neurons

Abnormal sensations associated with hyperalgesia

- Hyperpathia – increased or exaggerated pain intensity with minor stimulation
- Allodynia – non-noxious sensory stimulation is perceived as painful
- Dysesthesia – unpleasant sensation at rest or movement
- Paresthesia – unpleasant often shock-like or electrical sensation precipitated by touch or pressure (e.g. CRPS-II causalgia)

A-fiber nociceptors mediate secondary hyperalgesia to punctate stimuli through a second pathway.

The concerted actions of excitatory amino acids (EAAs) and neurokinin (NK) on facilitatory nociceptive pathways is the pharmacological crux of the phenomenon of secondary hyperalgesia. Most models of secondary hyperalgesia are single-neuron models in which a critical neuron, namely the nociceptive projection neuron, is sensitized by the combined interaction of EAAs and neurokinins [5–7]. Excitatory amino acids such as glutamate (Glu) and aspartate are responsible for fast synaptic transmission and rapid neuronal depolarization. Glutamate is released by all primary afferents while substance P is found only in nociceptors. Excitatory amino acids activate AMPA and kainite (KAR) receptors that regulate Na^+ and K^+ ion influx and intraneuronal voltage. Increasesd Na^+ ion flux facilitates priming and activation of NMDA receptors. Spinal and supraspinal NMDA receptors increase intraneuronal Ca^{2+} ion influx, the major requisite for the development of long-term potentiation (LTP). Sensitization of CNS neurons also underlies the transition from acute to persistent pain (Figure 5.4). Central sensitization can be divided into transcription-dependent and transcription-independent processes. Transcription-independent sensitization reflects neurochemical and electrical alterations that follow acute traumatic and experimentally induced pain. It includes stimulus-dependent neuronal depolarization, and stimulus-independent long-term potentiation. Transcription-dependent sensitization describes delayed-onset, long-lasting, noxious facilitation that follows genomic activation, transcription of mRNA and subsequent translational modifications. Activation of NMDA and NK-1 receptors and continued influx of Ca^{2+} leads to enhanced production of cAMP, protein kinases, and phosphokinases [8]. Phosphokinases and other nuclear activators initiate transcriptional processes over a period of several hours to several days. Key translational events include up-regulation of non-constitutive enzymes and proteins including superoxide dismutase, nitric oxide synthetase, and cyclooxygenase-2. These enzymes are responsible for production of the irritative and lytic mediators, superoxide, nitric oxide, and prostaglandins, which sensitize neuronal cell membranes, synaptic contacts, and associated glial cells.

The activation of spinal extracellular signaling-regulated kinase-1 and -2 (ERK1, ERK2) is also required for secondary hyperalgesia [8]. Noxious activation of ionotropic, metabotropic, and tyrosine kinase receptors in dorsal horn neurons activates protein kinase A (PKA) and protein kinase C (PKC), leading to the production of ERK. Hyperalgesia after thermal stimulation is mediated by non-NMDA receptors. The thermal stimulus model demonstrates distinct protein kinase involvement downstream from spinal non-NMDA receptor activation. Jones et al. [9]

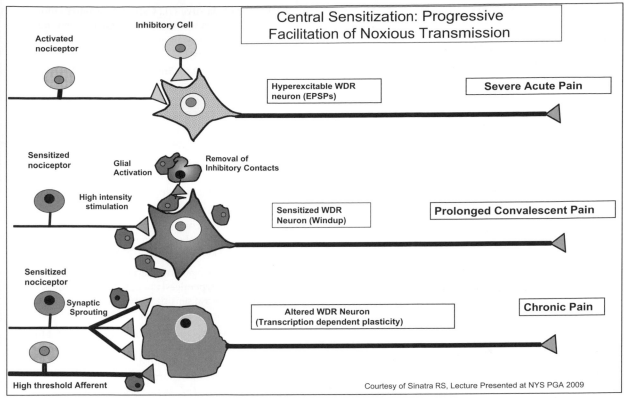

Figure 5.4. Following tissue injuries and release of noxious mediators, peripheral nociceptors become sensitized and fire repeatedly, stimulating second-order WDR cells in the dorsal horn (upper figure). The cells also become electrically sensitized and demonstrate excitatory postsynaptic potentials (EPSPs). Inhibitory interneurons and descending inhibitory fibers modulate and central sensitization by suppressing nociceptor release of noxious transmitters as well as the excitability of WDR cells. Continued barrage of noxious impulses further sensitizes second-order transmission neurons in dorsal horn, via a process termed "wind-up" (middle figure). The resulting process of central sensitization results in secondary hyperalgesia and spread of the hyperalgesic area to nearby uninjured tissues. In certain settings ongoing intracellular calcium influx and transcription-dependent changes lead to neurochemical/neuroanatomical plasticity, prolonged neuronal discharge and increased pain intensity and persistence (lower figure).

found that incision-induced sensitization also involves activation of protein kinases. These investigators confirmed that spinal calcium/calmodulin-dependent protein kinase II (CaMKII) mediates secondary hyperalgesia and spontaneous pain behavior after plantar incision.

Clinical implications

The recognition and control of nociceptor transduction and development of primary hyperalgesia are key to reducing the intensity and duration of acute pain. Nociceptor sensitization leads to reductions in noxious thresholds, increased pain disability, and delayed rehabilitation. The physiological response to transduction and the initiation of nociception can be limited or eliminated by peri-operative administration of non-opioid analgesics and anti-inflammatory agents (e.g. NSAIDS, steroids). Although opioids can inhibit

the release of substance P from primary afferent nerves, this class provides limited analgesic effects when nociceptors are sensitized by prostaglandins, bradykinin, and other inflammatory mediators. The development of TRPV-1 inhibitors and extended-duration local anesthetics may provide a safe and effective means to reduce acute pain for an extended duration of time, and eliminate the untoward effects of primary hyperalgesia. Central sensitization appears to play an important role in the persistence of pain even when the original injury has abated. The temporal sequence from the initial traumatic event to the development of chronic pain involves plasticity changes and can occur rapidly particularly in settings of analgesic undermedication (Figure 5.5). As ongoing pain signals bombard the dorsal horn, connections to WDR neurons begin to sprout and the number of NMDA receptors at the postsynaptic membrane is increased.

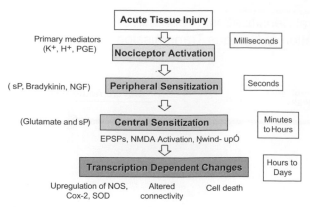

Figure 5.5. Temporal sequence of hyperalgesic and plasticity changes that follow acute tissue injury.

WDR endings grow into the areas where pain-receiving nerve cell bodies are located. The enlarged receptive field can now conduct non-noxious inputs, an effect that may be potentiated by the sprouting of A-beta fibers. The result of these changes is that non-noxious afferents (mechanical and proprioceptive) are now perceived as painful stimuli and can contribute towards maintaining sensitization even after the resolution of the primary injury. The current use of adjuvants for neuropathic pain includes many agents (calcitonin, ketamine, calcium channel blockers, etc.) that work to block or reduce facilitative pathways [10]. It is also appreciated that all patients with similar injuries do not develop persistent pain. This suggests that there is a certain level of genetic variability that may account for differences in clinical outcomes.

References

1. Treede RD, Magerl W. Modern concepts of pain and hyperalgesia: beyond the polymodal C-nociceptor. *News Physiol Sci* 1995;**10**:216–228.

2. Ferreira J, da Silva GL, Calixto JB. Contribution of vanilloid receptors to the overt nociception induced by B2 kinin receptor activation in mice. *Br J Pharmacol* 2004;**141**(5):787–794.

3. Wang H, Ehnert C, Brenner GJ, Woolf CJ. Bradykinin and peripheral sensitization. *Biol Chem* 2006;**387**(1):11–14.

4. Couture R, Harrisson M, Vianna RM, Cloutier F. Kinin receptors in pain and inflammation. *Eur J Pharmacol* 2001;**429**(1–3):161–176.

5. Serra J, Campero M, Bostock H, Ochoa J. Two types of C nociceptors in human skin and their behavior in areas of capsaicin-induced secondary hyperalgesia. *J Neurophysiol* 2004;**91**(6):2770–2781.

6. Simone DA, Ochoa J. Early and late effects of prolonged topical capsacin on Vanilloid receptors. *Pharmacol Rev* 1999;**51**:159–212.

7. Ziegler EA, Magerl W, Meyer RA, Treede R-D. Secondary hyperalgesia to punctate mechanical stimuli. Central sensitization to A-fibre nociceptor input. *Brain* 1999;**122**:2245–2257.

8. Walker SM, Meredith-Middleton J, Lickiss T, Moss A, Fitzgerald M. Primary and secondary hyperalgesia can be differentiated by postnatal age and ERK activation in the spinal dorsal horn of the rat pup. *Pain* 2007;**128**(1–2):157–168.

9. Jones TL, Lustig AC, Sorkin LS. Secondary hyperalgesia in the post-operative pain model is dependent on spinal calcium/calmodulin-dependent protein kinase II activation. *Anesth Analg* 2007;**105**:1650–1656.

10. Warncke T, Stubhaug A, Jorum E. Top of form ketamine, an NMDA receptor antagonist, suppresses spatial and temporal properties of burn-induced secondary hyperalgesia in man: a double-blind, cross-over comparison with morphine and placebo. *Pain* 1997;**72**(1–2): 99–106.

6

Pain pathophysiology

Alireza Sadoughi

Introduction

Pain is produced by stimuli that usually cause damage to tissues. It is in the best interest of an organism to detect potential damage to the body so it can take appropriate steps to avoid being harmed. The presence of pain usually forces immobilization of the injured area and prevents additional tissue damage from taking place and allows for the healing and repair processes to occur. Without the aid of the body's response to tissue damage, survival would be difficult.

Pathological pain is considered abnormal given that there is no protective value to the organism. This is a "morphism" in the nervous system that involves plasticity in both the peripheral and central nervous systems. It affects the way the nervous system detects the type of stimuli from the environment – a shift from a normally protective physiological mechanism to an abnormal and possibly pathological mechanism. Consequently, this justifies the concept that pain should be considered a disease process on its own.

This chapter will outline mechanisms of physiological nociceptive pain resulting from inflammation and from injury and its impact on the nervous system. The effects of stress hormone release on the cardiovascular system and other key target organs will also be discussed.

Central nervous system pathophysiology

Hyperalgesia

Pain is a complex process involving both the peripheral nervous system (PNS) and the central nervous system (CNS). Peripheral nociceptors are able to distinguish between noxious and innocuous stimuli and can translate the intensity of the stimulus from the frequency of impulse firing. The second-order neurons in the spinal-thalamic tract transmit noxious impulses from the spinal cord to the thalamus. From here axons within the thalamocortical system contact cells in sensory and limbic cortex responsible for conscious pain sensation. While nociceptive pain is elicited by noxious stimulation of sensory endings, pathological pain results from injury to tissue and neurons in the nervous system, which ceases to serve a protective function and instead degrades health and functional capability. Evidence exists that chronic pathological pain results from a combination of mechanisms, including neural "memories" of previous pain. Examples of neuropathic pain include carpal tunnel syndrome, post-herpetic neuralgia, diabetic neuropathy, and central pain syndrome [1–3]. There is a direct relationship between the intensity of the stimulus and the degree of pain sensation after application of a stimulus to the body. Enhanced noxious perception following peripheral tissue injury is termed hyperalgesia. Primary hyperalgesia defines increases in noxious sensitivity observed in areas around the site of tissue damage. The endings of the peripheral nociceptors become sensitized and more responsive to any applied stimulus. sh95:STARTSecondary hyperalgesia reflects the sensitization of second-order dorsal horn cells that receive input from primary afferent fibers. Allodynia is the phenomenon of pain sensation from a non-painful, normally innocuous stimulus despite tissue healing. Essentially, it is a disease of the nervous system where an area that normally is not sensitive to pain, upon touch, becomes vulnerable to substantial pain sensations. This process involves both peripheral and central sensitization [1–3].

Central sensitization

Central sensitization describes changes that occur in the central nervous system in response to repeated nerve stimulation. Following repeated stimulation, levels of neurotransmitters and brain electrical signals change as neurons develop a "memory" for responding to those signals. Frequent stimulation results in a stronger brain memory, so that the brain will respond more rapidly and effectively when experiencing the same stimulation in the future. The resulting changes in brain wiring and the responses are referred to as nerve plasticity. The sensitization can only occur with repeated stimuli and activation. For example, even after removal of a herniated disc, pain may continue. There are many important factors in building this sensitization including temporal summation, inflammatory response, production of new nerve fibers, and receptor up-regulation.

Temporal summation refers to a central spinal mechanism where repetitive noxious stimulations results in the sensation of increased pain in humans. It is due to the "second" pain from the C fibers, which is more dull and strongly related to chronic pain conditions. Ongoing C-fiber nociceptive impulses lead to increased glutamate release and repeated NMDA receptor activation of the STT neurons. This NMDA activation, along with SP release, results in a build-up of intracellular calcium ion (Ca^{2+}). Calcium influx induces two activities, activation of nitric oxide (NO) synthase as well as a Ca^{2+}-induced PKC. NO can affect the nociceptor terminals and enhance the release of sensory neuropeptides (in particular, SP) from presynaptic neurons, thereby contributing to the development of hyperalgesia and maintenance of central sensitization; whereas PKC induces sensitization of NMDA receptors by phosphorylation that leads to increased stimulation as well as reducing sensitivity to the opioid receptors, allowing an increased response to pain.

As discussed earlier, the inflammatory response of tissue damage also has a key role in central sensitization. The induction of COX-2 and the production of PG promotes an increase in presynaptic transmitter release but more importantly causes direct depolarization postsynaptically in the dorsal horn roots by removing the glycine receptor block and causing excitability. Furthermore, the widespread induction of COX-2 within the central nervous system can exacerbate pain and change appetite, mood, and sleep, and produce the general symptoms of illness.

In addition, after nerve and tissue destruction, regenerative sprouts "rewire" the afferent sensory system, where non-noxious stimuli can cause pain (allodynia). Schwann cells in damaged nerves produce increased mRNA for NGF and their receptors for regenerative events. Damaged axons often express adrenoreceptors, which cause discharges in response to circulating epinephrine and norepinephrine (NE).

These neurotrophins also may cause aberrant regeneration, such as the ingrowth of sympathetic postganglionic axons into dorsal root ganglia. It may also cause the ingrowth of large myelinated afferents into lamina II, forming abnormal connections in the nociceptive processing circuits within the dorsal horn (which may further explain allodynia). These sprouts develop active sodium channels that become sites of tonic impulse generation, known as ectopic foci. These impulses occur in primary nociceptive axons in the absence of noxious stimuli.

Loss of spinal inhibitory mechanisms

Spinal endogenous inhibitory systems serve as opposing compensatory influences and are gaining recognition for their powerful capacity to restrain allodynia and hyperalgesia. These include numerous G protein-coupled receptors (μ- and δ-opioid, α_2- adrenergic, purinergic A1, neuropeptide Y1 and Y2, cannabinoid CB1 and CB2, muscarinic M2, γ-aminobutyric acid type B, metabotropic glutamate type II–III, somatostatin) and perhaps nuclear receptors (peroxisome proliferator-activated receptor gamma). Excessive down-regulation or defective compensatory up-regulation of these systems may contribute to the maintenance of neuropathic pain. An increasing number of pharmacotherapeutic strategies for neuropathic pain are emerging that mimic and enhance inhibitory neurotransmission in the dorsal horn. In addition, inhibitory interneurons often stop functioning during severe conditions of neuropathic pain. This is hypothesized to result from denervation of input from A-beta afferent (deafferentation) or glutamate excitotoxicity.

Peripheral nervous system pathophysiology

Peripheral sensitization occurs due to activation of silent receptors, increased nociceptor receptors and neurotransmitters, abnormal functioning of non-pain receptors, and down-regulation of inhibitory neurotransmitters. Nerve growth factor (NGF), which is a survival factor in the nervous system, is produced during inflammation of tissue and it increases the synthesis of SP and CGRP through activating TrKA receptors. In normal tissue, there are silent nociceptors that are insensitive to mechanical or thermal stimuli; however, in the presence of inflammation, SP lowers the threshold of synaptic excitability resulting in the unmasking of normally silent interspinal synapses and the sensitization of second-order spinal neurons. Activation of silent nociceptors produces ongoing pain even though the stimulus has been removed. Furthermore, SP can extend long distances in the spinal cord and sensitize dorsal horn neurons at a distance from the initial input locus. This results in an expansion of receptive fields and the activation of WDR neurons by non-nociceptive afferent impulses. Neuropeptides, specifically SP, also act on G protein-coupled receptors such as the neurokinin-1 (NK-1) receptor, which results in slow synaptic currents that change the level of excitability of the postsynaptic cell. These G protein-coupled receptors can cause an increase in transmission from the primary afferent fiber to the second-order cell and again to the transmission of the signal to higher centers.

Inflammation produces up-regulation of genes and increased expression of TRPV1 and other sensory nerve-specific sodium channels in response to injury and inflammatory mediators. NGF decreases the threshold to noxious stimulation resulting in hyperalgesia as well as an increase in neurotransmitters such as SP and brain-derived neurotrophic factors that can amplify the input to spinal cord. The input to sodium channels may be blocked by lidocaine, mexiletine, and anticonvulsants.

Another important factor in peripheral sensitization is through A-beta afferent fibers. Normally, nonpainful sensations are detected by specialized corpuscle structures and free nerve endings that transduce mechanical stimuli via large myelinated A-beta afferent fibers. However, injured A-beta fibers in damaged tissue paradoxically begin to express SP and CGRP. These abnormal receptors have a low threshold and they release SP in the dorsal horn and cause hyperexcitability.

Neurogenic inflammation

Inflammatory cells surround the areas of tissue damage and produce cytokines and chemokines that usually act as mediators in the process of healing and tissue regeneration. However, these agents are also irritants and change the properties of the primary sensory neurons surrounding the area of trauma.

Cyclooxygenase (COX) plays an important role in both peripheral and central sensitizations. In normal, non-inflamed skin, there is no cyclooxygenase-2 (COX-2). COX-2 is a protein that acts as an enzyme and it catalyzes the production of prostaglandins. However, hours after peripheral inflammation, COX-2 increases massively and it leads to the production of prostaglandins. As a result of this induction of COX-2, a surge of prostaglandins are produced and act on very specific receptors called EP receptors. These EP receptors are G protein-coupled receptors that begin a cascade of intracellular signal transductions in the peripheral terminals. In particular, they activate two kinases, protein kinase A (PKA) and protein kinase C (PKC). The first is a cyclic AMP-dependent kinase, and the latter is a calcium-activated protein kinase. These kinases phosphorylate some of the transducing proteins, causing increased sensitivity to stimuli such as heat, reducing their threshold of activation. They also phosphorylate sodium channels that are expressed in the membrane, causing a hyperexcitable state. This state is reached by enhancing the tetrodotoxin (TTX) resistant Na^+ channels. There has been a study that demonstrated knockout of these channels caused pronounced mechanical hypoalgesia in mice.

CGRP and SP also cause vasodilatation. Hence, they induce vasodilatation, plasma extravasation and other effects, e.g. attraction of macrophages and degranulation of mast cells. This may result in the release of other mediators, which can produce further sensitization of primary afferent fibers, activation of primary afferent fibers, or sensitization or activation of nearby primary afferent nociceptors. There would be vasodilatation in the presence of heat, redness, and swelling from plasma extravasation. NGF also has the ability to act on mast cells directly to activate and sensitize sensory endings by mast cell degranulation [8].

Humoral and hormonal responses to poorly controlled pain

A large number of pathophysiological responses have been characterized in patients suffering pain following acute traumatic injuries. These responses developed teleologically and provide important survival benefits in young healthy individuals following life-threatening injuries. However, these same responses may significantly increase post-surgical morbidity in high-risk patients (Table 6.1).

Catecholamine responses

Poorly controlled pain is associated with clinically significant humoral/hormonal alterations. These include enhanced sympathoadrenal and neuroendocrine

Table 6.1. The acute injury response: potential benefits versus disadvantages in post-surgical settings

Beneficial effects after severe injury	Adverse effects in high-risk patients
1. Maintenance of intravascular volume and mean arterial pressure	1. Hypertension, hypervolemia, increased risk of arterial pressure hemorrhage, stroke
2. Maintenance of cardiac output and cerebral perfusion	2. Tachycardia, arrhythmias, myocardial ischemia, perfusion congestive heart failure
3. Enhanced hemostasis	3. Hypercoagulable state, increased risk of arterial and deep venous thrombosis
4. Substrate mobilization, enhanced energy production	4. Hyperglycemia, negative nitrogen balance
5. Immobilization. minimizing further tissue injury	5. Reduction in respiratory volume and flow rates hypoxia, pneumonia
6. Learned avoidance	6. Anxiety, fear, demoralization, prolonged convalescence
7. Nerve plasticity and regeneration	7. Nerve plasticity with development of chronic pain

Modified from: Ghori M, Sinatra RS. The pathophysiology of pain. In: Sinatra RS, Viscusi G, de Leon-Casasola O, Ginsberg B., eds., *Acute Pain Management*. Cambridge University Press, 2008.

responses that can have negative effects on key target organs [8–12]. The stress response to surgical or accidental trauma has been described as a general adaptation syndrome focused upon tissue repair and improved survival. The sympathetic-adrenal response to traumatic injury evolves in three stages. The initial alarm stage or "fight-flight reaction" allows rapid withdrawal from the traumatic event and maintains blood flow to critical organs, and later an "exhaustion stage" limits mobility and favors tissue repair. Following extensive tissue injury, nociceptive impulses stimulate sympathetic cells in the hypothalamus and preganglionic neurons in the anterior lateral horn. Once stimulated, catecholamines released by these cells initiate cardiac inotropic and chronotropic responses, increase peripheral vascular resistance, and redistribute blood flow away from peripheral tissues and viscera to the heart and brain [9–11]. These initially advantageous effects can become deleterious in time, particularly in at-risk or debilitated patients where myocardial activity and the work of breathing may exceed the oxygen and metabolic supplies. In general, highest elevations in plasma catecholamines are observed following extensive procedures and in younger individuals [10–12]. Pathophysiological changes associated with increased sympathetic tone and altered regional perfusion include the following: (1) an increased incidence of post-surgical hypertension, which ranges from 5% following minor, uncomplicated procedures to approximately 50% in patients recovering from more extensive vascular surgery; (2) increased peripheral vascular resistance, which is associated with increased in contractility and myocardial

oxygen consumption, as the organism attempts to maintain or augment cardiac output.

Neuroendocrine responses

In patients experiencing severe pain, nociceptive impulses traveling up the spinal cord via the midbrain reticular formation activate hypothalamic centers and initiate the neuroendocrine stress response [20–23]. These well-described changes, termed the "stress response to injury", are characterized by an increased secretion of catabolic hormones including cortisol, glucagon, growth hormone, catecholamines, and inhibition of anabolic mediators such as insulin and testosterone [9,10]. These mediators increase substrate mobilization, resulting in hyperglycemia and a negative nitrogen balance. Associated metabolic changes including gluconeogenesis, glycogenolysis, proteolysis and breakdown of lipid stores provide the injured organism with short-term benefits of enhanced energy production. The negative nitrogen balance observed in patients experiencing severe trauma-related pain has been related to release of adrenocorticotropic hormone (ACTh), increased secretion of glucocorticoids, and an altered insulin:glucagon ratio [9,10]. Plasma levels of beta-endorphin and the posterior pituitary-derived octapeptide, arginine vasopressin (AVP), rise dramatically and remain elevated for up to 5 days following extensive surgical trauma [10–12]. Increased secretion of AVP is responsible for post-surgical fluid retention, plasma hypoosmolarity, and oliguria. Prolonged negative nitrogen balance is associated with impaired wound healing and immunocompetence. Increased protein breakdown and diminutions in protein synthesis may inhibit cell division, production of collagen, and acute-phase/leukocytic responses. Such inhibition results in stress-induced lymphopenia, granulocytosis, decreased natural killer and T-cell activity, and impaired synthesis/release immunoglobulins [11–14]. In animal models, and initial clinical trials, invasive surgery and poorly controlled pain are associated with profound immune suppression and increased risk of tumor metastasis [14,15]. Diminished cellular and humoral immunity may predispose debilitated individuals and those with preexisting immune disorders to post-operative infections.

The pathophysiological impact of poorly controlled pain on key target organs

Cardiac and vascular effects

In high-risk populations, peri-operative cardiac ischemia is most likely to occur following surgery, most commonly between post-operative days 1 and 3 [16]. While a variety of factors may contribute to the development of post-operative myocardial ischemia, the above-mentioned responses to poorly controlled pain appear to play a prominent role [9,16]. Catecholamine-induced tachycardia, enhanced myocardial contractility, increased afterload, and hypervolemia, secondary to enhanced release of AVP and aldosterone, are well-characterized factors responsible for increased oxygen demand. Increased oxygen demand, together with hypervolemia, may precipitate ischemia and acute cardiac failure, especially in patients with poorly compensated coronary artery and/or valvular heart disease [9,16–18]. In a setting where myocardial oxygen requirements are increasing, oxygen supply may be diminished because of coronary artery thrombosis and alterations in pulmonary function. Coronary artery blockage may result from: (1) high circulatory levels of catecholamines and increased coronary sympathetic tone; (2) stress-induced increases in plasma viscosity and platelet-induced thrombosis; and (3) coronary vasospasm secondary to platelet aggregation and release of serotonin [17–19]. Catecholamines, angiotensin, and other factors associated with surgical pain may increase platelet activation and accelerate coagulation. Increased platelet-fibrinogen activation may be especially deleterious in patients with atherosclerotic vascular disease, since increased plasma viscosity, platelet

aggregation, and platelet release of vasoconstrictive factors may significantly reduce blood flow in critically stenosed vessels [9,10]. Enhanced sympathetic tone and intense vasospasm may also compromise distal graft patency and skin flap viability [10,11].

Pulmonary effects

Pulmonary alterations associated with poorly controlled pain include atelectasis secondary to hypoventilation and pulmonary edema resulting from stress-induced hypervolemia [20–22]. The magnitude of symptoms is influenced by the extent of the injury, location (thoracic and upper abdominal injuries), effectiveness of pain management, and the physical status of the patient. In contrast to resting pain, the intensity of effort-dependent pain markedly increases with inspiration and cough. The pain stimulus is also hyperalgesic in that severe discomfort and reflexive muscle splinting may be noted at many dermatomes above and below the site of injury. Chest wall and upper abdominal hyperalgesia are responsible for several pathophysiological alterations including musculoskeletal and diaphragmatic dysfunction, and impaired gas exchange. The classic pulmonary response to upper abdominal surgical pain includes an increased respiratory rate and decreased tidal volume (TV), vital capacity (VC), forced expiratory volume (FEV_1), and functional residual capacity (FRC) [22–24]. Significant reductions in VC are evident within the first 3 hours, and declines to 40–60% of pre-operative values have been reported. Following upper abdominal surgery, reductions in FRC and FEV_1 are detrimental, and are most pronounced at 24 hours; thereafter, values gradually return to near normal levels by post-operative day 7. As FRC declines, resting lung volume approaches closing volume, resulting in atelectasis, ventilation/perfusion mismatch, and hypoxemia. Following thoracotomy, alterations in chest wall motion reduce lung compliance and increase the work of breathing [20–22,24]. Splinting secondary to poorly controlled pain exaggerates this process by further decreasing respiratory effort. If pneumonia or ARDS occurs, the risk of prolonged hospitalization and mortality increases.

Venous thrombotic effects

In the setting of intense pain and increased sympathetic tone, perfusion of injured tissues is reduced and may result in impaired wound healing, increased muscle

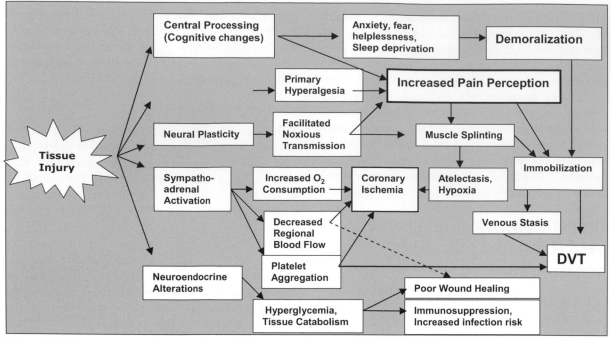

Figure 6.1. Pathophysiological impact of poorly controlled pain. Adapted from: Ghori M, Sinatra RS. The pathophysiology of pain. In: *Acute Pain Management*, Sinatra RS, Viscusi G, de Leon-Casasola O, Ginsberg B. (eds), 2008. Cambridge University Press.

spasm, and visceral-somatic ischemia and acidosis [8–10]. Inadequately controlled pain can predispose patients to post-surgical deep venous thromboses (DVT) and pulmonary embolism. As previously discussed, catecholamines and angiotensin released in response to surgical stress may result in platelet-fibrinogen activation and the development of a hypercoagulable state. Severe pain is commonly associated with an impaired ability to ambulate and decreased venous flow, and development of DVT. Thrombotic fragments can embolize and travel to the pulmonary arteries, resulting in varing degrees of ventilation perfusion mismatch and hypoxia. Pulmonary emboli incite the local release of vasoactive and inflammatory cytokines, worsening hypoxia symptoms within a short period of time. If not recognized and promptly treated this complication is associated with a 20–30% mortality [8–10].

Emotional and quality of life effects

Finally, poorly controlled and ongoing noxious perception can exacerbate emotional distress, increase patient anxiety and lead to persistent pain states [25]. Poorly controlled pain is associated with reduced morale, and learned helplessness. Patients are com-

monly troubled by sleep disturbances that negatively impact on mood and motivation to participate in rehabilitation [26,27]. Sleep quality and duration appear to be most impaired in patients reporting pain scores greater than 5 on a 0–10 scale. Many patients require anxiolytics and sedatives to experience limited intervals of sleep and generally awake experiencing increased pain. The widespread pathophysiological impact of poorly controlled pain is outlined in Figure 6.1.

References

1. *Bonica's Management of Pain*, 3rd ed. Philadelphia: Lippincott Williams & Wilkins, 2001.

2. Firestein G. *Kelley's Textbook of Rheumatology*, 8th ed. Philadelphia: W.B. Saunders, 2008.

3. Jensen T. Pathophysiology of pain: from theory to clinical evidence. *Eur J Pain Supp* 2008;**2**:13–17.

4. Gottschalk A, Smith DS. New concepts in acute pain therapy: preemptive analgesia. *Am Fam Physician* 2001;**63**:1979–1984.

5. Schaible H. *Pathophysiology of Pain*. Heidelberg: Langenbecks Archives of Surgery, 2004, pp. 237–243.

6. Samad TA. Interleukin-1ß-mediated induction of Cox-2 in the CNS contributes to inflammatory pain hypersensitivity. *Nature* 2001;**410**:471–475.

7. Woolf CJ, Shortland P, Coggeshall RE. Peripheral nerve injury triggers central sprouting of myelinated afferents. *Nature* 1992;**355**:75–78.

8. Cousins MJ. Acute pain and the injury response: immediate and prolonged effects. *Reg Anesth* 1989;**16**:162–176.

9. Kehlet H. Surgical stress: the role of pain and analgesia. *Br J Anaesth* 1989;**63**:189–195.

10. Breslow MJ. Neuroendocrine responses to surgery. In Breslow MJ, Miller CF, Rogers MC, eds. *Perioperative Management*. St Louis: Mosby-Year Book, 1990.

11. Lyons A, Kelly JL, Rodick ML, et al. Major injury induces increased production of interleukin-10 by cell of the immune system with a negative effect on infection resistance. *Ann Surgery* 1997;**226**:450–460.

12. Dubois M. Surgical stress in humans is accompanied by an increase in plasma beta-endorphin immunoreactivity. *Life Sci* 1981;**29**:1249–1254.

13. Redmond HP, Watson RW, Houghton K, et al. Immune function in patients undergoing open versus laproscopic surgery. *Arch Surg* 1994;**129**:1240–1246.

14. Allendorf JD, Bessler M, Kaylow ML, et al. Increased tumor establishment after laparotomy vs laparoscopy in a murine model. *Arch Surg* 1995;**130**:649–653.

15. Georges C, Lo T, Alkofer B, et al. The effects of surgical trauma on colorectal liver metastasis. *Surg Endoscopy* 2007;**21**:1817–1819.

16. Badner NH, Knoll RL, Brown JE, et al. Myocardial infarction after non cardiac surgery. *Anesthesiology* 1998;**88**:572–578.

17. Breslow MJ, Jordan DA, Christopherson R, et al. Epidural morphine decreases post-operative hypertension by attenuating sympathetic nervous system hyperactivity. *JAMA* 1989;**261**:3577–3581.

18. Freeman LJ, Nixon PG, Sallabank P, et al. Psychological stress and silent myocardial ischemia. *Am Heart J* 1987;**114**:477–482.

19. Willerson JT, Golino P, Eidt J, et al. Specific platelet mediators and unstable coronary artery lesions, *Circulation* 1989;**80**:198–205.

20. Moulton AL, Greenburg AG. The pulmonary system. In O'Leary JP, ed. *The Physiologic Basis of Surgery*. Philadelphia: Williams & Wilkins, 1993, pp. 512–514.

21. Sinatra RS, Ennevor S. Pain management following thoracic and upper abdominal trauma. In Rosenberg AD, ed. *International Trauma Anesthesia and Critical Care Society*. Baltimore, 1999.

22. Duggan J, Drummond GB. Activity of lower intercostal muscle function after upper abdominal surgery. *Anesth Analg* 1987;**66**:852–855.

23. Beecher HK. The measured effect of laparotomy on the respiration. *J Clin Invest* 1933;**12**:639–650

24. Ali J, Weisel RD, Layug AB. Consequences of post-operative alterations in respiratory mechanics. *Am J Surg* 1974;**128**:376–382.

25. Kehlet H, Woolf CJ. Persistent postsurgical pain: risk factors and prevention. *Lancet* 2006;**367**(9522):1618–1625.

26. Pavlin J, Chen C, Penaloza DA, Buckley P. A survey of pain and other symptoms that affect the recovery process after discharge from an ambulatory surgery unit. *J Clin Anesth* 2004;**16**:200–206.

27. Wu C, Naqibuddin M, Rowlingson AJ, et al. The effect of pain on health related quality of life. *Anesth Analg* 2003;**97**:1078–1085.

Neuropathic pain

Ho Dzung and Oscar A. de Leon-Casasola

Background

Neuropathic pain (NP) is defined by the International Association for the Study of Pain as "pain initiated or caused by a primary lesion or dysfunction in the nervous system".

For both diagnostic and therapeutic purposes, NP has been divided in two large groups: peripheral and central. Table 7.1 details the common causes and types of neuropathic pain.

Diagnosis is based on medical history; review of systems; physical and particularly neurological examination; motor and sensory examination (see below); and appropriate laboratory studies, including blood and serological tests, magnetic resonance imaging, and electrophysiological studies [1,2]. Sensory symptoms include paresthesia (abnormal sensation, either evoked or spontaneous), dysesthesia (evoked or spontaneous unpleasant, abnormal sensation), hyperalgesia (increased response to a normally painful stimulus), and allodynia (painful response to a non-noxious stimulus), hypoesthesia and hypoalgesia (loss of sensitivity to stimulation in general, and painful stimuli in particular). Sensory and perception abnormalities associated with neuropathic pain are described in Table 7.2. Different scales and questionnaires have been developed in an attempt to demonstrate discriminative features between neuropathic pain and non-neuropathic pain and various tools are available to screen for neuropathic pain [3]. A 30% reduction in pain scores using such scales is deemed clinically important [4].

Sensory examination should include touch, pinprick, pressure, cold, heat, and vibration assessment [5]. Responses are graded as normal, decreased, or increased to determine whether negative or positive sensory phenomena are involved. The stimulus-evoked (positive) pain types are classified as dysesthetic, hyperalgesic, or allodynic, and according to the dynamic or static character of the stimulus [6,7]. A more sophisticated neurophysiological test is the quantitative sensory testing (QST), which uses a battery of standardized mechanical and thermal stimuli [8]. When present, allodynia or hyperalgesia can be quantified by measuring intensity, threshold for elicitation, duration, and area. More detailed information on the assessment of pain, quantitative sensory testing, and measures of neuropathic pain is available [8–13].

Pharmacological management of neuropathic pain

Medications that are Food and Drug Administration (FDA)-approved for the treatment of NP include carbamazepine (trigeminal neuralgia); gabapentin (PHN); pregabalin (diabetic peripheral neuropathy [DPN]; PHN), duloxetine (PHN), and the 5% lidocaine patch (PHN). Thus, a significant portion of drug therapy used for neuropathic pain is off-label. Guidelines and systematic reviews on the pharmacological management of neuropathic pain are available [14–21] and are summarized in Figure 7.1.

In general, patients with peripheral NP are treated with the following algorithm.

1. A 5% lidocaine patch is used initially. If there is no response, or there is inadequate pain control, then a tricyclic antidepressant (TCA) is added to the therapeutic protocol, assuming there is no contraindication for it use. Alternatively a dual reuptake inhibitor (serotonin-norepinephrine) may also be used.

2. Alternative choices for TCAs include amitriptyline, nortriptyline, or desipramine. All of these agents have been shown to be effective in the treatment of neuropathic pain. Consequently, the choice is based on the drug's side-effect profile. In this regard, desipramine is not associated with sedation, as it lacks antihistaminic effects. Moreover, the incidence of anticholinergic effects is lower when compared to amitriptyline. Alternatively, nortriptyline may be used if lack of

Table 7.1. Types of neuropathic pain

Peripheral

- Acute and chronic inflammatory demyelinating polyradiculopathy
- Alcoholic
- Chemotherapy-induced peripheral neuropathy
- Complex regional pain syndrome type I and II
- Entrapment neuropathies (e.g. carpal tunnel syndrome)
- HIV sensory neuropathy
- Post-surgical (e.g. postmastectomy pain or post-thoracotomy pain)
- Idiopathic sensory
- Nerve compression, including tumor infiltration
- Nutrition deficiency-related
- Diabetic
- Phantom limb pain
- Post-herpetic neuralgia
- Post-radiation plexopathy
- Radiculopathy (cervical, thoracic, lumbar)
- Toxin-related
- Trigeminal neuralgia
- Post-traumatic

Central neuropathic pain

- Compressive myelopathy
- HIV myelopathy
- Multiple sclerosis-related
- Parkinson's disease-related
- Post-ischemic myelopathy
- Post-radiation myelopathy
- Post-stroke pain
- Post-traumatic spinal cord injury
- Syringomyelia

sleep is a problem because it will produce sedation comparable to amitriptyline, but very little anticholinergic effects. Moreover, nortriptyline will not block the baroreceptor reflex, making it an excellent choice for patients with diabetic peripheral neuropathy. Patients are started on 25 mg at bedtime and titrated up to 100 mg PO at bedtime on a weekly basis if needed.

3. If there is no response, or there is inadequate pain control, then an anticonvulsant such as gabapentin or pregabalin is added to the therapeutic protocol. For gabapentin, patients are started at 300 mg PO TID, and the dose is titrated on 300 mg increments weekly, until a dose of 1200 mg PO TID is reached. For pregabaline, patients are started at 50 mg PO TID and the dose is titrated on 50–100 mg increments weekly, until a maximum dose of 300 mg PO TID is reached. Patients are likely to experience sedation and dizziness with these drugs. However, titration continues until the maximum dose is reached, or severe side effects such as hallucinations, ataxia or severe myoclonic jerks are seen.

4. If no adequate clinical response is achieved with a combination of these three agents, then an opioid is indicated as a fourth-line agent. The opioid and the dose will vary with the patient's general condition and attention to drug–drug interactions plays an important role in the election of the drug.

5. If no efficacy is seen with this pharmacological algorithm, or severe side effects impair one's ability to titrate the medications to the target level, then invasive techniques are indicated (see below).

Patients with central neuropathic pain are managed with the same algorithm, except that 5% lidocaine patch is not used as the first-line agent.

Practice guidelines from the American College of Occupational and Environmental Medicine also address various diagnostic and treatment issues related to neuropathic pain, including drug therapy and some of the other interventions discussed below (i.e. psychological services, rehabilitation, electrical stimulation therapies and interdisciplinary pain management programs) [22].

Nonpharmacological management of neuropathic pain

Nonpharmacological approaches include physical modalities (physical therapy, massage, exercise, ice, heat and ultrasound therapy), psychological interventions, and electrical stimulation; in some cases, more invasive neuromodulatory or neurosurgical interventions may be needed as well.

Rehabilitation

Rehabilitation involves the restoration of lost function. All chronic illness, including persistent pain, results in loss of function or dysfunction. Rehabilitation

Table 7.2.

Term	Definition
Allodynia	Pain due to non-noxious stimuli (clothing, light touch) when applied to the affected area. May be mechanical (e.g. caused by light pressure), dynamic (caused by nonpainful movement of a stimulus), or thermal (caused by nonpainful warm, or cool stimulus)
Analgesia	Absence of pain in response to stimulation that would normally be painful
Anesthesia	Loss of normal sensation to the affected region
Dysesthesia	Spontaneous or evoked unpleasant abnormal sensations
Eudynia	Symptom-based pain provoked by an identifiable injury or noxious stimulus
Hyperalgesia	Exaggerated response to a mildly noxious stimulus applied to the affected region
Hyperpathia	Delayed and explosive response to a noxious stimulus applied to the affected region
Hypoesthesia	Reduction of normal sensation to the affected region
Maldynia	Maladaptive pain that persists in the absence of ongoing tissue damage or injury
Neuralgia	Pain in the distribution of a nerve or nerves
Neuropathic pain	Pain initiated or caused by a primary lesion or dysfunction in the nervous system
Neuropathy	A disturbance of function or pathological change in a nerve: in one nerve, mononeuropathy; in several nerves, mononeuropathy multiplex; if diffuse and bilateral, polyneuropathy
Nociceptor	A receptor preferentially sensitive to a noxious stimulus or to a stimulus that would become noxious if prolonged
Pain	An unpleasant sensory and emotional experience associated with actual or potential tissue damage, or described in terms of such damage
Paresthesias	Nonpainful spontaneous abnormal sensations
Phantom pain	Pain from a specific site that no longer exists (e.g. amputated limb) or where there is no current injury
Referred pain	Occurs in a region remote from the source

is essential in order to restore function and wellness. Rehabilitation is not limited to physical rehabilitation. It includes occupational, vocational, pharmacological, social, and other forms of rehabilitation. Modalities range from passive (massage, stretching) to active (exercise, dancing). Therapy must be properly supervised and should be progressive in order to restore function with minimal distress. It is important to avoid iatrogenic trauma and exacerbation of pain.

Psychological interventions

Specific psychological traits or experiences affect an individual's response to pain and suffering. These include fear, attention and vigilance to pain, catastrophizing and worry, avoidance of pain-inducing activity, mood disorders, anger and hostility, self-denigration, differences in the ability to achieve control in the face of distress and disability, and the ability to comprehend the factors exacerbating pain [23]. These psychological factors must be addressed in managing patients afflicted with persistent pain [24].

Behavioral treatments are designed to identify social and environmental factors that provoke pain behaviors or the lack of wellness behaviors. Withdrawal of attention (i.e. from spouse or caregiver) to pain behaviors is encouraged and avoidance behaviors (on the part of the patient) are discouraged through the use of reinforcers and punishments [25,26]. Behavioral approaches also employ self-regulatory treatments for chronic pain that teach patients to control certain bodily responses through relaxation, hypnosis and/or biofeedback. Time-contingent instead of pain-contingent drug use may be a part of this strategy as well, although this approach does not work especially well in patients who experience spontaneous, paroxysmal pain. Graduated activity exposure or pacing is another behavioral strategy used in chronic pain conditions to help patients regulate and gradually increase their activity level.

Cognitive therapy consists primarily of education and is generally employed in conjunction with behavioral therapy (see below). It demands patient participation and transfers the responsibility from an external

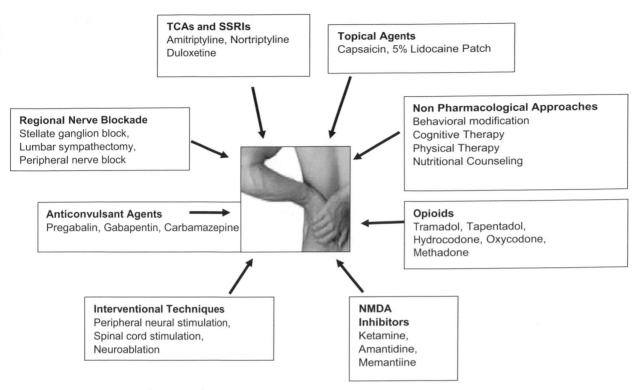

Figure 7.1. Treatment options for neuropathic pain.

to an internal locus of control, attempting to make the patient aware of the implications of pain and to better align expectations of treatment.

Cognitive-behavioral therapy (CBT) represents a selected combination and integration of treatments aimed at reducing or extinguishing the influence of the factors that reinforce or maintain patients' maladaptive behaviors, beliefs and patterns of thought [27]. Often the first stage in CBT is to educate and provide a credible rationale for treatment by addressing the causes and consequences of pain. This can assist in understanding the perpetuation of pain, disability and distress, and in challenging erroneous beliefs, fears, and maladaptive avoidance behavior. Patients are taught to develop insights into the nature of self-defeating patterns of thinking and develop ways of challenging the premises from which these thoughts develop. This can lead to reversal of symptom-contingent declines in activity; crafting achievable goals that can be reinforced; and fostering anger management, stress reduction, and development of self-relaxation responses. Published randomized controlled trials provide good evidence for the effectiveness of CBT or behavioral therapy for certain chronic pain conditions (e.g. back pain, fibromyalgia) in adults [28,29].

Multidisciplinary treatment

Behavioral medicine is generally embedded in a comprehensive, multimodal pain treatment program. Patients who suffer from chronic pain may experience higher rates of comorbid psychiatric disorders (e.g. depression, anxiety), as well as sleep disturbances. Effective treatment of these conditions must be part of the management plan.

Comprehensive treatments aim to eliminate maladaptive pain-related behaviors, achieve pain control, and improve coping through use of the above-noted techniques in combination with an interdisciplinary team approach to improve psychological functioning, reduce disability, and achieve rehabilitation [30]. A multimodal approach requires the combined efforts of: (1) a physician(s) knowledgeable in pharmacological and/or interventional procedures; (2) a psychiatrist or other mental health professional to diagnose and treat psychiatric conditions that may result from, cause, or exacerbate pain and suffering; referral for

33

biofeedback, cognitive-behavioral techniques, group therapy, and counseling are warranted early in the course of treatment in patients with psychosocial impairment; (3) a physical therapist or rehabilitation specialist to assess physical conditioning requirements; physical therapy referral is useful for neuromuscular rehabilitation, gait and prosthetic device assessment, therapeutic exercise instruction, desensitization (especially in patients with allodynia and hyperalgesia), and electrical stimulation trials (if warranted); and (4) nurses knowledgeable about these approaches who serve to improve team function, and provide valuable assistance in sustaining patient optimism and participation.

Several studies have evaluated the clinical and cost-effectiveness of multidisciplinary pain centers, generally supporting their efficacy on multiple outcome criteria [31–34]. A recent systematic review of multidisciplinary treatments for chronic pain showed they were effective in patients with chronic low back pain and fibromyalgia, but exhibited less robust effects in patients with chronic pain of mixed etiology [35].

Interventional management of neuropathic pain

When systemic or topical pharmacotherapy and other non-invasive approaches provide inadequate relief in patients with NP, interventional approaches may be used, including sympathetic blockade with local anesthetics, intraspinal drug delivery, spinal cord stimulation, peripheral subcutaneous nerve stimulation, or stimulation of specific central nervous system structures, and various neuroablative procedures (e.g. dorsal rhizotomy, neurolytic nerve block, intracranial lesioning). Neuroablative procedures are not reversible and should be reserved for carefully and properly selected patients with intractable pain.

Nerve blocks

The interruption, interference, or blockade of painful stimuli has been used in the management of pain for several decades. Acute, chronic, and post-operative pain can be diminished with various types of regional anesthesia or specific nerve blocks. In the setting of chronic pain management, various peripheral nerve blocks can be diagnostic, prognostic, or therapeutic in nature. Nerve blocks are generally most useful when a specific nerve or limb is affected. Neural blockade may help differentiate a peripheral source of pain from a neuroma or entrapped nerve root, identify sources of referred pain, or assist in distinguishing somatic from visceral pain.

Sympathetic ganglion blocks are widely employed for diagnostic and therapeutic purposes: e.g. diagnosis of sympathetically maintained pain; neuropathic pain, including phantom limb pain; complex regional pain syndrome; and ischemic pain. If analgesia is afforded with local anesthetic blockade, chemical or thermal neurolysis may be used in an attempt to provide long-term relief. Many case reports, case series, and retrospective reviews have been published, but few prospective placebo-controlled, blinded studies exist [36]. Controlled evidence supports the use of neurolytic blocks in patients with low back pain, head, neck and shoulder pain, fibromyalgia, complex regional pain syndrome, and cancer pain. The strongest evidence exists for celiac plexus/splanchnic neurolytic blockade for cancer pain and lumbar sympathetic block or neurolysis for reflex sympathetic dystrophy and lower extremity ischemic pain [36,37].

Neurostimulation

In the past 25 years, the field of pain management has increasingly incorporated technologies of neurostimulation as part of the treatment algorithm for patients with maldynia. Methodological problems are encountered in blinding, recruitment, and assessment in nearly all published trials of these interventions. Nevertheless, patients entered in these trials have generally suffered for extended periods, and many have reported substantial relief.

Transcutaneous electrical stimulation (TENS) for chronic pain

TENS is used in a variety of clinical settings to treat a range of acute and chronic pain conditions and has become popular with patients and healthcare professionals of different disciplines. By applying peripheral stimuli (rubbing, vibration, heat, cold) or, in the case of TENS, electrical stimulation directly over the area of pain, sensory information from larger-diameter (non-pain-carrying) afferents is activated, and affects the processing of pain impulses within the dorsal horn of the spinal cord. TENS is generally believed to be a safe and relatively non-invasive intervention that can be used to alleviate many different types of pain, including neuropathic pain (primarily diabetic peripheral neuropathy) [38]. However, systematic reviews have concluded there is insufficient evidence to draw any conclusions about the effectiveness of TENS for the treatment of chronic pain in adults, or in the treatment of chronic lumbar back pain [39,40].

Spinal cord stimulation

Spinal cord stimulation (SCS) is a form of therapy used to treat certain types of chronic pain. An array of stimulating metal contacts is positioned in the dorsal epidural space. An electrical field is generated through connection of the contacts with an electrical generator. The leads can be implanted by laminectomy or percutaneously, and the source of power is supplied by an implanted battery or by an external radio-frequency transmitter. The resulting field presumably stimulates DRG axons and dorsal column fibers [41,42]. The goal is to create a field of (tolerable) paresthesias that overlap and cover the anatomic distribution of pain reported by the patient. A temporary trial of stimulation, most commonly performed with percutaneous lead placement, is required to identify patients who might benefit.

A comprehensive set of practice parameters on the use of spinal cord stimulation in the treatment of chronic neuropathic pain has been developed [42]. Indications include failed back surgery syndrome, complex regional pain syndrome, peripheral neuropathic pain, phantom limb/post-amputation syndrome, recalcitrant PHN, root injury pain, and spinal cord injury or lesions. It also is being used in the management of pain associated with multiple sclerosis, pain due to ischemic peripheral vascular disease, and interstitial nephritis.

Motor cortex stimulation is reserved for the treatment of complex central and neuropathic pain syndromes that have proven refractory to medical treatment, including post-stroke pain, deafferentation pain, and some neuropathic pain states of peripheral origin.

Summary and conclusion

Neuropathic pain is distinct from normal, nociceptive pain triggered by noxious stimuli. It is believed to be triggered by persistent nociceptive stimuli or frank nerve injury. These conditions activate a series of adaptive and, eventually, maladaptive changes in the function and properties of pain-carrying fibers and other sensory neurons, including phenotypic changes and alterations in gene expression, as well as the fundamental properties of specific neurons and sensory

pathways. Likewise, NP involves not only neuronal pathways, but also Schwann cells, satellite cells in the DRG, components of the peripheral immune system, spinal microglia, and astrocytes. As such, it is a multidimensional process that warrants consideration as a chronic degenerative disease not only affecting sensory and emotional processing, but also producing an altered brain state, based on both functional imaging and macroscopic measurements.

Despite recent advances in understanding of the pathology related to nervous system injury, the management of NP remains a challenge. Patients who have substantial disability and psychosocial problems, and who have not benefited from conventional pain treatments, are often referred to multidisciplinary pain clinics. These multimodal programs aim to eliminate maladaptive pain-related behaviors, achieve pain control, and improve coping through biopsychosocial techniques in combination with an interdisciplinary team approach to improve psychological functioning, reduce disability, and achieve rehabilitation. These programs have largely been validated in patients with chronic noncancer pain or certain mixed pain states, but not in patients with NP per se. A number of interventional approaches, including nerve blocks, spinal cord stimulation, and cortical stimulation, may be required when patients do not respond adequately to medical, psychological, and pharmacological management.

References

1. Backomja MM, Galer BS. Pain assessment and evaluation of patients who have neuropathic pain. *Neurol Clin* 1998;**16**:775–789.

2. Baron R. Mechanisms of disease: neuropathic pain – a clinical perspective. *Nat Clin Pract Neurol* 2006;**2**: 95–105.

3. Bennett MI, Bouhassira D. Epidemiology of neuropathic pain: can we use the screening tools? *Pain* 2007;**132**:12–13.

4. Farrar JT, Young DP, LaMOreaux L, Werth JL, Poole RM. Clinical importance of changes in chronic pain intensity measured on an 11-point numerical pain rating scale. *Pain* 2001;**94**:149–158.

5. Baron R. Mechanisms of disease: neuropathic pain – a clinical perspective. *Nat Clin Pract Neurol* 2006;**2**:95–105.

6. Rasmussen PV, Sindrup SH, Jensen TS, Bach FW. Symptoms and signs in patients with suspected neuropathic pain. *Pain* 2004;**110**:461–469.

7. Watkins LR, Milligan ED, Maier SF. Glial activation: a driving force for pathological pain. *Trends Neurosci* 2001;**24**:450–455.

8. Baron T, Tolle R. Assessment and diagnosis of neuropathic pain. *Curr Opin Support Palliat Care* 2008;**2**:1–8.

9. Horowitz SH. The diagnostic workup of patients with neuropathic pain. *Anesthesiol Clin* 2007;**25**:699–708.

10. Breivik H, Borchgrevink PC, Allen SM, et al. Assessment of pain. *Br J Anaesth* 2008;**101**:17–24.

11. Jensen TS, Hansson PT. Chapter 34. Classification of neuropathic pain syndromes based on symptoms and signs. *Handb Clin Neurol* 2006;**81**:517–526.

12. Galer BS, Jensen MP. Development and preliminary validation of a pain measure specific to neuropathic pain; the Neuropathic Pain Scale. *Neurology* 1997;**48**:332–338.

13. Krause SJ, Backonja MM. Development of a neuropathic pain questionnaire. *Clin J Pain* 2003;**19**:306–314.

14. Attal N, Cruccu G, Haanpaa M, et al. EFNS guidelines on pharmacological treatment of neuropathic pain. *Eur J Neurol* 2006;**13**:1153–1169.

15. Finnerup NB, Otto M, McQuay HJ, Jensen TS, Sindrup SH. Algorithm for neuropathic pain treatment: an evidence based proposal. *Pain* 2005;**118**:289–305.

16. Khaliq W, Alam S, Puri N. Topical lidocaine for the treatment of postherpetic neuralgia. *Cochrane Database Syst Rev* 2007;**2**:CD004846.

17. Mason L, Moore RA, Derry S, Edwards JE, McQuay HJ. Systematic review of topical capsaicin for the treatment of chronic pain. *BMJ* 2004;**328**:991–994.

18. Saarto T, Wiffen PJ. Antidepressants for neuropathic pain. *Cochrane Database Syst Rev* 2007;**4**:CD005454.

19. Dworkin RH, O'Connor AB, Backonja M, et al. Pharmacologic management of neuropathic pain: evidence-based recommendations. *Pain* 2007;**132**:237–251.

20. Moulin DE, Clark AJ, Gilron I, et al. Pharmacological management of chronic neuropathic pain – consensus statement and guidelines from the Canadian Pain Society. *Pain Res Manag* 2007;**12**:13–21.

21. Sultan A, Gaskell H, Derry S, Moore RA. Duloxetine for painful diabetic neuropathy and fibromyalgia pain: systematic review of randomised trials. *BMC Neurol* 2008;**8**:29.

22. Chronic pain. In *Practice Guidelines*, revised ed. Chicago, IL: American College of Occupational and Environmental Medicine, 2008.

23. Eccleston C. Role pf psychology in pain management. *Br J Anaesth* 2001;**87**:144–152.

24. Turk D, Okifuji A. Psychological factors in chronic pain. Evolution and revolution. *J Clin Consult Psychol* 2002;**70**:678–690.

25. Okifuji A, Ackerlind S. Behavioral medicine approaches to pain. *Anesthesiol Clin* 2007;**25**:709–719.

26. Osborne TL, Raichle KA, Jensen MP. Psychologic interventions for chronic pain. *Phys Med Rehabil Clin N A* 2006;**17**:415–433.

27. Daniel HC, van der Merwe JD. Cognitive behavioral approaches and neuropathic pain. *Handbook Clin Neurol* 2006;**81**:855–868.

28. Morley S, Eccleston C, Williams A. Systematic review and meta-analysis of randomized controlled trials of cognitive behavior therapy and behavior therapy for chronic pain in adults, excluding headache. *Pain* 1999;**80**:1–13.

29. Hoffman BM, Paps R, Chatkoff DK, Kerns RD. Meta-analysis of psychological interventions for chronic low back pain. *Health Psychol* 2007;**26**:10–12.

30. Jensen MP, Turner JA, Romano JM, et al. Coping with chronic pain: a critical review of the literature. *Pain* 1991;**47**:249–283.

31. Flor H, Fydrich T, Turk DC. Efficacy of multidisciplinary pain treatment centers: a meta-analytic review. *Pain* 1992;**49**:221–230.

32. Gatchel RJ, Okifuji A. Evidence-based scientific data documenting the treatment and cost-effectiveness of comprehensive pain program for chronic non-malignant pain. *J Pain* 2006;**7**:779–793.

33. Turk DC. Clinical effectiveness and cost-effectiveness of treatments for patients with chronic pain. *Clin J Pain* 2002;**18**:355–365.

34. Gallagher RM. Rational integration of pharmacologic, behavioral, and rehabilitation strategies in the treatment of chronic pain. *Am J Phys Med Rehabil* 2005;**84**(3 Suppl):S64–S76.

35. Scascighini L, Toma V, Dober-Soieklman S, Sprott H. Multidisciplinary treatment for chronic pain: a systematic review of interventions and outcomes. *Rheumatology* **47**:670–678.

36. Day M. Sympathetic blocks: the evidence. *Pain Practice* 2008;**8**:98–109.

37. Markman JD, Philip A. Interventional approaches to pain management. *Med Clin North Am* 2007;**91**:271–286.

38. Hansson P, Lundberg T. Transcutaneous electrical nerve stimulation, vibration and acupuncture as pain-relieving measures. In Wall PD, Melzack R, eds. *Textbook of Pain*, 4th ed. Edinburgh: Churchill Livingstone, 1999, pp. 1341–1351.

39. Nnoaham KE, Kumbang J. Transcutaneous electrical nerve stimulation (TENS) for chronic pain. *Cochrane Database Syst Rev* 2008;**3**.

40. Khadilkar A, Milne S, Brosseau L, et al. Transcutaneous electrical nerve stimulation for the treatment of chronic low back pain: a systematic review. *Spine* 2005;**30**:2657–2666.

41. Lazorthes Y, Verdie JC, Sol JC. Spinal cord stimulation for neuropathic pain. *Handb Clin Neurol* 2006;**81**:887–899.

42. North R, Shipley JS. Practice parameters for the use of spinal cord stimulation in the treatment of chronic neuropathic pain. *Pain Med* 2007;**8**(Suppl 4):S200–S275.

**Section 1
Chapter**

Pain Definitions

Genetics and pain

Keith A. Candiotti and Claudia R. Fernandez Robles

Introduction

Human beings differ widely in their rating and experience of painful stimulation. There are large variations in interindividual sensitivities to noxious pain, susceptibility to acute or chronic pain (even among patients with the same medical condition), and individual responses to analgesics. These individual responses arise from a multitude of factors, including environmental elements and genetic variations or polymorphisms [1–5]. Understanding the factors that contribute to patient-related variability in pain behavior and responses to analgesics is critical for the effective treatment of patients and management of their pain. This chapter will review some important pain polymorphisms and how they can influence the pain behavior of patients.

Genetic factors (Table 8.1)

Mu opioid receptor (MOR)

The mu receptor OPRM1 is the primary target site for opioid medications. The gene for this receptor is located on chromosome 6 and is a significant factor in the variability of how a patient responds to opioids. The most common single nucleotide polymorphism

(SNP), or basepair change, of the MOR gene consists of a change of adenine to guanine in the 118 position that leads to a substitution of the amino acid asparagine for aspartate. This substitution affects the function of the receptor by increasing its binding affinity for β-endorphins and subsequently affects the action of opioids at the receptor site [1–3].

Carriers of the G118 MOR variant, when compared with homozygous carriers of the A118 allele (wild type), have a decreased clinical response to opioids. Klepsad et al. [1] found that chronic pain patients, homozygous for the variant G118 allele, required more morphine (225±143 mg/day) to achieve pain control when compared with heterozygous patients (A/G, 66±50 mg/day) and patients having the homozygous wild-type A/A (97±89 mg/day). While imparting resistance to the analgesic properties of morphine it was also noted that patients who were homozygous for G/G, and who had renal failure, better tolerated the accumulated levels of morphine-6-glucoronide and vomited less than non-carriers. In yet another study, patients who were G/G homozygotes and were undergoing a total knee arthroplasty consumed significantly more morphine in the first 24 and 48 hours (22.3 ± 10.0 mg and 40.4 ± 22.1 mg respectively) compared to A/A homozygous (16 ± 8 mg and 25.3 ±15.5mg) [3].

Table 8.1. Genetic modulation and clinical response to analgesics

	Good medication response or pain resistance	Poor medication response or pain sensitivity
OPRM1	Carriers of the variant A118 allele	Carriers of the variant G118 allele
COMT	Carriers of val/val genotype	Carriers met/met genotype
CYP2D6	Extensive metabolizers	Poor metabolizers
MCR1	Carriers of two MCR1 alleles	Non-carriers of MCR1 alleles
GCH1	Carriers of the CGH1 haplotype	Non-carriers of CGH1 haplotype
ABCB1	Homozygous T/T carriers	Homozygous C/C carriers

OPRM1, Mu opioid receptor; COMT, catechol-O-methly transferase; CYP2D6, cytochrome 2D6; MC1R, melanocortin-1-receptor; GCH1, guanosine triphosphate cyclohydrolase-1; ABCB1, ATP-binding cassette, sub-family B, member 1.

ATP-binding cassette, sub-family B, member 1 (ABCB1)

Another important determinant of opioid bioavailability is the efflux transporter P-glycoprotein ABCB1 encoded by ABCB1/MDR1 gene. ABCB1 can limit the entry of morphine and its metabolites into the brain and actively pump drugs out of the central nervous system. Campa et al. [4] demonstrated an example of the cumulative effect of polymorphisms in the ABCB1/MDR1 and OPRM1 genes by studying the SNP C3435T in the ABCB1/MDR1 gene and for the A118G SNP in the OPRM1 gene in patients undergoing morphine therapy. They reported that ABCB1 homozygous T/T carriers had significantly greater pain relief from morphine than subjects who were homozygous wild-type C/C carriers. Additionally, OPRM1 homozygous A/A subjects had a significantly greater decrease in pain than homozygous patients with the OPRM1 G/G genotype. Finally, when the two SNP were studied together, homozygous patients for OPRM1 A/A and ABCB1/MDR1 T/T were found to be best responders when compared with patients who were heterozygous for the OPRM1 and ABCB1/MDR1 SNPs.

Catechol-O-methyltransferase (COMT)

COMT is an enzyme that acts as a key modulator of the dopaminergic and adrenergic system. Recent studies have demonstrated the importance of this enzyme in the regulation of pain perception [6,7]. The gene encoding for this enzyme, located on chromosome 22, contains a common functional polymorphism in codon 158 that causes a substitution of valine for methionine (val158met). This substitution results in decreased thermostability of the enzyme and a 3–4-fold reduced activity, leading to a decrease in the degradation of dopamine, and, as a consequence, an increase in norepinephrine and epinephrine levels which appear to lead to exaggerated levels of pain.

Three different COMT haplotypes have been identified:

The val/val genotype has the highest activity of the COMT enzyme and patients are referred to as low pain sensitivity (LPS) patients.

The met/met genotype has the lowest activity of the COMT enzyme and patients are referred to as high pain sensivity (HPS) patients.

Patients having the heterozygous genotype have an intermediate COMT activity and are considered to have average pain sensivity (APS).

In a study of cancer patients [6] it was noted that homozygous carriers of the LPS genotype required less morphine (95 ± 99 mg/day) for relief of cancer pain than heterozygous patients (117 ± 10 0mg/day) and HPS patients (155±160 mg/day). In addition to their phenotypic pain behavior, it was also noted that LPS patients exhibit greater cortisol responses to naloxone administration and had higher brain concentrations of μ receptors.

Cytochrome CYP2D6

Cytochromes (CYP) are significant phase I metabolizing enzymes. Of the various CYP enzymatic pathways CYP2D6 has gained much attention in relation to codeine, oxycodone, tramadol, and hydrocodone metabolism. The variable clinical response to these particular opioids can to a great extent be explained by polymorphisms of the gene encoding for the CYP2D6 enzyme [8,9].

There are approximately 100 CYP2D6 allelic variants identified; however, there are basically four metabolizer states: poor metabolizers (PM), who have two inactive genes and have no enzymatic activity; intermediate metabolizers (IM), who have less than normal activity, usually one inactive and one low-activity gene; extensive metabolizers (EM), who have one or two wild-type genes; and ultrarapid metabolizers (UM), who possess more than two wild-type genes and increased enzymatic activity. These genetic variations may account for the differences in intrinsic clearance of 70-fold between EM and PM for codeine O-demethylation, 10-fold for dihydrocodeine and oxycodone and 200-fold for hydrocodone.

Using codeine as an example of the effects of a metabolizer state, patients who lack enzymatic activity (PM) will not be able to convert codeine to its most active metabolite, morphine, and thus patients will get little if any analgesic benefit from the drug. In contrast, it has been reported that ultrarapid metabolizers (UM) may convert codeine to morphine too quickly, resulting in an excessive dose of morphine even when giving only a standard dose of codeine. A true codeine overdose is probably due to multiple factors since it is not commonly reported and the CYP2D6 UM can be as high as approximately 30% in some populations.

CYP2D6 has also recently been demonstrated to be a rate-limiting enzyme in the production of cellular morphine in humans. It has been suggested that CYP2D6 UM might have increased pain tolerance due to potentially increased cellular morphine production. In one association study performed on surgical patients it was noted that those patients possessing a CYP2D6 UM state required less morphine in the acute post-operative period when compared with other CYP2D6 metabolizer groups [8].

Interleukin-1

The cytokine interleukin-1 (IL-1) acts as a major initial inducer of a proinflammatory state. Two structurally different forms (IL-1α and IL-1β) exist, both of which bind to the same receptor protein (IL-1R). A third component of the IL-1 complex is the IL-1 receptor antagonist (IL-1RA), which binds to the IL-1R but does not activate it. IL-1RA plays an important role in inflammation due to the fact that it down-regulates IL1-α and IL1-β thereby decreasing the inflammatory response and subsequently pain. Recent evidence suggests that the degree and severity of surgery-induced inflammation may be significantly influenced by genetic

polymorphisms of IL-1RA [2,10,11]. In a study performed in women undergoing transabdominal hysterectomy, a polymorphism in the IL-1RA gene, which leads to higher levels of IL1-RA, was associated with decreased morphine consumption [2]. In another study, conducted in patients with painful knee osteoarthritis, an injection of 150 mg of IL-1RA intra-articularly resulted in a significant improvement in pain scores (-20.4 ± 23.3 mm [$p = 0.008$]) on a visual analog scale [10].

Melanocortin-1-receptor (MC1R)

Melanocortin-1-receptor (MC1R) is one of the key proteins involved in regulating skin and hair color. Humans having a mutation in this gene typically will have a reddish hair color and fair skin. The protein is located on the plasma membrane of melanocytes. Several SNPs have been identified which result in a loss of function of MC1R due to impaired G protein coupling. Studies have shown that subjects carrying a non-functional MC1R have 1.3-fold higher tolerance to electrical pain stimuli, and they are more sensitive to thermal pain stimuli and more resistant to the analgesic effect of subcutaneous lidocaine when compared to control subjects with a functional MC1R gene [12,13].

MC1R variants appear to modulate opioid efficacy in a sex-specific manner. Women carrying two non-functional MC1R alleles demonstrated a greater benefit from the analgesic effects of the κ-opioid agonist pentazocine than women carrying only one or none of the MC1R variant or men with the same MC1R genotype. Mogil et al. [12] reported that inactivation of MC1R increased the analgesic effects of morphine-6-glucuronide. The effect in this case was noted to be gender-independent. Finally, it has also been reported that female patients carrying the MC1R variants associated with red hair also require more anesthetic agents to achieve a comparable MAC level compared to women with dark hair [13].

Guanosine triphosphate cyclohydrolase-1 (GCH1)

GCH1 is the rate-limiting enzyme in the production of tetrahydrobiopterin (BH4). It has been reported that excessive BH4 is associated with the development of neuropathic pain following injury. Polymorphisms in GCH1 that decrease function have been reported to be associated with decreased pain levels. This is noted to be especially true in subjects carrying a series of 15 polymorphisms in the GCH1 gene. For example,

Lötsch et al. [14] reported that the need for the initiation of opioid pain medication was delayed in homozygous carriers of this haplotype compared to heterozygotes or non-carriers, indicating that it imparts some degree of pain resistance.

Uridine diphosphate-glucuronosyltransferase 2 family polypepetide B7 (UGT)

Opioids such as morphine, buprenorphine, and codeine are mainly glucuronidated by UGT. In the case of morphine UGT metabolizes it to form morphine-6-glucoronide (M6G) and morphine-3-glucoronide (M3G); M6G acting as an opioid agonist and MG3 demonstrating anti-analgesics effects. Polymorphisms in the UGT2B7 gene have been linked to variability in the level of morphine and its metabolites. In a study performed on Japanese patients with cancer, patients with the UGT2B7*2 variant allele had a lower frequency of nausea when compared to subjects without the allele [15]. While variants of UGT have been noted to affect drug levels and metabolites it is unclear whether they have direct analgesic consequences.

Conclusion

Genetic variations appear to play a much bigger role in inter-individual pain responses than was once thought. This section is not meant to be a comprehensive review of genetics and pain but is intended to point out the significance of these factors in the pain phenotype. While many patients are often given labels relative to their pain behavior it seems likely that much of this phenotypic behavior is not truly within their control and may in fact be due to their individual genetics. It is important for the practitioner to keep in mind that resistance to opioids may not be due to acquired tolerance but rather genetic resistance [16,17]. When managing patients it would seem reasonable that if a treatment was not successful in the past or less than acceptable it should not be repeated. Overall, by keeping in mind that the genetics of a patient may be affecting their pain phenotype caregivers may be able to deliver more individualized and effective care.

References

1. Klepstad P, Rakvåg T, Kaasa S. The 118A_G polymorphism in the human opioid receptor gene may increase morphine requirements in patients with pain caused by malignant disease. *Acta Anaesthesiol Scand* 2004;**48**:1232–1239.

2. Bessler H, Shavit Y. Post-operative pain, morphine consumption, and genetic polymorphism of IL-1β and IL-1 receptor antagonist. *Neurosci Lett* 2006;**404**:154–158.

3. Chou WY, Yang LC. Association of m-opioid receptor gene polymorphism (A118G) with variations in morphine consumption for analgesia after total knee arthroplasty. *Acta Anaesthesiol Scand* 2006;**50**: 787–792.

4. Campa D et al. Association of ABCB1/MDR1 and OPRM1 gene polymorphisms with morphine pain relief. *Clin Pharmacol Ther* 2008; **83**;559–566.

5. Candiotti K, Yang Z. The impact of CYP2D6 genetic polymorphisms on post-operative morphine consumption. *Pain Med* 2009;10, No5.

6. Rakvag TT, Klepstad P, Baar C, et al. The Val158Met polymorphism of the human catechol-O-methyltransferase (COMT) gene may influence morphine requirements in cancer pain patients. *Pain* 2005;**116**:73–89.

7. Zubieta JK, Heitzeg MM, Smith YR. COMT val158met genotype affects mu-opioid neurotransmitter responses to a pain stressor. *Science* 2003;**299**:1240–1243.

8. Foster A, Mobley E, Wang Z. Complicated pain management in a CYP450 2D6 poor metabolizer. *Pain Practice* 2007;**4**:352–356.

9. Reynolds K, Ramey-Hartung B, Jortani S. The value of CYP2D6 and OPRM1 pharmacogenetic testing for opioid therapy. *Clin Lab Med* 2008;**28**:581–598.

10. Chevalier X. Safety study of intraarticular injection of interleukin 1 receptor antagonist in patients with painful knee osteoarthritis: a multicenter study. *J Rheumatol* 2005;**32**:7.

11. Edwards R. Genetic predictors of acute and chronic pain. *Curr Rheumatol Rep* 2006; **8**:411–417.

12. Mogil JS, Ritchie J, Smith SB, et al. Melancortin-1 receptor gene variants affect pain and mu-opioid analgesia in mice and humans. *J Med Genet* 2005;**42**:583–587.

13. Stamer U. Genetic factors in pain and its treatment *Curr Opin Anaesthesiol* 2007;**20**:478–484.

14. Lötsch J, Geisslinger G, Tegeder I. Genetic modulation of the pharmacological treatment of pain. *Pharmacol Ther* 2009;**124**:168–184.

15. Fujita K, Ando Y, Yamamoto W, et al. Association of UGT2B7 and ABCB1 genotypes with morphine-induced adverse drug reactions in Japanese patients with cancer. *Cancer Chemother Pharmacol* 2010;**65**:251–258.

16. Compton P, Geschwind D. Association between human m-opioid receptor gene polymorphism, pain tolerance, and opioid addiction. *Am J Med Genet Part B (Neuropsychiatric Genetics)* 2003;**121B**:76–82.

17. Somogyi A, Barratt D, Coller J. Pharmacogenetics of Opioids. *Clin Pharmacol Ther* 2007;**81**:429–444.

9 Persistent post-operative pain

Peter G. Lacouture

Introduction

Some have defined persistent pain as a disease entity unto itself. Persistent post-operative pain has challenged pain management specialists for decades; it is only in the past several years that it has received significant attention. The continuation of pain and pain disability beyond the immediate post-operative period often results in medical (interventional and pharmacological), economic (healthcare utilization, loss of productivity) and psychological (depression, anxiety) complications.

Definition

In order to better understand the information that follows, a clear definition of the entity that we call persistent post-operative (post-surgical) pain needs to be defined. Precision does not currently exist; however, we will follow one of the original attempts in 1999 to describe this condition as:

- pain that develops after a surgical procedure
- pain that is present for at least 2 months
- pain where other causes are excluded
- pain that is excluded if it exists from a pre-surgical problem

Obviously, the task of defining a pure condition or "syndrome" is not within the scope of this chapter. However, the limitations of the data from the literature must be appreciated.

Historical background

Chronic post-surgical pain was probably first described in 1944 by army surgeons who noted persistent intercostal pain in soldiers who had undergone thoracotomy procedures for trauma. Nearly half a century later in 1991, this condition was once again described in patients following thoracic surgery. However, it was not until 1998 that researchers published papers recognizing this condition and expanding its presence beyond thoracic surgery. At that time the term coined was chronic post-surgical pain. While this complication of surgery was well-recognized, the methodology to properly study this issue was not well-developed. However, attention to this condition increased and one researcher stated that chronic pain associated with inguinal hernia repair was the most serious and long-term problem with these surgeries. The "condition" was then defined as persistent post-operative pain. While any injury may lead to chronic painful conditions, it is the post-surgical patients that are the focus of this chapter. Clinical and scientific articles on this subject continue to grow to include many surgical procedures including thoracotomy, hernia repair, breast cancer surgery, joint replacement, abdominal surgery (hysterectomy, cholecystectomy, C-section) and amputation [1,2].

Epidemiology

The incidence of persistent post-operative pain varies not only with the operations involved but also with the methodologies utilized to collect and evaluate data. Table 9.1 presents the results of one such epidemiological exploration focusing on the incidence of this condition with selected surgical procedures.

While incidence rates are not precise because of the methodological variability used to gather this information, they do provide insight into the presence of this condition. The numbers reported from the UK and USA suggest the operations noted are surgical procedures that place patients at risk. The estimated incidence of persistent post-operative pain in these patients, based on more than 7 million operations, ranges from 6% for cesarean section to upward of 85% in amputation. While this rate with amputation could be anticipated (often because of existing pathologies), the incidence in hernia (up to 35%), mastectomy (up to 50%) and thoracotomy (up to 65%) can be of concern.

Table 9.1.

Type of operation	Incidence of chronic pain	No. of ops in UK in 2005–6	No. of ops in USA in 1994
Total operations		7 125 000	22 629 000
Mastectomy	20–50%	18 000	131 000
Cesarean section	6%	139 000	858 000
Amputation	50–85%	15 000	132 000
Cardiac surgery	30–55%	29 000	501 000
Hernia repair	5–35%	75 000	689 000
Cholecystectomy	5–50%	51 000	667 000
Hip replacement	12%	61 000	
Thoracotomy	5–65%		660 000

(With permission from Macrae 2008 [1].)

Significance

One of the most significant factors related to the importance of addressing this post-operative condition is the observation that the number of surgical procedures that are at risk has increased markedly over the decade. Subsequently, if we do not address the pathways and treatments of these chronic pains, the prevalence will probably increase. In turn, the physical, social and economic burden will also increase. In one study with post-thoracotomy patients, persistent post-operative pain limited normal daily activities in more than 50% of these patients and sleep disturbances were reported in 25–30% of this population. These disruptions are often driven by inadequate pain control.

In summary, persistent post-operative pain is a term that has its origin in the middle of the twentieth century, but it has been largely ignored as a significant issue with impact on patient comfort, social interactions and financial complications. The approach of this chapter is to help shed light on the operative procedures that have been linked to this chronic condition and define pathological mechanisms where possible. Identifying risk factors and predicting those who will develop this post-operative complication will be considered. Finally, treatments, both preventative and post-surgical, will be examined and future directions in this field of pain research identified.

Mechanisms

As with our understanding of the epidemiology of this condition, our understanding of the mechanism(s) involved is incomplete. To add complexity to the identification of these mechanisms is the belief that the pathways involved vary with the operative procedure, the skill of the surgeon, the patient's pain threshold, etc. Many of the changes seen in these patients are believed to be either neuropathic or inflammatory or probably both. In addition, visceral pain pathways have been proposed to play an important role in the development of this condition. As always, outcomes are complicated by the fact that there is no single mechanism that is operative in these patients. In general, mechanisms can be described by pain processes, structures and neuronal plasticity.

Pain processes

The three classic pain processes are believed to be involved in the evolution of persistent post-operative pain: nociceptive, inflammatory, and neuropathic. Nociceptive high-threshold receptors are first to respond to the incision made for the operation. These receptor activities can largely be reduced once the local tissue disruption is limited or removed. The next in the sequence of events involves a complicated cascade of events as the tissue responds with inflammatory mediators. These cytokines, chemokines and other tissue factors act by reducing the thresholds of nociceptors in the injured tissue (peripheral sensitization), ultimately resulting in CNS changes (central sensitization). These changes can go on for days if left unchecked. The neuropathic changes are the final act. Acute pain from the initial injury results in changes in the spinal cord and brain. The seminal event driving these changes is nerve injury (see below). Spontaneous pain, dysasthesia, hypersensitivity, allodynia, hyperalgesia, and hyperpathia develop.

Structures

Nerve

Peripheral changes

It is widely assumed that traumatic injury to the nerve is the major cause of post-operative neuropathic pain, but it is probably more complicated than this suggestion. It is also likely that the particular procedure and sensory systems in the surgical field contribute. Additionally, in some patients, continuous inflammatory responses, such as after inguinal hernia repair, drive the chronic response. However, it is the role of peripheral nociceptor sensitization that seems to be at the center of this issue.

In thoracotomy studies, damage to the intercostal nerves sustained from direct pressure, stretching and ischemia may contribute; however, some investigators have shown little relationship between nerve injury and chronic pain after 3 months.

In investigations following mastectomy, damage to the intercostobrachial nerve was believed to contribute to this condition, but one study demonstrated post-mastectomy syndrome with patients who had the intercostobrachial nerve spared. In a prospective, randomized, controlled trial with this nerve being spared in one group and sacrificed in another, while sensory deficit was less in the preserved group, there was no difference in the two groups at 3 months but interestingly the symptoms were worsened more in the group with the nerve preserved. While it is clear that nerve disruption obviously contributes to chronic involvement, it is equally clear that there are other processes involved.

In amputation patients, the peripheral changes evolve around the completely disrupted afferent nerve from the extremity. Following the injury/surgery, the neurons show retrograde degeneration and eventually terminal swelling and sprouting leading to neuroma formation. Ectopic discharges from these terminals lead to spontaneous pain due to the electrical properties of the cell membrane probably related to changes in sodium and potassium channels. Mechanistically it is interesting to note that local anesthetics reduce the stump pain, but not the phantom limb pain, suggesting involvement of proximal pathways. This possible pathway lies in the dorsal root ganglia, possibly regulated by sympathetic sprouting.

The spinal cord

Once again we can gain insights into persistent post-operative pain through the amputation model. Changes have been suggested to occur in several areas of the dorsal horn neurons whereby repeated firing of ectopic discharges from the damaged nerve result in a destruction of inhibitory GABA-containing neurons and a subsequent hyperexcitable spinal cord. Furthermore, down-regulation of the opioid receptors in the region and up-regulation of the cholecystokinin system contributes to hyperexcitability.

Central changes

Central sensitization often expressed as hyperalgesia and allodynia has always been considered a factor in the development of this chronic pain state. Experimental data from animals and humans support the thought that the continuous afferent barrage from the periphery generates and maintains sensitization of central neurons. Furthermore, studies examining the difference between neuraxial block over general anesthesia confirms this observation.

With persistent post-operative pain following amputation there is extensive change in the brainstem, thalamus and cortex. Axonal sprouting in the cortex has been shown in monkeys to lead to reorganizational changes, as have changes in the thalamus. In general, there are meaningful changes in cortical reorganization resulting in responses from surrounding areas not normally associated with the site of the injury. In addition, alterations in sensory and motor feedback result from incongruence between these two systems.

Non-nerve

Within the surgical field, there are many structures which may be damaged including muscle, vascular components, tendons, ligaments, etc. More recently, investigators feel that persistent post-operative pain may contain a visceral component generated by the non-neuronal tissues involved.

Neuronal plasticity

Whether affected pathways are peripheral or central, neuronal plasticity is certainly a key neuropathic component involved in persistent post-operative pain. A schematic representation is shown in Figure 9.1 in anatomical terms (central and peripheral).

Plasticity of neuronal tissue is generally divided into two types: reversible changes in the nerve programming

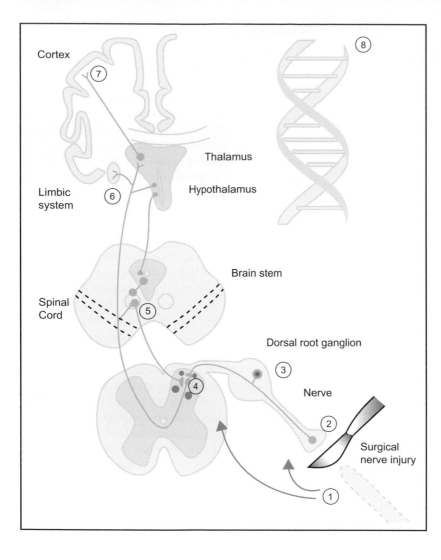

Figure 9.1. Sites and mechanisms responsible for chronic postsurgical neuropathic pain. (1) Denervated Schwann cells and infiltrating macrophages distal to nerve injury produce local and systemic chemicals that drive pain signaling. (2) Neuroma at site of injury is source of ectopic spontaneous excitability in sensory fibres. (3) Changes in gene expression in dorsal root ganglion alter excitability, responsiveness, transmission, and survival of sensory neurons. (4) Dorsal horn is site of altered activity and gene expression, producing central sensitisation, loss of inhibitory interneurons, and microglial activation, which together amplify sensory flow. (5) Brainstem descending controls modulate transmission in spinal cord. (6) Limbic system and hypothalamus contribute to altered mood behavior, and autonomic reflexes. (7) Sensation of pain generated in cortex (past experiences, cultural inputs, and expectations converge to determine what patient feels). (8) Genomic DNA predispose (or not) patient to chronic pain and affect their reaction to treatment. (With permission from Kehlet et al., 2006 [2].)

during inflammation and less reversible changes in the nerve structure related to nerve injury. The early reversible phase occurs during inflammation and is characterized by hypersensitivity. Inflammatory mediators such as by-products of the arachidonic acid cascade are released and lead to initial peripheral sensitization (primary hyperalgesia). This in turn leads to intracellular signaling through various ion channels which increases nerve excitability. Once healing is complete, this type of heightened nerve response generally abates. However, the changes that follow this initial phase are far more troublesome. The barrage of nerve input from the site of the injury results in a synaptic plasticity in the spinal cord that amplifies the pain signals. These signals are transmitted via the dorsal horn upward to the brainstem, thalamus and cortex. The sprouting of neurons that result leads to simple sensory input being magnified

to severe levels. To augment this action in the dorsal horn there is an altered gene transcription of the sensory nerves that increases excitatory transmitters and reduces inhibitory transmitters. Interestingly, these early changes can be reversed. However, if the central sensitization is significant and does not reverse, a normally innocuous stimulus activates pain pathways. This central sensitization is described as a normal sensory input that results in sensitivity spread beyond the site of injury (secondary hyperalgesia).

Unlike the plasticity orchestrated by inflammation, primary injured sensory neurons and their neighbors begin to fire spontaneously, further increasing central sensitization and peripheral tactile allodynia. In addition to changes in sodium channel function there is an up-regulation of voltage-gated calcium channels contributing to the negative central sensitization secondary to nerve injury. Neuroimmune effects then create changes at the distal end of the injured nerve axon releasing substances such as TNF-alpha that create more disturbances in the spinal cord, enhancing hypersensitivity. In addition, activated microglia responding in the synaptic junctions of the dorsal horn contribute to pain hypersensitivity. These changes continue for days, but while some are reversible, some are not, including the loss of sensory neurons resulting in a permanent CNS lesion. This largely peripheral effect increases to involve genetic changes in the dorsal horn. The damage is predominantly within the inhibitory pathways which usually buffer incoming sensory input. These changes continue upward until significant changes occur in the cortex.

Despite the complexities, it is of great value to attempt to dissect the important pathways that are probably involved in the generation of this chronic state. Whatever the pathway involved determining the major contributor (inflammatory, neuropathic and/or visceral) will help define the most successful treatment approach.

Operative procedures

There is a risk of persistent post-operative pain with any surgery and the list is growing. However, some of these operative procedures have received more scrutiny and investigation than others.

Thoracic surgery

Several studies have examined the incidence of chronic post-thoracotomy pain and suggest that this condition exists in 44–67% of patients. Reasons for thoracic surgery may be many, but two surgical approaches are defined: open chest (sternal or intercostal) or laparotomy (video-assisted thoracoscopy). While studies vary in their methods of evaluation, all seem to agree that there is significant risk of developing persistent post-operative pain following these procedures. One study investigated the possibility that the less invasive thoracoscopy would produce less persistent post-operative pain and found that the prevalence was approximately equal in both (40–47%). This study also suggested that only half of the pain suggested a neuropathic element and that a visceral element may also play a role. This finding, if borne out in future studies, suggests that intercostal nerve damage is not the only operative in this chronic painful condition and that a visceral component with more extensive surgery and/or pleurectomy may complicate the picture.

Inguinal hernia repair

Inguinal hernia repair forms the basis of a common surgical procedure (2800 per million people in the USA) in relatively healthy individuals to further explore the nature and incidence of persistent post-operative pain. While in the 1980s persistent post-operative pain was considered somewhat rare, by the 1990s it was estimated that upward of 50% of patients experienced this pain. In a review of 40 studies on this subject, the overall incidence ranged from 15 to 53%. Pain was reported in 63% at 1 year and 54% after 2 years. Patients with moderate to severe pain (12%) reported persistent pain at 2 years. In another study a cumulative prevalence of 30% at 3 years was reported, with 33% of these patients reporting moderate to unbearable pain. In 17 trials comparing laparoscopic to open repair techniques, eight trials reported less persistent pain with laparoscopic, four trials reported more with laparoscopic and five trials found no difference. It is interesting that the less invasive techniques may not demonstrate a lower incidence of this chronic condition. Three studies evaluated mesh and non-mesh repairs, with two of these studies reporting less persistent post-operative pain with mesh repair. From these studies, patients at risk of developing this condition were those with recurrent hernia, those with pre-operative pain, those with a visible bulge before surgery, those with high pain scores post-operatively and those with outpatient surgeries. A definitive interpretation of all these data is difficult because of the lack of consistent methodology among the studies.

Breast surgery

The majority of the information in this area relates to cancer-related breast surgery. While chronic post-operative pain following breast cancer surgery was also considered rare, many studies have indicated that the incidence of this condition was over 50%. However, the impact of emotional states and follow-up treatment (chemotherapy and/or radiation) makes precise attribution to the surgical procedure difficult. Can we learn from the type of surgery in the breast cancer patient; i.e. is it radical (mastectomy) or is it conserving (lumpectomy)? Unfortunately, the incidence of this persistent post-operative pain has not varied greatly with these two substantially different procedures, mastectomy (23–56%) and breast conserving (35–61%). This again reflects a similar observation seen with thoracic and inguinal hernia surgery that less invasive approaches still carry significant risk of developing this chronic condition. It is of interest to note that a study comparing the incidence in high volume (43%) with low volume (56%) hospitals was similar. Risk factors for the development of persistent post-operative pain include age (suggesting that younger patients are at greater risk), but this may be complicated by the fact that these patients in general have a poorer prognosis. Additionally, chemotherapy and radiation have been possibly linked to a greater risk. The presence of pre-operative pain and the severity of post-operative pain have also been shown to increase the risk of developing persistent post-operative pain. Finally, psychosocial factors such as distress may increase the risk for this condition. Additionally, there is a need for quality studies comparing cancer and non-cancer populations. In one such study, the incidence reported with mastectomy with reconstructive implant was 53%, but 31% with a simple mastectomy and only 22% for breast reduction.

Abdominal hysterectomy

Little is known about persistent post-operative pain in relation to gynecological procedures; however, hysterectomy is one of the more common surgical procedures. In a 2008 review, only eleven studies were found, defined and analyzed. Pain was commonly reported as a pre-operative symptom and pain 1–2 years after surgery ranged from 4.7 to 31.9%. Epidemiological studies with this procedure suggested that the rate was 14.7% in the USA and 24% in the UK. Pre-operative pain was associated with a higher risk of having pelvic pain on follow-up and it was suggested that this preexisting pain may have sensitized nerve pathways and contributed to the development of chronic pain. Interestingly, the presence of chronic pain was similar whether surgery was trans-abdominal or trans-vaginal. Furthermore, pre-operative depression resulted in a higher incidence of this postoperative pain.

Amputation

While persistent post-operative pain was believed to be low following amputation (2%), phantom limb pain occurs in anywhere from 50 to 80% of amputees. It is suggested to be independent of age, but it is more prevalent if the amputation is conducted in adulthood vs. childhood. It is also independent of gender or site of amputation. Most studies show no relationship with health status and this condition exists whether the amputation is for trauma or medical reasons. Onset is early, with 76% of patients developing pain within the first few days after amputation; however, it can be delayed for months or years. There are a series of mechanisms involved in the generation of phantom limb pain including changes in the periphery, the spinal cord and the brain. The first events are likely to involve the periphery (deafferentation) and spread to the DRG (ectopic discharges and sprouting), to the dorsal horn (central sensitization) and then to various areas of the brain (brainstem and cortical reorganization). Clearly, neuroplastic changes develop at all sites.

Cesarean section

One of the operative procedures that continues to grow in western countries from 9% in 1980 to 12% in 1990 to 22–24% in 2002 is cesarean section. A study of women post-cesarean section in 2004 found that nearly 20% reported chronic pain 3 months after surgery and 12% at 6 months. Interestingly, it has been suggested that the frequency of chronic pain is higher in patients receiving general anesthesia vs. those receiving spinal anesthesia. This finding has many pointing to the need to block the continuous barrage from afferent pathways which leads to central sensitization (hyperalgesia and allodynia). In these studies the level of immediate post-operative pain was positively correlated with the incidence of persistent post-operative pain.

Overall, persistent post-operative pain exists with many operative procedures and the incidence varies, but its impact may be based on the number of these operations performed. It is of particular interest to note that the theoretically less invasive procedures still result in this chronic condition. One would suggest that there is much more for us to learn about this condition and how to standardize evaluations defining cause and effect. In general, however, research methodologies need to improve in order to better understand the operative risks and how to minimize their impact.

Risk factors

Patient factors

Many factors related to the individual patient carry importance in affecting the risk of developing persistent post-operative pain. These include age, psychosocial variables, pre-operative and post-operative experiences with pain, and genotype.

Interestingly, with breast cancer surgery and inguinal hernia repair increasing age has been reported to decrease the risk of developing persistent post-operative pain. With mastectomy, younger patients may have larger tumors, poorer response to therapy and poorer prognosis, leading to an incidence of 65% in those 30–49 years old, 40% in those 50–69 years old and 26% in those over 70 years old. In fact, it has been approximated that with inguinal hernia and breast cancer surgery the risk decreases by 5% with each year increase of age. A similar relationship was also reported with thoracic surgery. Juxtaposed to these observations, phantom limb pain seems more common when the amputation occurred in adulthood and less frequent in children.

While there are many studies that examine psychosocial variables in acute post-operative pain, there are fewer that examine these factors related to persistent post-operative pain. To make things worse, the results are often contradictory! One study in thoracotomy patients, possibly compromised by small numbers, showed no relationship between depression and anxiety in patients with or without persistent post-operative pain. However, in a trial with breast cancer surgery, one year after surgery, while pre-operative anxiety levels had returned to normal in patients with or without persistent post-operative pain, depression remained high in those with persistent post-operative pain. In another investigation, fear of surgery was associated with a negative outcome for persistent post-operative pain. However, in these studies, catastrophizing was not identified as a risk factor. Furthermore, is seems the psychosocial factors that are predictive for acute pain are generally not predictive for persistent post-operative pain.

Pre-operative screening has been employed in an attempt to identify those at risk. In one study with patients S/P thoracotomy, testing for diffuse noxious inhibitory control (DNIC) demonstrated its value. A logistic regression revealed that DNIC and acute post-operative pain intensity were independent predictors of persistent post-operative pain.

Pre-operative and acute post-operative pain has been considered to play an important role in this condition. Pre-operative pain has been demonstrated in several trials on inguinal hernia repair to be related to the development of persistent post-operative pain. Similar suggestions for this relationship were determined in post-amputation and breast cancer studies. However, a correlation for total hip arthroplasty was not observed. One of the variables that has been discussed is the impact of acute post-operative pain. Severe pain post-operatively has been identified as a consistent risk factor for developing this chronic pain condition. One investigation with thoracotomy even suggested that early post-operative pain was the only factor that significantly predicted long-term chronic pain. These post-operative pain investigations have included inguinal hernia repair, breast cancer surgery, total hip arthroplasty and cesarean section.

Surgical/medical factors

While it is clear that the type of surgical procedure has significant impact on the development of persistent post-operative pain, the duration of surgery (longer than 3 hours) was observed to correlate with the development of chronic pain. The duration could be a risk factor because longer operations may reflect more serious disease, complications of the surgery and final outcomes. Additionally, the surgical technique also weighs heavily on the incidence of persistent post-operative pain. The surgical procedure has also been examined with different types of breast cancer surgery (see above). With inguinal hernia repair there was no clear relationship with type of procedure and persistent post-operative pain; however, with cholecystectomy the open procedure had a higher incidence than the laparoscopic procedure. With thoracic surgery, the less invasive video-assisted thoracoscopy failed to show a lower incidence of persistent post-operative pain.

While the skill of the surgeon is likely to play a role, it is difficult to measure. Nevertheless, one study evaluating breast surgery for cancer found that the incidence of persistent post-operative pain was less in high-volume specialists than with lower-volume less experienced practitioners. However, this is in contrast to the report that there was no difference between high-volume and low-volume hospitals. Findings with different operations including amputation (traumatic vs. disease), thoracic surgery (esophageal disease vs. lung cancer), and hernia surgery (initial vs. revision) are equivocal.

Anesthetic and analgesic use has also been evaluated as a possible contributor to persistent post-operative pain. One study has suggested that properly used regional anesthetic techniques can reduce the incidence of chronic post-thoracotomy pain. In another study evaluating patients undergoing thoracotomy procedures, it was shown that nearly 50% of the patients taking opioid analgesics prior to surgery developed persistent post-operative pain, but only 5% of those not receiving opioids prior to surgery.

One of the areas of recent interest with anesthetics and analgesics focuses on the theory that ascribes pain before and after the operative procedure to result from sensitizing of the nervous system which contributes to the development of persistent post-operative pain. Preclinical research suggests that post-operative control of acute pain may significantly reduce the incidence of this condition. However, a major difference to be addressed is the fact that animals tested in these trials are pain-free before the operation where patients may have pain and therefore already sensitize key pain pathways. Several trials suggest a benefit to post-operative pain control including abdominal hysterectomy, cesarean section, thoracotomy and iliac crest harvesting. However, there are other trials which show no benefit. Also, multimodal therapy has been attempted, but results are inconsistent. Despite these failures, it would seem that the correct combination, at the correct time, for the correct duration of control would have a positive impact on reducing persistent post-operative pain.

Finally, concomitant therapy with radiotherapy or chemotherapy may have a measureable negative impact on persistent post-operative pain. In a study of women following surgery for breast cancer, there was an increased risk of persistent post-operative pain with radiotherapy.

Genetic factors

Several investigators have suggested that certain patients many be genetically predisposed to developing chronic pain following nerve injury. This theory has been supported by laboratory studies with mice. These studies have investigated several models of neuropathic pain. Conditions that could predispose patients include fibromyalgia, migraine, IBS, irritable bladder and Raynaud's syndrome. In a hernia population, a history of backache, IBS or headache was positively associated with the development of this chronic condition. Also, in a study in women following abdominal hysterectomy, a possible genetic link to fibromyalgia was proposed. This is a new and growing area of research that is likely to offer significant insight into this condition in the future.

Predicting persistent post-operative pain

Predicting the occurrence of persistent post-operative pain begins with an understanding of the surgical procedure (and specific techniques) described above,

as well as the risk factors described above. However, can we develop an algorithm or scoring system to identify those patients at increased risk of developing this potentially debilitating condition? While the answer to this question is not complete at this time, it is promising. In 2003 a scoring system based on age, sex, type of injury, extent of post-operative pain and level of anxiety was developed. Additionally, investigations into pre-operative sensitivity to heat and cold stimuli in knee surgery, cholecystectomy and cesarean section suggest positive correlations with severe post-operative pain experiences. Since the intensity of post-operative pain has been linked to persistent post-operative pain, understanding those likely to have severe pain following surgery may help eliminate this finding in those patients. In even more advanced thinking, pain-protecting or pain-producing gene haplotypes identified by SNPs could contribute to our understanding of this condition and guide our intervention. These steps are not fully validated; however, they are steps that must be taken and repeated.

Management

Prevention

Is an ounce of prevention worth a pound of treatment?

Certainly the first "ounce of prevention" would begin with describing to the patient pre-operatively that with all surgery there is tissue damage by its nature and sometimes disruption of nerve function. Probably one of the easiest and often most productive approaches to avoiding the development of this condition is to stabilize the psychological component. Patients who wish to blame the surgeon often have behavioral problems with their pain and are poor responders to other treatment modalities. One study found that patients who believe they were injured in surgery had lower pain thresholds, deconditioning and reduced activity. It is important to manage these behaviors pre-operatively in order to minimize the confusing input from psychological dimensions.

Probably the most obvious way to reduce the development of persistent post-operative pain is to utilize surgical techniques that avoid damage to major nerves. In inguinal hernia repair, laparoscopic procedures as opposed to open procedures where possible can possibly reduce the risk of nerve injury. In addition, lightweight mesh may reduce the inflammatory response following surgery; although, as noted above, some believe these measures are not effective. In mastectomy, preservation of the intercostobrachial nerve has been suggested to reduce chronic pain. Also sentinel node biopsy can indicate that further axillary dissection is not necessary, thereby further protecting the intercostal nerve structure. Similarly, minimally invasive thoracoscopy may spare the intercostal innervations. Stretch and retraction with open thoracotomy has also been shown to increase the risk of damaging the intercostal nerve. The utilization of intercostal suture techniques may help avoid nerve compression. Other anatomical approaches such as using a posterolateral approach for thoracotomy may reduce the impact of nerve disruption, although not all agree with these suggestions.

Treatment

Preemptive/preventative

Preemptive approaches to control post-operative pain have been studied in many trials with many approaches. To date, the results have been mixed, but have generally been disappointing. Part of this finding may be that we need to understand more about the pain mechanism and the type and duration of pre-treatment efforts. This approach is complicated by research that demonstrates an inflammatory and neuropathic component to post-surgical pain. While local anesthetics may be effective in reducing the barrage from injured nerves and subsequent development of central plasticity, does their effect last long enough? In addition, the inflammatory component may need more aggressive therapy lasting longer through the healing period. Some research indicates that the changes leading to plasticity may not occur until well after the surgical procedure, indicating that not only the mechanism of treatment but also the timing of treatment is important. Furthermore, new treatments may be needed to specifically address the biological cascades and events that result in this persistent post-operative condition. Currently, much of the approach to treating these patients lends itself to the focused development of multimodal approaches.

Post-operative

Other than the preventative approaches taken above, the most effective treatment is the aggressive management of post-operative pain. Some of the most significant information suggests that severe post-operative pain is associated with a higher incidence of persistent post-operative pain. While a perfect cause and effect link is not available, we have strong suggestions that aggressive and well-structured peri-operative pain

management is pivotal. A recent study in post-cesarean patients found that patients with persistent post-operative pain exhibited a stronger recall of uncontrolled post-operative pain. While the results are somewhat equivocal, it would appear that the effectiveness and duration of treatment is more important than the timing (preemptive) of treatment. Many believe that our inadequate treatment and anticipation of acute pain contributes on a psychological level to the development of persistent post-operative pain. Most suggest that a balanced multi-modal approach may best address the myriad of mechanisms contributing to this condition. These strategies are largely driven by differentiating neuropathic from non-neuropathic origins.

Opioids

Clearly nociceptor activity plays a role in post-surgical pain. The most effective treatment of classic nociceptor pathways is mu-agonist opioids. There are many to select from and the decision is largely based on the severity of post-operative pain and the anticipated duration of nociceptive firing.

COX-1/COX-2 inhibitors

These are commonly used interventions that have merit because of the significant role that inflammation plays in this condition. However, the NSAIDs that inhibit the constitutive cyclooxygenase (COX-1) are not as likely to be effective as are the agents that inhibit the inducible cyclooxygenase (COX-2), which is more responsible for inflammation. Furthermore, they are effective in visceral pain, significantly potentiate opioids and inhibit central prostaglandins responsible in part for central sensitization.

Alpha-2 receptor agonist

The discovery of the alpha receptor in the regulation of many of the centrally mediated pain responses has made these agents an interesting option. Development of central sensitization, wind-up leading to allodynia and hyperalgesia has been significantly attenuated by these agonists. They have also been shown to significantly potentiate opioids and local anesthetics.

Ketamine (NMDA antagonists)

While the NMDA antagonists commercially available have not been extremely effective, the antagonism of glutamate is likely to play an important role in the neuropathic elements of this condition. Newer agents targeted at several receptors in the glutamate family may be available in the future, which could have significant impact on this chronic condition.

Local anesthetics

The use of injectable and topical local anesthetics may have a palliative role in treatment of the immediate post-operative period, resulting in more effective treatment of pain. Generally, these agents have short durations of action; however, continuous infusions and potentially longer-acting agents (3–5 days) have merit. While somewhat less effective, patches and creams may be beneficial in some patients.

Multimodal

Given the complexity of persistent post-operative pain, it is likely that a multifaceted approach to different pathological mechanisms is needed. Since the origins of the pain differ with differing surgical procedures, the first approach would be to consider the needs following differing surgeries. Since inflammation has been suggested to play a significant role in this condition, the utilization of a COX-2 inhibitor is logical; however, we will need anti-inflammatory agents in the future that have a more pronounced and targeted effect. Tricyclic antidepressants are commonly used in some analgesic cocktails because they act through serotonin and noradrenaline to modulate neuropathic elements. Other membrane-stabilizing drugs such as gabapentin, topiramate, tiagabine, etc. work in concert to block ion channels and glutamate release. Approaches using ketamine or other NMDA antagonists could help blunt central plasticity. Combining this approach with a longer-acting local anesthetic could prove effective. Once again, it is paramount to address the multiple pain pathways involved post-operatively.

New targets

There are a number of new developments in the treatment of inflammatory and neuropathic pain that are in development (see Chapter 108: Novel targets for new analgesics). This includes the advancement of neurotrophic factors (NGF, BDNF, etc.) and other cytokines. Also the ion channel modulators (sodium, calcium, and potassium) show promise. Several receptor-driven products including the purinergic receptors (P2X4 and P2X7) and the glutamate receptors (NMDA, AMPA, and the mGluR family) may have utility.

Epilogue – future directions

The approach for the future in managing this disruptive post-operative condition starts with prevention.

Improvement in surgical techniques to reduce nerve and other tissue disruption will be important. The role of inflammation discussed above should always be aggressively addressed and newer anti-inflammatory treatments developed. Next is the need to better understand and manage post-operative pain. Longer-acting local anesthetics can interrupt the sensory afferents to reduce neuronal sensitization. Application of growth factors such as neurotropic factors may help prevent transcriptional changes in the sensory nerves. Prevention of microglial activation has been suggested to help protect DRG and dorsal horn structures. Ion channel (sodium, potassium, calcium) agents that modify nerve transmission and those that modulate glutamate transporters and reduce caspases decrease excitotoxicity. Maybe one of the more significant advances is in the area of research. We must try and design studies that consistently capture information that properly characterizes the procedure, the pain and the persistence. Procedure-specific parameters should be developed, as should studies with pre-operative, intra- and post-operative and extended (> 3 months) assessments.

There is little debate that persistent post-operative pain is an important phenomenon for us to consider and better understand. As in many areas of science and medicine, there is much to be learned from identifying those at risk to provide treatment to minimize the personal, healthcare, and psychological burdens. While disagreement exists as to description, quantification, differentiation, and management of these patients, it is this spirit that propels us forward to produce more research in this area from the bench (pathways, genetics) to the bedside (pre- and post-operative and less disruptive surgical procedures).

References

1. Macrae WA. Chronic post-surgical pain: 10 years on. *Br J Anaesth* 2008;**101**:77–86.

2. Kehlet H, Jensen TS, Woolf C. Persistent post-surgical pain: risk factors and prevention. *Lancet* 2006;**367**:1618–1625.

3. Brandsborg B, Nikolajsen L, Kehlet H, Jensen TS. Chronic pain after hysterectomy. *Acta Anaesthesiol Scand* 2008;**52**:327–331.

4. Flor H, Nikolajsen L, Jensen TS. Phantom limb pain: a case of maladaptive CNS plasticity. *Nature Rev Neurosci* 2006;**7**:873–881.

Pain Definitions

10 Analgesic gaps

Sunil J. Panchal

Introduction

Despite significant efforts to improve acute pain management through the development and implementation of pain management guidelines and acute pain services in many hospitals, acute post-operative pain management remains inadequate. A number of variables have been cited as causes of undermedication, including educational deficits, over-reliance on opioid analgesic monotherapy, inadequate patient assessment and technology-related failures. Goals of the clinical practice guideline established by the Agency for Healthcare Research and Quality (formerly the Agency for Health Care Policy and Research) include reducing the incidence and severity of post-operative pain and improving patient satisfaction and comfort to optimize pain management [1]. Other organizations have also tried to address the under-treatment of pain in the acute pain setting through evidence-based clinical practice guidelines and position statements, such as the International Association for the Study of Pain; the American Pain Society; American Society of Anesthesiologists (ASA); and the American Academy of Pain Medicine [2]. Yet, a review of the literature found that a significant proportion of patients receiving post-operative analgesia still experienced moderate-to-severe pain following surgery. A survey of 250 adults who had undergone surgical procedures was performed in which questions were asked about the severity of post-surgical pain, treatment, satisfaction with pain medication, patient education, and perceptions about post-operative pain and pain medications. Approximately 80% of patients experienced acute pain after surgery. Of these patients, 86% had moderate, severe, or extreme pain, with more patients experiencing pain after discharge than before discharge. Experiencing post-operative pain was the most common concern (59%) of patients [3]. These findings were very similar to a survey performed a decade earlier [4]. This continuing problem has a significant impact on patient outcomes, as management of acute post-operative pain is often suboptimal, leading to delayed recovery, prolonged hospital stays, and increased patient distress and anxiety [5]. At the same time it is important to recognize that while opioid analgesics effectively control acute pain, they also can cause life-threatening side effects [6]. Analgesics are the most common class of drugs associated with preventable adverse drug events (ADE) [7], which are defined as "injuries resulting from medical intervention related to a drug", and may involve either the appropriate or inappropriate use of a drug.

One contributor to the inadequate management of post-operative pain may be the occurrence of analgesic gaps, defined as periods during which the patient does not have access to analgesia. Patients may experience analgesic gaps while being transported from one location to another, such as from the OR to the PACU or ICU, or the PACU to hospital bed, for common examples. Patients may also experience analgesic gaps when waiting for nursing staff to administer bolus doses of opioid via the intravenous (IV) or intramuscular (IM) route, or during the transition from one analgesic modality to another, such as transitioning from patient-controlled epidural analgesia (PCEA) to IV-PCA [8,9]. In a study by Ng and colleagues, the analgesic gap was defined as the shortfall of pain management during patients' transition from post-surgical epidural analgesia or IV-PCA to oral analgesics. A period of inadequate analgesia occurred in 40 (45%) of 89 post-operative patients within the first 2 days after surgery and in 17 (17%) of 22 patients with high pain scores after IV-PCA was discontinued. In a survey of 115 patients 24 hours after IV-PCA was discontinued per standard guidelines, Chen and coworkers found that 38 (33%) patients requested that IV-PCA be restarted, mostly because they believed that it would be more effective than the prescribed oral analgesic [10]. To avoid this analgesic gap, it is critical to consider the timing of discontinuing IV or epidural therapy in the patient's recovery, use equianalgesic

51

conversions, and allowing time for oral therapy to take effect before stopping any technology-supported pain therapies. Above all, patients should be frequently assessed for interruptions in pain control.

The incidence of analgesic gaps may vary depending on the analgesic delivery system used to administer analgesia. For instance, systems that are complex, invasive, or involve multiple steps for analgesic administration may have a higher frequency of technology failures or system-related events (SREs, defined as problems related to the analgesic system that must be addressed by healthcare providers) that may result in interruptions in pain control. Patient-controlled analgesia (PCA) modalities may help to minimize analgesic gaps, since they allow patients to control their pain according to their personal analgesic needs. IV-PCA is routinely used to manage post-operative pain and is often considered the "gold standard" for acute pain management. However, analgesic administration using IV-PCA requires manual programming of the infusion pump, which introduces the potential for programming errors.

IV-PCA systems are also prone to patient errors and system malfunctions. In some cases these issues occur at a frequency great enough to cause the US Food and Drug Administration (FDA) to take action by issuing a recall due to a design defect that caused some of the infusion pumps to disrupt analgesic therapy [11]. Furthermore, the complexity of the IV-PCA system may increase the risk of SREs, due to problems with the infusion pump, IV line, or other components of the system.

Panchal and coworkers evaluated the incidence of analgesic gaps resulting from SREs for patients using the fentanyl iontophoretic transdermal system (ITS), a non-invasive PCA system, or morphine IV-PCA for post-operative pain management [12]. For morphine IV-PCA, infiltration of the IV line was the most frequently reported SRE that resulted in an analgesic gap. Infiltration at the catheter site is a problem commonly encountered with IV-related procedures, and may result in IV line failure and/or a subcutaneous depot of opioid, leading to inadequate and ineffective delivery

Table 10.1. Frequency of SREs resulting in an analgesic gap

	Fentanyl ITS	Morphine IV-PCA
Type of SRE	($n = 647$)	($n = 658$)
Infiltration	none	17
Device malfunction or failure	26	11
Line pulled out	none	8
Low or dead battery	none	8
Alarm going off	none	7
Incorrect programming /dosing	none	5
Line leaking	none	4
Incompatible medication in line	none	4
Edema	none	4
Patient/family tampering	none	3
Could not locate button	4	3
Patient had difficulty with use	3	2
Air in the line	none	1
Phlebitis	none	1
Pain at the site	none	1
Itching	1	none
Erythema	1	none
Other	6	16
Total	41	98

SRE, system-related event; ITS, iontophoretic transdermal system; IV-PCA, intravenous PCA.

of analgesic, as well as pain and discomfort (Table 10.1). Incorrect programming and dosing errors occurred with morphine IV-PCA in the two studies included in this analysis. Many of the SREs encountered with morphine IV-PCA are not possible with fentanyl ITS, as the system does not require IV access or dose adjustment. Device malfunctions or failures accounted for most of the SREs that occurred with the fentanyl ITS; however, manufacturer diagnostics found no problem with the system in 35% of these cases. Such a result may be attributed to nurses' unfamiliarity with this novel analgesic delivery system. In other words, nurses may have mistakenly diagnosed a malfunctioning or failing unit when there was no problem. Improved nurse training after product availability is likely to decrease the rate of system failures.

Use of the fentanyl ITS may require fewer resources to address SREs and resulting analgesic gaps, including decreased time spent by nurses and other healthcare providers. Technological advances that reduce the staff time and resource consumption required for analgesic administration may be an important consideration in determining preferred analgesic modalities.

Another study by Hankin and colleagues evaluated 2009 IV-PCA-related reports filed with the FDA (MAUDE database) during a 2-year index period (2002–2003), the majority of which could be classified as possibly preventable (those classified as possible operator errors, patient-related events, or device safety events) [13]. Given that published accounts of IV-PCA problems have historically focused on operator error and patient tampering [14–16], the authors were surprised to find that device safety events (i.e. device malfunctions) were the suspected cause of nearly 80% of reported events (75% of these reportedly attributable to defective switches, display boards, or motors) (Table 10.2). It is noteworthy that nearly two-thirds (64.9%) of these device malfunctions were duplicated and confirmed upon inspection by the manufacturer. Of those device malfunctions that were not confirmed, about half are under continued evaluation by the manufacturer and nearly one-quarter were never received by the manufacturer. Only 159 suspected device malfunctions (representing 10% of the total events in this category) were conclusively cleared of defects upon manufacturer inspection.

Although operator errors were less frequent than device malfunctions, these events were associated with the most severe consequences, including six deaths, two occurrences of respiratory arrest, and 50 cases in which naloxone was administered. Device safety events were associated with no deaths or instances of respiratory arrest or depression, and only four occurrences of naloxone administration. This seems to suggest that operator errors were more likely than device malfunctions to result in the over-delivery of medications, which is the most dangerous consequence of an IV-PCA-related event. In contrast, device safety events usually resulted in under-delivery of medications, thereby creating analgesic gaps.

In consideration that there are approximately 50 000 device-related reports that are submitted annually to the FDA, IV-PCA-specific reports identified during this 2-year review represent 2% of total device-related reports. The total number of events identified in this analysis probably underestimates the true number of IV-PCA-related events as there are substantial barriers to event reporting, including fear of potential liability, assumptions that information provided will not be meaningful to others, and concern regarding the complexity and time required to complete narrative reports. Indeed, researchers estimate that only 1.2–7.7% of actual adverse events are ever reported [17–20], suggesting that the true rate of IV-PCA-related events that occurred during this two-year index period ranged from 13 948 (1074 divided by 7.7%) to 89 500 (1074 divided by 1.2%). This is the first study to comprehensively examine FDA reports of IV-PCA-related problems since event reporting became required by both industry and healthcare facilities. It is clear that IV-PCA pumps are inherently complex devices that may be especially susceptible to both operator error and device malfunction. Continued in-depth study of adverse events involving these devices can help identify innovations in device design and testing to reduce the occurrence of preventable adverse events, as well as analgesic gaps.

Conclusion

Analgesic gaps are a significant component as to why patients are under-treated in regard to acute pain, and occur from a variety of causes. In order to mitigate this problem and improve patient outcomes, it is important for institutions to take a comprehensive approach. It is necessary to address transition issues such as patient location changes, as well as transitions from one analgesic therapy to another. This will

Table 10.2. Frequency of reported events by possible causes, results of manufacturer testing, and adverse event patient outcomes

Reported event and possible cause (per narrative text)	Total reported		Results of manufacturer testing				Adverse event		
			Sent and tested by mfg	Possible cause confirmed by mfg					
	n	%	n	n	% of tested	% of total	n	% of total reported	AE type (n)
Device safety									
Defective reed switch	516	32.5	437	409	93.6	79.3		0.0	
Defective motor	488	30.7	428	384	89.7	78.7	1	0.2	N(1)
Battery, display board, software	214	13.5	129	84	65.1	39.3	2	0.9	U(1), B(1)
Defective support assembly	114	7.2	96	80	83.3	70.2		0.0	
Faulty alarm system	48	3.0	29	22	75.9	45.8		0.0	
Failure to deliver drug on demand	38	2.4	1	0	0.0	0.0	1	2.6	NoΛ(1)
Defective patient pendant	29	1.8	20	19	95.0	65.5	2	6.9	N(2)
Defective mechanism board	23	1.4	12	4	33.3	17.4		0.0	
Defective or loose 5 mL switch and/or EOS alarm	19	1.2	19	14	73.7	73.7		0.0	
Faulty syringe injector assembly	6	0.4	1	1	100.0	16.7	1	16.7	N(1)
Other	95	6.0	19	15	78.9	15.8	1	1.1	NoA(1)
Total	1590	100.0	1191	1032	86.6	64.9	8	0.5	
Operator error									
PCA pump programming error	106	80.9	58	39	67.2	36.8	54	50.9	D(3), N(38), RA(1), S(5), U(4), RD(3)
Failure to clamp or unclamp tubing	6	4.6	2	0	0.0	0.0	1	16.7	N(1)

Table 10.2. (*cont.*)

Reported event and possible cause (per narrative text)	Total reported		Results of manufacturer testing				Adverse event		
			Sent and tested by mfg	Possible cause confirmed by mfg					
	n	%	*n*	*n*	% of tested	% of total	*n*	% of total reported	AE type (*n*)
Pharmacy error	6	4.6	2	0	0.0	0.0	4	66.7	D(1), N(1), RA (2)
Improperly connected to patient	4	3.1	1	0	0.0	0.0	2	50.0	S(1), N(1)
Improperly loading syringe or cartridge	4	3.1	0	0	0.0	0.0	0	0.0	
Medication prescription error	3	2.3	0	0	0.0	0.0	2	66.7	D(2)
Battery improperly inserted	2	1.5	2	1	50.0	50.0	0	0.0	
Total	131	100.0	65	40	61.5	86.8	63	48.1	
Patient-related									
Intentional tampering with device	8	66.7	3	1	33.3	12.5	4	50.0	N(4)
Family members operating demand button	4	33.3	3	0	0.0	0.0	0	0.0	
Total	12	100.0	6	1	16.7	8.3	4	33.3	
Indeterminate									
Inaccurate amount of drug delivered	13	5.5	2	0	0.0	0.0	3	23.1	BL(1), BR(1), N(1)
Over-delivery of drug	165	70.2	57	1	1.8	0.6	48	29.1	C(1), D(7), DZ(1), N(31), RA(1), D(2), S(1), U(4)
Under-delivery of drug	57	24.3	22	0	0.0	0.0	0	0.0	
Total	235	100.0	81	1	1.2	0.4	51	21.7	

B, battery fell on patient; BL, blood backed up into catheter; BR, catheter broke off in patient; C, coma; D, death; DZ, dizziness; N, naloxone/narcan; NoA, no analgesia delivered; RA, respiratory arrest; D, respiratory depression; S, sedation; U, unspecified.

require understanding of the pharmacokinetic differences of various therapeutic options, as well as maintaining the availability of the therapy that is to be discontinued until the new treatment option is confirmed to be effective. Analysis of the technologies utilized and understanding of the ways that failure of analgesic delivery can occur would allow strategies to be created to cope with these issues. It is also important to be open to new technologies that may simplify and thereby eliminate some factors that contribute to analgesic gaps.

References

1. Agency for Health Care Policy and Research (AHCPR) Public Health Service. *Acute Pain Management: Operative Medical Procedures and Trauma*. Clinical Practice Guideline No.1. AHCPR Pub. No. 92–0032. Rockville, MD: AHCPR, 1992.

2. American Society of Anesthesiologists Task Force on Acute Pain Management, Ashburn MA, Caplan RA, Carr D, Connis R, Ginsberg B, Green C, Lema M, Nickinovich DG, Rice LJ. Practice guidelines for acute pain management in the perioperative setting: an updated report by the American Society of Anesthesiologists Task Force on Acute Pain Management. *Anesthesiology* 2004;**100**:1573–1581.

3. Apfelbaum JL, Chen C, Mehta SS, Gan TJ. Postoperative pain experience: results from a national survey suggest postoperative pain continues to be undermanaged. *Anesth Analg* 2003;**97**:534–540.

4. Warfield CA, Kahn CH. Acute pain management. Programs in U.S. hospitals and experiences and attitudes among U.S. adults. *Anesthesiology* 1995;**83**(5):1090–1094.

5. Joshi GP, Ogunnaike BO. Consequences of inadequate postoperative pain relief and chronic persistent postoperative pain. *Anesthesiol Clin North Am* 2005;**23**:21–36.

6. American College of Physicians. Common side effects of opioids. In *ACP Observer*: American College of Physicians, 2004.

7. Bates DW, Cullen DJ, Laird N, et al. Incidence of adverse drug events and potential adverse drug events. Implications for prevention. ADE Prevention Study Group. *JAMA* 1995;**274**:29–34.

8. Ng A, Hall F, Atkinson A, Kong KL, Hahn A. Bridging the analgesic gap. *Acute Pain* 2000;**3**:194–199.

9. Smith G, Power I. Audit and bridging the analgesic gap. *Anaesthesia* 1998;**53**:521–522.

10. Chen PP, Chui PT, Ma M, Gin T. A prospective survey of patients after cessation of patient-controlled analgesia. *Anesth Analg* 2001; **92**(1):224–227.

11. Baxter Healthcare Corp. signs consent decree with FDA; agrees to correct manufacturing deficiencies. Available at: http://www.fda.gov/bbs/topics/NEWS/2006/NEW01402.html. Accessed October 3, 2006.

12. Panchal SJ, Damaraju CV, Nelson WW, Hewitt DJ, Schein JR. System-related events and analgesic gaps during postoperative pain management with the fentanyl iontophoretic transdermal system and morphine intravenous patient-controlled analgesia. *Anesth Analg* 2007;**105**(5):1437–1441.

13. Hankin CS, Schein J, Clark JA, Panchal S. Adverse events involving intravenous patient-controlled analgesia. *Am J Health Syst Pharm* 2007; **64**(14): 1492–1499.

14. Ashburn MA, Love G, Pace NL. Respiratory-related critical events with intravenous patient-controlled analgesia. *Clin J Pain* 1994;**10**:52–56.

15. Brown SL, Bogner MS, Parmentier CM, et al. Human error and patient-controlled analgesia pumps. *J Intraven Nurs* 1997;**20**:311–316.

16. Callan CM. An analysis of complaints and complications with patient-controlled analgesia. In Ferrante FM, Ostheimer GW, Covino BG, eds. *Patient-controlled Analgesia*. Oxford, UK: Blackwell Scientific Publications, 1990, pp. 139–150.

17. Cullen DJ, Bates DW, Small SD, et al. The incident reporting system does not detect adverse drug events: a problem for quality improvement. *Jt Comm J Qual Improv* 1995;**21**:541–548.

18. Jha AK, Kuperman GJ, Teich JM, et al. Identifying adverse drug events: development of a computer-based monitor and comparison with chart review and stimulated voluntary report. *J Am Med Inform Assoc* 1998;**5**:305–314.

19. Classen DC, Pestotnik SL, Evans RS, et al. Computerized surveillance of adverse drug events in hospital patients. *JAMA* 1991;**266**: 2847–2851.

20. Gardner S, Flack M. *Designing a medical device surveillance network*: FDA Report to Congress; 1999.

11

Multimodal analgesia (sites of analgesic activity)

Bryan S. Williams and Asokumar Buvanendran

Introduction

Clinicians are confronted with an array of medications for the treatment of pain conditions, and with the pharmacological armamentarium available most pain states can be treated effectively. The prevalence of chronic pain in the general population has been estimated to range from 10% to over 40% [1–3], with 25 million Americans suffering from acute pain from injury or surgery and 75 million suffering with chronic pain [4]. Despite the ever-expanding number of medications indicated for various pain conditions, there still remains an unmet need for chronic pain management [5]. Harden and Cohen [5] identify four possible reasons for unmet analgesia in chronic pain, which include inadequate diagnosis and appreciation of the mechanisms involved; inadequate management of comorbid conditions; incorrect understanding or selection of treatment options; or use of inappropriate outcome measures. With respect to the mechanism involved, equally important is the mechanism by which the medications have their analgesic effect. The diversity of pain mechanisms, patient responses and diseases necessitates a mechanistic approach to pain management; based on current understanding of the peripheral and central mechanisms involved in nociceptive transmission providing newer options for clinicians, to manage pain effectively treatment must be individualized [6].

Several strategies have been adopted in order to avoid the shortcomings of the unmet need of chronic pain management, including multimodal pain management and mechanistic approaches. The former, multimodal pain management, was introduced more than a decade ago as a technique to improve analgesia and reduce the incidence of opioid-related adverse events. This concept can be applied to chronic pain management utilizing our understanding of the mechanism by which injury occurs and the mechanism of action of the medications used to treat pain conditions

[7]. Multimodal techniques reduce the total dose of any one medication by attending to analgesic requirements through various receptor modulations. Multimodal analgesia is achieved by combining different analgesics that act by different mechanisms, resulting in additive or synergistic analgesia, reducing adverse effects of the sole administration of individual analgesics [7].

Therapeutic strategies aimed at selecting treatments by targeting the putative mechanisms of pain (mechanism-based strategies) have been proposed [8, 9]. The signs of neuropathic pain (heat hyperalgesia, mechano-hyperalgesia, mechano- and cold allodynia) may have different pathophysiological mechanisms. Evidence from animal models indicates that distinct signs of neuropathic pain respond differently to various drugs [10]. Targets are being identified by pharmaceutical investigation for the discovery of highly specific small molecules as potential novel analgesics. The discovery of targets specific to particular pain mechanisms will soon enable therapy to be targeted specifically at those mechanisms [11].

In this chapter, we will review the analgesic sites of action as a mechanistic and multimodal approach to pain medicine and chronic pain management. The mainstay of pain management has been opioid therapy, but, with the increasing knowledge of pain mechanisms, adjuvant medications are gaining a more prominent role in chronic pain management.

Opioids

Endorphins and enkephalins are endogenous opioids that are released from the periaqueductal gray matter and nucleus raphe magnus, respectively, and travel within the central nervous system (CNS) descending pain-control systems [12]. Exogenous opioid agonists mimic the activity of enkephalins and endorphins at the central descending pathways of the pain-processing loop [13]. Opioid receptors are found at pre- and postsynaptic sites of the ascending pain transmission system in the dorsal horn of the spinal cord, the brainstem, thalamus, and the cortex. Opioid receptors are also found in the midbrain periaqueductal gray, the nucleus raphe magnus, and the rostral ventral medulla, which comprise the descending inhibitory system modulating spinal pain transmission [14]. There are at least three opioid receptors, mu (μ), kappa (κ), and delta (δ), which are located at the dorsal horn of the spinal cord, the dorsal root ganglion and peripheral nerves [15]. These opioid receptors are guanine (G) protein-coupled. Opioid activation mediates the reduction in neurotransmitter (e.g. glutamate, substance P and calcitonin gene-related peptide) release from the presynaptic membrane secondary to the inhibition of voltage-gated calcium channels (Figure 11.1.). This is accomplished by the reduction in the second messenger cyclic adenosine monophosphate (cAMP). Additionally, the mode of action of opioids is via activation of opioid receptors in second-order pain transmission cells preventing the ascending transmission of the pain signal at the central terminals of C fibers in the spinal cord, and activating opioid receptors in the periphery to inhibit the activation of the nociceptors as well as inhibit cells that may release inflammatory mediators [16,17]. Postsynaptically, opioids cause inhibition of adenyl cyclase and activation of inwardly rectifying potassium currents resulting in neuronal hyperpolarization [18,19]

Opioids have been the mainstay of analgesia and by interacting at the aforementioned receptors these medications produce reliable analgesia, but these medications should only be a part of an analgesic regimen. Adjuvant medications should be employed in any multimodal analgesic regimen, enhancing analgesia.

NSAIDs, acetaminophen and COX-2 inhibitors

Nonsteroidal anti-inflammatory drugs (NSAIDs) are among the most widely used analgesic medications in the world because of their ability to reduce pain and inflammation [7,20,21]. They are structurally diverse, but all have antipyretic, anti-inflammatory and analgesic or anti-hyperalgesic properties. NSAIDs have a peripheral and central role of action [7,22,23]. Cell injury induces the production of phospholipids with conversion to arachidonic acid and the cyclooxygenase (COX) enzyme converts arachidonic acid to prostaglandins. Peripherally, prostaglandins (PGE_1 and PGE_2) are not important mediators of pain transmission, but they contribute to hyperalgesia by sensitizing nociceptive sensory nerve endings to other mediators (histamine and bradykinin) and by sensitizing nociceptors to respond to non-nociceptive stimuli, such as touch [22,24,25]. In the periphery NSAIDs prevent the sensitization of peripheral nociceptors, diminishing prostaglandin formation, and centrally hyperalgesia evoked by spinal action of substance P and N-methyl-D-aspartate [25,26]. Centrally, prostaglandins are capable of enhancing pain transmission by increasing substance P and glutamate, increasing nociceptive transmission at second-order neurons and inhibiting the release of descending inhibitory neurotransmitters [25,27–29]. To this end, the mechanism of action of the NSAIDs is inhibition of prostaglandin production by either reversible or irreversible acetylation of cyclooxygenase.

Acetaminophen (paracetamol) probably produces its analgesic effect by inhibiting central prostaglandin synthesis with minimal inhibition of peripheral prostaglandin synthesis [30,31]. Often labeled as an NSAID, acetaminophen and NSAIDs have important differences such as acetaminophen's weak anti-inflammatory effects and its generally poor ability to inhibit COX in the presence of high concentrations of peroxides, as are found at sites of inflammation [30,31], nor does it have

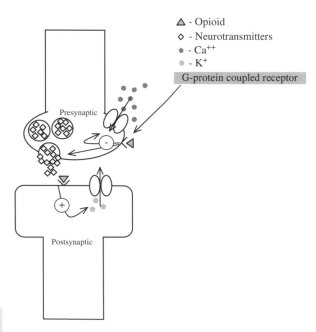

△ - Opioid
◇ - Neurotransmitters
● - Ca^{++}
⬤ - K$^+$
G-protein coupled receptor

Presynaptic

Postsynaptic

Figure 11.1. Opioid receptor agonist.

an adverse effect on platelet function [32] or the gastric mucosa [30].

Non-selective NSAIDs inhibit both cyclooxygenase 1 and 2 and with increased COX-1 selectivity the tendency is towards gastrointestinal toxicity [33]. It is the COX-2 isoform that is induced by pro-inflammatory stimuli and cytokines causing fever, inflammation and pain and thus the target for anti-inflammation by NSAIDs [34]. The COX-1 isoform is constitutive, causing hemostasis, platelet aggregation, and the production of prostacyclin, which is gastric mucosal protective. The inhibition of COX-1 isoform may be responsible for the adverse effects related to the non-selective NSAIDs [35]. COX-2 inhibitors (celecoxib, rofecoxib and valdecoxib) were approved for use in the USA and Europe, but both rofecoxib and valdecoxib were withdrawn from the market due to their adverse event profile. Recently parecoxib and etoricoxib have been approved in Europe but still await approval in the USA. The newest drug in the class, lumiracoxib, is under consideration for approval in Europe and the USA. Upon administration most of the coxibs are distributed widely throughout the body, with celecoxib possessing an increased lipophilicity enabling transport into the CNS. Lumiracoxib is more acidic than the others, which may favor its accumulation at sites of inflammation. Despite these subtle differences, all of the coxibs achieve sufficient brain concentrations to have a central analgesic effect [36]. The estimated half-lives of these medications vary (2 to 6 hours for lumiracoxib, 6 to 12 hours for celecoxib and valdecoxib, and 20 to 26 hours for etoricoxib). Likewise the relative degree of selectivity for COX-2 inhibition is lumiracoxib = etoricoxib > valdecoxib = rofecoxib >> celecoxib [31].

Local anesthetics

One of the first uses of local anesthetics (LA) for anesthesia was in the late nineteenth century with William Halsted reporting a mandibular block and brachial plexus block using cocaine [37,38]. The chemical structure of local anesthetics in clinical use consists of an aromatic (lipophilic) benzene ring linked to an amino group (hydrophilic) via either an ester or an amide intermediate chain. The intermediate link classifies the local anesthetic as either an ester (procaine, chloroprocaine, tetracaine, and cocaine) or an amide (lidocaine, prilocaine, mepivacaine, bupivacaine, etidocaine, and ropivacaine).

Local anesthetics exert their action by binding to sodium channels in nerve cell membranes and inhibiting the influx of sodium ions [39]. The limited influx of sodium ions reduces the rate of rise of the action potentials, increases the threshold for electrical excitability and slows impulse conduction [40]. The action potential fails to reach the threshold level and no impulses are conducted if sufficient sodium channels are blocked. Local anesthetics, therefore, do not affect the resting membrane potential, but rather affect the formation and propagation of the action potential.

At peripheral nerves the reduction in sodium influx leads to a decrement in action potential formation and propagation. In animal studies a reduction in action potential by 50% is necessary for observable loss of neuronal function and exposure length of the nerve fiber is important in conduction blockade [41]. At central neuraxial administration of LA similar mechanisms to those previously discussed occur at the level of the spinal nerve roots. Additionally, at the dorsal horn, LA possibly exert action at sodium and potassium channels in ventral and dorsal horn neurons [41]. Furthermore local anesthetics may exert action at neurotransmitters or neuropeptides such as substance P or γ-aminobutyric acid (GABA) by either directly binding to receptors or by altering local pharmacokinetics of endogenous agonists [41].

Anticonvulsants

The anticonvulsants are a diverse class of medications that modulate multiple sites such as calcium channels, sodium channels, GABA, and glutamate. The class includes medications such as gabapentin, pregabalin, topiramate, carbamazepine, lamotrigine phenytoin, valproic acid, and others. Several studies have shown this class of medications to be effective in a number of chronic pain states [42–45]. Two of the more widely used anti-epileptics drugs (AEDs) are the gabapentenoid membrane stabilizers gabapentin and pregabalin. Gabapentin, 1-(aminomethyl)cyclohexane acetic acid, is a structural analog of the neurotransmitter GABA, initially synthesized to mimic the chemical structure of the GABA, but is not believed to bind directly to GABA receptors or have any effect on the uptake or breakdown of GABA. The analgesic mechanism of action for gabapentin remains unknown, although possible mechanisms include the modulation or binding to the 21 subunits of the $\alpha_2\delta$ voltage-dependent calcium channels [46,47]. Gabapentin binds to the $\alpha_2\delta$ subunit and modulates calcium influx at the presynaptic nerve

59

terminal, reducing the release of several neurotransmitters, including glutamate, norepinephrine, and substance P [48–50] (Figure 11.2). Gabapentin blocks the tonic phase of nociception, and it exerts a potent inhibitory effect in several animal modes of neuropathic pain such as mechanical hyperalgesia, mechanical allodynia, thermal hyperalgesia, and thermo-allodynia [51,52]. Pregabalin, when compared to gabapentin, has greater lipid solubility and binds to the $\alpha_2\delta$ subunit with six times greater affinity than gabapentin [48,53], thus improving diffusion across the blood–brain barrier, better pharmacokinetic properties, and fewer drug interactions, due in part to an absence of hepatic metabolism [54].

NMDA-receptor antagonists

The N-methyl-d-aspartate (NMDA) receptors are one of the main mediators of excitatory neurotransmission and through inhibition of NMDA receptors, which are thought to play a crucial role in the generation and maintenance of chronic pain, NMDA receptor antagonists can be administered to produce analgesia. The receptor is a ligand-gated ion channel, which permits the influx of calcium and sodium and the efflux of potassium across the postsynaptic membrane. The NMDA receptor activation is dependent on the binding of both glutamate and the co-agonist glycine. Glutamate is a major excitatory neurotransmitter in the brain and spinal cord, exerting its effects postsynaptically. The receptor can be modulated by a number of antagonists, including competitive antagonists at the glutamate and glycine binding sites and noncompetitive NMDA receptor channel blockers (e.g. ketamine, memantine, magnesium) [55]. NMDA receptor activation triggers a cascade of events including a significant increase in intracellular calcium and activation of protein kinases and phosphorylating enzymes. NMDA receptor stimulation will also increase the production of spinal phospholipase and induce the production of nitric oxide synthetase. Inhibition at the NMDA receptor prevents the influx of calcium and activation of protein kinases and phosphorylating enzymes (Figure 11.3). Ketamine, currently the most potent clinically available

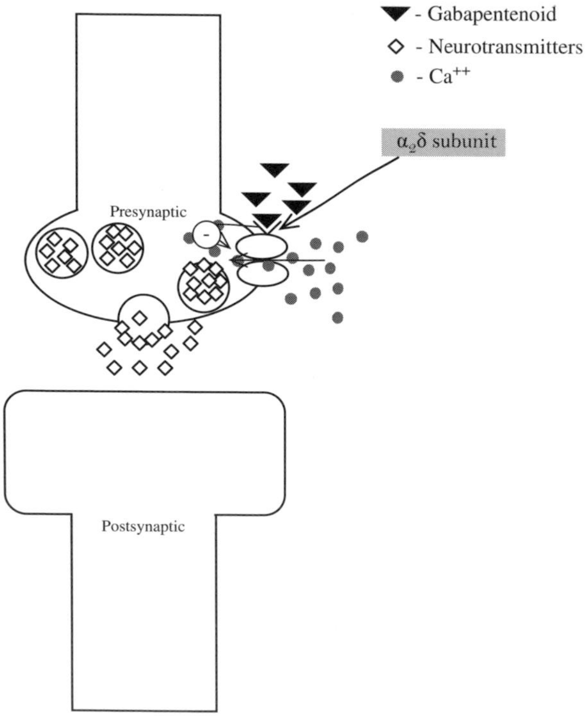

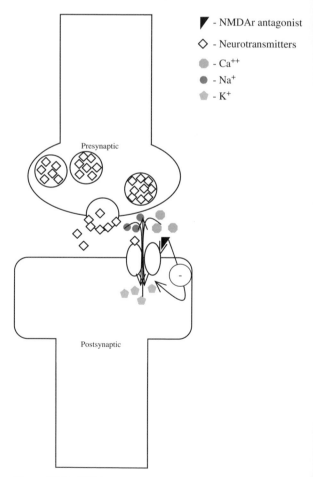

Figure 11.2. Gabapentenoid receptor agonist.

Figure 11.3. NMDA receptor antagonist.

NMDA antagonist [56], has been studied in the treatment of acute and chronic pain [57]. The NMDA receptor has a crucial role in excitatory synaptic transmission, plasticity, and neurodegeneration in the central nervous system [58] and has become an avenue to modulate the excitatory effects of glutamate.

Ketamine not only functions as an antagonist at NMDA receptors, but also blocks non-NMDA glutamate receptors, binds weakly to opioid receptors, antagonizes muscarinic cholinergic receptors, facilitates $GABA_A$ signaling, and possesses local anesthetic and possibly neuroregenerative properties [59–61]. Animal studies have identified NMDA receptors on unmyelinated and myelinated axons in peripheral somatic tissues [62,63] and local injections of glutamate or NMDA result in nociceptive behaviors that can be attenuated by peripheral administration of NMDA receptor antagonists [58,64–66]. The peripheral administration of ketamine enhanced the local anesthetic and analgesic actions of bupivacaine used for infiltration anesthesia [58,67] and inhibited the development of primary and secondary hyperalgesia after experimental burn injuries [58,68].

Antidepressants

Tricyclic antidepressants (TCA) have an analgesic effect that is demonstrated to be independent of their antidepressant effect [69]. The pharmacological actions of tricyclic antidepressants can be linked to their effect as a calcium channel antagonist, sodium channel antagonist, their NMDA receptor antagonist effect, but particularly the presynaptic reuptake inhibition of the monoamines such as serotonin and norepinephrine (Figure 11.4) [70,71]. The tricyclic antidepressants have no effect on dopamine reuptake but may have some indirect dopaminergic action by the adrenergic effect and desensitization of dopamine D_2 receptors [70]. Additionally, TCAs have been reported to bind to opioid receptors, but their binding affinity is probably too low to be relevant in humans at therapeutic drug concentrations [72]. More specifically, the analgesic effect is believed to occur primarily through reuptake inhibition of norepinephrine rather than serotonin at spinal dorsal horn synapses, with secondary activity at the sodium channels [73,74]. Within the class of tricyclic antidepressants, variation exists between the inhibition of norepinephrine and serotonin. The tertiary amine agents (e.g. amitriptyline and imipramine) demonstrate a balance in their ability to inhibit norepinephrine and serotonin, while the secondary amines (e.g. nortriptyline and desipramine) favor the inhibition of norepinephrine. The secondary amines appear to be as effective as the tertiary agents in treating neuropathic pain and produce markedly fewer side effects [75,76].

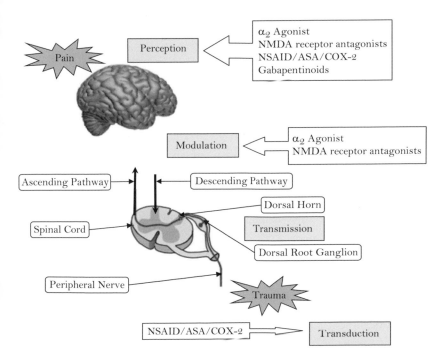

Figure 11.4. Site of action of adjuvant medications.

Serotonin-norepinephrine reuptake inhibitors (SNRIs) (e.g. duloxetine, venlafaxine and desvenlafaxine) inhibit the reuptake of both serotonin and norepinephrine and are referred to as dual inhibitors or "selective serotonin norepinephrine inhibitors". The SNRIs' lack of anticholinergic side effects results in a distinct advantage over traditional TCAs [13,77,78]. For example, duloxetine is a potent, balanced inhibitor of serotonin and norepinephrine reuptake [79]. Venlafaxine inhibits serotonin reuptake at lower dosages and inhibits both serotonin and norepinephrine reuptake at higher dosages [70,80].

Alpha-2-adrenergic agonists

The analgesic activity of α_2-agonists may be mediated by both supraspinal and spinal mechanisms. The central α_2-adrenoceptors in the locus coeruleus (supraspinal site) and in the substantia gelatinosa of the dorsal horn of the spinal cord are a primary site of action by which the antinociceptive effect occurs [81–83]. Clonidine induces analgesia primarily by stimulating presynaptic and postsynaptic α_2-adrenergic receptors in the dorsal horn of the spinal cord [84,85], which inhibit substance P release [86] and decrease dorsal horn neuronal firing [87,88]. Dexmedetomidine is eight times more specific for α_2-adrenoceptors than clonidine [89]. As an α_2-agonist the actions of dexmedetomidine are suggested to be mediated through postsynaptic α_2-adrenoceptors which activate pertussis toxin-sensitive G proteins [90], thereby increasing conductance through potassium ion channels [91].

Summary

The knowledge of medications' mechanism of action and receptor modulation may provide a conceptual framework for rational medication choice. A mechanistic approach and multimodal medication administration utilizing the synergistic effects of the aforementioned medications may provide the most effective analgesic regimen. Figure 11.4 represents the pain pathway and the site within the pathway where the medications have their effect.

References

1. Mantyselka PT, Turunen JH, Ahonen RS, et al. Chronic pain and poor self-rated health. *JAMA* 2003;**290**(18):2435–2442.

2. Verhaak PF, Kerssens JJ, Dekker J, et al. Prevalence of chronic benign pain disorder among adults: a review of the literature. *Pain* 1998;**77**(3):231–239.

3. Bouhassira D, Lanteri-Minet M, Attal N, et al. Prevalence of chronic pain with neuropathic characteristics in the general population. *Pain* 2008;**136**(3):380–387.

4. McCarberg BH, Nicholson BD, Todd KH, et al. The impact of pain on quality of life and the unmet needs of pain management: results from pain sufferers and physicians participating in an Internet survey. *Am J Ther* 2008;**15**(4):312–320.

5. Harden N, Cohen M. Unmet needs in the management of neuropathic pain. *J Pain Symptom Manage* 2003;**25**(5 Suppl):S12–17.

6. Pyati S, Gan TJ. Perioperative pain management. *CNS Drugs* 2007;**21**(3):185–211.

7. Kehlet H, Dahl JB. The value of "multimodal" or "balanced analgesia" in postoperative pain treatment. *Anesth Analg* 1993;**77**(5):1048–1056.

8. Attal N, Cruccu G, Haanpaa M, et al. EFNS guidelines on pharmacological treatment of neuropathic pain. *Eur J Neurol* 2006;**13**(11):1153–1169.

9. Baron R. Mechanisms of disease: neuropathic pain – a clinical perspective. *Nat Clin Pract Neurol* 2006;**2**(2):95–106.

10. Gallagher RM. Management of neuropathic pain: translating mechanistic advances and evidence-based research into clinical practice. *Clin J Pain* 2006;**22**(1 Suppl):S2–8.

11. Woolf CJ, Max MB. Mechanism-based pain diagnosis: issues for analgesic drug development. *Anesthesiology* 2001;**95**(1):241–249.

12. Brookoff D. Chronic pain: 2. The case for opioids. *Hosp Pract (Minneap)* 2000;**35**(9):69–72, 75–66, 81–64.

13. Namaka M, Gramlich CR, Ruhlen D, et al. A treatment algorithm for neuropathic pain. *Clin Ther* 2004;**26**(7):951–979.

14. Benzon HT, Raja SN, Molloy RE, et al. Chapter 10 in *Essentials of Pain Medicine and Regional Anesthesia*, 2nd ed. Philadelphia: Elsevier, Churchill Livingstone, 2005.

15. Benzon HT, Rathmell JP, Wu CL, et al. *Raj's Practical Management of Pain*, 4th ed. Philadelphia: Mosby Elsevier; 2008, pp. 597–611.

16. McCleane G, Smith HS. Opioids for persistent noncancer pain. *Med Clin North Am* 2007;**91**(2):177–197.

17. Brunton L, Lazo J, Parker K. Chapter 21 in *Goodman & Gilman's The Pharmacological Basis of Therapeutics*, 11th ed. New York: McGraw-Hill, 2006.

18. Cohen SP, Dragovich A. Intrathecal analgesia. *Med Clin North Am* 2007;**91**(2):251–270.

19. Ocana M, Cendan CM, Cobos EJ, et al. Potassium channels and pain: present realities and future opportunities. *Eur J Pharmacol* 1 2004;**500**(1–3): 203–219.

20. Baum C, Kennedy DL, Forbes MB. Utilization of nonsteroidal antiinflammatory drugs. *Arthritis Rheum* 1985;**28**(6):686–692.

21. Laine L. Approaches to nonsteroidal anti-inflammatory drug use in the high-risk patient. *Gastroenterology* 2001;**120**(3):594–606.

22. McCormack K. The spinal actions of nonsteroidal anti-inflammatory drugs and the dissociation between their anti-inflammatory and analgesic effects. *Drugs* 1994;47 Suppl. **5**:28–45; discussion 46–27.

23. Cashman JN. The mechanisms of action of NSAIDs in analgesia. *Drugs* 1996;52 Suppl. **5**:13–23.

24. Bjorkman R. Central antinociceptive effects of non-steroidal anti-inflammatory drugs and paracetamol. Experimental studies in the rat. *Acta Anaesthesiol Scand Suppl* 1995;**103**:1–44.

25. Benzon HT, Raja SN, Molloy RE, et al. Chapter 16 in *Essentials of Pain Medicine and Regional Anesthesia*, 2nd ed. Philadelphia: Elsevier, Churchill Livingstone, 2005.

26. Malmberg AB, Yaksh TL. Hyperalgesia mediated by spinal glutamate or substance P receptor blocked by spinal cyclooxygenase inhibition. *Science* 1992;**257**(5074):1276–1279.

27. England S, Bevan S, Docherty RJ. PGE2 modulates the tetrodotoxin-resistant sodium current in neonatal rat dorsal root ganglion neurones via the cyclic AMP-protein kinase A cascade. *J Physiol* 1996;**495**(Pt 2): 429–440.

28. Ahmadi S, Lippross S, Neuhuber WL, et al. PGE(2) selectively blocks inhibitory glycinergic neurotransmission onto rat superficial dorsal horn neurons. *Nat Neurosci* 2002;**5**(1):34–40.

29. Vasko MR. Prostaglandin-induced neuropeptide release from spinal cord. *Prog Brain Res* 1995;**104**:367–380.

30. Graham GG, Scott KF. Mechanism of action of paracetamol. *Am J Ther* 2005;**12**(1):46–55.

31. Brunton L, Lazo J, Parker K. Chapter 26 in *Goodman & Gilman's The Pharmacological Basis of Therapeutics*, 11th ed. New York: McGraw-Hill, 2006.

32. Munsterhjelm E, Munsterhjelm NM, Niemi TT, et al. Dose-dependent inhibition of platelet function by acetaminophen in healthy volunteers. *Anesthesiology* 2005;**103**(4):712–717.

33. FitzGerald GA, Patrono C. The coxibs, selective inhibitors of cyclooxygenase-2. *N Engl J Med* 2001;**345**(6):433–442.

34. Vane JR, Botting RM. Mechanism of action of nonsteroidal anti-inflammatory drugs. *Am J Med* 1998;**104**(3A):2S–8S; discussion 21S–22S.

35. Lanza FL. A review of gastric ulcer and gastroduodenal injury in normal volunteers receiving aspirin and other non-steroidal anti-inflammatory drugs. *Scand J Gastroenterol Suppl* 1989;**163**:24–31.

36. Buvanendran A, Kroin JS, Tuman KJ, et al. Cerebrospinal fluid and plasma pharmacokinetics of the cyclooxygenase 2 inhibitor rofecoxib in humans: single and multiple oral drug administration. *Anesth Analg* 2005;**100**(5):1320–1324, table of contents.

37. Hadzic A. *Textbook of Regional Anesthesia and Acute Pain Management*, 1st ed. New York: McGraw Hill, 2007, pp. 105–120.

38. Keys T. *The History of Surgical Anesthesia: Wood Library, Museum of Anesthesiology*; 1996.

39. Butterworth JF, Strichartz GR. Molecular mechanisms of local anesthesia: a review. *Anesthesiology* 1990;**72**(4):711–734.

40. Brunton L, Lazo J, Parker K. Chapter 14 in *Goodman & Gilman's The Pharmacological Basis of Therapeutics*, 11th ed. New York: McGraw-Hill, 2006.

41. Benzon HT, Raja SN, Molloy RE, et al. Chapter 67 in *Essentials of Pain Medicine and Regional Anesthesia*, 2nd ed. Philadelphia: Elsevier, Churchill LIvingstone, 2005.

42. Backonja M, Beydoun A, Edwards KR, et al. Gabapentin for the symptomatic treatment of painful neuropathy in patients with diabetes mellitus: a randomized controlled trial. *JAMA* 1998;**280**(21):1831–1836.

43. Freynhagen R, Strojek K, Griesing T, et al. Efficacy of pregabalin in neuropathic pain evaluated in a 12-week, randomised, double-blind, multicentre, placebo-controlled trial of flexible- and fixed-dose regimens. *Pain* 2005;**115**(3):254–263.

44. Rull JA, Quibrera R, Gonzalez-Millan H, et al. Symptomatic treatment of peripheral diabetic neuropathy with carbamazepine (Tegretol): double blind crossover trial. *Diabetologia* 1969;**5**(4):215–218.

45. Keskinbora K, Pekel AF, Aydinli I. Gabapentin and an opioid combination versus opioid alone for the management of neuropathic cancer pain: a randomized open trial. *J Pain Symptom Manage* 2007;**34**(2):183–189.

46. Gee NS, Brown JP, Dissanayake VU, et al. The novel anticonvulsant drug, gabapentin (Neurontin), binds to the alpha2delta subunit of a calcium channel. *J Biol Chem* 1996;**271**(10):5768–5776.

47. Tiippana EM, Hamunen K, Kontinen VK, et al. Do surgical patients benefit from perioperative gabapentin/pregabalin? A systematic review of efficacy and safety. *Anesth Analg* 2007;**104**(6):1545–1556, table of contents.

48. Gajraj NM. Pregabalin: its pharmacology and use in pain management. *Anesth Analg* 2007;**105**(6):1805–1815.

49. Fink K, Dooley DJ, Meder WP, et al. Inhibition of neuronal Ca(2+) influx by gabapentin and pregabalin in the human neocortex. *Neuropharmacology* 2002;**42**(2):229–236.

50. Maneuf YP, Hughes J, McKnight AT. Gabapentin inhibits the substance P-facilitated K(+)-evoked release of [(3)H]glutamate from rat caudial trigeminal nucleus slices. *Pain* 2001;**93**(2):191–196.

51. Tremont-Lukats IW, Megeff C, Backonja MM. Anticonvulsants for neuropathic pain syndromes: mechanisms of action and place in therapy. *Drugs* 2000;**60**(5):1029–1052.

52. Field MJ, McCleary S, Hughes J, et al. Gabapentin and pregabalin, but not morphine and amitriptyline, block both static and dynamic components of mechanical allodynia induced by streptozocin in the rat. *Pain* 1999;**80**(1–2):391–398.

53. Jones DL, Sorkin LS. Systemic gabapentin and S(+)-3-isobutyl-gamma-aminobutyric acid block secondary hyperalgesia. *Brain Res* 1998;**810**(1–2): 93–99.

54. Shneker BF, McAuley JW. Pregabalin: a new neuromodulator with broad therapeutic indications. *Ann Pharmacother* 2005;**39**(12):2029–2037.

55. Rang H, Dale, MM, Ritter, JM. *Amino Acid Transmitters. Pharmacology*. Edinburgh: Harcourt, 2001, pp. 470–482.

56. Kiefer RT, Rohr P, Ploppa A, et al. Efficacy of ketamine in anesthetic dosage for the treatment of refractory complex regional pain syndrome: an open-label phase II study. *Pain Med* 2008;**9**(8):1173–1201.

57. Himmelseher S, Durieux ME. Ketamine for perioperative pain management. *Anesthesiology* 2005;**102**(1):211–220.

58. Petrenko AB, Yamakura T, Baba H, et al. The role of N-methyl-D-aspartate (NMDA) receptors in pain: a review. *Anesth Analg* 2003;**97**(4):1108–1116.

59. Kohrs R, Durieux ME. Ketamine: teaching an old drug new tricks. *Anesth Analg* 1998;**87**(5):1186–1193.

60. Cohen SP, Verdolin MH, Chang AS, et al. The intravenous ketamine test predicts subsequent response to an oral dextromethorphan treatment regimen in fibromyalgia patients. *J Pain* 2006;**7**(6):391–398.

61. Himmelseher S, Pfenninger E, Georgieff M. The effects of ketamine-isomers on neuronal injury and regeneration in rat hippocampal neurons. *Anesth Analg* 1996;**83**(3):505–512.

62. Carlton SM, Hargett GL, Coggeshall RE. Localization and activation of glutamate receptors in unmyelinated axons of rat glabrous skin. *Neurosci Lett* 1995;**197**(1):25–28.

63. Coggeshall RE, Carlton SM. Ultrastructural analysis of NMDA, AMPA, and kainate receptors on unmyelinated and myelinated axons in the periphery. *J Comp Neurol* 1998;**391**(1):78–86.

64. Jackson DL, Graff CB, Richardson JD, et al. Glutamate participates in the peripheral modulation of thermal hyperalgesia in rats. *Eur J Pharmacol* 1995;**284**(3):321–325.

65. Zhou S, Bonasera L, Carlton SM. Peripheral administration of NMDA, AMPA or KA results in pain behaviors in rats. *Neuroreport* 1996;**7**(4):895–900.

66. Lawand NB, Willis WD, Westlund KN. Excitatory amino acid receptor involvement in peripheral nociceptive transmission in rats. *Eur J Pharmacol* 1997;**324**(2–3):169–177.

67. Tverskoy M, Oren M, Vaskovich M, et al. Ketamine enhances local anesthetic and analgesic effects of bupivacaine by peripheral mechanism: a study in post-operative patients. *Neurosci Lett* 1996;**215**(1):5–8.

68. Warncke T, Jorum E, Stubhaug A. Local treatment with the N-methyl-D-aspartate receptor antagonist ketamine, inhibit development of secondary hyperalgesia in man by a peripheral action. *Neurosci Lett* 1997;**227**(1):1–4.

69. Dworkin RH, Backonja M, Rowbotham MC, et al. Advances in neuropathic pain: diagnosis, mechanisms, and treatment recommendations. *Arch Neurol* 2003;**60**(11):1524–1534.

70. Sindrup SH, Otto M, Finnerup NB, et al. Antidepressants in the treatment of neuropathic pain. *Basic Clin Pharmacol Toxicol* 2005;**96**(6):399–409.

71. Colombo B, Annovazzi PO, Comi G. Medications for neuropathic pain: current trends. *Neurol Sci* 2006;**27** Suppl. **2**:S183–189.

72. Hall H, Ogren SO. Effects of antidepressant drugs on different receptors in the brain. *Eur J Pharmacol* 1981;**70**(3):393–407.

73. Sawynok J, Esser MJ, Reid AR. Antidepressants as analgesics: an overview of central and peripheral mechanisms of action. *J Psychiatry Neurosci* 2001;**26**(1):21–29.

74. Gordon DB, Love G. Pharmacologic management of neuropathic pain. *Pain Manag Nurs* 2004;**5**(4 Suppl. 1): 19–33.

75. Jackson KC, 2nd. Pharmacotherapy for neuropathic pain. *Pain Pract* 2006;**6**(1):27–33.

76. McQuay HJ, Tramer M, Nye BA, et al. A systematic review of antidepressants in neuropathic pain. *Pain* 1996;**68**(2–3):217–227.

77. Sindrup SH, Bach FW, Madsen C, et al. Venlafaxine versus imipramine in painful polyneuropathy: a randomized, controlled trial. *Neurology* 2003;**60**(8):1284–1289.

78. Mattia C, Paoletti F, Coluzzi F, et al. New antidepressants in the treatment of neuropathic pain. A review. *Minerva Anestesio* 2002;**68**(3):105–114.

79. Wong DT, Bymaster FP. Dual serotonin and noradrenaline uptake inhibitor class of antidepressants potential for greater efficacy or just hype? *Prog Drug Res* 2002;**58**:169–222.

80. Dworkin RH, O'Connor AB, Backonja M, et al. Pharmacologic management of neuropathic pain: evidence-based recommendations. *Pain* 2007;**132**(3):237–251.

81. Buerkle H, Yaksh TL. Pharmacological evidence for different alpha 2-adrenergic receptor sites mediating analgesia and sedation in the rat. *Br J Anaesth* 1998;**81**(2):208–215.

82. Buvanendran A, Kroin JS. Useful adjuvants for post-operative pain management. *Best Pract Res Clin Anaesthesiol* 2007;**21**(1):31–49.

83. Unnerstall JR, Kopajtic TA, Kuhar MJ. Distribution of alpha 2 agonist binding sites in the rat and human central nervous system: analysis of some functional, anatomic correlates of the pharmacologic effects of clonidine and related adrenergic agents. *Brain Res* 1984;**319**(1):69–101.

84. Eisenach JC, Dewan DM, Rose JC, et al. Epidural clonidine produces antinociception, but not hypotension, in sheep. *Anesthesiology* 1987;**66**(4):496–501.

85. Detweiler DJ, Eisenach JC, Tong C, et al. A cholinergic interaction in alpha 2 adrenoceptor-mediated antinociception in sheep. *J Pharmacol Exp Ther* 1993;**265**(2):536–542.

86. Kuraishi Y, Hirota N, Sato Y, et al. Noradrenergic inhibition of the release of substance P from the primary afferents in the rabbit spinal dorsal horn. *Brain Res* 1985;**359**(1–2):177–182.

87. Fleetwood-Walker SM, Mitchell R, Hope PJ, et al. An alpha 2 receptor mediates the selective inhibition by noradrenaline of nociceptive responses of identified dorsal horn neurones. *Brain Res* 1985;**334**(2):243–254.

88. Owen MD, Fibuch EE, McQuillan R, et al. Post-operative analgesia using a low-dose, oral-transdermal clonidine combination: lack of clinical efficacy. *J Clin Anesth* 1997;**9**(1):8–14.

89. Coughlan MG, Lee JG, Bosnjak ZJ, et al. Direct coronary and cerebral vascular responses to dexmedetomidine. Significance of endogenous nitric oxide synthesis. *Anesthesiology* 1992;**77**(5):998–1006.

90. Salonen M, Reid K, Maze M. Synergistic interaction between alpha 2-adrenergic agonists and benzodiazepines in rats. *Anesthesiology* 1992;**76**(6):1004–1011.

91. Bhana N, Goa KL, McClellan KJ. Dexmedetomidine. *Drugs* 2000;**59**(2):263–268; discussion 269–270.

12

A stepwise approach to pain management

Raymond S. Sinatra

The traditional three-step approach

Up to 70% of patients with cancer experience moderate to severe pain during their illness. In an effort to better manage malignancy-related pain, the World Health Organization (WHO) in 1986 developed a stepwise approach to analgesic dosing [1–3]. The WHO three-step "ladder" correlated analgesic selection and dosing in relation to the intensity of the pain complaint (Figure 12.1) The ladder classified cancer pain into three levels of severity: mild, moderate, and severe [1,2]. Patients with mild pain were assigned to the lowest step or rung of the ladder (step 1) and were to be treated with non-opioid analgesics. If pain persisted and progressed to moderate intensity, the patient was advanced to step 2 and treated with "weak" opioid analgesics such as codeine, propoxyphene, tramadol, oxycodone, and hydrocodone. Advancement to step 2 was often problematic since weak opioids are associated with the same risks of adverse effects, tolerance, and diversion/abuse as more potent agents. For this reason, many clinicians consider step 2 to be a "large" step when compared to those that precede and follow it (Figure 12.2).

Patients may be advanced to step 3 of the ladder in situations where pain has progressed to severe or very severe intensity, and is inadequately controlled with weak opioids. At this step, potent opioids including morphine, hydromorphone, oxymorphone, and transdermal delivered (TDS) fentanyl are commonly prescribed. In general, sustained-release opioids are provided daily or twice daily for baseline pain control with immediate-release opioids taken as needed for breakthrough pain. Total daily opioid dose is increased as required, thereby allowing patients to gain freedom from pain.

While simplistic in nature, the WHO analgesic ladder was considered to be a successful therapeutic advance as it provided an organized approach to pain assessment and management on a global scale [3]. The major drawback associated with the WHO stepwise approach was the fact that approximately 20–25% of patients did not respond to morphine or other potent opioids, and continued to suffer severe pain [3–5].

A stepwise analgesic care plan would be expected to be even less effective for long-term chronic pain management, and controversy exists as to whether opioids should be prescribed to patients with musculoskeletal pain or benign disease-related pain [4,5]. Some caregivers argue that prescription of step 2 and 3 opioids may be the only way to provide effective pain relief, while others worry that such therapy may lead to lifelong dependencies, which can be particularly problematic in younger patients. Despite acceptance of a stepwise approach to chronic pain, many primary care physicians and surgeons remain uncomfortable prescribing opioids, while at the same time they lack a clear understanding of pain processing and the benefits of multimodal analgesia. Other educational deficits, including patient assessment, determination of need, initiation of opioid therapy, and how to treat adverse effects, often lead to undermedication, intolerability, and inadequate management of chronic pain. Comorbid conditions, including obesity, sleep apnea, and chronic obstructive pulmonary disease, and mental health issues such as anxiety, depression, and post-traumatic stress, further complicate pain management and reduce caregiver comfort in prescribing opioids [4,5].

Rationale for a four-step approach

With the advent of anesthesiology and multi-specialty-based pain clinics and caregiver specialization in interventional pain management, a four-step analgesic approach was developed to more effectively treat patients with benign and malignancy-related chronic pain (Figure 12.3). The first three steps of this care plan are similar to the WHO analgesic ladder; however, a new fourth step, termed the interventional step, utilizes invasive techniques that are placed and managed by pain specialists. Interventional therapy

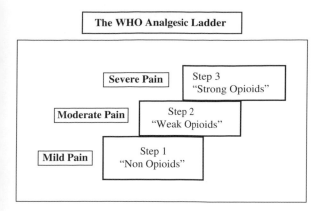

Figure 12.1.

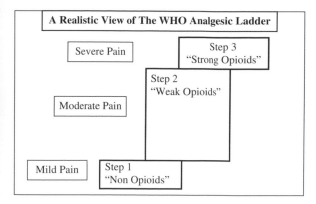

Figure 12.2.

includes implantable analgesic pumps, peripheral and epidural stimulators, regional and neuraxial steroids, and neurolysis. Such therapy may provide measurable reductions in pain intensity and opioid sparing effects that are particularly beneficial to highly tolerant patients, the elderly, and those suffering intolerable dose-related adverse events

The current four-step approach for chronic pain management is initiated and maintained in a manner that is the exact opposite to analgesic treatment plans employed for post-operative pain (Figure 12.4). In acute settings, the intensity of pain is most severe during the first 24–72 h following surgery or traumatic injury. During this period pain is optimally controlled using step-4 interventional techniques including neuraxial analgesia and continuous peripheral neural blockade. Analgesic benefits are greatest in high-risk patients and those recovering from the most painful of procedures, and must be balanced by the fact that these techniques are more invasive, require skill and specialization for placement, are associated with risk

of bleeding/infection, and are more expensive than treatment with oral/IV opioids. As the patient recovers, interventional therapy is discontinued and the patient is advanced downward to step 3, and treated with intravenous PCA or strong parenteral opioids. As bowel function returns, the patient may be advanced downward to step 2 and treated with oral opioid plus acetaminophen compounds for several days to weeks depending upon the surgical procedure. Thereafter, residual discomfort may be treated with step-1 non-opioid analgesics, until complaints of pain resolve entirely.

In chronic pain settings, patients follow the opposite clinical course characterized by progressive increases in pain intensity. Progression of disease and associated discomfort is best controlled by upward steps in analgesic dose, and potency, as well as increasing complexity and invasiveness of analgesic delivery. The major difference between the WHO three-step ladder and the four-step approach is that the latter care plan recognizes that not all patients can gain adequate pain relief with opioids, despite proportionate increases in dose. The WHO ladder was designed for malignancy-related chronic pain and palliation in patients not expected to survive beyond several months to a year [1,2,5,6]. This care plan is often unacceptable and inappropriate for individuals suffering intractable benign pain that may last for many years. For these patients, interventional techniques offer an analgesic alternative that can often minimize risks of excessive sedation and cognitive deficits while improving functionality and quality of life.

The four-step approach to chronic pain management: common sense guidelines

Optimal pain management is initiated following a thorough screening of the patient. In addition to history and diagnostic imaging, a focused yet detailed physical examination is necessary to evaluate the pain complaint [7]. The caregiver must not only localize the site(s) involved and the intensity of discomfort but should also characterize associated symptoms as being either somatic, visceral, inflammatory neuropathic, myelopathic or mixed pain. Pain complaints are rarely the same and these clinical findings are key to formulating analgesic prescriptions and developing a treatment plan.

Whenever possible chronic pain management should begin on step 1 with non-opioid analgesics.

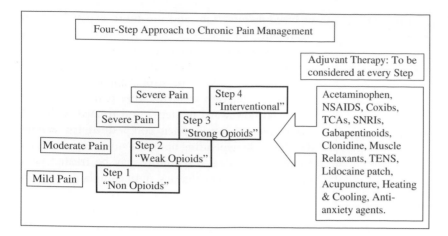

Figure 12.3.

Four-Step Approach to Chronic Pain Management

Adjuvant Therapy: To be considered at every Step

Severe Pain — Step 4 "Interventional"

Severe Pain — Step 3 "Strong Opioids"

Moderate Pain — Step 2 "Weak Opioids"

Mild Pain — Step 1 "Non Opioids"

Acetaminophen, NSAIDS, Coxibs, TCAs, SNRIs, Gabapentinoids, Clonidine, Muscle Relaxants, TENS, Lidocaine patch, Acupuncture, Heating & Cooling, Anti-anxiety agents.

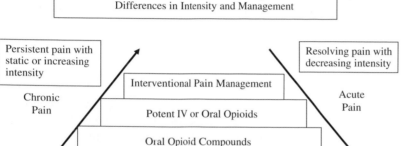

Figure 12.4.

Acute and Chronic Pain: Temporal Differences in Intensity and Management

Persistent pain with static or increasing intensity

Resolving pain with decreasing intensity

Chronic Pain

Acute Pain

Interventional Pain Management

Potent IV or Oral Opioids

Oral Opioid Compounds

Non Opioid Analgesics

No Analgesics

Caregivers should always use the lowest effective analgesic dose administered by the simplest route and consider a multimodal approach rather than relying on high-dose monotherapy. The caregiver should maintain patients on step 1 as long as is possible by adding pharmacological adjuvants, physical therapy, emotional and psychological support, and non-pharmacological and non-traditional analgesic techniques.

When opioids are deemed necessary to establish or maintain effective pain control, caregivers often face a controversial dilemma regarding whether "weak" or "potent" agonists should be employed. Conventional stepwise care plans recommend that caregivers prescribe weaker agents including tramadol, buprenorphine, hydrocodone, and oxycodone, while maximizing their effectiveness with non-opioid analgesics and adjuvants. New thinking suggests that step-2 opioids should not be prescribed at all for malignancy-related pain, as these agents are associated with less uniform pain control, adverse events and rapid dose escalation [5,6,8]. Instead, caregivers should consider prescribing more potent step-3 agents in low dose, and preferably as extended-duration tabs or transdermal patches. The correct solution is to adjust opioid potency and dose according to the current severity of pain complaint. For example, patients initially presenting with excruciating or rapidly progressing pain should be given the option to bypass step 2 and take an "analgesic elevator" to step 3 [8]. In contrast, patients requiring minimal analgesic supplementation may gain effective relief for an extended period of time, with occasional "as needed" doses of step-2 agonists. If, or when, pain intensity increases and step-2 opioid dosing is either ineffectual or excessive, advance to step 3 is appropriate.

Whether short-acting or sustained-release/extended-duration preparations, or their combination, are most useful for step-3 analgesia is generally based on patient need. Patients who complain of occasional episodes of severe breakthrough pain are best treated with rapid-acting short-duration opioids, while those with constant discomfort or frequent episodes of pain appreciate the convenience and uniformity of relief provided by extended-duration opioids. The fact that extended-duration formulations produce steady-state concentration with fewer peak-and-trough levels may also reduce the incidence of annoying AEs such as nausea or somnolence.

Patients treated with extended-duration opioids may experience breakthrough pain which can be controlled with immediate-release, short-acting opioids; however, if three or more PRN doses are used daily, the dose of extended-duration opioid should be increased by 10–25%. With regard to ongoing dose escalation and total opioid dose, the caregiver should think long term, and consider a daily maximum dose that should not be exceeded. This is a very controversial aspect of chronic pain management and there are few guidelines. In general, the maximum allowable dose is determined by caregiver experience and level of comfort, as well as other variables including adverse effects and intolerability, patient age, expected duration of need (weeks, months, years, decades), and risk of abuse and diversion.

Patients treated with potent opioids often experience reductions in analgesic efficacy related to tolerance development. As dosing escalates, many patients experience intolerable adverse events that limit the overall analgesic effectiveness of the agent originally prescribed. In these individuals, opioid rotation to a different agonist may be useful. The success of rotation has been related to differences in opioid receptor subtypes, greater mu receptor affinity and differences in metabolism, that may allow a new opioid to re-establish analgesic efficacy with greater tolerability.

Patients exceeding the maximum opioid daily dose and those exhibiting intolerability and increased adverse events despite rotation are candidates for step-4 interventional therapy [9,10]. Techniques that may be offered include spinal and peripheral neural stimulation, which provides effective non-pharmacological modulation of pain transmission. Intrathecal infusions of morphine or hydromorphone either alone or in combination with local anesthetics offer powerful pain control as well as significant reductions in total opioid dose. Intrathecal dosing is particularly useful for patients suffering benign and malignancy-related thoracic, abdominal, and pelvic pain. Other techniques, including neurolysis, intrajoint and epidural steroids, and blockade or destruction of sympathetic ganglia or celiac plexus, can dramatically reduce opioid dose requirements while restoring functionality and quality of life [10]. Following successful intervention, pain scores may decline dramatically; however, opioids employed at step 3 should in most cases be continued to further improve overall analgesic effectiveness, although significant dose reductions may be achievable.

To further optimize analgesic effectiveness and reduce opioid burden, non-opioid analgesics employed at step 1 should be continued whenever possible, as patients are advanced to steps 2, 3 and 4. In addition, analgesic adjuvants including central norepinephrine reuptake inhibitors, gabapentanoids, and NMDA receptor inhibitors should be prescribed particularly for patients with high-grade opioid tolerance and neuropathic pain. Finally, pharmacological, nonpharmacological, and non-traditional therapeutic techniques including use of anxiolytics and antidepressants, heat/cold applications, topical analgesics, transcutaneous electrical neural stimulation (TENS), acupuncture, and massage could be included at every step of the ladder.

Moving toward a flexible approach to pain managment

The previously described three- and four-step ladders are widely employed for managing malignancy-related and other terminal pain states; however, the time has come to rethink and possibly discard these traditional stepwise approaches [6,8,9]. Application of flexible and more individualized treatment plans would be particularly beneficial for patients suffering benign chronic pain. For these individuals, care plans that include non-opioid-based multimodal analgesia and early application of interventional pain management may be superior to progressive increases in opioid dosing [10,11]. For example, an elderly female with pain related to spinal stenosis can often gain superior pain relief with greater safety and analgesic tolerability by avoiding steps 2 and 3 and moving directly to an interventional step-4 technique such as epidural steroid injections. For patients with chronic low back pain and chronic pelvic pain, early use of spinal stimulation, neurolysis, and intrathecal analgesic techniques may improve functionality and quality of life while avoiding the sedative effects of step-3 opioids. Even in patients with malignancy-related pain, evidence suggests that substituting interventional procedures for high doses of potent opioids offers more effective analgesia and possibly a more prolonged survival rate [11].

Patients entering a flexible pain management care plan can be treated with a mixture of peripheral and central-acting non-opioid analgesics as well as psychological support, physical therapy, and non-traditional analgesic techniques. Entry-level analgesics would include NSAIDs and COX-2 inhibitors for patients suffering inflammatory pain, as well as acetaminophen, lidocaine transdermal patch and clonidine for patients complaining of somatic pain. Muscle relaxants should always be prescribed for skeletal muscle spasm and associated discomfort. Norepinephrine reuptake inhibitors including tricyclic antidepressants, SNRIs (duloxetine), alpha-2 delta subunit ion channel blockers (gabapentin, pregabalin), and

transdermal local anesthetic patches may be prescribed for patients presenting with neuropathic pain (Figure 12.5).

Instead of being considered as a "last resort", interventional pain management can be employed at an early stage of care. Patients are carefully assessed and, if deemed to be clinically appropriate, offered interventional procedures including neurolysis, spinal stimulation, and intrathecal infusions. Such therapy, while invasive and expensive, would be encouraged in settings where patients might benefit from improved pain relief and significant opioid-sparing effects.

If, and when, additional opioid-mediated analgesia is required, supplementation with dual-acting analgesics such as tramadol and tapentadol can be provided. Although the clinical usefulness of "weaker" opioids in the management of cancer pain has been challenged, these agents offer dosing versatility for either moderate or severe discomfort and should be considered as entry-level supplements for patients with benign chronic pain. Tramadol is a relatively weak unscheduled analgesic that can provide useful supplementation of multimodal analgesic regimens and can help control moderate breakthrough pain. In

Figure 12.5.

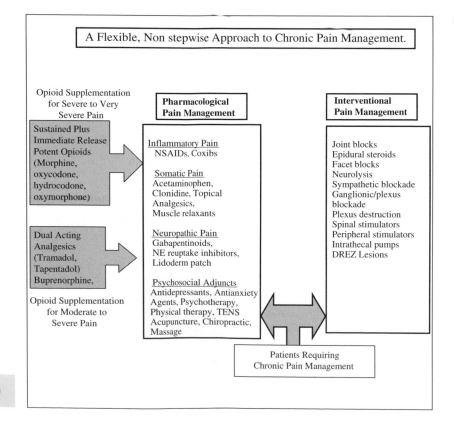

contrast, tapentadol is a more powerful schedule II agent that binds mu opioid receptors and blocks norepinephrine reuptake. Tapentadol 50–100 mg provides analgesic efficacy comparable to oxycodone 10–15 mg with an unexpectedly lower incidence of adverse events [12]. Currently tapentadol has approval for acute pain or acute breakthrough pain in patients with chronic pain. A sustained-release tapentadol preparation is being developed for around the clock treatment of chronic pain. Tapentadol's improved tolerability profile may overcome an important barrier to optimal chronic pain management; that being the fact that patients are often unwilling to take effective medications because they don't like how they make them feel. Nevertheless, the added cost of tapentadol may restrict its use as a first-line opioid analgesic. In that case, judicious use of hydrocodone and oxycodone plus acetaminophen compounds may also be considered.

In opioid-naive patients, supplemental opioids should be prescribed for control of breakthrough incident pain and pain during sleep, not for constant pain. A potential advantage of flexible pain management plans that employ combinations of multimodal and interventional analgesia is that many patients may require only minimal to moderate amounts of opioid supplementation in order to maintain effective relief [10,13].

For patients presenting with excruciating pain or those experiencing progressive increases in discomfort despite receiving multimodal and interventional therapy, supplementation with potent sustained- and immediate-release opioids may be indicated. Dosing should not be restricted, but instead titrated according to the individual patient's needs. There are many options, including oral administration of sustained-release morphine, oxycodone, and oxymorphone as well as fentanyl transdermal patch [14]. Extended-release oxymorphone has been well tested in patients with chronic low back pain where it provides uniform and durable pain relief. Methadone in low dose has also been advocated as a method of reducing dose escalation of the primary opioid being administered. In palliative care settings and for individuals suffering intractable pain, parenteral opioids and infusions of ketamine may also be provided [15].

Flexible chronic pain management care plans would best be initiated at earlier stages of complaint rather than after progression of symptoms and development of disability. Individuals suffering longstanding poorly controlled pain develop central sensitization and neural plasticity changes that may be difficult to overcome. These alterations facilitate noxious transmission and are associated with development of pain behaviors, sleep deprivation, de-conditioning, fatigue, and weight gain, which negatively influence the patient's ability to return to work or resume a normal quality of life. The early application of analgesic adjuvants and interventional pain management may restore CNS homeostasis and hopefully break the cycle of sensitzation, plasticity, and intractable noxious transmission and perception. Other clinical benefits that may be achieved include a significant reduction and possibly elimination of opioids and their associated adverse events, and improvements in functionality and rehabilitation.

This is an exciting time for both primary caregivers and pain specialists as a number of new analgesics are emerging that will complement existing non-opioid regimens and further ensure the success of opioid-avoidance care plans. While there is no analgesic "silver bullet" on the horizon, peripherally acting agents in development, including anti-nerve growth factor, TRPV-1 inhibitors, and peripherally selective mu and kappa agonists, promise not only high analgesic efficacy but also improved patient safety and greater tolerability than opioids and other central-acting agents.

The ultimate goal of flexible chronic pain management is to achieve a balance of patient safety and meaningful pain relief, not a stepwise plan to eliminate all pain at the cost of therapeutic intolerability. The patient must not be led to believe that "you take this pill and you will feel much better". Instead, the patient agrees to, and actively participates in, a multidisciplined flexible care plan that includes interventional therapy, vigorous physical therapy, and psychological support. The therapeutic goals are to limit chronic pain disability and restore physical and psychological functionality, while avoiding excessive opioid dependency.

In summary, a stepwise approach to pain management, while useful for many patients, may not be appropriate for all. The application of a flexible multimodal care plan and appropriate opioid supplementation can, in most settings, offer patients freedom from severe chronic pain and return to baseline quality of life. Therapy should always be individualized and provided in a logical order based on potential benefits, associated risks, adverse events, and overall cost.

References

1. World Health Organization. *Cancer Pain Relief.* Geneva: World Health Organization, 1986.

2. World Health Organization. *Cancer Pain Relief,* 2nd ed. Geneva: World Health Organization, 1996.

3. Foley KM. 2006. Appraising the WHO Analgesic Ladder on Its 20th Anniversary. www.whocancerpain.

4. Adams NJ, Plane MB, Fleming MF, Mundt MP, Saunders LA, Stauffacher EA. Opioids and the treatment of chronic pain in a primary care sample. *J Pain Symptom Manage* 2001;**22**:791–796.

5. Portenoy RK. Opioid therapy for chronic nonmalignant pain: a review of the critical issues. *J Pain Symptom Manage* 1996;**11**:203–217.

6. Nicholson B. Responsible prescribing of opioids for the management of chronic pain. *Drugs* 2003;**63**:17–32.

7. Brunton S. Approach to assessment and diagnosis of chronic pain. *J Fam Pract* 2004;**53**:S3–10.

8. Eisenberg E, et al. *J Clin Oncol* 1994;**12**:2756–2765.

9. Justins D, Seimaszko O. Rational use of neural blockade for the management of chronic pain. *Pain 2002- An updated Review, Refresher Course Syllabus.* Seattle: IASP Press, 2002.

10. JA Turner, JD Loeser, KG Bell. Spinal cord stimulation for chronic low back pain: a systematic literature synthesis. *Neurosurgery* 1995;**37**:1088–1095.

11. Wong GY, Schroeder DR, Carns PE, et al. Effect of neurolytic celiac plexus block on pain relief, quality of life, and survival in pancreatic cancer. *JAMA* 2004;**291**:1092–1099.

12. Hartrick C, Van-Hove I, Stegmann J, et al. Efficacy and tolerability of tapentadol immediate release and oxycodone immediate release in patients awaiting primary joint replacement. *Clin Ther* 2009;**31**:260–271.

13. Mercadante S. The use of anti-inflammatory drugs in cancer pain. *Cancer Treat Rev* 2001;**27**:51–61.

14. Farrar JT, Cleary J, Rauck R, Busch M, Nordbrock E. Oral transmucosal fentanyl citrate: randomized, double-blinded, placebo-controlled trial for treatment of breakthrough pain in cancer patients. *J Natl Cancer Inst* 1998;**90**:611–616.

15. Hocking G, Cousins MJ. Ketamine in chronic pain management: an evidence-based review. *Anesth Analg* 2003;**97**:1730–1739.

Opioids and opioid receptors

Raymond S. Sinatra

Introduction

Opioids are a class of central-acting analgesics that provide powerful dose-dependent relief of moderate to severe pain [1–3]. They include compounds with variable pharmacokinetics and pharmacodynamics, no cardiac or hepato-renal toxic effects, no ceiling effect for achievable pain relief, and are approved for oral, nasal, parenteral, transdermal, and neuraxial administration. Opioid analgesics include natural derivatives of opium such as morphine, substituted semisynthetics such as oxycodone and hydrocodone, complex synthetics including meperidine, fentanyl, and methadone, and endogenous ligands such as enkephalin (Figure 13.1) [1–3].

Morphine, named after Morpheus, the god of dreams, was isolated in the 1850s, and termed "God's own medicine" by Sydenham [1,2]. The use of morphine and intravenous syringes during the US Civil War (1860s) greatly improved pain management; however, misuse and overuse led to excessive rates of dependency and addiction. Fears of opioid addiction were responsible for the establishment of the US Narcotic Control Acts of the early 1900s which limited opioid distribution and use [1,4,5]. Over the last two decades, regulatory easements and greater medical acceptance have dramatically increased opioid dosing for patients suffering moderate to severe pain [4]. Nevertheless, because of highly publicized cases of diversion and abuse, the pendulum has started to swing back toward increasing restriction, as evidenced by high-profile court cases and FDA/DEA statements discouraging high-dose opioid prescriptions [5]. The benefits and liabilities of opioid analgesics are outlined in Table 13.1.

Opioid receptors

Opioids interact with specific transmembrane G protein-coupled binding sites termed opiate or opioid receptors. These receptors are located primarily in spinal dorsal horn, central gray, medial thalamus, amygdala, limbic cortex and other regions of the central nervous system (CNS) that process affective and suffering aspects of pain perception [1–3]. Conversely, opioid receptors are not concentrated in the somatosensory cortex or other regions responsible for pain localization [1–3,6]. Opioid receptors serve as binding sites for endogenous ligands including endorphin and the enkephalins, which naturally modulate pain transmission and perception [1,6]. Naturally occurring opiates and synthetic opioids have structural/chemical similarities that enable them to bind and activate opioid receptors resulting in powerful, dose-dependent, analgesia (Figure 13.2). Opioids provide highly selective analgesia in that they reduce or eliminate the suffering aspects of pain while preserving noxious localization [6,7]. Analgesic selectivity is also related to the fact that opioids block noxious sensation without affecting other forms of sensory perception such as light touch, pressure, and temperature [1,2,6].

Four principal opioid receptor subtypes, designated as mu, kappa, delta, and sigma, have been characterized [1,2]. A newer receptor classification system utilizes labels OPR_1, OPR_2 and OPR_3, which correspond to mu, kappa, and delta receptors respectively [1,3,8]. Mu receptors (OPR_1) mediate supraspinal analgesia, as well as respiratory depression, nausea and vomiting, miosis and bowel hypomotility. Mu receptors also mediate euphoria and physical and psychological dependence, and are responsible for the increased release of prolactin and growth hormone [1,2].

Kappa receptors (OPR_2) are believed to mediate spinal analgesia, visceral analgesia, and sedation, but have minimal effect on respiration [1–3]. Peripheral kappa receptors have been identified in the GI tract, skin, muscle, and connective tissues, and provide analgesic, antineuropathic, and anti-inflammatory effects [1]. Kappa receptors localized in the kidney are associated with antidiuresis and oliguria [1,2]. Delta

73

The Essence of Analgesia and Analgesics, ed. Raymond S. Sinatra, Jonathan S. Jahr and J. Michael Watkins-Pitchford. Published by Cambridge University Press. © Cambridge University Press 2011.

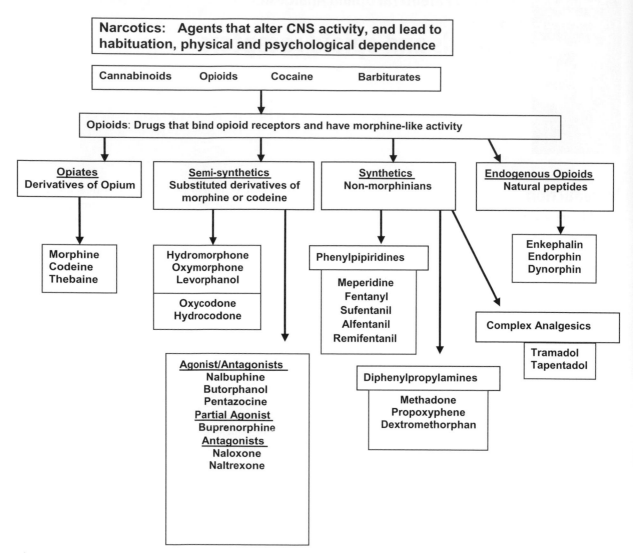

Figure 13.1. An overview of commonly administered opioid analgesics including naturally occurring, semisynthetic, synthetic, and endogenous compounds.

receptors (OPR_3) are not as well characterized but appear to facilitate mu receptor activity and enhance spinal and supraspinal analgesia. The primary ligand for delta receptors is enkephalin [1]. An additional, poorly characterized, receptor subtype designated the sigma-1 receptor is activated by pentazocine. Sigma-1 receptors are no longer considered true opioid receptors since ligand binding is not antagonized by naloxone and other opioid antagonists. Sigma-1 receptors are believed to mediate opioid-related dysphoria, hallucinations, and confusion.

Of all subtypes, the mu receptor has been most studied [1,2,8]. Mu receptors are located at pre- and postsynaptic contacts between nociceptive cells and function to limit release of noxious transmitters and reduce neuronal excitation. The mu receptor complex is activated following precise stereospecific attachment of agonist chemical groups, including a negatively charged hydroxyl group, the phenolic ring, and tertiary nitrogen to complementary regions on the extra-membrane binding site [1–3]. Receptor activation is followed by secondary activation of intracellular G proteins and an associated effector protein complex. Effector proteins inhibit adenylate cyclase and influence the activity of phosphokinases and other second messengers [9]. These alterations decrease cAMP, limit potassium and calcium ion flux, and hyperpolarize nociceptive cells (Figure 13.2) [1,9].

Table 13.1. Opioid analgesics

Benefits

1. Rapid onset of analgesia for moderate, severe and very severe pain

2. Highly effective analgesia (no analgesic dose ceiling)

3. Selective analgesia: reduction in pain suffering, minimal effects on pain localization

4. No effects on key organs: cardiac, renal, hepatic, and hemostatic safety

5. Multiple agents and routes of administration are available

6. Relatively inexpensive (morphine, oxycodone)

Drawbacks

1. Annoying adverse effects: nausea, pruritus, sedation, constipation

2. Clinically significant adverse effects: illeus, bowel obstruction, severe vomiting, confusion, dysphoria

3. Life-threatening effects: airway obstruction, respiratory depression, respiratory arrest

4. Social effects: dose escalation, physical dependence, diversion and abuse, addiction

5. May be expensive (sustained-release opioids, oral buccal preparations)

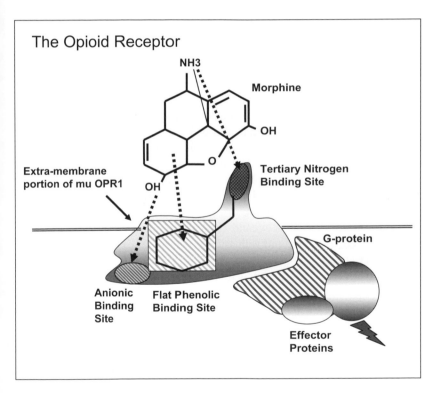

Figure 13.2. A schematic of the extramembranous portion of the mu opioid receptor and its interaction with morphine and associated effector proteins. Morphine and other opioid agonists attach to specific portions of the receptor including an anionic site, a flattened surface site which accepts the phenolic group, and a tertiary nitrogen attachment site. Attachment at the tertiary nitrogen binding site appears to be important for receptor activation and subsequent activation of the G protein. G proteins in turn activate other effector proteins within the complex that influence second messengers and neuronal ion flux. Opioid antagonists bind with high affinity to portions of the receptor; however, a bulky methyl or allyl group added to the tertiary nitrogen prevents receptor activation.

Opioid pharmacokinetics

Physiochemical and structural differences between opioid agonists can influence affinity and binding kinetics at mu receptors, as well as their ability to activate G proteins and other transducer molecules [1,3]. Receptor binding affinity influences agonist association/disassociation kinetics as well as pharmacological onset and duration of activity. The intrinsic efficacy of a given opioid agonist is related to its ability to activate coupled G proteins [1,3]. In general, potent opioids such as fentanyl and sufentanil have greater intrinsic efficacy at mu receptors than naturally occurring opiates such as morphine and codeine. In clinical settings, pharmacokinetic variables such as lipid solubility, degree of ionization and volume of distribution play key roles in determining agonist potency, onset of effect, and analgesic duration [1–3]. Analgesic onset is determined by the ability of an agonist to enter the CNS compartment and distribute into gray matter where receptors are primarily localized. Drugs that are highly lipophilic and un-ionized easily enter the CNS and have a very rapid onset of effect. In contrast, ionized hydrophilic opioids such as morphine have difficulty penetrating the blood–brain barrier (BBB) and have a delayed onset [1–3]. Opioid analgesic potency, or the amount of drug required to achieve an analgesic effect, is closely related to the octanol-water coefficient (lipophilicity vs. hydrophilicity) and intrinsic efficacy of the agonist. As a rule, highly lipophilic opioids have significantly greater potency than less lipophilic or hydrophilic agents [1,3].

Analgesic duration is related to several factors including receptor dissociation kinetics, redistribution, and elimination kinetics and volume of distribution. Lipophilic opioids including fentanyl and sufentanil have dose-related durations of activity. With low doses, duration is limited by rapid T1/2 alpha redistribution kinetics. With higher doses, duration correlates with T1/2 beta metabolism/elimination kinetics, which is dependent upon enterohepatic reuptake, hepatic blood flow and extraction, and protein binding. Since T1/2 beta kinetics are time- and enzyme-dependent, administration of higher doses can markedly extend analgesic duration [1–3]. Morphine and methadone have unique attributes that also affect analgesic duration. Morphine's hydrophilic properties slow BBB egress and favor its sequestration in the CSF. These factors prolong its duration despite declines in plasma morphine concentration. The formation of active metabolites (morphine-6-glucuronide) also tends to increase its duration of effect [1,3]. Methadone's large volume of distribution leads to accumulation and a progressive prolongation in analgesic duration with repeated doses. After achievement of steady state, drug sequestered in peripheral compartments is taken up by the vasculature and maintains minimal effective plasma concentrations [1].

Opioid tolerance and hyperalgesia

Continued patient exposure to opioid analgesics leads to tolerance development and clinical manifestations such as physical dependence. Tolerance is defined as the progressive increases in dose required to maintain a desired pharmacological effect, and is characterized by a shift to the right in the classic dose-response curve [1–3,9,10]. This physiological adaptation is observed in patients prescribed opioids for pain management, as well as those abusing this class of drug. Endocytosis of mu opioid receptors counteracts receptor desensitization and opioid tolerance by inducing fast reactivation and recycling. Opioid agonists have differing abilities to initiate endocytosis and regulate surface receptor concentrations [10]. Development of tolerance is delayed with opioids having high endocytotic efficacy; however, these compounds are associated with a more rapid onset of physical dependence [1,2].

Physical dependence is a normal and commonly observed phenomenon in opioid-tolerant patients. Upon abrupt discontinuation of opioids, the cAMP pathway is further up-regulated and parasympathetic tone is markedly increased [1,9]. Patients experience unpleasant, but rarely life-threatening, withdrawal symptoms termed "the abstinence syndrome", which includes sweating, shaking, cramping, and diarrhea.

Psychological dependence includes drug-seeking behavior and drug administration for purposes other than pain control. Addiction is a term describing an extreme form of psychological dependence where patients demonstrate impaired control, craving, compulsive use, and continued use despite harm. Although opioid addiction is driven primarily by psychological maladaptations, such behavior is also reinforced by physical dependence and fears of withdrawal [1–3,9]. Unlike physical dependence, opioid addiction is rarely observed in patients suffering moderate to severe acute pain.

A second clinical alteration observed in patients treated with opioids is termed "opioid induced hyperalgesia" [11]. This phenomenon is characterized by paradoxical increases in pain intensity (hyperesthesia), the development of new pain complaints, and alterations in pain characteristics (allodynia) in response to continued administration or increased dosing of opioid analgesics.

Opioid-induced hyperalgesia (OIH) is most often observed in tolerant patients, but has also been observed in naive individuals exposed to rapid-acting short-duration opioids including remifentanil and alfentanil. Mechanisms responsible for opioid-induced analgesia are not completely understood; however, glutamate-induced activation of NMDA receptors and upregulation of cholecystokinin (CCK) and dynorphin, which have anti-analgesic excitatory effects, have been proposed [1,11]. Excitatory effects of opioid metabolites (morphine-3-glucuronide, hydromorphone-3-glucuronide) may also play a role in the development and progression of OIH.

Historically, it was believed that patient responses to opioid agonists were similar; nevertheless, measurable inter-individual variability in efficacy, tolerability, and incomplete cross-tolerance are commonly observed. In recent years, opioid receptor pharmaco-genomic research has uncovered significant mu receptor polymorphisms with over 20 different genetic variants detected [1,8,12]. Differences in mu opioid receptor gene (ORM1) expression do not affect ligand binding kinetics at the extracellular membranous portion of the receptor, but appear to influence subsequent activation of associated proteins and second messengers [1,8,12]. Genetic variability of the catechol-O-methyltransferase (COMT) gene also influences morphine dose requirements. Finally, polymorphisms of the transporter P-glycoprotein (ABCB1) system also influence opioid clearance from cerebrospinal fluid [1].

Opioid classification

According to their binding affinities and intrinsic activity at receptor subtypes, opioids are classified as either agonists, partial agonists, mixed agonist–antagonists or complete antagonists [1–3]. Opioid agonists include compounds such as morphine, hydromorphone or fentanyl that bind receptors with moderate to high affinity, activate G proteins and are capable of producing a maximal response following receptor activation. Partial agonists such as buprenorphine bind mu receptors with higher affinity than morphine but activate the receptor and associated G proteins incompletely. The analgesic efficacy curve of partial agonists is bell-shaped, such that low doses provide increasing levels of analgesia to a point after which additional doses either do not increase pain relief or slightly diminish it [1,2].

Agonist–antagonist-type opioids include butorphanol and nalbuphine. These compounds bind mu and kappa receptor subtypes but differ in activation efficacy. Generally they behave as agonists at kappa receptors and antagonists at mu. At low doses, the analgesic properties of mixed agonist–antagonists are comparable to those of weak agonists, such as propoxyphene and codeine; however, at higher doses no additional analgesia is achieved [1–3]. This phenomenon, termed "the analgesic ceiling effect", restricts their use to patients with mild to moderate pain.

Antagonists such as naloxone and naltrexone bind to all receptor subtypes with high affinity but do not activate the receptor and G proteins. Antagonists competitively block the activity of agonists by preventing or displacing their binding to the receptor. Although antagonists provide no direct analgesic effects, when administered in low doses they may alter receptor conformation and increase the intrinsic efficacy of opioid agonists [1,2]. Dose-response curves for opioid agonists, mixed agonists and antagonists are presented in Figure 13.3.

Parenteral opioid therapy

Since oral analgesics generally have low bioavailability, delayed onset, and are poorly tolerated during the immediate post-operative period, parenterally (IV) administered opioids are commonly prescribed for pain management. There are several situations where parenteral opioids are employed. (1) They are useful for patients advancing from IV-PCA or

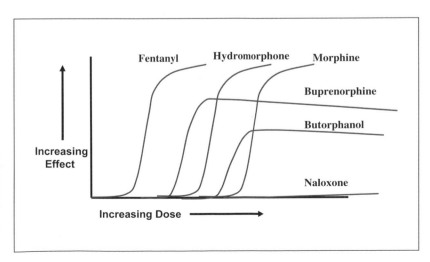

Figure 13.3. Dose-response curves of commonly employed agonists, partial agonists, mixed agonist–antagonists, and antagonists. Pure agonists are able to achieve maximum effect; however, dose requirements are dependent upon potency. Mixed agonist–antagonists and partial agonists may have higher potency than agonists at low doses; however, analgesic efficacy is limited and maximum effect is not achieved. Antagonists have high affinity and can competitively displace agonists; however, they have no efficacy.

epidural opioid-based analgesia, who have moderate to severe discomfort, but have yet to tolerate oral diets. Parenteral dosing is of particular importance in patients who are nauseous or vomiting, who might not absorb oral agents. (2) Several subsets of patients including the elderly, the cognitively impaired and overly dependent individuals are poor candidates for IV-PCA and may achieve better pain control with intravenous/intramuscular opioids administered by the clock or PRN. In these individuals, parenteral opioid requirements during early post-operative intervals may be used to provide a conversion guide for oral analgesic dosing that follows. Opioid-dependent patients with significant tolerance development may require both IV-PCA or parenteral opioid infusions for baseline pain management, in addition to epidural or regional blockade for surgical pain.

Morphine remains the standard parenteral opioid analgesic for control of acute pain following surgical and traumatic injuries [1,2]. Ten milligrams of parenteral morphine is generally recommended as a starting dose for acute pain management in patients over 50 kg. Onset of analgesia with IV morphine is noted within 5–15 minutes while its duration ranges from 1–3 hours depending upon dose administered. Hydromorphone, oxymorphone, and, to a lesser extent, meperidine offer therapeutic alternatives for patients experiencing inadequate pain control with morphine or intolerant of its adverse effects. In post-operative settings, hydromorphone offers a more rapid onset, higher analgesic potency and greater tolerability than morphine [13]. Oxymorphone has been available for over 40 years and is currently marketed as a 1 mg vial for acute pain management. Oxymorphone's onset to peak effect is more rapid than morphine's and its overall analgesic efficacy is superior [14]. IV oxymorphone may be effectively employed in the PACU for patients experiencing very severe pain. Parenteral doses of methadone are also advocated for patients with opioid tolerance and others suffering severe acute pain that is poorly responsive or unresponsive to morphine and hydromorphone [15]. Methadone may be employed in low doses as an adjuvant or as primary therapy [15,16].

Fentanyl is best administered in patients with marked hemodynamic instability or well-documented allergies to naturally occurring or semisynthetic morphinians [1–3,17]. The quality of analgesia provided by IV fentanyl infusions is excellent and equivalent to comparable doses administered epidurally, but with less pruritus [17]. The analgesic effectiveness of parenteral opioids may be potentiated with small doses of anticholinergic/antihistaminics such as phenergan and vistaril; however, increased levels of sedation should be expected [1,2,3]. Other complications associated with parenteral opioids include respiratory depression, nausea and vomiting, pruritus and bowel dysfunction.

Oral analgesic dosing

Once patients are able to tolerate a liquid diet they may be advanced to oral opioids, which should be continued during the convalescent and rehabilitative periods following surgery. Oral administration offers a safe, convenient, non-invasive and cost-effective method of controlling acute pain that should always be considered in patients who continue to experience moderate to severe pain.

Oral opioids including morphine, meperidine, hydrocodone, and oxycodone and compounded preparations containing acetaminophen, aspirin, and ibuprofen provide effective relief for patients complaining of moderate to severe pain. Orally administered morphine and meperidine are poorly absorbed and undergo significant entero-hepatic metabolism [1,2]. When compared to parenteral dosing, onset is delayed, duration is less predictable and dose requirements are increased. In this regard equianalgesic oral morphine and meperidine doses are 2–3 times higher than parenteral requirements. Oxycodone is more reliably absorbed than morphine. Following oral administration, both oxycodone and hydrocodone have a rapid and predicable onset at 35 min, a peak effect at 60 min, and duration of 3.5–4 h [1,18,19].

Sustained-release opioid preparations including morphine (MS-Contin®) and oxycodone (Oxycontin®) and oxymorphone (Opana® ER) offer several advantages including less frequent administration intervals, avoidance of peak and trough plasma levels and greater analgesic uniformity. These preparations provide 8–12 hours of pain relief and are best suited for patients suffering chronic pain and prolonged post-operative pain [1,2,20].

An additional opioid preparation that may be considered for patients who cannot tolerate oral analgesics but continue to experience brief episodes of severe pain is the fentanyl oralet (Actiq®). Fentanyl oralet releases between 100–400 µg of fentanyl within 15 minutes with high bioavailability. While not approved for acute pain management, this preparation is effective when given 20–30 minutes prior to short painful procedures such as closed reduction, dressing changes, or chest tube placement [21].

Less potent opioid analgesics such as tramadol and codeine may be prescribed to patients recovering from dental and ENT surgeries and medical procedures associated with mild to moderate pain [22]. A compounded form of tramadol (Ultracet®) provides greater effectiveness than tramadol alone. Ultracet is an oral multimodal analgesic containing tramadol plus acetaminophen, approved for the short-term management of acute pain. A newly released "dual acting" analgesic, tapentadol (Nucynta), activates mu opioid receptors and also inhibits norepinephrine reuptake. Its analgesic efficacy is equivalent to oxycodone; however, it has a better tolerability profile, causing less nausea, vomiting, constipation and pruritus [23].

Short-acting oral opioids agents such as morphine immediate release (IR), hydrocodone IR, hydromorphone IR, oxycodone IR, and oxymorphone IR may be favored initially because they are easy to titrate [24]. These agents are best employed in opioid-naive patients, recovering from uncomplicated procedures that require relatively limited durations of treatment. Following extensive surgery with severe discomfort and prolonged and painful convalescence, sustained-release opioids may be considered. Short-acting opioids are characterized by a rapid rise and fall in serum opioid levels, whereas serum levels of sustained-release opioids increase slowly to therapeutic levels, remain there for an extended period, and then decline slowly [25]. (Opioid analgesics and dosing recommendations are summarized in Table 13.2.)

Table 13.2. Dosing guidelines for oral and parenteral opioids

Opioid	Route	Dose (mg)	Onset	Duration	Comments
Morphine	(PO)	(15–45)	45 min	4–5 h	Poor oral effect
Morphine	(IV)	(5–15)	10 min	3.5–4 h	Histamine release
Meperidine	(PO)	(1–300)	45 min	3.5 h	Toxic metabolite
Meperidine	(IV)	(75–125)	10 min	3 h	Useful for visceral pain
Hydrocodone	(PO)	(7.5–15)	35 min	4–6 h	Similar to oxycodone
Oxycodone	(PO)	(5–15)	30 min	4–6 h	Good oral analgesic
Codeine	(PO)	(30–70)	45 min	3.5 h	High side-effect profile
Methadone	(PO)	(7.5–15)	10–20 min	6–8 h	Prolonged elimination
Methadone	(IV)	(5–7.5)	5–10 min	6–8 h	Difficult to titrate
Hydromorphone	(PO)	(7.5–15)	35 min	4–6 h	Well tolerated
Hydromorphone	(IV)	(1–3)	10–15 min 3.5–4 h	3.5–4 h	Useful for severe pain
Oxymorphone	(PO)	(5–15)	30 min	4–6 h	Poor oral bioavailability
Oxymorphone	(IV)	(0.5–2)	5–10 min	4 h	Useful for severe pain
Fentanyl	(PO)	(2–400 µg)	5–10 min	60 min	Rapid onset
Fentanyl	(IV)	(1–150 µg)	3–5 min	30 min	Very rapid onset
Tramadol	(PO)	(1–200 mg)	40 min	4–6 h	For mild-moderate pain
Tapendadol	(PO)	(50–100 mg)	32 min 4–6 h	4–6 h	Dual-acting analgesic

Opioid-related adverse events

In settings of acute pain, most opioid-related adverse events are transient and tend to resolve with ongoing treatment [1–3,26]. Common adverse events associated with parenteral and orally administered opioids and their active metabolites include nausea, vomiting, sedation, pruritus and constipation [26]. In sensitive individuals the incidence and severity of these adverse events may be so annoying and distressing that patients self-limit or discontinue opioid dosing and suffer poor pain control. Patients recovering from abdominal and gynecological surgery are generally at risk of opioid-induced bowel dysfunction and ileus, mandating that such therapy be supplemented with stool softeners, bulk laxatives, and occasional enemas. Most opioid-related AEs are dose-dependent, which is why it is important to initiate therapy with the lowest effective dose and to utilize a multimodal analgesic approach. Some opioid-related AEs are often treated symptomatically, for example prescribing an antiemetic for nausea or laxatives and/or a peripheral mu antagonist for constipation [27]. Other side effects, such as sedation and pruritus, are typically addressed by decreasing the opioid dose rather than by treating the symptom. In addition to dose reductions, other strategies that can be employed to minimize opioid-related AEs include changing the route of administration, switching to a different opioid or providing multimodal pharmacological therapy [28].

Future directions with oral and parenteral opioids for acute pain

In the near future improved and more selective opioid analgesics may be developed that better suit individual patient needs [29]. Rapidly disintegrating and readily absorbed lingual and buccal preparations avoid gastric absorption and first-pass hepatic and offer advantages of convenience and rapid analgesic onset. While originally developed for breakthrough chronic pain these routes of delivery may become available for acute pain management. Nasal and pulmonary delivered opioid preparations offer similar advantages as well as convenience, and may displace the need for IV dosing and possibly IV-PCA in patients who remain NPO [30]. The use of the active and better-tolerated morphine metabolite, morphine-6-glucuronide, may become available as an alternative to morphine [31]. Kappa agonists are being developed that can activate peripheral receptors yet do not penetrate the blood–brain barrier. These selective peripheral agonists provide analgesia without central effects such as excessive sedation, euphoria, and respiratory depression. They offer the promise of effective relief of visceral pain (Ob-GYN, GU-renal colic), with low risk of mu-mediated respiratory depression.

Opioids with lower risk of diversion and abuse

Opioids formulated in crush-resistant, water-insoluble tablets may provide a lower risk for diversion, adulteration, and abuse (snorting, injecting). Tablets containing mixtures of an agonist plus an antagonist that is released if the tablet is adulterated are also being studied.

References

1. Gutstein HB, Akil H. Opioid analgesics. In Hardman JG, Limbird LE, Gilman AG, eds. *Goodman & Gilman's The Pharmacological Basis of Therapeutics*, 10th ed. New York: McGraw-Hill, 2002, pp. 569–619.

2. Way WL, Fields HL, Schumaker MA. Opioid analgesics. In Katsung BG, ed. *Basic & Clinical Pharmacology*, 9th ed. Lange Medical Books/McGraw-Hill, 2004.

3. Pasero C, Portenoy RK, McCaffery M. Opioid analgesics. In McCaffery M, Pasero C, eds. *Pain Clinical Manual*. St. Louis, MO: Mosby, 1999, pp. 161–299.

4. Joint Commission on Accreditation of Healthcare Organizations. JCAHO Standards for Pain Management [referenced from the Comprehensive Accreditation Manual for Hospitals, Update 3, 1999 (effective January 1, 2001)]. Available at: http://www.texmed.org/has/prs/pop/jps.asp.

5. Gilson AM, Joranson DE. U.S. policies relevant to the prescribing of opioid analgesics for the treatment of pain in in patients with addictive disease. *Clin J Pain* 2002;**18**:S91–98.

6. Bonica JJ. Biochemistry and modulation of nociception and pain. In Bonica JJ, ed. *The Management of Pain*, 2nd ed. Philadelphia: Lea and Febiger, 1990, pp. 94–121.

7. Beecher H. Pain in men wounded in battle. *Ann Surg* 1946;**123**:96–105.

8. Pan YX, Xu J, Bolan E, Moskowitz HS Pasternak GW. Identification of four novel exon 5 splice variants of the mouse mu opioid receptor gene. *Mol Pharmacol Fast Forward* 2005; **68**:866–875.

9. Nestler EJ, Aghajanian GK: Molecular and cellular basis of addiction. *Science* 1997;**278**:58–63.

10. Zastrow M, Svingos A, Haberstock H, et al. Regulatory endocytosis of opioid receptors: cellular mechanisms and proposed role in physiological adaptation to opiate drugs. *Curr Opin Neurobiol* 2003;**13**:348–353.

11. Angst MS, Clark JD. Opioid-induced hyperalgesia: a qualitative systematic review. *Anesthesiology* 2006;**104**:570–587.

12. Ross JR, et al. *Pharmacogenetics J* 2005;**5**:324–336. *Goodman & Gilman's Pharmacology*, 11th ed. New York: McGraw-Hill, 2006.

13. Mahler DL, Forrest WH. Relative analgesic potencies of morphine and hydromorphone in post-operative pain. *Anesthesiology* 1975;**42**:602–607.

14. Sinatra RS, Harrison DM, Hyde N. Oxymorphone revisited. *Semin Anesthesiol* 1988;**7**:209–215.

15. Peng PW, Sandler AN. Fentanyl for post-operative analgesia: a review. *Anesthesiology* 1999;**90**:576–599.

16. Marco CA, Plewa MC, Buderer N, Black C, Roberts A. Comparison of oxycodone and hydrocodone for the treatment of acute pain associated with fractures: a double-blind, randomized, controlled trial. *Acad Emerg Med* 2005;**12**:282–288.

17. Stambaugh JE, Reder RF, Stambaugh MD, Stambaugh H, Davis M. Double-blind, randomized comparison of the analgesic and pharmacokinetic profiles of controlled- and immediate-release oral oxycodone in cancer pain patients. *J Clin Pharmacol* 2001;**41**:500–6.

18. Opana ER(R) (Oxymorphone extended-release capsules, Endo Pharmaceuticals Incorporated, Chadds Ford, Pennsylvania). Full prescribing information, 2005.

19. Mitra S, Sinatra RS. Perioperative management of acute pain in the opioid-dependent patient. *Anesthesiology* 2004;**101**:212–227.

20. Shir Y, Rosen G, Zeiden A, Davidson M. Methadone is safe for treating hospitalized patients. *Canad J Anesthesia* 2001;**48**:1109–1113.

21. Sinatra RS. Treatment guidelines and unpublished observations. Yale University Pain Management Service, 2007.

22. Sinatra RS, Sramcik J. Tramadol: its use in pain management. In Hines RL, ed. *Anesthesiology Clinics of North America,* vol. 2. Philadelphia: W.B. Saunders, 1998, pp. 53–69.

23. Hartrick C, Van-Hove I, Stegmann J, et al. Efficacy and tolerability of tapentadol immediate release and oxycodone immediate release in patients awaiting primary joint replacement. *Clin Ther* 2009;**31**: 260–271.

24. Ginsberg B, Sinatra RS, Adler LJ, Crews JC, Hord AH, Laurito CE, Ashburn MA. Conversion to oral controlled-release oxycodone from intravenous opioid analgesic in the post-operative setting. *Pain Med* 2003;**4**(1):31–38.

25. McCarberg BH, Barkin RL. Long-acting opioids for chronic pain: pharmacotherapeutic opportunities to enhance compliance, quality of life, and analgesia. *Am J Ther* 2001;**8**:181–186.

26. Wheeler M, Oderda GM, Asburn MA, Lipman AG. Adverse events associated with post-operative opioid analgesia: a systematic review. *J Pain* 2002;**3**:159–180.

27. Thomas J, Karver S, Austin Cooney G, et al. Methylnaltrexone for opioid-induced constipation in advanced illness. *NEJM* 2008;**358**:2332–2343.

28. Marret E, Kurdi O, Zufferey P, Bonnet F. Effects of nonsteroidal antiinflammatory drugs on patient-controlled analgesia morphine side effects: meta-analysis of randomized controlled trials. *Anesthesiology* 2005;**102**:1249–60.

29. National Institutes of Health. *The NIH Guide: New Directions in Pain Research I.* Washington DC: U.S. Government Printing Office, 1998.

30. Mather LE, Woodhouse A, Ward ME, Farr SJ. Pulmonary administration of aerosolised fentanyl: Pharmacokinetic analysis. *Br J Anaesth* 1998; **46**:37–43.

31. Romberg R, van Dorp E, Hollander J, et al. A randomized double-blind placebo-controlled pilot study of morphine-6-glucoronide for post-operative pain relief after knee replacement surgery. *Clin J Pain* 2007;**23**:197–203.

14

Morphine – oral and parenteral

Joseph Rosa and Swati Patel

Generic Names: morphine, morphine sulfate

Trade/Proprietary Names: oral – Morphine Sulfate Immediate Release Tablets™, Morphine Sulfate Oral Solution™, OMS Concentrate, Roxanol™ Concentrated Oral Solution, Oramorph™; parenteral – Min-I-Jet-Morphine Sulfate Injection™, Morphine Sulfate Add-Vantage™, Select-A-Jet Morphine Sulfate Injection™, Infumorph™

Drug Class: opioid analgesic

Manufacturers: Purdue Pharma, One Stamford Forum, Stamford, CT; Roxane Laboratories, 1809 Wilson Rd, Columbus, OH; Baxter Healthcare, One Baxter Parkway, Deerfield, IL; Richwood-Shire Pharmaceuticals, 5 Riverwalk, Citywest Business Campus, Dublin 24, Ireland

Chemical Structure: see Figure 14.1

Chemical Name: 7,8-didehydro-4,5-∂-epoxy-17-methylmorphinan-3,6-∂-diol sulfate

Introduction

Morphine is the principal alkaloid of opium, and remains the standard of comparison, and the most widely employed opioid agonist worldwide for acute and chronic pain management. It is available in a variety of dosing formulations; however, its major sites of administration are via oral and parenteral routes.

Major and minor sites of action

As the principal opiate analgesic, morphine exerts its pharmacological effects on the central nervous system and the gastrointestinal tract with its primary actions of therapeutic value being analgesia and sedation. Clinically it has moderate analgesic potency, a slow onset to peak effect, and an intermediate duration of activity. Morphine is a hydrophilic drug that has difficulty penetrating the blood–brain barrier and

reaching sites of activity in the brain and spinal cord. Morphine's analgesic effects involve at least three anatomical areas of the CNS: the periaquaductal gray matter, the ventromedial medulla and spinal cord. Morphine is a mixed agonist that binds to and activates mu, kappa and delta receptor subtypes [1]:

- µ – moderates supraspinal analgesia and respiratory depression
- κ – modulates spinal analgesia and sedation
- σ – associated with dysphoria, hallucinations, and respiratory and vasomotor stimulation

Receptor interactions

Morphine interacts primarily with the mu (µ) receptor. The mu receptor binding sites of morphine are very discretely distributed in the brain with high densities in the posterior amygdala, hypothalamus, thalamus, caudate nucleus, and putamen [1,2]. The mu receptors are also found on the terminal axons of primary afferents within the laminae I and II (substantia gelatinosa) of the spinal cord and in the spinal nucleus of the trigeminal (fifth cranial) nerve. Morphine appears to increase the patient's tolerance of pain and decreases the perception of suffering. It also causes mood alterations including euphoria, dysphoria, drowsiness, and mental clouding. Morphine depresses various respiratory centers, depresses the cough reflex, and causes miosis. It may cause nausea and vomiting by stimulating the chemoreceptor trigger zone (CTZ). Gastrointestinal effects include increased tone and decreased propulsive power of smooth muscle of the GI tract, resulting in constipation and an increase in the tone of the biliary tract, potentially worsening biliary colic. It decreases pancreatic, biliary, and gastric secretions. Morphine increases the tone of the urinary tract smooth muscle, which may result in urinary retention and may reduce urine formation by increasing the release of ADH (antidiuretic hormone). Morphine may result in histamine release to varying

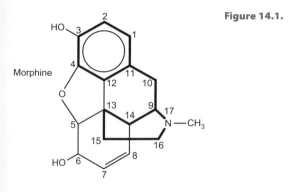

Figure 14.1.

Morphine

degrees and may, in some patients, cause orthostatic hypotension.

Metabolic pathways, drug clearance and elimination

After parenteral administration the typical $t_{1/2}$ for morphine is 2.1–2.6 hours. Metabolism occurs in the liver via conjunction with glucuronic acid and the majority of this morphine 3-glucuronide compound is excreted in the urine by glomerular filtration. Approximately 90% of excretion occurs within 24 hours of the last dose, with 7–10% being excreted in the feces, the largest portion of which is through the biliary system, as conjugated morphine [1–3]. The onset of analgesia after SQ or IM administration is 10–30 min, with a peak effect after SQ of 50–90 min, after IM of 30–60 min, and after IV of approximately 20 min. Duration of analgesia is 3–6 h. Morphine is relatively ineffective in the injection form taken orally as it undergoes extensive first-pass by the intestinal mucosa and liver.

Indications

Surgical acute pain: oral and parenteral doses of morphine are used commonly for the relief of moderate to severe post-operative surgical pain.

Medical pain: morphine is the drug of choice for the relief of pain due to myocardial infarction. Relief of ischemic pain decreases sympathetic nervous system activity thus reducing myocardial oxygen demand. Morphine is used in patients with acute pulmonary edema for its cardiovascular effects and to decrease air hunger. Morphine can be used to treat the pain of sickle cell disease with crisis. Morphine can be used to treat the pain of Guillain-Barré syndrome, osteoarthritis and obstetric pain. Morphine's sedative effects can be utilized in the intubated and ventilated patient.

Chronic non-malignancy pain: morphine can be used for moderate to severe chronic pain especially in terminally ill patients.

Cancer pain: morphine can be used for the treatment of moderate to severe cancer pain.

Somatic visceral and neuropathic pain: morphine can be useful in the treatment of pain that has a somatic visceral or neuropathic component or origin.

Contraindications

Absolute: known hypersensitivity to morphine

Relative: asthma, hypercarbia, paralytic ileus, respiratory depression, heart failure secondary to chronic lung disease, cardiac arrhythmia, intracranial mass associated with increased intracranial pressure, acute alcoholism, delirium tremens, obstructive sleep apnea.

Common doses

Oral: the usual adult dosage of morphine is 10–30 mg as conventional tablets, capsules or solutions. Dosages should be adjusted with sustained- or extended-release proportions accordingly. It is suggested to initiate oral morphine therapy with an immediate-release proportion as titration is more easily achieved. The patient can then be switched to an extended- or sustained-release proportion. The initial dosage of the extended- or sustained-release proportion should be based on the total immediate-release dosage.

Parenteral: the usual adult subcutaneous (SQ) or intramuscular (IM) dose of morphine sulfate is 10 mg every 4 hours as necessary; dosage may range from 5 to 20 mg every 4 hours as needed depending on patient response and requirement. The IV dosage is 2.5–15 mg injected IV slowly every 4–5 minutes in adults. SQ or IM dose in children is 0.1–0.2 mg/kg every 4 hours as needed. IV dosage of 0.05–0.1 mg/kg may be given slowly in children. In patients with acute MI morphine may be given to relieve anxiety and pain associated with myocardial ischemia. Dosages of 2–15 mg can be administered parentally and repeated as needed. When morphine sulfate is administered via patient-controlled analgesia (PCA) dosage should be adjusted according to the severity of the pain and the patient's response. When morphine is administered by continuous infusion for relief of severe, chronic pain associated with primary or metastatic cancer the dose (individualized according to response and tolerance of the patient) should be started at 0.8–10 mg/h. Dosing guidelines for morphine are presented in Table 14.1.

83

Table 14.1.

Indication	Route					
	Adult dose			Pediatric dose		
	Oral[a]	Parenteral[b]		Oral	Parenteral	
		IM/SQ	IV		IM/SQ	IV
Standard/ post-operative pain	10–30 mg immediate release (IR)	5–20 mg q4h	2–15 mg q5min	Safety and efficacy of extended release oral formulation not studied in pts under 18 yrs of age	0.1–0.2 mg/kg q4h	0.05–0.1 mg/ kg q3h
Acute MI			2–10 mg slowly			
Cancer pain	10–30 mg q4h (IR)	2–20 q4h	2–10 mg		0.1–0.2 mg/kg q4h	0.05–0.1 mg/kg
	30 mg q24h (extended release Avinza)					
Mechanically ventilated, sedation			0.07–0.5 mg/kg per h			0.01–0.03 mg/kg per h
			0.01–0.15 mg/kg q1–2h			

[a]Conversion from oral to parenteral morphine sulfate: the estimated daily requirement is one-third of the total daily oral requirement; with the starting dose at 1/2 the calculated dose.
[b]Conversion from parenteral to oral morphine sulfate: three times the estimated total daily parenteral requirement may be sufficient in chronic use settings.
Dose adjustments:
Renal impairment: moderate failure (GFR 10–50 mL/min), 75% of normal dose; severe failure (GFR less than 10 mL/min) 50% of normal.
Liver impairment: alter dose in cirrhotic patients.
Neonates: increase dosing frequency to every 4–6 h.

Potential advantages

Ease of use: morphine and all the other injectable opioids are very easy to use. One major advantage of morphine that leads to its ease of use is the multiple routes of administration (IV, IM, SQ, IT epidural, intraventricular, rectal, oral, and inhalational). Morphine can easily be titrated to sedation levels, pain scores, and respiratory rate.

Tolerability: morphine and all the other injectable opioids are well tolerated in most patients. There are some exceptions to be discussed.

Cost: morphine as a generic drug is very inexpensive.

Monotherapy: morphine is commonly used as the sole analgesic agent.

Potential disadvantages

Toxicity: morphine is not known to have mutagenic or carcinogenic potential at non-narcotic doses in animals. However, mutagenicity and carcinogenicity have not been established in humans.

Pregnancy, fertility and lactation

Pregnancy: there are no adequate controlled studies to date in humans regarding the effects of morphine in pregnancy. Morphine should only be used when the benefits to the mother and fetus outweigh the risks.

Fertility: morphine is not known to impair fertility at non-narcotic doses in animals; however, the effects of morphine on human fertility have not been established.

Lactation: morphine should be used with caution in nursing women since the drug has been reported to distribute into milk.

Drug interaction

Morphine should be administered cautiously and in reduced dosages when other CNS depressants are used, including other narcotic analgesics, barbiturates, benzodiazepines, antihistamines, phenothiazines, TCAs, tranquilizers, major or minor, or in the presence of alcohol. Morphine sulfate may compete with other drugs such as cimetidine, mephenesin, meprebamate, and clanrolene for hepatic glucuronidation. The concomitant use of centrally acting muscle relaxants and opioid analgesics can cause exacerbations in respiratory depression, hypotension, and profound sedation. Concomitant use of morphine and esmolol has been reported to result in increased esmolol serum levels.

Multimodal analgesia

Morphine can be used in combination with other opioids to decrease the dose of morphine or with other non-opioids for an opioid-sparing effect and, depending on the agent, an additive or synergistic effect is seen. Opioid-sparing drugs include NSAIDs, TCAs, sedative-hypnotics, analytics and agents such as neurontin. Some believe that cross-tolerance between morphine and hydromorphone is incomplete, making alternating morphine and hydromorphone in rotation beneficial.

Drug-related adverse events and common side effects

Cardiovascular: <5% incidence of each of the following: bradyarrhythmia, cardiac arrest secondary to respiratory or cardiac depression hypertension, hypotension (probably secondary to histamine release). Morphine is noted to have the greatest potential for histamine release compared with other opioids, possibly leading to a <5% chance of orthostatic hypotension, circulatory depression, palpitations, shock, syncope, and tachycardia and a 5–10% chance of peripheral edema.

Dermatological: pruritus (up to 80% incidence is primarily seen with neuraxial injection), 5–10% incidence of rash, sweating, and urticaria. Recurrent herpes simplex virus I or II reactivation may be seen with neuraxial delivery.

Endocrine, Metabolic: alterations in thermoregulation and hypogonadism.

Gastrointestinal: abdominal pain <5–10%, biliary colic <5%, constipation <10%, diarrhea 5–10%, feed-ing problems primarily in preterm infants. Loss of appetite 5–10%, nausea and vomiting 7–70%, xerostomia 5–10%.

Neurological effects: asthenia 5–10%, confusion <5%, dizziness 6%, headache 10%, insomnia 5–10%, lightheadedness, myoclonus, parasthesia 5–10%, somnolence >10%, CNS excitation, and Meniere's disease. Seizures may be associated with high doses. Use with extreme caution in patients with increased ICP as a further increase may occur.

Psychological effects: anxiety <6%, delirium, depression, dysphoria, euphoria, hallucinations, auditory and visual, psychosis.

Renal effects: nephrotoxicity, urinary retention 5–10%.

Reproductive effects: sexual dysfunction; prolonged use can result in repression of male secondary sexual characteristics, and disruption of ovulation, amenorrhea and depression of lactation.

Respiratory effects: cough suppression; may suppress productive cough leading to pneumonia, dyspnea 5%, irregular breathing, and pulmonary edema. Respiratory depression with timing dependent upon route of administration (neuroaxial, epidural 5–12 hours; intrathecal 4–11 hours; IV, SQ 90 min; IM, 30 min; IV, 10 min).

Treatment of adverse events

Naloxone is the drug of choice for reversal of respiratory depression.

Nausea and vomiting can be treated with ondansetron, metoclopramide, droperidol, steroids, etc.

Pruritus from histamine release may be treated with benadryl or other antihistamines. Can also be treated with low-dose nalaxone (0.2 mg) or low-dose propofol (10 mg).

References

1. AHFS Drug Information, 2009.
2. *Goodman and Gilman's The Pharmacological Basis of Therapeutics*, 11th ed. New York: McGraw Hill, 2006.
3. Drugedex Evaluations.
4. Baxter Package Insert Doc, 2003.

Oral and Parenteral Opioid Analgesics

Morphine sulfate controlled-release

Parisa Partownavid

Generic Names: morphine sulfate controlled-release tablet; morphine sulfate extended-release capsule

Trade/Proprietary Names: MS Contin®, Avinza®, Kadian®

Drug Class: opioid analgesic, Schedule 2

Manufacturers: Purdue Pharma, One Stamford Forum, Stamford, CT; King Pharmaceuticals, Inc., Bristol, TN; Alpharma Pharmaceuticals LLC, One New England Avenue, Piscataway, NJ 08854

Chemical Structure: MS Contin and Kadian, see Figure 15.1; Avinza, see Figure 15.2

Introduction

Of the commonly used opioids, morphine remains the gold standard for the treatment of severe pain. Extended-release morphine is available in tablet and capsule formulations. One of the first controlled-release systems for the oral administration of morphine is MS Contin tablet, which is a combination matrix consisting of a hydrophilic granular system inserted in a hydrophobic matrix. Upon ingestion, gastric fluid dissolves the tablet surface and hydrates the hydrophilic polymer to produce a gel layer through which morphine is released at a rate determined by the type of hydrophilic polymer, hydrophobic matrix or their ratio. Various dosage strengths require different ratios of polymers to ensure dose proportionally.

Capsule formulations contain pellets or beads consisting of an inert core, surrounded by a morphine layer and a polymer coat. Following administration, fluid in the gastrointestinal tract diffuses through the polymer coat to release the morphine. The nature of the inert core and the thickness of the polymer coat control the rate of dissolution of morphine while transiting through the gastrointestinal tract in a pH-dependent fashion.

One capsule formulation, Avinza, contains both immediate-release and extended-release beads of morphine for once-daily oral administration. Upon ingestion, 10% of the beads release their morphine content immediately while the residual beads gradually release their morphine content over the next 24 hours. Another capsule formulation is Kadian, which is indicated for every 12 hours or 24 hours dosing. Unlike Avinza it does not contain immediate-release morphine.

Mode of activity

Morphine is a naturally occurring alkaloid from the opium poppy seed. Modern formulations employ synthetic morphine. Major and minor sites of morphine activity include spinal and supraspinal opioid receptors. Morphine binds to and activates mu, kappa and delta receptor subtypes.

Receptor interactions: morphine is a pure opioid agonist at mu, and is a weak agonist for kappa.

Metabolic pathway

Absorption: morphine is released from MS Contin and Kadian somewhat more slowly than from Avinza and immediate-release oral preparations. Following oral administration of a given dose of morphine, the amount ultimately absorbed is essentially the same whether the source is controlled-release or an immediate-release formulation. Because of pre-systemic elimination (i.e. metabolism in the gut wall and liver) only about 40% of the administered dose reaches the central compartment. Following the administration of immediate-release oral morphine products, approximately 50% of the absorbed morphine reaches the systemic circulation within 30 minutes. However, following the administration of MS Contin or Avinza, this extent of absorption occurs after 1.5 hours, and with Kadian on average after 8 hours

Metabolism: most of the metabolism of the opioids occurs in the liver. Although a small fraction (less

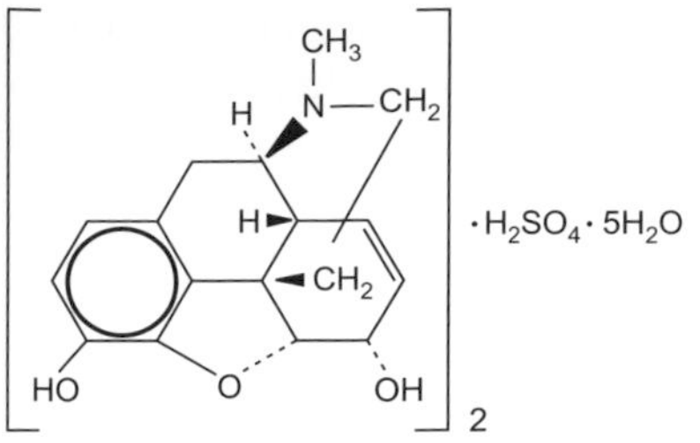

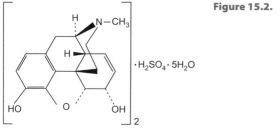

Figure 15.1.

Figure 15.2.

than 5%) of morphine is demethylated, virtually all morphine is converted to glucuronide metabolites including morphine-3-glucuronide, M3G (about 50%) and morphine-6-glucuronide, M6G (about 5 to 15%). M3G has no significant analgesic activity. M6G has been shown to have opioid agonist and analgesic activity in humans.

Excretion: approximately 10% of morphine dose is excreted unchanged in the urine. Most of the dose is excreted in the urine as M3G and M6G. A small amount of the glucuronide metabolites is excreted in the bile and there is some minor enterohepatic cycling. Seven to 10% of administered morphine is excreted in the feces.

As with any drug, caution should be taken to guard against unanticipated accumulation if renal and/or hepatic function is seriously impaired.

Indications (approved/non-approved)

Controlled-release oral formulation of morphine sulfate is indicated for the management of moderate to severe pain when a continuous, around-the-clock opioid analgesic is needed for an extended period of time. These formulations are not intended for use as a PRN analgesic.

Surgical acute pain: the only indication for postoperative use of the controlled-release oral formulation of morphine sulfate is if the patient is already receiving the drug prior to surgery or if the postoperative pain is expected to be moderate to severe and persist for an extended period of time.

Controlled-release oral formulation of morphine sulfate is not indicated for pain in the immediate postoperative period (the first 12–24 hours following surgery) in patients not previously taking the drug, because its safety in this setting has not been established.

Controlled-release oral formulation of morphine sulfate is also not indicated for pain in the postoperative period if the pain is mild, or not expected to persist for an extended period of time.

Medical pain: controlled-release oral formulation of morphine sulfate is indicated for relief of moderate to severe pain in patients who require potent opioid analgesics over periods more than few days.

Chronic non-malignancy pain: controlled-release oral formulation of morphine sulfate could be administered in a more convenient schedule than immediate-release oral morphine products, and significantly improves pain control at a lower daily opioid dose, with less rescue doses for breakthrough pain.

Cancer pain: controlled-release oral formulation of morphine sulfate is a well-recognized oral agent for the treatment of cancer pain.

Contraindications

Absolute: controlled-release oral formulation of morphine sulfate is contraindicated in patients with known hypersensitivity to morphine.

Relative: in any situation where opioids are contraindicated. This includes patients with respiratory depression, and in patients with acute or severe bronchial asthma or hypercarbia. Morphine is contraindicated in any patient who has or is suspected of having a paralytic ileus, renal and hepatic impairment.

Common doses

The controlled-release nature of the formulation allows it to be administered on a more convenient schedule than conventional immediate-release oral morphine products. However, MS Contin does not release morphine continuously over the course of a dosing interval. The administration of single doses of MS Contin on an every 12 hours dosing schedule will result in higher peak and lower trough plasma levels than those that occur when an identical daily dose of morphine is administered using conventional oral formulations on a q4h regimen. The clinical significance of greater fluctuations in morphine plasma level has not been systematically evaluated.

For patients who have not received narcotics before, the starting dose should be the lowest, and the patient needs to be monitored for side effects such as respiratory depression. The dose may gradually be increased until pain relief is obtained.

Conversion from parenteral to oral morphine: because of inter-subject variation and cross-tolerance, it is better to underestimate the 24-hour oral morphine requirement than to overestimate. Estimates of the oral to parenteral potency of morphine vary. Some authors suggest that a dose of oral morphine only three times the daily parenteral morphine requirement may be sufficient in chronic use settings. In patients whose daily morphine requirements are expected to be less than or equal to 120 mg per day, the 30 mg tablet strength is recommended for the initial titration period. Once a stable dose regimen is reached, the patient can be converted to the 60 mg or 100 mg tablet strength, or an appropriate combination of tablet strengths, if desired.

MS Contin tablets are available in the following strengths: 15 mg, 30 mg, 60 mg, 100 mg, 200 mg; 100 mg and 200 mg tablets are for use in opioid-tolerant patients

Avinza capsules are available as 30 mg, 45 mg, 60 mg, 75 mg, 90 mg, and 120 mg doses. The fumaric acid (a component of Avinza capsules that promotes absorption of the drug within the gastrointestinal tract by acting as an osmotic agent and a local pH modifier) limits the daily dose of Avinza to a maximum of 1600 mg, because of the potential for renal toxicity from high doses of fumaric acid.

Kadian capsules are available in 20 mg, 30 mg, 50 mg, 60 mg, and 100 mg doses. Dosing guidelines for controlled release morphine preparations are presented in Table 15.1.

Potential advantages

Ease of use, tolerability: controlled-release oral formulations of morphine sulfate provide significant pain relief, ensure uniform blood concentrations, offer less frequent dosing, fewer adverse side effects, and flexible titration with different dosing strengths.

As monotherapy: controlled-release oral morphine is generally not used as monotherapy.

As used for multimodal analgesia: controlled-release oral morphine is prescribed to control the basal pain, and needs to be supplemented by immediate-release oral morphine for breakthrough pain.

Kadian capsules have the advantage of being swallowed whole, or opened and contents sprinkled on a small amount of apple sauce or administered through a 16 French gastrostomy tube. Avinza may be opened too and the entire bead content sprinkled on a small amount of apple sauce, but the beads should not be chewed, crushed, or dissolved due to the risk of acute overdose.

Cost: MS Contin is relatively economical, is available as a generic too, and is widely available at most hospitals.

Avinza and Kadian are costly and currently not available in generic form. The first patent for Avinza

Table 15.1.

Drug	Dose	Interval	Breakthrough pain	General considerations
MS Contin	If daily requirement dose expected to be less than 60 mg: start 15 mg tablet	8–12 h	May need to be supplemented with immediate-release medication	Not to be broken, chewed, dissolved, or crushed
Avinza	In opioid-naive patients: start 30 mg, increments not greater than 30 mg every 4 days	24 h	5–15% of total daily dose given in form of immediate-release	The capsule may be opened and bead contents sprinkled on a small amount of apple sauce. Capsule or beads not to be chewed, crushed, or dissolved
Kadian	In opioid-naive patients: start 20 mg, increments not greater than 20 mg every other day	12–24 h	May need to be supplemented with immediate-release medication	The capsule may be opened and contents sprinkled on a small amount of apple sauce or administered through a 16 French gastrostomy tube

will expire in November 2017, and for Kadian it expired in March 2010.

Potential disadvantages

Toxicity: acute overdosage with morphine can be manifested by respiratory depression, somnolence progressing to stupor or coma, skeletal muscle flaccidity, cold and clammy skin, constricted pupils, rhabdomyolysis progressing to renal failure, and sometimes bradycardia, hypotension, and death.

Drug interactions: morphine has additive effects when used in conjunction with alcohol, other opioids, or illicit drugs that cause central nervous system depression because respiratory depression, hypotension, and profound sedation or coma may result.

Agonist/antagonist analgesics (i.e. pentazocine, nalbuphine, and butorphanol) should be administered with caution to a patient who has received or is receiving morphine sulfate. In this situation, mixed agonist/antagonist analgesics may reduce the analgesic effect of morphine sulfate and/or may precipitate withdrawal symptoms in these patients.

Morphine decreases the metabolism of tricyclic antidepressants, leading to toxicity.

Drug-related adverse events

Common/serious adverse events: the severe adverse reactions include respiratory depression, apnea, respiratory arrest, circulatory depression, hypotension, cardiac arrest, and shock.

Most common adverse events: constipation, lightheadedness, dizziness, sedation, nausea, vomiting, sweating, dysphoria, and euphoria.

Less common adverse events: weakness, headache, agitation, tremor, uncoordinated muscle movements, seizure, alterations of mood, muscle rigidity, transient hallucinations, disorientation, visual disturbances, insomnia, increased intracranial pressure, dry mouth, biliary tract spasm, laryngospasm, anorexia, diarrhea, cramps, taste alteration, constipation, ileus, intestinal obstruction, dyspepsia, increases in hepatic enzymes, flushing of the face, chills, tachycardia, bradycardia, palpitation, faintness, syncope, urine retention or hesitance, amenorrhea, reduced libido and/or potency, pruritus, urticaria, edema, diaphoresis, antidiuretic effect, paresthesia, bronchospasm, muscle tremor, blurred vision, nystagmus, diplopia, miosis, anaphylaxis.

Treatment of adverse events

In the treatment of morphine overdosage, primary attention should be given to the re-establishment of a patent airway and institution of assisted or controlled ventilation. Supportive measures (including oxygen, vasopressors) should be employed in the management of circulatory shock and pulmonary edema accompanying overdose as indicated. The pure opioid antagonists, such as naloxone, are specific antidotes against respiratory depression, which results from opioid overdose. Naloxone should be administered intravenously, however; because its duration of action is relatively short, and considering the long duration of action of the controlled-release form of morphine sulfate, the patient must be carefully monitored until spontaneous respiration is reliably re-established. If the response to naloxone is suboptimal or not sustained, additional naloxone may be administered, as needed, or given by continuous infusion to maintain alertness and respiratory function; however, there is no information available about the cumulative dose of naloxone that may be safely administered.

For the treatment of nausea and vomiting ondansetron or metoclopramide is often useful. For management of constipation one should consider that tolerance does not usually develop for the constipating effects of opioids. Laxatives and/or stool softeners should be used prophylactically from the beginning of opioid therapy. Agents that increase gastrointestinal propulsion should not be used as it may increase the risk of bowel perforation, if the patient has ileus and impacted stool.

References

1. Trescot AM, Helm S, Hansen H, et al. Opioids in the management of chronic non-cancer pain: an update of American Society of the Interventional Pain Physicians' (ASIPP) guidelines. *Pain Physician, Opioids Special Issue* 2008;**11**:S5–S62.

2. Holgado MA, Iruine A, Alvarez-Fuentes J, Fernandez-Arevalo M. Development and in vitro evaluation of controlled release formulation to produce wide dose interval morphine tablets. *Eur J Pharm Biopharm* 2008;**70**(2):544–549.

3. Pergolizzi J, Böger RH, Budd K, et al. Opioids and the management of chronic severe pain in the elderly: consensus statement of an international expert panel with focus on the six clinically most often used World Health Organization step III opioids (buprenorphine, fentanyl, hydromorphone,

methadone, morphine, oxycodone). *Pain Practice* 2008;**8**(4):287–313.

4. Rosenblum A, Marsch LA, Joseph H, Portenoy RK. Opioids and the treatment of chronic pain: controversies, current status, and future directions. *Exp Clin Psychopharmacol* 2008;**16**(5):405–416.

5. Sasaki J, Weil A, Ross E, Nicholson B. Effectiveness of polymer-coated extended-release morphine sulfate capsules in older patients with persistent moderate to severe pain: a subgroup analysis of a large, open-label, community-based trial. *Curr Ther Res* 2007;**68**(3):137–150.

**Section 2
Chapter**

Oral and Parenteral Opioid Analgesics

16

Combination agonist–antagonist opioid analgesics

Jeff Gudin

Generic Names: morphine plus naltrexone, oxycodone plus naloxone, oxycodone plus naltrexone

Trade/Proprietary Names: Embeda™, OXN™ Oxytrex™

Drug Class: opioid analgesic

Manufacturers: King Pharmaceuticals, 501 Fifth Street, Bristol, TN; Purdue Pharma Inc, One Stamford Forum, Stamford, CT; Pain Therapeutics Inc., 2211 Bridgepointe Parkway Suite 500, San Mateo, CA

Chemical Structures: morphine, see Figure 16.1; naltrexone, see Figure 16.2; oxycodone, see Figure 16.3; naloxone, see Figure 16.4

Chemical Names:
morphine: (5α,6α)-7,8-didehydro-4,5-epoxy-17-methylmorphinan-3,6-diol
naltrexone: 17-(cyclopropylmethyl)-4,5α-epoxy-3,14-dihydroxymorphinan-6-one
oxycodone: 4,5α-epoxy-14-hydroxy-3-methoxy-17-methylmorphinan-6-one
naloxone: 10,17-dihydroxy-4,12-oxa-4-azapentacyclooctadeca-18-trien-14-one

Introduction

During the last decade a dramatic rise in abuse of prescription opioids has occurred in the USA and other countries. In testimony presented to Congress in 2008 on trends in unintentional drug overdose, the CDC identified opioid pain relievers as a driver for recent large increases in deaths. They called on drug manufacturers to modify opioid analgesics; to make them more difficult to tamper with, and/or combine them with agents that block the effect of the opioid, if it is dissolved and injected [1]. These are complex problems requiring multi-faceted solutions including hardening of the tablet, combining the opioid with an antagonist drug, or adding an irritant chemical that would prevent nasal or parenteral misuse. This chapter will describe combination agonist plus antagonists that have recently become available or that are in development.

Opioid analgesics are one of the few classes of medications available to treat severe levels of pain. Adding another drug to an opioid (compounding) may enhance analgesia, minimize adverse effects, reduce opioid tolerance and/or potentially deter overuse or abuse. Most astute clinicians recognize that concerns about abuse and addiction should not prevent the proper management of pain. In response,

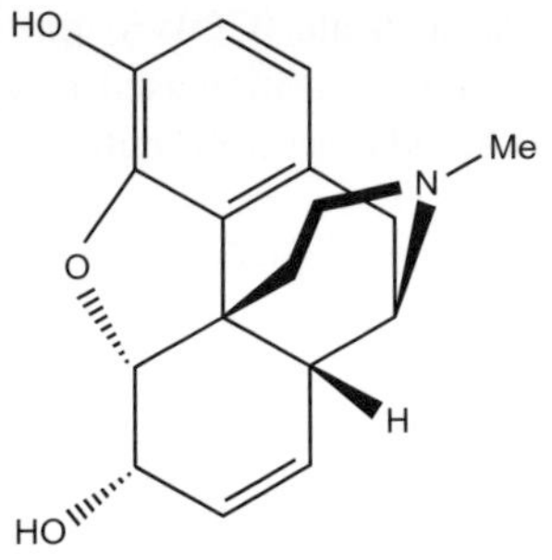

Figure 16.1.

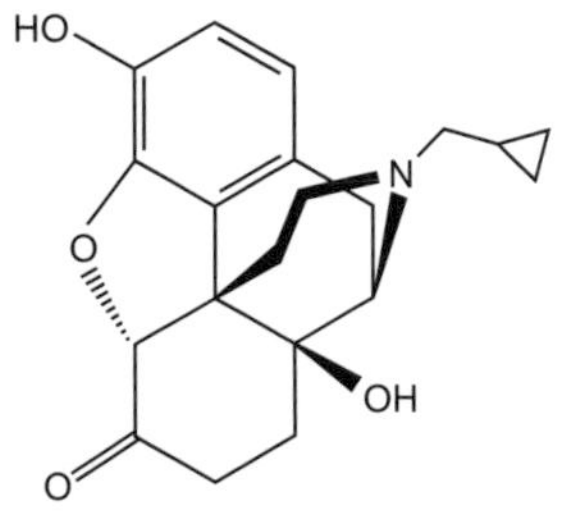

Figure 16.2.

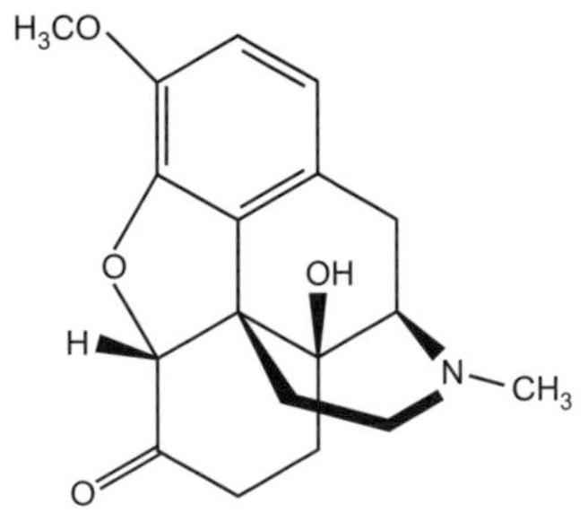

Figure 16.3.

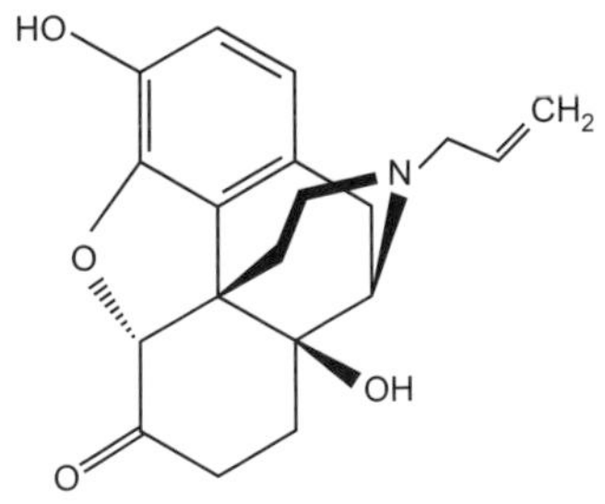

Figure 16.4.

Table 16.1. Facts regarding opioid adulteration and abuse in 2005

1. 5.2 million Americans used prescription pain relievers for nonmedical purposes each month
2. Each day approximately 2500 teens try abusing prescription painkillers for the first time
3. 5.2% of high school seniors abused long-acting oxycodone
4. 9.6% of high school seniors abused hydrocodone products
5. More than three in five say prescription pain relievers are easy to get from parents' medicine cabinets
6. Total cost of opioid abuse = $9.5 billion in 2005 dollars

Summarized from References 3, 4, and 5.

Abuse data collected by NIDA/SAMHSA [3,4] indicate that abusers will crush, chew or dissolve an extended-released opioid formulation to convert the drug to an immediate-release, more desirable and abusable form. Oral consumption and nasal administration (snorting) are reported to be the most common modes of illicit prescription abuse by teenagers. Data taken from 109 prescription drug abusers entering a treatment facility in central Kentucky showed that the most commonly abused opioids were hydrocodone (78%) and oxycodone-containing products (69%) [2]. Most respondents reported altering the delivery system of prescribed sustained-release opioid tablets by either chewing or crushing. Following crushing the adulterated drug was administered by snorting, subcutaneous skin popping or IV administration. This form of adulteration and misuse is also true for short-acting drugs [4,5]. Some facts regarding opioid adulteration and abuse are presented in Table 16.1.

Opioid agonist–antagonist combinations

Opioid antagonists reverse the subjective and analgesic effects of opioid agonists by binding competitively at the mu opioid receptor. Naloxone is an opioid antagonist administered intravenously in cases of overdose or in low doses to reverse some bothersome, adverse effects of opioid analgesics. Naltrexone is available as an orally administered opioid antagonist and is used most commonly to oppose the potential effects of opioids or block cravings from alcohol and other substances. Combining opioids in an attempt to deter misuse is not a new concept. Talwin™ Nx was created in an attempt to curb the injection of the drug pentazocine by adding naloxone.

much focus has been placed on appropriate prescribing and risk stratification of these controlled substances. One area of study and industry support has been the development of "tamper-resistant" combination opioids with the potential to deter abuse. Many of these conceptual and developed products utilize the opioid antagonists naloxone and naltrexone as a key ingredient in their formulations.

91

The amount of naloxone present in Talwin Nx (0.5 mg per tablet) has no action when taken orally and does not interfere with the pharmacological action of pentazocine. However, this amount of naloxone given by injection has profound antagonistic action to the opioid analgesics.

When considering new novel combination agents, we must ensure that their primary function, efficacy and safety are met. There are no guidelines set for the development of "tamper-proof" or "abuse deterrent" agents. Obviously they must first undergo rigorous phase I, II and III trials to confirm the pharmacokinetics, efficacy and safety of the primary (opioid) ingredient. Then the pharmacokinetic and pharmacodynamic properties of the additional added agents (i.e. antagonists) must be assessed, when the preparation is either taken whole or tampered with.

Morphine plus naltrexone combination

Currently, the only FDA-approved controlled-release opioid/naltrexone combination is Embeda™. This preparation of sustained-release (SR) morphine contains a sequestered antagonist that is released only upon tampering. Embeda™ contains pellets of an extended-release oral formulation of morphine sulfate surrounding an inner core of naltrexone hydrochloride and is indicated for the management of moderate to severe pain when a continuous, around-the-clock opioid analgesic is needed for an extended period of time. The morphine/naltrexone ratio is 25:1 (4%), with the largest available dosage form being 100/4 mg. Crushing, chewing, or dissolving combined morphine/naltrexone (Embeda™) will result in the uncontrolled delivery of the opioid and pose a significant risk to the abuser that could result in overdose and death; it will also result in the release of naltrexone, which may precipitate withdrawal in opioid-tolerant individuals.

Combined morphine/naltrexone capsules have shown comparable analgesia, adverse effects and bioequivalence to a similar morphine sulfate extended-release capsule product (Kadian™) with regard to rate and extent of plasma morphine absorption [8]. In the clinical efficacy trial in patients with pain due to osteoarthritis, change in the weekly BPI average pain score was statistically significantly superior for those treated with Embeda as compared to placebo. A review of the Subjective Opiate Withdrawal Scales (SOWS) and Clinical Opiate Withdrawal Scale (COWS) and adverse event profile did not detect an increased risk of opioid withdrawal for combined morphine/naltrexone compared to placebo [8].

Combined morphine/naltrexone capsules are to be swallowed whole or the contents of the capsules sprinkled on apple sauce and the pellets in the capsules are not to be crushed, dissolved, or chewed. A pK study of combined morphine/naltrexone crushed vs. whole was done to compare the plasma concentrations and relative bioavailability of morphine, naltrexone, and the major naltrexone metabolite (6-β-naltrexol). Plasma morphine levels from crushed morphine/naltrexone capsules showed no extended-release properties. While concurrent administration of high-fat food decreased the rate and extent of morphine absorption from combined morphine/naltrexone, the total bioavailability or sequestration of naltrexone was not affected. An alcohol effects study examined the bioavailability of combined morphine/naltrexone when dosed under fasting conditions with 4%, 20% and 40% alcohol compared to water. The rate and extent of bioavailability and total exposure to morphine (AUC, C_{max}) were not affected when the drug was administered concomitantly with either 4% or 20% alcohol, when compared to administration with water. When combined morphine/naltrexone was administered with 40% alcohol (240 mL over 15 minutes), the rate and extent of bioavailability (C_{max}) doubled and the t_{max} was 5 hours earlier, when compared to administration with water. The total systemic exposure to morphine (AUC) was not affected [9].

Abuse liability

"Abuse liability" is the potential for a drug to produce positive effects that will reinforce a pattern of misuse, abuse, or diversion. To date, there is no evidence that the naltrexone component of combined morphine/naltrexone will prevent or deter abuse. Novel abuse liability trials have been developed to assess the effects of combined morphine/naltrexone when tampered with. The pharmacodynamic effect of naltrexone in the setting of crushed morphine/naltrexone capsules was examined in two clinical trials: an oral and an intravenous abuse liability trial [8]. These were conducted in nondependent recreational opioid abusers, as dependent, daily or habitual users would probably experience a withdrawal syndrome when exposed to the naltrexone component with crushed morphine/naltrexone capsules.

The oral abuse liability study was a randomized double-blind four-way crossover trial comparing 120 mg oral morphine delivered in the following routes: placebo, MSIR (immediate release), Embeda™ whole, and Embeda™ crushed [8]. The greatest drug liking scores were for MSIR. Overall, 87.5% of subjects had some degree of reduced drug liking after receiving crushed morphine/naltrexone, while 12.5% had no reduction in drug liking. There was considerable individual variability in the degree of reduction in drug liking, ranging between 10 and 50%. Similarly, 69% of subjects showed some decrease in euphoria with crushed morphine/naltrexone compared to IR morphine and 31% of subjects did not report a reduction in euphoria. There was similar individual variability in the degree of reduction in euphoria.

In addition to the oral abuse study above, an intravenous abuse liability study was performed. This was a randomized double-blind, placebo-controlled, three-way crossover trial in nondependent recreational opioid-users administered placebo, 30 mg of IV morphine alone or 30 mg of IV morphine in combination with 1.2 mg of IV naltrexone to simulate parenteral use of crushed capsules containing morphine/naltrexone [8]. The primary objective was to determine the relative drug liking and euphoric effects of IV morphine alone compared to IV morphine plus naltrexone following single bolus doses. Pharmacodynamic measures were assessed by subjective responses to the Drug Effects Questionnaire (DEQ) Question #5 "How high are you now?" The combination of morphine with naltrexone resulted in 71% of subjects reporting a reduction in euphoria compared to morphine alone. Note that the intravenous injection of crushed morphine/naltrexone may result in serious injury and death due to a morphine overdose or an embolic event. Intravenous injection of crushed morphine/naltrexone may precipitate a severe withdrawal syndrome in opioid-dependent patients.

The clinical significance of the degree of reduction in drug liking and euphoria reported in these studies has not yet been established. To reiterate, there is no evidence that the naltrexone in combined morphine/naltrexone reduces its abuse liability.

Future combinations

Although only available currently as an SR morphine combination, other naltrexone-containing analgesic products are in development. Multiple companies are researching combination oxycodone/naltrexone products, including Purdue Pharma's combined oxycodone/naloxone (OXN™) and Pain Therapeutics Inc.'s combined oxycodone/naltrexone preparation (Oxytrex®). Animal and phase 3 human data indicate that these combinations of oxycodone and either naloxone or naltrexone minimize the development of physical dependence and analgesic tolerance while prolonging analgesia. They may also reduce opioid-induced bowel dysfunction, since released antagonist might inhibit mu receptors in the gut. Oxytrex™ is in late-stage clinical development for the treatment of moderate-to-severe chronic pain. To evaluate the safety and efficacy of the oxycodone/naltrexone combination, three clinical studies have been conducted, one in healthy volunteers and the other two in patients with chronic pain. The putative mechanism of ultra-low-dose naltrexone is to prevent an alteration in G-protein coupling by opioid receptors that is associated with opioid tolerance and dependence. Opioid agonists are initially inhibitory but become excitatory through constant opioid receptor activity. The agonist/antagonist combination of Oxytrex may reduce the conversion from an inhibitory to an excitatory receptor, thereby decreasing the development of tolerance and physical dependence.

References

1. CDC Report to Congress on opioid analgesic overdose. March 12, 2008.

2. Passik SD, Hays L, Eisner N, Kirsh KL. Psychiatric and pain characteristics of prescription drug abusers entering drug rehabilitation. *J Pain Palliat Care Pharmacother* 2006;**20**(2):5–13.

3. Substance Abuse and Mental Health Services Administration Office of Applied Studies. Rockville, MD: 2008. Results from the 2007 National Survey on Drug Use and Health: National Findings DHHS Publication No. SMA 07–4293. http://www.oas.samhsa.gov/NSDUHlatest.htm. Published September 2008. Accessed October 30, 2008.

4. Office of National Drug Control Policy. National Youth Anti-Drug Media Campaign: Campaign Overview Fact Sheet. http://www.mediacampaign.org/newsroom/press08/fs_012408.pdf. Published January 24, 2008. Accessed February 26, 2008.

5. Johnston LD, O'Malley PM, Bachman JG, Schulenberg JE. *Secondary School Students*. Bethesda, MD: National Institute on Drug Abuse; 2007. Monitoring the Future: National Survey Results on Drug Use, 1975–2006; vol I. NIH Publication

07–6205. http://www.monitoringthefuture.org/pubs/monographs/vol1_2006.pdf. Published September 2007. Accessed February 26, 2008.

6. The Partnership for Drug Free America. The Partnership Attitude Tracking Study – Teens 2005 (PATS). http://www.drugfree.org/Files/Full_Teen_Report. Published May 15, 2006. Accessed February 26, 2008.

7. Birnbaum HG, White AG, Reynolds JL, et al. Estimated costs of prescription opioid analgesic abuse in the United States in 2001. *Clin J Pain* 2006;22(8).

8. Embeda™ *package insert*, King Pharmaceuticals.

9. Embeda™: *Alcohol effect study (Study 103) Data on File*, King Pharmaceuticals.

Section 2 Chapter

17

Oral and Parenteral Opioid Analgesics

Meperidine

Ellen Flanagan and Brian Ginsberg

Generic Name: meperidine, pithidine, pethanol

Trade Name: Demerol™

Class of Drug: opioid analgesic (Schedule II)

Manufacturers: Abbott Laboratories, Hospital Products Division, Abbott Park, IL 60064; Sanofi-Aventis U.S. LLC, 55 Corporate Drive, Bridgewater, NJ 08807

Chemical Structure: see Figure 17.1

Chemical Name: ethyl 1-methyl-4-phenylpiperidine-4-carboxylate; $C_{15}H_{21}NO_2$

Description

Meperidine is a synthetic phenylpiperidine-based opioid analgesic, with structural similarities to fentanyl and sufentanil. It was first synthesized in 1939 as an anticholinergic agent and subsequently on routine screening its analgesic effect was demonstrated [1,2]. Meperidine's analgesic activity is primarily mediated by binding and activating mu opioid receptors and secondarily via activation of alpha 2 adrenergic and delta opioid receptors. In clinically relevant concentrations, meperidine is a potent agonist at the α_{2B} adrenoceptor.

Major and minor sites of action

Sodium channel blocker

Meperidine reversibly blocks voltage-gated Na^+ currents with a half-maximum inhibiting concentration (IC_{50}) of 112 μM. Clinically, meperidine shows a dose-dependent blockade of both the sensory and motor fibers of the ulnar nerve after infiltration. Two percent meperidine blocks both sensory and motor activity at the hypothenar muscle. Intrathecal doses of meperidine 50 mg can provide short-duration spinal anesthesia.

Anticholinergic

Meperidine has no spasmolytic effects but an anticholinergic effect, displacing the dose-response curve for carbacholine to the right, indicating competitive antagonism. Only chemically induced spasm of guinea pig large intestine is relaxed by direct application of meperidine solution, possibly due to meperidine's local activity.

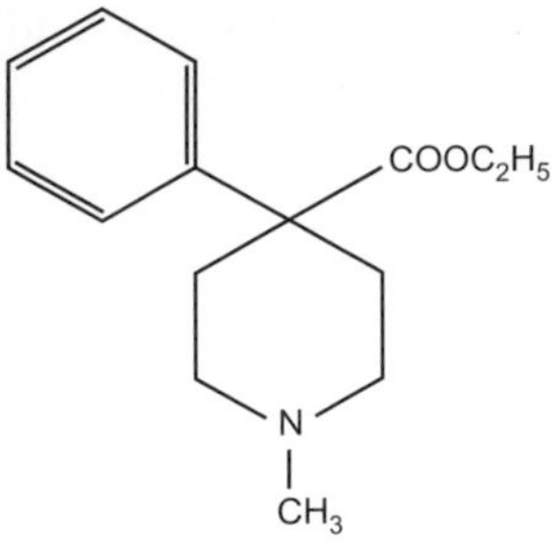

Figure 17.1.

Opioid receptor

Meperidine binds to the mu opioid receptor to promote analgesia. Animal studies demonstrate counterclockwise hysteresis between the blood level of meperidine and analgesia, reflecting a delay while meperidine crosses the blood–brain barrier. At meperidine's EC_{50}, it induces less stimulation of the mu opioid receptor and had less efficacy than morphine, fentanyl or sufentanil. In contrast to other opioids, meperdine is not a substrate for P glycoprotein (P-gp), which mediates the efflux of opioids across the blood–brain barrier, impacting the onset, magnitude, and duration of analgesic response. Genetic variability and pharmacological agents do not influence the flux of meperidine across the blood–brain barrier.

Alpha-2-adrenergic receptors

Recent data have provided convincing evidence in mice that meperidine reduces the thermoregulatory temperature threshold primarily by activation at the alpha-2-adrenoreceptor and that this mechanism is probably independent of the mu opioid receptor, as evidenced by the lack of effect of naloxone.

In an elegant series of experiments, knockout mice have been used to determine the specific alpha adrenergic receptor subtype responsible for the thermoregulatory effects of meperidine [3]. Wild-type and knockout mice with deletions of either the alpha 2a, alpha 2b or alpha 2c adrenoreceptor were studied after meperidine treatment in the presence or absence of atipamezole, an alpha 2 receptor antagonist. Wild-type and alpha 2b or 2c knockout mice treated with meperidine exhibited decreased thermoregulatory threshold temperatures antagonized, that is prevented, by atipamezole. In contrast, thermoregulatory thresholds in alpha 2a knockout

mice were unaffected by meperidine. It was demonstrated that the alpha 2a receptor is probably the primary mechanism responsible for the meperidine-induced decrease in thermoregulatory threshold [3]. While these data are derived from mice rather than humans, and the primary mechanism of thermoregulation differs between species, these data are intriguing.

Metabolic pathways, drug clearance and elimination

Meperidine is metabolized by two different pathways, primarily by hepatic carboxylesterase to meperidinic acid, an inactive metabolite which is glucuronated and then excreted. In addition, meperidine undergoes N-demethylation via the cytochrome P450 system to normeperidine. Normeperidine formation in human liver microsomes is mainly catalyzed by CYP2B6 and CYP3A4, with a minor contribution from CYP2C19. Normeperidine is further metabolized to either normeperidinic acid by carboxylesterase or by microsomal hydroxylation to N-hydroxynormeperidine followed by renal elimination. Normeperidine has half the analgesic potency of meperidine but two to three times the potency as a CNS excitatory agent. Signs and symptoms of normeperidine-related CNS excitation include irritability, tremors, myoclonus, muscle twitches, shaky feelings and generalized seizures [1,3]. Elevated levels of normeperidine occur with prolonged administration of high doses of meperidine and decrease excretion.

After oral administration, the levels of normeperidine are increased compared to systemic administration. In hepatic disease, the reduced hepatic clearance of meperidine results in increased absorption necessitating a reduction in dose. Following intramuscular administration of meperidine, the elimination half-life ($t_{1/2}\beta$) is 3.6 hours (3.1–4.1 hours). Intramuscular absorption is highly variable with a two-fold variation in blood levels in the same patient and a wider five-fold intra-patient variability. The $t_{1/2}\beta$ is 111.4 hours in cirrhotic patients (range 8.3–18.7), but the levels of normeperidine are reduced. The elimination half-life of meperidine and normeperidine are prolonged in patients with renal failure. The $t_{1/2}\beta$ elimination half-life of normeperidine is anywhere from 14–21 h to 24–48 h and as long as 34 h in renal failure [3].

Indications

Surgical acute pain

Fifty milligrams of meperidine shows no superiority over placebo but a 100 mg dose is comparable to 10–15 mg morphine. Following IM administration, onset of analgesia occurs within 10–15 minutes and peak effects occur within 1 hour. In a comparison of three doses of meperidine compared to three equipotent doses of morphine delivered via PCA, meperidine demonstrated equivalent analgesia at rest but morphine was superior with activity. These data have been replicated by others. In children, PCA morphine produced significantly better pain scores than meperidine with no difference in the side-effect profiles [1]. Low doses of meperidine, 12.5 mg, are used effectively to treat post-operative shivering and the shivering induced by an infusion of amphotericin.

Medical pain

Renal colic

Meperidine has been used extensively to treat renal colic [1–3]. There is some evidence which suggests that meperidine may produce less smooth muscle spasm than equianalgesic doses of morphine. A comparison of meperidine with ketorolac, in the management of renal colic, demonstrated that the NSAID had a more rapid onset of action and fewer side effects than meperidine. Similarly, a comparison of 1 mg hydromophone to 50 mg of meperidine, also used to treat renal colic, demonstrated the need for fewer breakthrough medications (hydromophone 31% vs. meperidine 68%), fewer IV pyelograms (28% vs. 54%), fewer hospital admissions (25% vs. 49%) and improved analgesia.

Migraine

Meperidine is commonly used in the management of migraine but ketorolac is as effective as an analgesic with fewer side effects reported with the NSAID.

Rigors

Rigors, or involuntary shivering, are a poorly understood but common post-operative complication. Shivering is also associated with fever seen in malignancy and amphotericin or granulocyte infusions. Numerous investigations have proven the efficacy of meperidine for the prophylaxis and abortive treatment of shivering with treatment of established shivering slightly more effective than prophylaxis. Clearly, the evidence supports the use of meperidine for the treatment of post-operative shivering.

Meperidine appears to have the greatest effect on shivering when compared to the analgesic equivalents of fentanyl and sufentanil. Using a non-shivering thermogenesis mouse model, it was demonstrated that intraperitoneal injection of meperidine led to a decrease in threshold of non-shivering thermogenesis as measured by expiratory carbon dioxide and body temperature [3]. Meperidine's effect was abolished if mice were subsequently treated with atipamezole, an alpha-2 antagonist. Control mice injected with saline maintained a normal threshold of non-shivering thermogenesis that was unaffected by further treatment with atipamezole.

Chronic nonmalignant pain

Sickle cell disease

Since oral meperidine results in higher levels of normeperidine than equipotent doses of intravenous or intramuscular meperidine, its use has been limited to the management of acute pain of sickle cell disease and precludes the use of oral meperidine in the management of chronic pain that is associated with sickle cell disease. A literature review found an incidence of seizures in the sickle cell population of 1 to 12% and questions have been raised regarding the role of meperidine and its metabolite normeperidine in precipitating seizures [3]. A pain protocol using morphine or hydromorphone coupled with increased access to outpatient clinics decreased ED visits, hospitalizations, and increased utilization of a more stable primary care clinic setting by patients with sickle cell disease. Appropriate pharmacological treatment of sickle pain entails the use of non-opioid analgesics, opioid analgesics (excluding meperidine) and adjuvants singly or in combination depending on the severity of pain.

Bilary spasm

All opioids increase the phasic wave frequency of the sphincter of Oddi, which may impair filling of the sphincter and increase pressure. All studies to date have shown no statistical difference in the mean basal pressure between morphine and meperidine [1].

Contraindications

Absolute

The absolute contraindication to the use of meperidine is a history of a serotonergic crisis in the past and renal failure.

Relative

Relative contraindications to the use of meperidine include other anti-serotonin drugs, renal dysfunction and seizures.

Common doses/uses

Oral

Approximately 50% of oral meperidine is absorbed into the systemic circulation (range 41 to 61%). After oral administration the onset of analgesia is within 15 minutes and peak effects occur in 60–90 minutes [1,3]. In hepatic disease, with reduced hepatic clearance, the absorption of meperidine is increased from the gastrointestinal tract, necessitating a reduced dose.

Parenteral

Following subcutaneous or IM administration, onset of analgesia occurs within 10–15 minutes and peak effects occur within 1 hour [1,3]. Meperidine binds to both albumen and alpha-1-acid glycoprotein (AAG). The AAG level is dependent on the stress response and levels increase with trauma and infection. Further variability may be induced by eyrthocyte binding. Following intramuscular administration of meperidine the elimination half-life ($t_{½}\beta$) is 3.6 hours (3.1–4.1 hours). The average parenteral dose of meperidine is 1–1.5 mg/kg.

Neuraxial

The epidural dose of meperidine has ranged from 20 to 150 mg with an infusion rate of 5–20 mg/h. The onset of action occurs in 5 minutes after a bolus and the analgesia lasts 4 to 8 hours. Meperidine, 10 to 30 mg, has been used for subarachnoid bolus with an anticipated analgesia of 10 to 24 hours [1,3].

Potential advantages

Meperidine may offer advantages for relief of visceral pain [1–3].

Potential disadvantages

Potential disadvantages associated with meperidine are primarily related to the neurotoxic effects of its metabolite, normeperidine.

Studies in rats have determined that subcutaneous doses of both meperidine and normeperidine lower the seizure threshold. In contrast, after intracerebroventricular (ICV) administration, meperidine raised the threshold while normeperidine lowered it. Naloxone antagonized this anticonvulsant effect of ICV-administered meperidine and enhanced the proconvulsant effect of normeperidine. Neurotoxic symptoms can range from muscle twitching and jerking to full tonic-clonic seizures. Symptoms are worsened with parenteral doses approaching 1 g/day, in patients with underlying seizure disorders, pre-eclampsia, and acute renal failure.

Adverse events

Respiratory effects

The respiratory depressant effect of meperidine exceeds that of morphine. Naloxone reverses the respiratory depression seen with relative overdoses of meperidine.

Euphoria

In human volunteers meperidine causes dose-related subjective effects such as "sedated", "coasting or spaced out", or "feel drug effect" that persisted for 4 or 5 hours. These subjective effects were associated with drug liking.

Drug-related adverse events

Serotonin crisis

Meperidine is thought to inhibit both the 5-HT2A receptors and norepinephrine (NE) reuptake mechanism which may precipitate a serotonin syndrome, a toxic state secondary to excessive serotonin agonism of the CNS [3,4]. This adverse drug reaction occurs most commonly in patients who are using single or multiple medications that increase postsynaptic serotonin levels. Inherited deficiencies in the metabolism of serotonin may contribute to the development of the syndrome. Hypertension, atherosclerosis, and hyperlipidemia are all associated with a reduction in endothelial MAO activity and thus a reduced capacity to metabolize serotonin may increase the risk of a serotonin crisis. The diagnosis of serotonergic crisis is made by the presence of tremor, hyperreflexia, spontaneous clonus or inducible clonus with agitation and diaphoresis, a temperature > 38°C and muscle rigidity.

Conclusions

Meperidine is an older opioid analgesic with typical annoying and occasionally serious adverse events such as respiratory depression. It is also associated with significant risks of cortical irritability and potential neurotoxicity. Meperidine may provide useful relief of visceral pain, post-operative shivering, and sickle cell crisis-related pain; however, because of its adverse event profile, its role in modern pain medicine is becoming increasingly limited [4].

References

1. Clark R, Wei E, Anderson P. Meperidine: therapeutic use and toxicity. *J Emerg Med* 1995;**13**:797–802.

2. Kranke P, Eberhart L, Roewer N, Tramer M. Pharmacological treatment of post-operative shivering: a quantitative systematic review of randomized controlled trials. *Anesth Analg* 2002;**94**:453–460.

3. Latta K, Ginsberg B, Barkin R. Meperidine: a critical review. *Am J Ther* 2002;**9**(1);53–68.

4. Raymo L, Camejo M, Fudin J. Eradicating analgesic use of meperidine in a hospital. *Am J Health Syst Pharm* 2007;**64**(11);1148–1152.

**Section 2
Chapter**

18

Oral and Parenteral Opioid Analgesics

Codeine and codeine compounds

Anjali Vira

Generic Name: codeine

Trade/Proprietary Names: Robafen AC®, Robitussin A-C® Syrup, Tylenol with Codeine (No. 2, No. 3, No. 4)®, Nurofen Plus®

Manufacturer: Roxane Laboratories Inc., 1809 Wilson Rd, Columbus, OH; Reckitt Benckiser plc, Slough, UK

Drug Class: opioid analgesic, opiate antitussive

Chemical Structure: see Figure 18.1

Chemical Name: methylmorphine, 3-methoxy-17-methylmorphinan-6-ol; $C_{18}H_{21}NO_3$

Description

Codeine is an opiate alkoloid that can be extracted from the opium poppy, *Papaver sominiforum*. It was first isolated in 1832 and remains a widely used oral opiate analgesic that has roughly one-tenth the potency of oral morphine [1]. Codeine is a useful antitussive and is a component of numerous cough-suppressant compounds. It is commonly prescribed for management of acute pain following dental surgery, minor general surgery and for relief of acute trauma. Codeine tablets are manufactured alone (Schedule II) or in combination with aspirin or acetaminophen (Schedule III). The combination of codeine

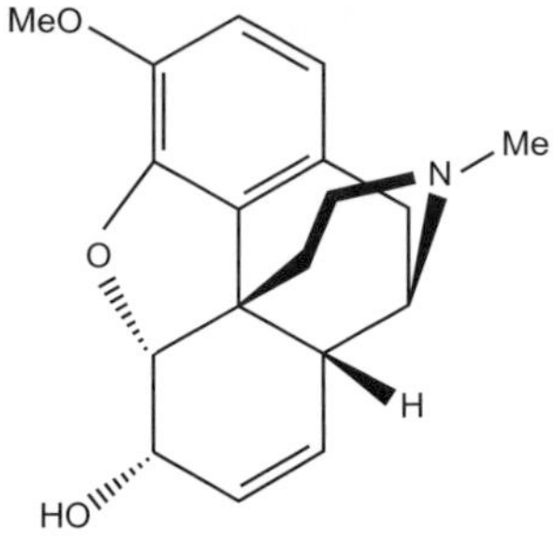

Figure 18.1.

plus ibuprofen (Nurofen Plus™) is available as a pain reliever in Europe and the UK. Codeine is medically prescribed for the relief of mild to moderate pain but is less effective for severe and very severe pain. Compared to morphine, codeine produces less analgesia, sedation, and respiratory depression. Codeine is the parent drug used for the production of dihydrocodeine and hydrocodone.

Mode of activity

Site of activity

Like other opioid agonists, codeine's major sites of action are localized to and mediated by supraspinal and spinal opioid receptors. Codeine has a low affinity for mu and kappa opioid receptors and its major effects are due to its conversion to morphine. Morphine binds mu opioid receptors with higher affinity, producing dose-dependent analgesia, as well as negative effects typical of mu receptor agonists such as respiratory depression, constipation, and nausea. Codeine also provides clinically useful central antitussive effects through a central mechanism that is not completely understood [1].

Metabolic pathways

Codeine is a prodrug that exerts most of its effects through two active metabolites, namely morphine and codeine-6-glucuronide. N-Demethylation of codeine into norcodeine by CYP3A4 and the glucuronidation of codeine are the main pathways for converting the molecule into inactive compounds, accounting for more than 80% of its clearance. O-Demethylation of codeine into morphine by the cytochrome P450 enzyme CYP2D6 represents a minor pathway of codeine metabolism accounting for less than 10% of clearance. Nevertheless, this pathway is essential in order to gain analgesic activity as it allows codeine to be converted to morphine. Because codeine itself is not an effective analgesic, individuals who are not able to convert codeine to morphine do not gain adequate analgesia [2]. Genetic polymorphisms of CYP2D6 are found in 10% of the Caucasian population and 2% of Asians. Lack of efficacy in these "poor metabolizers" should be recognized quickly and they should be switched to equianalgesic doses of an alternative opioid [2]. Conversely patients with induction of this enzyme system or others with phenotypic ultrarapid metabolism may experience opioid intoxication following exposure to small doses of codeine [3]. This situation may be worsened in patients with renal failure who have difficulty eliminating the G-6 metabolites of codeine and morphine. The concentration of O-demethylated metabolites can be as much as 45 times as high in persons with ultrarapid CYP2D6 metabolism as it is in those with poor metabolism. Codeine has a half-life of roughly 2.5–3 hours and has an oral bioavailability that is poor when compared to other oral narcotics such as oxycodone and methadone.

Indications

Codeine is approved to treat mild to severe acute and chronic pain, post-operative pain, irritable bowel syndrome, diarrhea, and cough. It is also commonly used as a post-procedure analgesic for patients recovering from dental procedures.

Contraindications

Absolute: hypersensitivity to codeine.

Relative: codeine and other narcotics should be used with caution in patients who have severe respiratory compromise as they can cause respiratory depression. Because 90% of oral codeine is renally cleared, patients with severe renal disease require prolonged monitoring for delayed respiratory depression and sedative effects of codeine. Care should be exercised in patients co-treated with drugs that either inhibit or up-regulate CYP2D6.

Common doses

Dosage should be adjusted according to the severity of the pain and the response of the patient. It may occasionally be necessary to exceed the usual dosage recommended below or employ a more potent opioid in cases of very severe pain or in patients who have developed opioid tolerance.

Oral: the recommended analgesic starting dose for adults is 30–60 mg every 3–4 hours (or 1 mg/kg every 3–4 hours as needed for children or adults weighing less than 50 kg). The recommended antitussive dose for adults and children over 12 years of age is 10–20 mg every 4–6 hours. Codeine is readily absorbed from the GI tract with the peak analgesic effects noted 45–60 minutes post administration

Nurofen Plus™ contains 12.8 mg of codeine and 200 mg of ibuprofen per tablet, and is prescribed as 1–2 tablets every 4–6 h as required. When prescribing codeine compounds, caregivers should calculate total daily exposure to acetaminophen, aspirin and ibuprofen to reduce risks of hepatotoxicity and gastrointestinal bleeding

Parenteral: the recommended starting dose of codeine is 60 mg every 2 h given as intramuscular or subcutaneous injection.

Potential advantages

Codeine is one of the few opioids that possess central antitussive effects. Furthermore codeine suppresses cough at doses that are significantly lower than the dose required to effect analgesia. The combination of antitussive effect and analgesia may be useful in patients suffering pain related to lung cancer and other terminal forms of lung and tracheal disease. The typical antitussive dose of codeine starts at 10 or 20 mg, which can be titrated to effect. At these lower antitussive but sub-analgesic doses, the unwanted side effects such as respiratory depression are low. Compared with other drugs codeine is relatively inexpensive.

Potential disadvantages

As discussed above, the analgesic effect of codeine depends greatly on its ability to be metabolized to morphine. In patients in whom large amounts of codeine have been administered without relief, the possibility of a polymorphism of the CYP2D6 enzyme must be considered. Medications that inhibit CYP2D6 may reduce or even completely block the conversion of codeine to morphine. These include selective serotonin reuptake inhibitors (SSRIs), cimetidine, and antidepressants such as buproprion. On the other hand agents that induce CYP450 isozymes, such as rifampin and dexamethasone, increase the conversion rate and increase the risk of adverse events.

As an oral drug, codeine is much less effective as an analgesic due to its large first-pass hepatic metabolism compared to morphine, hydrocodone and oxycodone. The plasma half-life of codeine is also shorter than many other orally available opiates such as morphine, hydromorphone, and oxymorphone. Like all opioids, continued use of codeine may result in tolerance development and physical dependence. However, when compared to potent mu agonists, codeine is less addictive and is associated with mild withdrawal symptoms.

Drug-related adverse events

Codeine is associated with the same adverse events that may occur with an opiate. Respiratory depression, sedation, nausea, constipation, and pruritus are all common side effects of codeine. These effects are especially pronounced in the elderly and may be more prolonged in any patient who is slow to clear the drug, such as patients with renal failure.

Conclusion

Codeine is an older opioid agonist that offers few analgesic advantages over newer derivatives such as hydrocodone and oxycodone, and appears to be associated with a higher incidence of annoying side effects, such as sedation, nausea, and vomiting. Since the drug must be metabolized to an active compound, codeine has a delayed analgesic onset, and may be associated with inadequate pain relief in patients who have CYP2D6 deficiencies.

References

1. Brunton LL. *Goodman and Gilmore's The Pharmacological Basis of Therapeutics*, 11th ed. New York: McGraw Hill, 2006, pp. 563–580.

2. Sindrup SH, Brosen K. The pharmacogenetics of codeine hypoalgesia. *Pharmacogenetics* 1995;**5**: 335–346.

3. Yue QY, Hasselstrom J, Svensson JO, Sawe J. Pharmacokinetics of codeine and its metabolites in Caucasian healthy volunteers: comparisons between extensive and poor hydroxylators of debrisoquine. *Br J Clin Pharmacol* 1991;**31**:635–642.

19

Oxycodone and oxycodone compounds

Mary Keyes

Generic Names: oxycodone, oxycodone plus acetaminophen compound, oxycodone plus aspirin compound

Proprietary Names: Roxicodone®, Roxicodone® oral solution, Intensol®: Oxy IR®, Oxyfast®, Oxydose®. Compounds: Percocet®, Percodan®, Endodan, Tylox®, Roxiprin®, Roxicet™, Percolone®, Combunox®.

Drug Class: opioid analgesic (Schedule II)

Manufacturers: Purdue Pharma, One Stamford Forum, Stamford, CT; Xanodyne Pharmaceutical, Newport, KY; Endo Pharmaceuticals, 100 Endo Boulevard, Chadds Ford, PA; Ortho McNeil Pharmaceutical, Raritan, NJ; Roxane Laboratories, Columbus, OH

Chemical Structure: see Figure 19.1

Chemical Name: 6-deoxy-7,8-dihydro-14-hydroxy-3-O-methyl-6-oxomorphine

Chemical Formula: $C_{18}H_2NO_4$; molecular wt 315

Introduction

Oxycodone is a semi-synthetic opioid analgesic related to codeine and derived from thebaine, an alkaloid found in opium. Although it has been in clinical use since 1917 (first manufactured in Germany), the use of oxycodone for the treatment of acute and chronic pain has grown remarkably in the past decade.

Mode of activity

Oxycodone is a mu-receptor-specific ligand, although with binding affinity less than that of morphine and methadone. Some animal studies have established that some portion of the antinociceptive properties of oxycodone are mediated through kappa receptors as well.

Oxycodone is structurally similar to codeine while pharmacodynamically comparable to morphine in onset and duration of action. It is approximately 1.5 times more potent than morphine with equivalent effectiveness in equianalgesic dosages. Oxycodone has high oral bioavailability (60%) compared with morphine (20–30%), which is the most notable difference between these drugs. It also explains why oxycodone has a rapid analgesic onset and onset-to-peak effect. In clinical practice oxycodone does not release significant amounts of histamine and may cause less sedation than equivalent doses of morphine.

As for all opioids, hepatic biotransformation is the primary route of metabolism for oxycodone. Methylation at position 3 in both oxycodone and codeine protects both drugs from rapid first-pass elimination. Approximately half of an oxycodone dose undergoes N-demethylation, producing noroxycodone, which has weak analgesic properties. The second pathway, which accounts for 10%, involves the isoenzyme CYP2D6 of the P450 cytochrome. The O-methylation that occurs results in the production of oxymorphone, a potent analgesic. The small quantities of oxymorphone produced have little clinical relevance. Inhibition of this pathway by other drugs likewise has little clinical relevance. The use of concomitant medications interacting with these pathways may affect the plasma levels of oxycodone, resulting in reduced analgesia or adverse events.

Oxycodone and its metabolites are eliminated by the kidneys. Dosage adjustments are required in patients with moderate to severe liver and kidney dysfunction, although to a lesser extent than with morphine. No dosing decrements are required in the elderly except for those who are debilitated.

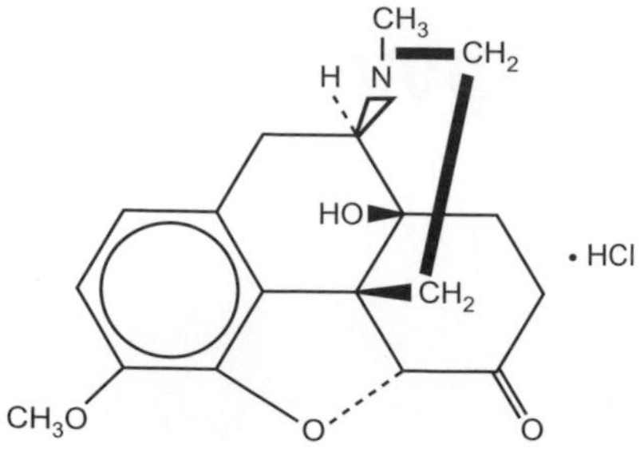

Figure 19.1.

Indications

Oxycodone is indicated for the treatment of moderate to severe pain that is either acute or chronic. It is effective for the treatment of pain caused by a variety of etiologies including malignancies, surgery, somatic, visceral, and neuropathic disease.

Patients having outpatient surgical procedures who experience moderate to moderately severe pain are frequently prescribed an oxycodone product as soon as oral intake is possible. The drug has high oral bioavailability and is well absorbed as either a tablet or elixir. Oxycodone oral solution is particularly useful to treat post-operative pain in children in the outpatient setting. Like many drugs used for children, oxycodone has not been approved for pediatric use by the FDA.

Oxycodone compounds that are combined with aspirin, acetaminophen, or ibuprofen are limited in dose by the amount of the non-opioid component. These combination products provide enhanced analgesic effect with fewer opioid side effects, and possibly better compliance because the patient does not need two separate medications. Use of oxycodone alone may be advantageous in those patients who are at risk for toxicity from NSAIDs or acetaminophen. The maximum daily dose of acetaminophen is 4000 mg in a person with no liver impairment.

Oxycodone IR (immediate release) is appropriate for use in acute pain as in the post-operative setting, acute injuries, or breakthrough pain. The onset of action is within 15 minutes, reaching peak blood levels at 1 hour with a 4 hour duration of action. The pharmacokinetics of morphine IR is similar.

Oxycodone CR (controlled release) is indicated for patients whose pain requires control around the clock on a longer term or chronic basis as in cancer, osteoarthritis, or during rehabilitation following major orthopedic surgery (refer to Chapter 21). Oxycodone CR and IR have equal analgesic efficacy

(10 mg of CR oxycodone b.i.d. is equivalent to 5 mg IR oxycodone q.i.d.).

Contraindications

True allergy to opioids is rare. Hypersensitivity to oxycodone or its non-opioid component in a combination product is an absolute contraindication.

Hepatic impairment

Oxycodone is extensively metabolized in the liver, impairing clearance in patients with significant hepatic dysfunction or failure. Usual doses should be reduced by 30–50% and adjusted accordingly. Compounds that include acetaminophen should be avoided.

Renal impairment

Elimination is prolonged in uremic patients due to increased volume of distribution and reduced clearance. Usual doses should be reduced by 50% and avoided for patients on hemodialysis.

Respiratory depression

Respiratory depression is the chief hazard from all opioid agonist drugs. Respiratory depression occurs most frequently in elderly or debilitated patients, usually following large initial doses in non-tolerant patients, or when opioids are given in conjunction with other agents that depress respiration.

Oxycodone should be used with caution in patients with significant chronic obstructive pulmonary disease or cor pulmonale, and in patients having decreased respiratory reserve, hypoxia, hypercapnia, or preexisting respiratory depression. In such patients, even usual therapeutic doses may decrease respiratory drive to the point of apnea.

Common doses/uses

Although parenteral preparations of oxycodone exist, in the USA oral formulations only are available. Controlled-release forms must be swallowed whole so as not to interfere with the controlled-release mechanism; chewing or cutting may lead to an overdose. Available oxycodone preparations are listed in Table 19.1.

Initial doses of oxycodone IR (all oxycodone is IR unless in the controlled-release formulation) are 5 to

Table 19.1.

Formulations	Strengths	Common brand names
Oxycodone	5 mg, 15 mg, 30 mg tablets	Roxicodone®
	5mg capsules	OxyIR®
Oxycodone/acetaminophen (mg)	5/325, 7.5/325, 10/325	Percocet®
	5/500, 7.5/500, 10/500	Tylox®
		Roxicet™
Oxycodone/aspirin (mg)	2.5/325, 5/325	Percodan®
		Endodan®
Oxycodone/ibuprophen (mg)	5/400	Combunox
		Roxiprin®
Oxycodone oral solution	1 mg/mL	Roxicodone®
		Percolone®
Oxycodone oral concentrate solution	5 mg/mL	Roxicodone Intensol®
		Oxyfast®
		Oxydose™
Oxycodone CR	10 mg, 15 mg, 20 mg, 30 mg, 40 mg, 60 mg[a], 80 mg[a], 160 mg[a]	OxyContin®

[a] 60, 80, 160 mg strengths to be used in opioid-tolerant patients only. The 160 mg tablets are no longer available in the USA.

15 mg every 4 hours. It is recommended to start with an immediate-release product and titrate to adequate pain relief. When pain control is achieved, the conversion to a controlled-release oxycodone is suggested to improve compliance and avoid fluctuating blood levels in patients with long-term pain management needs. The total daily dose is closely equivalent whether IR or CR. For example, oxycodone 20 mg q.i.d is equivalent to 40 mg oxycodone CR b.i.d. Some patients may require an additional dose of an IR product in between the b.i.d. dosing for breakthrough pain.

The pediatric dose published in the Harriet Lane Handbook is 0.05–0.15 mg/kg q 4–6 hours. It is useful in young children who cannot swallow capsules or tablets and in older pediatric patients having painful procedures, particularly tonsillectomies. (As stated above, oxycodone is not FDA approved for children.)

Potential advantages

Oxycodone provides rapid onset of analgesic effect following oral administration.

A number of studies have shown fewer hallucinations and less nausea and pruritus when oxycodone is compared to morphine. There is less inter-individual variability in plasma levels with oxycodone because of its higher and more predictable oral bioavailability.

Potential disadvantages

According to a US Veterans Administration study, oxycodone CR is a higher-priced option when compared to both morphine CR and methadone.

The use of oxycodone (as well as some other opioids) has been associated with causing the "serotonin syndrome" in susceptible patients taking antidepressants of the SSRI class.

Oxycodone may also decrease the bioavailability of cyclosporine in renal transplant patients.

Oxycodone compounds containing acetaminophen can be overprescribed and overused, increasing the risk of hepatotoxicity. The FDA has recommended removal of acetaminophen or a marked reduction in compounded dose.

Oxycodone compounds containing aspirin increase risks of gastric irritation and bleeding.

Oxycodone CR contains a relatively large dose of drug per tablet, which when chewed or crushed provides rapid release of the total dose.

Drug-related adverse events

Respiratory: the most serious adverse effect is respiratory depression, which may lead to apnea and respiratory arrest. Respiratory depression is treated with naloxone, preferably given intravenously, but it may be given intramuscularly, subcutaneously, or sublingually.

Gastrointestinal: constipation and nausea are common. Nausea may be treated with antiemetics, and frequently improves with ongoing therapy. Virtually all patients taking opioids become constipated and do not become tolerant to this side effect. Activation of mu receptors in the gastrointestinal tract slows peristalsis, which promotes further absorption of water and electrolytes in the colon. Patients should be treated prophylactically with stool softeners and/or laxatives. There is an oral oxycodone/naloxone prolonged-release tablet in clinical trials to counteract opioid-induced constipation, which is often debilitating.

Compounds containing acetaminophen or aspirin are associated with respective increases in risk of hepatotoxicity or gastrointestinal bleeding.

Nervous system: somnolence, dizziness, headache, and dry mouth are not uncommon. These adverse effects usually subside over time and can be minimized by slow titration of the dose.

Dermatological: pruritus occurs with all opioids, although less so with oxycodone due to its semisynthetic chemistry leading to less histamine release (as compared with morphine and codeine, which are natural opioids).

Psychiatric: paranoia, psychosis, and hallucinations have all been reported.

Conclusions

Oxycodone and compounds containing oxycodone are widely prescribed and more effective alternatives to codeine. The high oral bioavailability ensures a rapid and reliable analgesic effect, while the adverse event profile, particularly incidences of nausea and pruritus, is superior to codeine and provides improved tolerability.

References

1. Coluzi F, Mattia C. Oxycodone: pharmacological profile and clinical data in chronic pain management. *Minerva Anesthesiol* 2005;**71**:451–460.

2. Kalso E. Oxycodone. *J Pain Symptom Manage* 2005;29(5S).

3. Gallego OA, Baron GM, Arranz EE. Oxycodone: a pharmacologic and clinical review. *Clin Transl Oncol* 2007;**9**:298–307.

4. Mandema JW, Kaiko RF, Oshlack B, et al. Characterization and validation of a pharmacokinetic model for controlled-release oxycodone. *Br J Clin Pharmacol* 1996:**42**:747–756.

Opioid plus ibuprofen compounds

Kellie Park

Generic Name: hydrocodone + ibuprofen, oxycodone + ibuprofen

Proprietary Names: Vicoprofen™, Ibudone™, Reprexain™, Combunox™

Manufacturers:

Vicoprofen™: Abbot Labs, 100 Abbott Park Road, Abbott Park, IL 60064–3500

Combunox™: Forest Pharmaceuticals, 909 Third Avenue, New York, NY 10022

Ibudone™: ProEthic Pharmaceuticals, 530 Industrial Park Boulevard, Montgomery, AL

Reprexain™: Centrix Pharmaceuticals, 31 Inverness Center Parkway, Suite 270, Birmingham, AL 35242

Drug Class: opioid analgesic compound

Chemical Names: 4,5α-epoxy-3-methoxy-17-ethylmorphinan-6-one + 2-(4-isobutylphenyl) propionic acid; 4,5α-epoxy-14-hydroxy-3-methoxy-17-methylmorphinan-6-one + 2-(4-isobutylphenyl) propionic acid

Chemical Structures: hydrocodone, see Figure 20.1; oxycodone, see Figure 20.2; ibuprofen, see Figure 20.3

Introduction

Combination medications, including opioid plus NSAID preparations, are more effective than either drug alone for relief of acute pain, including post-surgical pain [1]. Vicoprofen™, hydrocodone plus ibuprofen, was developed in 1997. Combunox™, oxycodone plus ibuprofen, was developed in 2001 and approved for use in 2004 [2]. Reprexain™ also was marketed in 2004, while Ibudone™ was released in 2006. These combination medications were approved for use for approximately 7–10 days for relief of acute moderate to severe pain. They are not approved for chronic pain management.

Major and minor site of action/receptor interactions [3]

Hydrocodone and oxycodone are widely prescribed opioid analgesics that are agonists at the mu, kappa, and delta receptors in the central nervous system. The cellular changes that occur with agonism at the opioid receptors are still under investigation. However, it is known that mu opioid receptors are G protein-coupled receptors that decrease intracellular levels of cAMP. This decrease in intracellular cAMP inhibits the release of critical neurotransmitters and hormones including substance P, acetylcholine, GABA, somatostatin, and other substances that activate or sensitize nociceptors. Inhibition of neurotransmitter release causes a subsequent decrease in the perceived level of pain by the patient. Also, activation of opioid receptors modifies specific calcium channels at the surface of cells, which hyperpolarizes and decreases excitability of neurons.

Ibuprofen is an analgesic and antipyretic. Its mechanism of action is not fully determined. However, part of its effect is its inhibition of cyclooxygenase (COX) and the subsequent production of prostaglandin. Prostaglandins are lipid compounds that regulate a variety of tissue functions and also cause tissue inflammation. By inhibiting COX, ibuprofen limits prostaglandin production, which in turn limits tissue inflammation and associated pain.

Metabolic pathways/drug clearance and elimination [3]

Hydrocodone and oxycodone are metabolized similarly. Both are subject to a high degree of first-pass metabolism once absorbed from the GI tract. Both drugs are metabolized to more potent compounds in the liver;

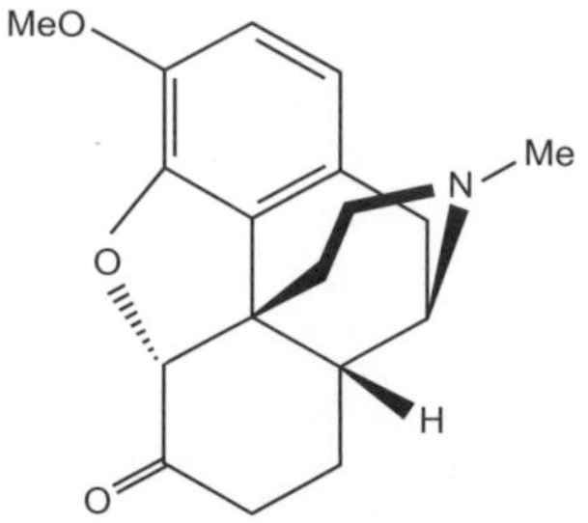

Figure 20.1.

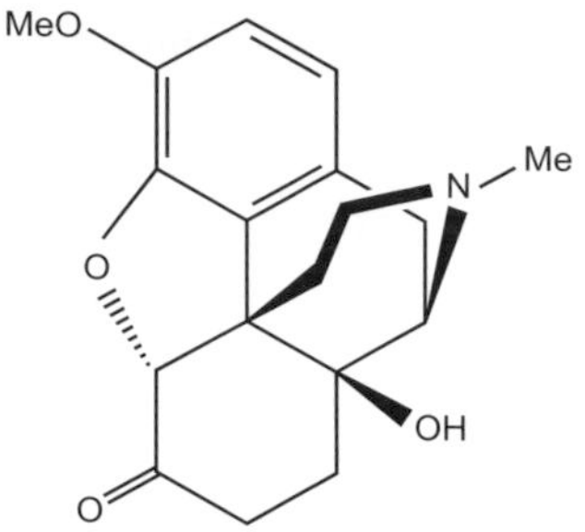

Figure 20.2.

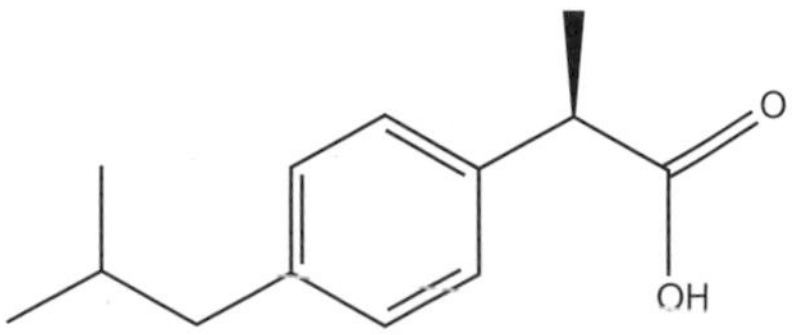

Figure 20.3.

they are demethylated by cytochrome P450 2D6 to hydromorphone and oxymorphone, respectively. Both parent drugs and their metabolites are conjugated in the liver, and both unconjugated and conjugated forms of the drug are excreted by the kidneys and are found in the urine. The approximate half-life of hydrocodone is 3.8 hours, while that of oxycodone is 3.5 hours. Ibuprofen is metabolized through hydroxylation, carboxylation, and glucuronidation. Metabolites are excreted by the kidneys. The primary metabolites are (+)-2-[p-(2hydroxymethyl-propyl)phenyl] propionic acid and (+)-2-[p-(2carboxypropyl)phenyl] propionic acid. Both conjugated and unconjugated metabolites are present in the urine. The approximate half-life of ibuprofen is 1.8 hours.

Indications (approved/non-approved)

Acute surgical pain

Both types of combination medications, hydrocodone/ibuprofen and oxycodone/ibuprofen, are used for pain associated with surgery and trauma in selected populations of patients [1]. They are approved for use for 7 to 10 days for moderate to severe pain. Treatment beyond 7 days is not approved nor is it recommended. Studies have clearly demonstrated that the combination of hydrocodone plus ibuprofen provides a more rapid onset than ibuprofen alone, and a more prolonged and powerful effect than hydrocodone/oxycodone alone.

Cancer

Data from studies on cancer pain treated with combination opioid plus NSAIDs are equivocal. NSAIDs with opioids have shown no improvement or limited improvement in pain control. However, the medications have not been approved for long-term therapy, which probably would be required for treatment of cancer pain. Further studies are needed to determine safety and efficacy of combination drugs in this patient population.

Chronic non-malignancy pain

Studies on treatment of chronic non-malignancy pain, such ash chronic low back pain, showed a measurable improvement in symptoms when patients took opioid plus NSAID combination drugs versus the drugs alone. As with cancer pain, the duration of treatment in the studies was short (8 days). It is reasonable to suspect that longer duration of therapy would be necessary in these patients. Therefore, further studies are needed to determine the safety and efficacy of longer duration therapies in this patient population.

Contraindications

Absolute contraindications for both opioids and NSAIDS include hypersensitivity reactions, such as development of shortness of breath, severe rash, etc. Oxycodone and hydrocodone are contraindicated in patients with risk for significant respiratory depression. Because of the inhibition of GI motility by narcotic medications, oxycodone and hydrocodone are contraindicated in the setting of paralytic ileus.

NSAIDs, including ibuprofen, are contraindicated in patients with active bleeding, ulceration, or perforated viscous. NSAIDs are contraindicated in the setting of acute or chronic renal dysfunction. NSAIDs have been shown to increase the risk of cardiovascular thrombotic events, myocardial infarction, and stroke, especially in patients with known cardiovascular disease or with known risk factors for cardiovascular disease. Patients should not take NSAIDS to treat pain in the peri-operative period prior to coronary artery bypass graft (CABG) surgery.

There are numerous relative contraindications to combination opioids and NSAIDs. They include but are not limited to a past medical history of GI bleeding, history of chronic renal disease, a history of abuse of drugs or other substances, a history of seizures related to head trauma, brain tumor, or increased intracranial pressure, or documented urinary retention with use of narcotics.

Common doses (oral)

Combination opioids and NSAIDs are provided in oral preparations. Vicoprofen is supplied as 7.5 mg hydrocodone plus 200 mg ibuprofen tablets. For acute moderate to severe pain 1 tablet should be taken every 4–6 hours. Ibudone is supplied as a 10 mg/200 mg tablet, while Reprexain is manufactured as 2.5 mg, 5 mg or 10 mg/200 mg combination tablets. Each is commonly prescribed as 1 tablet every 4–6 hours for acute moderate to severe pain. Combunox is 5 mg oxycodone and 400 mg ibuprofen, every 6 hours, with a maximum of four tablets daily. Combunox may offer advantages over other preparations since it contains a higher dose of ibuprofen (400 mg) equivalent to doses commonly prescribed for acute pain. It is recommended that therapy be limited to 7–10 days or less.

Potential advantages/disadvantages (opioid sparing/cost and side effects)

As indicated above, combination opioids and ibuprofen are a more effective treatment for pain in selected patients with moderate to severe pain. Marret et al. [7] recently described the results of a meta-analysis of the effect of nonsteroidal anti-inflammatory drugs (NSAIDs) on opioid dose and opioid-related adverse events. Their meta-analysis showed a significant 30% decrease in the incidence of post-operative nausea and vomiting (PONV) with morphine with the addition of NSAIDs. The authors attribute this reduction to the morphine-sparing effect of the NSAID addition on the basis of a documented linear relation between the incidence of PONV and morphine consumption in the post-operative period. Of interest, data collected from 2437 patients enrolled in randomized, double-blind, single-dose studies of the combination of oxycodone 5 mg/ibuprofen 400 (Combunox™) in the ambulatory surgery setting reveal similar results (Table 20.1). The combination of the NSAID ibuprofen (400 mg) with oxycodone 5 mg significantly enhanced analgesia while reducing the incidence of post-operative nausea and vomiting by nearly 50% compared with oxycodone 5 mg alone.

Reductions in the incidences of nausea and vomiting in these studies [5,6] with the combination of ibuprofen and oxycodone compared with oxycodone alone and oxycodone plus acetaminophen may be related to significant opioid-sparing effects. In addition, reductions in the incidence of nausea and vomiting may be related to NSAID-related inhibition of PGE synthesis. Several studies in animal models have shown that the emetic reflux in the medullary "vomiting center" is potentiated by the presence of prostaglandins. Opioids also exert their emetic effects by stimulating prostaglandin synthesis in the central nervous system. It is possible that co-administered doses of ibuprofen may suppress opioid-induced up-regulation of PGE sysnthesis and attenuate symptoms of nausea and vomiting.

Despite these advantages therapy with opioid plus ibuprofen combinations is limited at this time to short duration (7–10 days) because of risks associated with long-term NSAID use, including GI bleeding and renal injury. In fact, a recent paper in the *Journal of American Geriatrics Society* [6] describes updated warnings and recommendations for geriatric patients taking NSAIDs. They recommend a proton pump inhibitor or misoprostol (Cytotec) for GI prophylaxis and regular evaluation of renal, GI, and cardiac

Table 20.1. Incidence of nausea and vomiting in single-dose studies of oxycodone 5 mg/ibuprofen 400 mg [5]

Incidence of event, n (%)	Oxycodone 5 mg/ ibuprofen 400 mg (n = 923)	Oxycodone HCl 5 mg (n = 286)	Ibuprofen 400 mg (n = 913)	Placebo (n = 315)
Nausea	81 (8.8%)	46 (16.1%)	44 (4.8%)	21 (6.7%)
Vomiting	49 (5.3%)	30 (10.5%)	16 (1.8%)	10 (3.2%)

function. Also, it should be noted the recommendations state that patients taking aspirin for cardiac prophylaxis should not use ibuprofen. Overall, further studies are needed to determine whether long-term use is safe or efficacious.

References

1. Raffa RB. Pharmacology of oral combination analgesics: rational therapy for pain. *J Clin Pharm Ther* 2001;**26**:257–64.

2. Hydrocodone and Oxycodone. *Opioids: past, present and future.* http://www.opioids.com. Accessed November 26, 2009.

3. Hardman JG, Limbird LE, Gilman AG, eds. *Goodman and Gilman's The Pharmacological Basis of Therapeutics*, 10th ed. New York: McGraw-Hill, 2001, pp. 587–591, 711–712.

4. McNicol ED, Strassels S, Goudas L, Lau J, Carr DB. NSAIDS or paracetamol, alone or combined with opioids, for cancer pain. *Cochrane Database Syst Rev* 2005; **2**:CD005180.

5. Palangio M, Morris E, Doyle RT Jr, Dornseif BE, Valente TJ. Combination hydrocodone and ibuprofen versus combination oxycodone and acetaminophen in the treatment of moderate or severe acute low back pain. *Clin Ther* 2002;**24**(1):87–99.

6. Ferrell B, Argoff CE, Epplin J, Fine P, Gloth FM, Herr K, Katz JD, Mehr DR, Reid C, Reisner L. Pharmacological management of persistent pain in older persons. *J Am Geriatr Soc* 2009;**57**(8): 1331–1346.

7. Marret E, Kurdi O, Zufferey P, Bonnet F. The effect of NSAIDS on PCA morphine side effects: a meta-analysis. *Anesthesiology* 2005;**102**(6): 1249–1260.

Section 2 Chapter

21

Oral and Parenteral Opioid Analgesics

Oxycodone controlled-release

Amanda Barker, Justin Hata and Eric Hsu

Generic Name: oxycodone hydrochloride controlled-release tablets

Proprietary Name: OxyContin®

Drug Class: opioid analgesic, Schedule II

Manufacturer: Purdue Pharma L.P., One Stamford Forum, Stamford, CT

Chemical Structure: see Figure 21.1

Chemical Name: 4,5α-epoxy-14-hydroxy-3-methoxy-17-methylmorphinan-6-one hydrochloride

Chemical Formula: $C_{18}H_{21}NO_4HCl$; molecular wt 351.83

Introduction

OxyContin® (oxycodone hydrochloride controlled-release, Oxycodone CR) is an extended-duration oral opioid analgesic. It is formulated as a tablet with an outer more rapidly acting component and slower-release inner matrix that provides up to 12 hours of pain relief. Oxycodone CR offer prolonged and uniform analgesia avoiding trough effects observed with immediate-release oxycodone. Controlled-release oxycodone has abuse and diversion liability since the tablet can be easily crushed, and the entire 12 h dose administered nasally, leading to excessive acute effects and potential overdose [1].

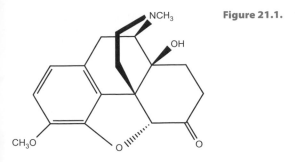

Figure 21.1.

Mode of activity

The pharmacological effect of OxyContin tablets is primarily related to the parent drug oxycodone. Oxycodone, like other opioid agonists, binds to and activates spinal and superspinal opioid receptors. Following activation, these receptors suppress pain transmission at pre- and postsynaptic sites along the noxious transmission pathway. For further discussion regarding oxycodone's mode of action see Chapter 19.

Metabolic pathways/drug clearance and elimination

OxyContin tablets are designed to provide controlled delivery of oxycodone over 12 hours. Oxycodone release from OxyContin tablets is pH-independent. Oxycodone is well absorbed from OxyContin tablets with an oral bioavailability of 60% to 87%. The relative oral bioavailability of OxyContin to immediate-release oral dosage forms is 100%. Steady-state levels are achieved within 24–36 hours in normal volunteers after repeated dosing in pharmacokinetic studies.

Oxycodone is extensively metabolized and eliminated primarily in the urine as both conjugated and unconjugated metabolites. The apparent elimination half-life of oxycodone following the administration of OxyContin was 4.5 hours compared to 3.2 hours for immediate-release oxycodone. About 60% to 87% of an oral dose of oxycodone reaches the central compartment in comparison to a parenteral dose. This high oral bioavailability is due to low pre-systemic and/or first-pass metabolism.

In normal volunteers, OxyContin tablets exhibit a biphasic absorption pattern with two apparent absorption half-lives of 0.6 and 6.9 hours, which describes the initial release of oxycodone from the tablet followed by a prolonged release [1,2].

Indications

Chronic non-surgical pain: OxyContin tablets are a controlled-release oral formulation of oxycodone hydrochloride indicated for the management of moderate to severe pain when a continuous, round-the-clock analgesic is needed for an extended period of time.

Acute surgical pain: OxyContin is only indicated for post-operative use if the patient is already receiving the drug prior to surgery. OxyContin may be considered if the post-operative pain is expected to be moderate to severe and persist for an extended period of time.

Neuropathic pain: patients with neuropathic pain, including post-herpetic neuralgia and diabetic neuropathy, have successfully been treated with oxycodone. Higher opioid doses may be needed for neuropathic pain. Data suggest that incorporation of opioids earlier on might be beneficial.

Somatic pain: treatment with OxyContin for patients with osteoarthritis, back pain and pre- and post-operative pain is well documented. Round-the-clock controlled-release oxycodone therapy seems to provide effective analgesia for patients with chronic, moderate to severe, osteoarthritis-related pain.

Visceral pain: myocardial ischemia, urinary colic, irritable bowel syndrome, and pancreatitis patients have received adequate pain relief with OxyContin.

Cancer pain: OxyContin has been shown to successfully manage cancer pain. OxyContin has been shown to provide equivalent analgesic efficacy compared to CR morphine.

Contraindications

Absolute: OxyContin is contraindicated in patients with known hypersensitivity to oxycodone, or in any situation where opioids are contraindicated. OxyContin is contraindicated in any patient who has or is suspected of having paralytic ileus.

Relative: a single dose greater than 40 mg, or total daily doses greater than 80 mg, are only indicated in opioid-tolerant patients.

Oxycodone CR should be used with caution in patients with certain co-morbidities:

General: morbid obesity

Psychiatric: patients with a history of drug abuse or acute alcoholism

Neurological: head trauma or elevated intracranial pressure, CNS depression/coma, patients with a history of seizures

Pulmonary: COPD, skeletal disorders which may restrict respiratory function

Endocrine: Addison's disease, thyroid dysfunction

Gastrointestinal: hepatic impairment, biliary tract impairment

Genitourinary: prostatic hyperplasia or urinary stricture, renal impairment

Obstetrics/gynecology: pregnancy (caution with prolonged use or high doses at term)

Dosage

Once therapy is initiated, pain relief and other opioid effects should be frequently assessed. Because steady-state plasma concentrations are approximated within 24 to 36 hours, OxyContin dosage adjustment may be carried out accordingly. The usual starting dose for opioid-naive patients or patients presenting with severe pain uncontrolled by weaker opioids is 10 mg twice daily. Dosing must be carefully monitored and titrated. For the majority of patients, the maximum dose is 200 mg twice daily. It is most appropriate to increase the q12h dose instead of decreasing dosing interval. There is no clinical information on dosing intervals shorter than q12h [2,3,4].

As a guideline, the total daily OxyContin dose usually can be increased by 25% to 50% of the current dose at each increase. If signs of excessive opioid-related adverse experiences are observed, the next dose may be reduced. If this adjustment leads to inadequate analgesia, a supplemental dose of immediate-release oxycodone may be given. Alternatively, non-opioid analgesic adjuvants may be employed. Dose adjustments should be made to obtain an appropriate balance between pain relief and opioid-related adverse experiences. During periods of changing analgesic requirements, including initial titration, frequent contact is recommended between the physician, other members of the health-care team, the patient, the caregiver and family.

Most patients given round-the-clock therapy with controlled-release opioids may need to have immediate-release medication available for exacerbations of pain or to prevent pain that occurs predictably during certain patient activities (incident pain). During chronic therapy, especially for non-cancer pain syndromes, the continued need for round-the-clock opioid therapy should be reassessed periodically (e.g. every 6 to 12 months) as appropriate.

When the patient no longer requires therapy with oxycodone CR tablets, doses should be tapered gradu-ally to prevent signs and symptoms of opioid withdrawal in physically dependent patients [3,4].

Potential advantages

A single-dose, double-blind, placebo- and dose-controlled study was conducted using OxyContin (10, 20, and 30 mg) in an analgesic pain model involving 182 patients with moderate to severe pain. Twenty and 30 mg of OxyContin were superior in reducing pain compared with placebo, and this difference was statistically significant. The onset of analgesia with oral OxyContin occurred within 1 hour in most patients.

Although early studies showed oxycodone CR and morphine CR to be essentially equivalent milligram for milligram, oxycodone CR has been shown to have a higher bioavailability than morphine, resulting in an equianalgesic ratio of approximately 2 mg oral oxycodone to 3 mg oral morphine. Because of its greater oral bioavailability, patients may require lower doses compared to morphine.

Comparison studies show that oxycodone CR has an improved side-effect profile compared to morphine with less occurrence of reactions, including nausea, vomiting, pruritus, and fewer hallucinations.

Potential disadvantages

Drug interactions: oxycodone hydrochloride is extensively metabolized to noroxycodone, oxymorphone, noroxymorphone, and their glucuronides. The major circulating metabolite is noroxycodone. Noroxycodone is reported to be a considerably weaker analgesic than oxycodone. Oxymorphone, although possessing analgesic activity, is present in the plasma only in low concentrations. The correlation between oxymorphone concentrations and opioid effects was much less than that seen with oxycodone plasma concentrations. The analgesic activity profile of other metabolites is not known. The formation of oxymorphone and noroxycodone is mediated by cytochrome P450 2D6 and cytochrome P450 3A4, respectively. In addition, noroxymorphone formation is mediated by both cytochrome P450 2D6 and cytochrome P450 3A4. Therefore, the formation of these metabolites can, in theory, be affected by other drugs. Oxycodone is metabolized in part by cytochrome P450 2D6 to oxymorphone, which represents less than 15% of the total administered dose. This route of elimination may be blocked by a variety of drugs (e.g. certain cardiovascular drugs including amiodarone and quinidine as well as polycyclic antidepressants). However, in a study involving 10 subjects using quinidine, a known inhibitor of cytochrome P450 2D6, the pharmacodynamic effects of oxycodone were unchanged.

Drug abuse and addiction

Oxycodone, like morphine and other opioids used in analgesia, can be abused and is subject to criminal diversion. Breaking, chewing or crushing oxycodone CR tablets eliminates the controlled delivery mechanism and results in the rapid release and absorption of a potentially fatal dose of oxycodone.

Review of case reports has indicated that the risk of fatal overdose is further increased when oxycodone CR is abused concurrently with alcohol or other CNS depressants, including other opioids.

This should be considered when prescribing or dispensing oxycodone CR in situations where the physician or pharmacist is concerned about an increased risk of misuse, abuse, or diversion.

Toxicity: oxycodone CR consists of a dual-polymer matrix, intended for oral use only. Abuse of the crushed tablet poses a hazard of overdose and death. This risk is increased with concurrent abuse of alcohol and other substances. With parenteral abuse, the tablet excipients, especially talc, can be expected to result in local tissue necrosis, infection, pulmonary granulomas, and increased risk of endocarditis and valvular heart injury.

How supplied

Oxycodone CR is supplied in 10 mg, 15 mg, 20 mg, 30 mg, 40 mg, 60 mg, 80 mg, and 160 mg tablet strengths for oral administration. A 40 mg tablet of OxyContin® by prescription costs approximately $4 – $400 for a 100-tablet bottle in a retail pharmacy. Street prices vary depending on geographic location, but generally OxyContin® sells for between 50 cents and $1 per milligram.

Drug-related adverse events

Use of OxyContin is associated with increased potential risks and it should be used only with caution in the following conditions: acute alcoholism; adrenocortical insufficiency (e.g. Addison's disease); CNS depression or coma; delirium tremens; debilitated patients; kyphoscoliosis associated with respiratory depression; myxedema or hypothyroidism; prostatic hypertrophy or urethral stricture; severe impairment of hepatic, pulmonary or renal function; and toxic psychosis.

Oxycodone CR should be used with caution and started in a reduced dosage (1/3 to 1/2 of the usual dosage) in patients who are concurrently receiving other central nervous system depressants including sedatives or hypnotics, general anesthetics, phenothiazines, other tranquilizers, and alcohol. Interactive effects resulting in respiratory depression, hypotension, profound sedation, or coma may result if these drugs are taken in combination with the usual doses of oxycodone CR.

Discussion

Previous registry data demonstrated that a subgroup of non-cancer patients reported extensive pain relief and tolerable side effects with oxycodone CR. There was only modest need for dose escalation throughout the long-term follow-up. However, with alarming rates of abuse in prescription drugs, oxycodone CR will continue to result in challenges to many healthcare providers. Physicians should be aware of potential patients who are seeking oxycodone CR for recreational use. Those individuals who become dependent on oxycodone CR may exhibit a trend from oral use to either snorting or intravenous administration [4]. A better sociocultural understanding is needed to manage these cases of oxycodone CR diversion. It is imperative to maintain a collaborative communication between the pain management society and the addiction treatment community [5].

References

1. Portenoy RK, Farrar JT, Backonja MM, Cleeland CS, Yang K, Friedman M, Colucci SV, Richards P. Long-term use of controlled-release oxycodone for noncancer pain: results of a 3-year registry study. *Clin J Pain* 2007;**23**(4):287–299.

2. Watson CPN, Babul N. Efficacy of oxycodone in neuropathic pain. A randomized trial in postherpetic neuralgia. *Neurology* 1998;**50**:1837–1841.

3. Mucci-LoRusso P, Berman BS, Silberstein PT, et al. Controlled-release oxycodone compared with controlled-release morphine in the treatment of cancer pain: a randomized, double-blind, parallel-group study. *Eur J Pain* 1998;**2**:239–249.

4. Aquina CT, Marques-Baptista A, Bridgeman P, Merlin MA. OxyContin use and misuse in three populations: substance abuse patients, pain patients, and criminal justice participants. *Postgrad Med* 2009;**121**(2):163–167.

5. Wunsch MJ, Cropsey KL, Campbell ED, Knisely JS. OxyContin abuse and overdose. *J Opioid Manage* 2008;**4**(2):73–79.

Hydrocodone bitartrate

Edward J. Park

Generic Names: hydrocodone (also dihydrocodeinone)

Proprietary Names: (1) combined with acetaminophen: (multiple different preparations in tablet, capsule, and elixir form) Vicodin™, Lortab™, Norco™, and numerous generic formulations; (2) combined with aspirin or ibuprofen: Damason-P™, Vicoprofen™

Drug Class: opioid analgesic compound (Class III)

Manufacturers: Abbott Laboratories, Abbott Park, IL; Watson Pharmaceuticals, Inc., 311 Bonnie Circle, Corona, CA; Mason Pharmaceuticals, 4425 Jamboree St, Suite 450, Newport Beach, CA; Nature's Bounty, 2100 Smithtown Avenue, Ronknokoma, NY; UCB Pharmaceuticals, Brussels, Belgium

Chemical Name: 4,5α-epoxy-3-methoxy-17-methylmorphinan-6-one

Chemical Structure: see Figure 22.1

Chemical Formula: $C_{18}H_{21}NO_3$; molecular wt 299.3

Introduction

First produced in 1920, hydrocodone is a semisynthetic hydrogenated ketone related to the phenanthrene derivative codeine. It is only available as an enteral agent in oral preparations. Hydrocodone bitartrate is currently approved in the USA only for use in fixed combinations with non-opioid medications as an analgesic or antitussive agent. Another preparation, hydrocodone polistirex, is used as an antitussive agent, again only in combination with non-opioid medications. Hydrocodone bitartrate forms a water-soluble crystalline powder; it is sensitive to light and typically stored at room temperature in a light-resistant fashion. Hydrocodone bitartrate in combination with acetaminophen is a less restricted opioid preparation (Schedule III) and is more easily prescribed in many States in the USA. Because of their relative ease in prescription and perceived safety and efficacy, compounds containing hydrocodone plus acetaminophen have become the most widely prescribed opioid analgesics in the USA.

Mode of activity

Major and minor sites of action

Like all other opioid agonists, hydrocodone interacts with endogenous opioid receptors found principally in the central nervous system and gastrointestinal tract. Analgesic properties are attributed to agonism at the receptors located primarily in the CNS at both the spinal and supraspinal levels, though peripheral opioid receptors may also mediate analgesia to an undefined extent. Through unclear mechanisms, perceptions of pain at the spinal cord and higher centers of the brain, as well as their attendant emotional responses, are altered. Neuronal transmission thresholds and response to noxious stimuli do not seem to be affected in involved afferent nerves.

Receptor interactions

With respect to opioid receptor subtypes, hydrocodone is thought to interact primarily with μ receptors, and the full significance of its distribution and agonism at other G protein-coupled opioid receptors (κ, δ, and σ subtypes) is not yet fully understood. Binding at the μ_1 receptor subtype is thought to mainly promote supraspinal analgesia, while agonism at the μ_2 receptor subtype mediates many of the untoward side effects of opioids, such as respiratory depression and decreased gastrointestinal motility. Spinal analgesia may be the result of interaction with δ receptors, while sedation and segmental spinal analgesia are thought to occur through modulation of κ receptors.

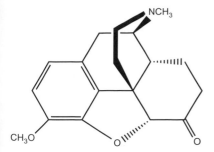

Figure 22.1.

Metabolic pathways

Hydrocodone bitartrate is administered orally, with excellent absorption from the gastrointestinal tract and a bioavailability of approximately 50–60%. Peak serum concentrations of hydrocodone occur after approximately 1.3 hours, with an elimination half-life of approximately 3.8 hours, in normal adults. It is probably metabolized mostly in the liver and primarily cleared via renal pathways. Similar to codeine and oxycodone, hydrocodone is known to undergo metabolism by the cytochrome P450 isoenzyme CYP2D6, genetic polymorphisms of which may explain some of the observed interindividual variation noted with its use. This enzyme converts hydrocodone to hydromorphone, which displays significantly more avid binding for μ receptors and may account for much of hydrocodone's clinical effect. Concurrent use of hydrocodone with medications known to induce or inhibit this isoenzyme may thus alter its efficacy and toxicity.

Indications (approved and non-approved)

As an analgesic agent, hydrocodone bitartrate is used for the symptomatic relief of temporary pain that is moderate to moderately severe, such as acute post-operative pain. It may also be appropriate for the symptomatic treatment of pain associated with acute medical disorders, particularly in the treatment of migraine headaches. For the treatment of chronic non-malignant pain, hydrocodone bitartrate preparations should only be used when non-opioid pharmacological and non-pharmacological modalities have been exhausted and fail to provide measurable symptomatic relief. In the management of severe chronic pain associated with cancer or other terminal illness, hydrocodone

may not be potent enough to offer effective pain relief compatible with adequate quality of life. As with all other opioid agonists, patients who are unable to tolerate the side effects of hydrocodone may benefit by switching to a different agent of the same class.

Currently, hydrocodone bitartrate is available in the USA only in combination with other agents, and its use is only indicated as an analgesic or antitussive agent. On October 1, 2007, only hydrocodone salts or esters prepared with other medications in fixed combinations approved by the Food and Drug Administration were allowed to be marketed by drug manufacturers. All other preparations, without valid new drug applications, would subject violating companies to enforcement actions and penalties. Manufacturing and distribution deadlines for unapproved combinations ranged from October 31, 2007, to March 31, 2008, though preparations manufactured and distributed before these dates were still available for sale for a short period of time that has since passed.

Contraindications
Absolute contraindications

Hydrocodone bitartrate is absolutely contraindicated in patients with known hypersensitivity reactions to hydrocodone. Commercial preparations may also contain sulfite compounds that can produce allergic reactions, including bronchospasm and anaphylaxis, in certain susceptible individuals, particularly asthmatic patients. In addition, the dye tartrazine is present in one preparation of hydrocodone bitartrate, combined with chlorpheniramine maleate and phenylephrine hydrochloride, that is used as an antitussive and expectorant agent (Vanex). Also known as FD&C yellow No. 5, tartrazine can cause asthmatic and other allergic reactions in some susceptible patients, especially those with aspirin sensitivities.

Relative contraindications

General precautions associated with the use of all opioid agonists should be observed with the use of hydrocodone bitartrate; respiratory depression and adverse CNS effects are primary concerns, and the use of hydrocodone should be individually tailored in those patients at risk for these complications, if undertaken at all. Particular attention is warranted in

113

patients who have undergone general anesthesia or are being concomitantly treated with other opioid agonists, anxiolytics, sedative-hypnotic agents, or other medications with CNS depressant properties. As with other opioid agonists, hydrocodone use may obscure the diagnosis and management of patients with acute abdominal processes and may possibly contribute to the development of ileus or bowel obstruction, especially in patients with impaired gastrointestinal motility or those taking anticholinergic medications. It should also be used in caution in patients with liver and kidney disease, as well as those at the extremes of age, as inadequate and/or impaired hepatic and renal function may contribute to toxic effects in smaller doses. Safety in pregnancy has not been clearly demonstrated, and whether hydrocodone redistributes into breast milk has not been elucidated. Therefore, its use should be limited in parturients and nursing mothers to clinical situations where its benefits outweigh the potential associated risks.

Common doses

For the symptomatic relief of moderate to moderately severe pain, hydrocodone should be administered in the smallest dose as infrequently as possible to achieve the desired treatment effect and minimize the development of tolerance and dependence. The usual adult dosage is 5 to 10 mg PO every 4 to 6 hours as necessary, with manufacturer recommendations on maximum daily total doses of 60 mg when combined with acetaminophen and 37.5 mg when combined with ibuprofen. Unlike when used as an antitussive, where the recommended dose for children 6 to 12 years of age is 2.5 mg PO every 4 to 6 hours as necessary with a daily maximum of 15 mg, there is no consensus pediatric recommendation for the use of hydrocodone bitartrate as an analgesic agent. Additionally, in both cases, there are no data on the efficacy and safety of its use in children under 6 years of age. However, some authors and clinicians recommend an analgesic pediatric starting dose, based on the hydrocodone component of various preparations, of 0.1 mg/kg every 4 to 6 hours as needed, similar to the pediatric dose of oxycodone.

Potential advantages

Given that all opioid agonists tend to produce relatively equivalent effects at equipotent doses, combining hydrocodone with other medications that achieve analgesia via different mechanisms of action, as with the commercially available preparations noted above, results in an additive but not synergistic cumulative effect that may result in lower overall total doses of each. This has been observed in studies evaluating post-operative analgesia following abdominal, gynecological, and obstetric surgeries, as well as in one study evaluating the treatment of postpartum pain. Additionally, since the physiological side effects of opioid agonists, as well as the other medications combined therewith, are also dose-dependent, the use of hydrocodone combined with other medications may also result in decreased incidences of these unwanted effects.

Potential disadvantages

Similar to other opioid agonists, the main disadvantage of hydrocodone is the possibility of clinically significant respiratory depression with its use, though this should never discourage clinicians from the appropriate treatment of either symptomatic acute or chronic pain. There should never be a ceiling to the maximum dose of an opioid agonist in the treatment of pain if its use is effective. However, given that hydrocodone is only available in fixed combinations with other medications that may demonstrate significant hepatic (acetaminophen), renal (ibuprofen and other NSAIDs), or other dose-related organ system toxicities at higher doses, its use is necessarily curtailed to the maximum acceptable and allowable doses of its co-administered agents.

Drug-related adverse events

The most common side effects of hydrocodone include CNS reactions (dizziness, lightheadedness, sedation) and GI disturbances (nausea and vomiting), both of which can be exacerbated in ambulatory versus recumbent patients and possibly ameliorated by adopting the supine position. Other adverse reactions include constipation, urinary retention, dysphoria and/or euphoria, rash, and pruritus. Patients should also be advised that the use of hydrocodone may impair the performance of certain daily activities that require increased physical coordination or mental acuity, such as driving or operating machinery. Because hydrocodone is only available in commercial preparations combining it with other medications, such as aspirin, ibuprofen, or acetaminophen, observation of the precautions associated with those adjunct agents is obviously also warranted.

References

1. Barkin RL. Acetominophen, aspirin, or ibuprofen in combination analgesic products. *Am J Ther* 2001; **8**(6):433–442.

2. Golianu B, Krane EJ, Galloway KS, Yaster M. Pediatric acute pain management. *Pediatr Clin North Am* 2000; **47**(3):559–587.

3. Lurcott G. The effects of the genetic absence and inhibition of CYP2D6 on the metabolism of codeine and its derivatives, hydrocodone and oxycodone. *Anesth Prog* 1999;**45**(4):154–156.

4. McEvoy GK, ed. AHFS Drug Information. *STAT!Ref Online Electronic Medical Library* 2009; Bethesda, MD: American Society of Health-System Pharmacists, 28:08.08, 48:08.

5. Tobias JD. Weak analgesics and nonsteroidal anti-inflammatory agents in the management of children with acute pain. *Pediatr Clin North Am* 2000;**47**(3):527–543.

Section 2 Chapter

Oral and Parenteral Opioid Analgesics

23 Hydromorphone (oral and parenteral)

Carsten Nadjat-Haiem and Joseph Rosa

Generic Names: hydromorphone, dihydromorphinone, dimorphone

Trade/proprietary Names: Dilaudid™, Dilocol™, HydroStat™, Liberaxim™, Opidol™, PMS Hydromorphone™, Sophidone™

Drug Class: opioid analgesic (Class II)

Manufacturers: Purdue Pharma, One Stamford Forum, Stamford, CT; Roxane Laboratories, 1809 Wilson Rd, Columbus, OH; Baxter Healthcare, One Baxter Parkway, Deerfield, IL; Abbott Laboratories, 100 Abbott Park Rd, Abbott Park, IL; Barr Laboratories, 223 Quaker Road, Pomona, NY; Richwood-Shire Pharmaceuticals, 5 Riverwalk, Citywest Business Campus, Dublin 24, Ireland

Chemical Structure: see Figure 23.1

Chemical Name: 4,5-α-epoxy-3-hydroxy-17-methyl morphinan-6-one

Chemical Formula: $C_{17}H_{19}NO_3$; molecular wt: 321

Introduction and description

Hydromorphone is a potent semi-synthetic phenanthrene-derived centrally acting opiate agonist. Hydromorphone is very lipid-soluble, which allows for rapid central nervous system penetration. Hydromorphone is second only to morphine in its use as an analgesic in the acute post-operative setting. It was first researched and synthesized in 1924 in Germany, and marketed by Knoll Pharmaceuticals in 1926 under the brand name Dilaudid™. Hydromorphone hydrochloride is a fine, white or essentially white, crystalline powder and is freely soluble in water and sparingly soluble in alcohol.

Mode of activity

Hydromorphone is a hydrogenated ketone derivative of morphine which is about seven to eight times as potent as the parent compound morphine. The duration of action is shorter or similar to morphine at about 4–5 hours. When administered orally or intramuscularly, it retains only about one-fifth the potency of an intravenous dose, and the onset of action is slower, but the duration of action is longer [1–3].

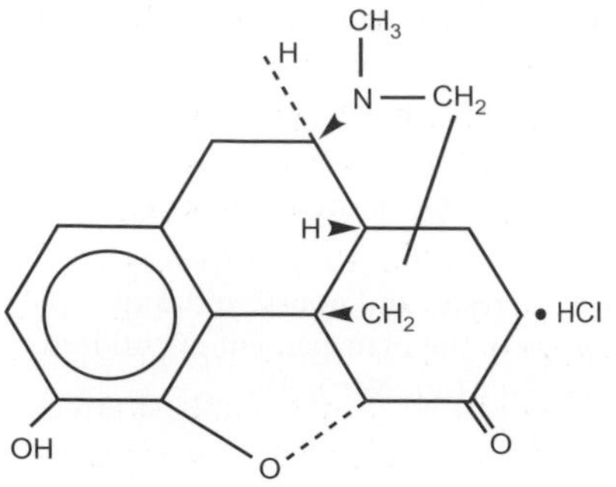

Figure 23.1.

Hydromorphone binds to mu and delta opiod receptors in the central nervous system. It has no effect at the kappa, sigma, or epsilon opioid receptors. Activity at the mu receptors causes analgesia, but also miosis, urinary retention, constipation, hyperthermia, and euphoria. Other side effects such as respiratory depression, pruritus, nausea, vomiting, and development of tolerance are due to binding at both mu and delta receptors. Hydromorphone, unlike other opioids, also has a direct depressant effect on the respiratory brainstem center and the cough center in the medulla.

Parenteral dosing results in initial pain relief in about 15 minutes and a duration of action of about 4 to 5 hours. Oral dosing causes initial pain relief after 30 minutes, a peak of relief after 60 to 90 minutes, and a duration of action of about 3 to 4 hours (up to over 13 hours with sustained-release formulation). Peak plasma levels after epidural administration were achieved after 8 minutes, while peaks after oral administration were reached after about an hour.

Oral hydromorphone has a bioavailability of 62% regardless of whether it is given as regular hydromorphone or extended-release capsules. Food has no effect on peak levels. The drug is 20% protein-bound. The two distribution half-lives are 1.3 and 14.7 minutes. The volume of distribution is 4 L/kg [1,2].

Hydromorphone is primarily conjugated in the liver. Its metabolites are dihydroisomorphine and dihydromorphine. Excretion via the kidneys occurs up to 13% as unchanged parent compound, and 22–51% as conjugated hydromorphone. Total body clearance is 1.66 L/min. The elimination half-life is about 2.5 hours for the immediate-release compound and the intravenously administered drug, and about 19 hours for the extended-release drug [1,4].

Indications

Hydromorphone is FDA-approved for the treatment of moderate to severe acute and chronic pain. A high-potency formulation is available for opioid-tolerant patients. Hydromorphone is used to treat pain secondary to cancer, myocardial infarction, burns, renal colic, biliary colic, surgery, and soft tissue and bone trauma. It is an excellent analgesic if given epidurally after cesarean section.

Off-label use has been reported for treatment of refractory erythromelalgia, and good pain relief is achieved with a combination of epidural hydromorphone and clonidine.

Contraindications

The only absolute contraindication is use in patients who have a hypersensitivity or allergy to hydromorphone.

Relative contraindications:

1. Acute or severe bronchial asthma, status asthmaticus
2. Depressed ventilatory function such as encountered in COPD, cor pulmonale, emphysema, and kyphoscoliosis
3. Intracranial lesions associated with increased intracranial pressure
4. Obstetrical analgesia
5. Known or suspected paralytic ileus
6. Respiratory depression in the absence of resuscitative equipment

Common doses

Reported epidural therapeutic doses for treatment of acute pain in adults are 0.5–1.5 mg diluted in normal saline to a total volume of 5–15 mL. This can be supplemented with a continuous infusion of 0.2 mg/h. The epidural hydromorphone needs to be preservative free, and the standard 2 and 4 mg/mL single dose vials fulfill this requirement. The spread of analgesia can be increased by increasing the diluent to 15 mL, and if epinephrine is added to the solution at 1:200 000 concentration, the onset of action is hastened and the duration of action is prolonged [5,6].

The intramuscular route for chronic cancer pain based on a timed regimen is given at a dose of 3–4 mg every 3–4 hours. Terminal cancer patients may have much higher requirements, and, as with all opioids, there is no ceiling effect. The dose for the acute treatment of pain is 1–2 mg IM every 4–6 hours. Tolerance to this regimen is typically evidenced by a reduction in duration of pain relief. A reduction in the duration of action indicates a developing tolerance to hydromorphone.

Hydromorphone can be administered intrathecally by an implanted infusion pump for the treatment of intractable cancer pain. Clonidine is an important adjunct when pain becomes refractory to increasing doses of hydromorphone.

Hydromorphone 0.2 mg/mL intravenously is used extensively for patient-controlled analgesia (PCA) in the treatment of acute pain. A typical bolus dose is 0.2 mg with a lock-out period of 6 minutes. When used on an as-needed basis hydromorphone is given at a dose of 1–2 mg every 4–6 hours. A lower initial dose should be used in opiate-naive patients. Doses can be escalated in refractory pain. Again, a decrease in the duration of pain-free periods suggests the development of tolerance to the analgesic effects of hydromorphone. Intravenous administration of hydromorphone should be slow over 2–3 minutes.

Oral hydromorphone is about one-fifth as effective as intravenous hydromorphone. Oral hydromorphone used for chronic pain is usually given at a dose of 2–4 mg every 3–4 hours, and as needed. Extended-release hydromorphone is usually reserved for opioid-tolerant patients. Care must be taken not to overestimate the initial dose when converting from another opioid. Capsules have to be swallowed whole, and alcohol use must be avoided due to the risk of rapid release of the drug. Dosing must be individualized, taking into account prior opioid treatment, medical conditions, risk of abuse, type of pain, concomitant medications, variability in opioid conversion, and balance between adequate pain management and adverse reactions. Standard conversion tables can be used when switching opioids, taking into account the duration of action of the prior opioid used. Of note, it is prudent to be conservative with the initial dose, and therefore one has to make allowance for medication for breakthrough pain. Oral hydromorphone therapy for acute pain in non-tolerant patients is usually initiated at a dose of 2–4 mg every 4 hours. Doses may need to be adjusted to achieve at least 3–4 hours' pain relief with a single dose.

Rectal hydromorphone is generally given for chronic pain at a dose of 3–6 mg every 3–4 hours, while the dosing schedule for acute pain is 3 mg every 6–8 hours.

Continuous subcutaneous infusion is an alternative for patients who are unable to take hydromorphone orally. Patients with inadequate subcutaneous tissue, severe heart disease, renal, metabolic, electrolyte, fluid, or coagulation abnormalities should not be considered. The starting dose over 24 hours should be the same as the oral one; however, the mean maintenance dose may be several times higher than the oral dose. The dose is increased by 25% to 50% every 24 to 48 hours until adequate pain control is achieved or side effects become intolerable. Programming of the pump should include available doses for breakthrough pain that are 25–50% of the hourly dose. Adverse reactions of this route of administration are subcutaneous edema, infection, and local inflammatory reactions. The site of injection should be changed frequently. Subcutaneous injections for acute pain are typically stated at 1–2 mg every 4–6 hours.

Pediatric dosing on a weight basis is similar to adult dosing. A typical intravenous dose for moderate to severe acute pain is 0.015 mg/kg, while the equivalent oral dose is 0.05–0.1 mg/kg.

Doses should be decreased for patients with moderate to severe renal and hepatic disease. Also, because of decreased hepatic, renal, and cardiac function and concomitant disease or drug therapy geriatric patients have to be dosed with caution. Other patients who may need lower doses are those who are debilitated, following gastrointestinal surgery, and patients with the following conditions: myxedema or hypothyroidism, adrenocortical insufficiency, CNS depression or coma, toxic psychoses, prostatic hypertrophy or urethral stricture, gall bladder disease, acute alcoholism, delirium tremens, or kyphoscoliosis.

Potential advantages

Hydromorphone is easily available and titrateable, inexpensive (except extended release), and well tolerated. It causes less pruritus than morphine. It is equivocal whether it causes less nausea in cases where substantial doses are administered. Hydromorphone can be used in a multimodal approach to treat both acute and chronic pain. It carries less risk of toxic metabolites when compared to morphine and meperidine in patients with renal disease. Overdoses are readily treated with the antagonist naloxone.

Potential disadvantages

Like all opioid drugs hydromorphone carries a risk of abuse and both psychological and physical dependence. It must be stressed that development of dependence is rare if the drug is used for indicated medical reasons. In acute pain situations the onset of action may be too slow to gain control of pain and may have to be bridged with faster-acting opioids such as fentanyl.

Drug-related adverse events

Hydromorphone can cause significant hypotension, especially if given IV or IM. The incidence and severity are significantly higher than with an equipotent dose of morphine sulfate. The incidence of hypotension when given IV can be decreased by slow administration over 2–3 minutes. Hydromorphone-induced histamine release may be responsible for pruritus, flushing of the face, and sweating. Allergic reactions are rare; pruritus, urticaria, and skin rashes are most common. Gastrointestinal tract issues include nausea, vomiting, and constipation. The risk of constipation is as high as 40%. Nausea and vomiting occur more frequently in ambulatory than recumbent patients. Hydromorphone may produce biliary tract spasm thereby increasing the intraluminal pressure of the common bile duct. This may disrupt surgical anastamoses. Patients with ulcerative colitis may experience increased colonic motility, which in the acute phase may lead to toxic dilatation. The most common central nervous system side effects are drowsiness and sedation, which occur in up to 60% of patients. There are reports of seizures and myoclonus in severely compromised cancer patients. Other central nervous system issues include confusion, agitation, dizziness, restlessness, paresthesia, sensory changes, vertigo, headache, mental clouding, tremor, weakness, myoclonus, anxiety, fear, euphoria, psychological dependence, and mood changes. Genitourinary side effects include oliguria, urinary retention, and ureteral and vesicular sphincter spasm. Respiratory side effects relate primarily to respiratory depression due to a direct effect on the brainstem. One milligram of hydromorphone has similar depressant effects to 10 mg morphine. This depression can be antagonized by titration of the opioid antagonist naloxone. It must be kept in mind that the duration of action of naloxone is shorter than that of hydromorphone, and therefore repeated doses of naloxone may be needed to avoid recurrence of respiratory depression, as well as vigilant monitoring of the patient. Respiratory control can also be affected by hydromorphone, leading to irregular and periodic breathing.

Hydromorphone should be used with caution if other central nervous system depressants are given concomitantly. These drugs are other opioids, general anesthetics, phenothiazine, tricyclic antidepressants, sedative-hypnotics, and other central nervous system depressants (including ethanol).

The FDA labels hydromorphone as a Category C. Hydromorphone readily crosses the placenta. The Thompson Lactation Rating states that infant risk is minimal.

References

1. Micromedex® Healthcare Series, DrugDex® Evaluations, Thompson Healthcare. Hydromorphone, 2009. http://www.thomsonhc.com/hcs/librarian/ND_T/HCS/ND_PR/Main/CS/4A9061/DUPLICATIONSHIELDSYNC/236166/ND_PG/PRIH/ND_B/HCS/SBK/2/ND_P/Main/PFPUI/JbY1nE2XnPyXj/PFActionId/hcs.common.RetrieveDocumentCommon/DocId/0531/ContentSetId/31#all.

2. Inturrisi C, Portenoy R, Stillman M, et al. Hydromorphone bioavailability and pharmacokinetic-pharmacodynamic relationships. *Clin Pharm Ther* 1988;**43**:162–169.

3. Ritschel WA. Absolute bioavailability of hydromorphone after oral and rectal administration in humans. *J Clin Pharmacol* 1987;**27**:647–653.

4. Babul N, Darke AC, Hagen N. Hydromorphone metabolite accumulation in renal failure. *J Pain Sympt Management* 1995;**10**(3):184–186.

5. Brodsky JB, Chaplan SR, Brose WG, Mark JBD. Continuous epidural hydromorphone for postthoracotomy pain relief. *Ann Thorac Surg* 1990;**50**:888–893.

6. Sinatra RS, Levin S, Ocampo CA. Neuroaxial hydromorphone for control of postsurgical, obstetric, and chronic pain. *Semin Anesth Periop Med Pain* 2000;**19**:108–131.

Oral and Parenteral Opioid Analgesics

Oxymorphone injectable

Balazs Horvath

Generic Name: oxymorphone hydrochloride

Proprietary Names: OPANA™ Injection; Numorphan™ Injection

Manufacturers: Endo Pharmaceuticals, Endo Corporate Headquarters, 100 Endo Boulevard, Chadds Ford, PA 19317; Bristol-Myers Squibb – Canada, Pharmaceutical Group, 2344 Alfred-Nobel Boulevard, Montreal, Quebec, H4S0A4

Class: Semi-synthetic opioid analgesic

Chemical Structure: see Figure 24.1

Chemical Name: 14-hydroxydihydromorphinone (4,5α-epoxy-3,14-dihydroxy-17-methylmorphinan-6-one hydrochloride)

Chemical Formula: $C_{17}H_{19}NO_4$; molecular weight: 337.80

Introduction

Oxymorphone hydrochloride is a potent, semi-synthetic opioid analgesic approved for control of moderate to severe pain. It is a white or slightly off-white, odorless powder, which is sparingly soluble in alcohol and ether, but freely soluble in water. The octanol/aqueous partition coefficient at 37°C and pH 7.4 is 0.98. Oxymorphone is a synthetic derivative of thebane, and its structural configuration is similar to morphine and other morphinians. Like other opioid analgesics, oxymorphone exerts its principal pharmacological effects by activating opioid receptors in the CNS and the gastrointestinal tract. Oxymorphone's principal therapeutic effect is analgesia, but it is also associated with dose-dependent sedation, euphoria, cognitive deficits, nausea and vomiting and respiratory depression. Following intravenous administration, 1 mg of injectable oxymorphone is approximately equivalent in analgesic activity to 10 mg of injectable morphine sulfate. Attesting to the high therapeutic efficacy of intravenous administration, 1 mg of injectable oxymorphone is equivalent to 10 mg of oral oxymorphone [1–4].

Historical overview

First approved by the US Food and Drug Administration (FDA) in 1959, oxymorphone was initially used in postanesthesia care units, intensive care units and in the emergency department for rapid relief of severe surgical pain, and on medical wards for chronic pain flare [4–6]. Sinatra and colleagues have previously reviewed the positive characteristics of the molecule that make it useful in these settings, including its rapid onset, clean profile, powerful analgesic effects, high specificity for the μ receptor, and increased penetrance to the central nervous system relative to morphine [5,6]. Given these advantages the preparation has been advocated for intra-operative anesthetic supplementation and for post-operative pain management for use with intravenous patient-controlled analgesia.

Eddy and coworkers [7] were first to compare the effectiveness of injectable oxymorphone with morphine in the same patients for relief of chronic cancer pain. Under these conditions 1.02 mg of oxymorphone hydrochloride is equivalent to 10 mg of morphine sulfate. These doses were not materially different with regard to peak effect or duration of analgesic effect. If the dose of oxymorphone was increased to 2.0 mg, the peak effect was increased and analgesia was somewhat better sustained, but the overall duration of effect was not greater than with 12.0 mg of morphine. The side effects of equipotent analgesic doses were slightly less for oxymorphone; at least there appeared to be less nausea and vomiting. As might be expected, increases in oxymorphone dose, compared in the same patients, increases the side effects and may be accompanied by severe respiratory depression in debilitated individuals, possibly to a greater extent than with morphine.

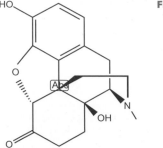

Figure 24.1.

Robinson et al. [8] noted that oxymorphone injectable was less likely to release histamine in dogs than equivalent doses of morphine. Since cardiovascular effects associated with histamine release (vasodilatation, hypotension) are minimal with oxymorphone this opioid may offer safety advantages for patients presenting with cardio- and cerebrovascular disease.

The safety and efficacy of fentanyl and oxymorphone, used as adjuncts in general anesthesia, were studied in 39 patients undergoing elective gynecological surgery of at least 2 hours duration [6]. It was found that less narcotic and recovery room analgesics were required in the oxymorphone-treated group. On the other hand, decreased naloxone requirements and a more rapid emergence suggested that fentanyl was a safer agent when administered in relatively unrestricted fashion.

Oxymorphone has also been evaluated for use as a post-operative analgesic [9,10]. Seventy-five patients ($n = 75$) recovering from elective cesarean delivery were randomly assigned to receive one of three opioid analgesics, oxymorphone, morphine or meperidine, via patient-controlled analgesia (PCA). After adjusting for potency, no differences in 24-h dose requirements were noted between treatment groups (NS). However, onset of analgesia was most rapid with oxymorphone. Oxymorphone was associated with a higher incidence of nausea and vomiting, whereas increased sedation and pruritus were noted with morphine. Whereas morphine is a more commonly utilized PCA analgesic, the excellent analgesia, low incidence of sedation, and high patient satisfaction provided by oxymorphone suggested a useful alternative [9].

In a follow-up clinical trial, the analgesic efficacy and adverse effects of morphine and oxymorphone in patients who received traditional PCA following cesarean delivery were compared with those in patients receiving the same agents via PCA plus basal opioid infusion (PCA + BI) [10]. Patients utilizing PCA + BI noted significant reductions in resting pain scores with oxymorphone and decreased pain during movement with both opioids when compared with individuals using PCA alone. There were no significant differences between treatment groups in 24-h dose requirements or patient satisfaction with therapy [10].

Oxymorphone has also been evaluated for subcutaneous administration. White [11] evaluated 120 patients undergoing major orthopedic, urological or gynecological procedures who were randomly assigned to receive either morphine or oxymorphone post-operatively using a patient-controlled analgesic (PCA) delivery system. The opioid analgesic was administered either intravenously (IV-PCA) or subcutaneously (SQ-PCA) during the 72-h study period. The average morphine and oxymorphone dose requirements were significantly higher with SQ-PCA when compared to IV-PCA. Post-operative analgesia scores and patient satisfaction were similar in all four PCA treatment groups. Thus SQ-PCA with either oxymorphone or morphine represents a clinically acceptable alternative to IV-PCA in the treatment of post-operative pain, particularly in patients with poor intravenous access.

Clinical pharmacology

Like other potent opioid agonists, oxymorphone provides dose-dependent analgesia, sedation, euphoria, and respiratory depression by binding and activating mu opioid receptors located in brain, brainstem and spinal cord. Activation of mu receptors in the medulla oblongata results in depression of the cough reflex and provocation of nausea and vomiting. Minor sites of action include the gastrointestinal tract where oxymorphone increases smooth muscle tone, decreases motility, and causes constipation.

Oxymorphone has minimal effects on peripheral vascular resistance and is associated with less histamine release than morphine. Oxymorphone's clearance and elimination kinetics are similar to hydromorphone. Average time to onset following IM and SQ administration is 5–15 minutes with a duration of action of 3.5 h. The drug is primarily metabolized in the liver, and is primarily conjugated with glucuronic acid. Oxymorphone is excreted primarily via the kidneys, renal, and with bile. Thirty-three to 38% of the drug is excreted as oxymorphone-3-glucuronide, with less than 1% excreted unchanged.

Oxymorphone is also produced as a metabolite of oxycodone – the liver metabolises oxycodone by means of O-demethylation and it is catalysed by cytochrome P450–2D6.

Indications

Relief of moderate to severe acute pain, surgical pain, medical pain, chronic non-malignancy pain, cancer pain and labor pain.

Contraindications

Known hypersensitivity to oxymorphone hydrochloride, morphine analogs such as codeine, or any of the other ingredients of OPANA, moderate or severe hepatic impairment and any situation where opioids are contraindicated such as: patients with respiratory depression (in the absence of resuscitative equipment or in unmonitored settings), acute or severe bronchial asthma, hypercarbia, and in any patient who has or is suspected of having paralytic ileus.

Common doses/uses

Acute pain management

Injectable oxymorphone may be employed as a substitute for morphine or hydromorphone intra-operatively and for post-surgical pain management. Subcutaneous or intramuscular oxymorphone should initially be administered as 1 mg to 1.5 mg doses repeated every 4 to 6 hours as needed. Intravenous oxymorphone can be administered in doses of 0.5 mg. In non-debilitated patients the dosages can be titrated to 1.5–2.5mg until satisfactory pain relief is obtained. Oxymorphone's rapid onset-to-peak effect offers clinical advantages for patients experiencing very severe pain. Onset is noted within 5 minutes, and, unlike fentanyl, the duration of effect may be prolonged for several hours [5]. Rather than spending time titrating morphine to

patients recovering from extremely painful procedures or those with high-grade opioid tolerance, 1–2 mg of IV oxymorphone can be administered to rapidly establish a powerful level of analgesia.

IV-PCA

PCA syringe concentration is generally 0.2–0.3 mg per mL. This requires that up to 10 ampoules be opened and diluted with saline to make up a standard 30 mL PCA syringe. Earlier clinical trials employed oxymorphone PCA doses of 0.3 mg with a 6–8 minute lockout interval [9,10]. This dose was associated with a high incidence of nausea and vomiting, particularly when a 0.3 mg/hour basal infusion was employed [11]. To reduce adverse events, we recommend lower doses of 0.1–0.2 mg every 6 min. PCA dosing guidelines for oxymorphone are presented in Table 24.1.

Labor analgesia

Injectable oxymorphone in doses of 0.5–1 mg may be administered for analgesia during labor. OPANA injection should be used with caution during labor. Sinusoidal fetal heart rate patterns may occur with the use of opioid analgesics. Opioids cross the placenta and may produce respiratory depression and psychophysiological effects in neonates. Neonates whose mothers received opioid analgesics during labor should be observed closely for signs of respiratory depression. A specific opioid antagonist, such as naloxone or nalmefene, should be available for reversal of opioid-induced respiratory depression.

It is not known whether oxymorphone is excreted in human milk. Because many drugs, including some opioids, are excreted in human milk, caution should be exercised when OPANA injection is administered to a nursing woman. Ordinarily, nursing should not be undertaken while a patient is receiving oxymor-

Table 24.1. Oxymorphone doses for IV-PCA

Route	Dose	Dose/Frequency	Note
IV-PCA (opioid-naive patients)	0.5–1.5 mg loading dose	0.1–0.2 mg every 6–8 min	May provide basal infusion of 0.1–0.2 mg/h[a]
IV –PCA (opioid-tolerant patients)	1.5–3 mg loading dose	0.3–0.5 mg every 6–8 min[b]	Provide basal infusion of 0.3–0.5 mg/h [b]

[a]May increase the incidence of nausea and vomiting.
[b]Higher doses may be required.

Table 24.2. Injectable oxymorphone dosing

Route	Dose	Frequency	Note
IV (opioid-naive patients)	0.5–1.5 mg	Every 4 hours	In opioid-naive patients, titrate the dose based on the patient's response to the initial dose, pain intensity and adverse reactions
IM/SC	1–1.5 mg	Every 4–6 hours	
IV (opioid-tolerant patients)	1.5–3 mg initial dose	Every 3–4 h	Cautious increase until satisfactory pain relief

General consideration: oxymorphone should be started at 1/3 to 1/2 of the usual dose in patients who are concurrently receiving other CNS depressants including sedatives or hypnotics, general anesthetics, phenothiazines, tranquilizers, and alcohol, because respiratory depression, hypotension, and profound sedation or coma may result. No specific interaction between oxymorphone and monoamine oxidase inhibitors has been observed, but caution in the use of any opioid in patients taking this class of drugs is appropriate.

phone because of the possibility of sedation and/or respiratory depression in the infant.

Conversion from oral OPANA to OPANA Injection

Oxymorphone's absolute oral bioavailability is very low, and is equivalent to 10% of that observed with intravenous dosing. Patients receiving oral doses of OPANA IR may be converted to OPANA Injection by administering one-tenth the patient's total daily oral oxymorphone dose as OPANA Injection in four or six equally divided doses. Patients receiving 10 mg oral oxymorphone (OPANA IR) every 4–6 hours (40 mg total daily dose) may be converted to injectable oxymorphone 1 mg every 4–6 hours or 4–5 mg total daily. Due to patient variability with regard to opioid analgesic response, upon conversion patients should be closely monitored to ensure adequate analgesia and to minimize side effects. Safety and effectiveness of OPANA Injection in pediatric patients below the age of 18 years have not been established. Intravenous dosing guidelines are presented in Table 24.2.

Preparations

Oxymorphone is available for oral, rectal, and parenteral administration. Oxymorphone injectable (OPANA Injection™) is available in 1 mL ampoules containing 1 mg/mL oxymorphone hydrochloride. In addition, each 1 mg/mL ampule contains 8.0 mg/mL sodium chloride. pH is adjusted with hydrochloric acid.

OPANA™ Injection: supplied as 1 mL ampoules (1 mg/mL)

Numorphan™ Injection; supplied in 1 mL or 5mL vials (1 mg/mL or 1.5mg/mL); also supplied as 5 mg suppositories

Price: approximately $2.00/1 mg

Drug interactions

Injectable oxymorphone is not associated with CYP450 PK drug–drug interactions at clinically relevant doses. No dose adjustments required for concomitant medications metabolized via the CYP450 pathway.

Drug-related adverse events

Serious adverse events: respiratory depression, similar to other potent injectable opioids particularly in elderly or debilitated patients. Predisposing conditions include hypoxia, hypercapnia, or decreased respiratory reserve such as asthma, chronic obstructive pulmonary disease or cor pulmonale, severe obesity, sleep apnea syndrome, myxedema, kyphoscoliosis, central nervous system (CNS) depression, or coma.

Major CNS depression may be observed in elderly, debilitated patients, with co-administration of opioid analgesics, general anesthetics, phenothiazines or other tranquilizers, sedatives, hypnotics, or other CNS depressants (including alcohol) and mild hepatic dysfunction.

References

1. OPANA Full Prescribing Information. *Chadds Ford, Pa: Endo Pharmaceuticals*; 2006

2. OPANA Injection: www.endo.com/pdf/products/opana_injection_PI.pdf.

3. Gimbel JS. Oxymorphone: a mature molecule with new life. *Drugs Today (Barc)* 2008; **44**(10):767–82. Review.

4. Prommer E. Oxymorphone: a review. *Support Care Cancer* 2006;**14**(2):109–115. Epub 2005 Nov 30.

5. Sinatra RS, Hyde NH, Harrison DM. Oxymorphone revisited. *Semin Anesth* 1988;**7**:209–215.

6. Sinatra RS, Harrison DM. A comparison of oxymorphone and fentanyl as narcotic supplements in general anesthesia. *J Clin Anesth* 1989;**1**:253–258.

7. Eddy NB, Lee LE. The analgesic equivalence to morphine and relative sideeffect liability of oxymorphone. *J Pharmacol Exp Ther* 1959;**125**(2):116–121.

8. Robinson EP, Faggella AM, Henry DP, Russell WL. Comparison of histamine release induced by morphine and oxymorphone administration in dogs. *Am J Vet Res* 1988;**49**(10):1699–1701

9. Sinatra RS, Lodge K, Sibert K, et al. A comparison of morphine, meperidine, and oxymorphone as utilized in patient-controlled analgesia following cesarean delivery. *Anesthesiology* 1989;**70**:585–590.

10. Sinatra R, Chung KS, Silverman DG, Brull SJ, Chung J, Harrison DM, Donielson D, Weinstock A. An evaluation of morphine and oxymorphone administered via patient-controlled analgesia (PCA) or PCA plus basal infusion in postcesarean-delivery patients. *Anesthesiology* 1989;**71**(4):502–507.

11. White PF. Subcutaneous-PCA: an alternative to IV-PCA for postoperative pain management. *Clin J Pain* 1990;**6**:297–300.

Section 2
Chapter

Oral and Parenteral Opioid Analgesics

25 Oxymorphone extended-release

Steven Levin and Imanuel Lerman

Generic Name: oxymorphone hydrochloride extended release

Proprietary Name: OPANA™ ER

Drug Class: opioid analgesic

Manufacturers: Endo Pharmaceuticals Inc., 100 Endo Boulevard, Chadds Ford, PA 19317; Novartis Consumer Health Inc., Lincoln, NE 68517

Chemical Structure: see Figure 25.1

Chemical Name: 4,5α-epoxy-3,14-dihydroxy-17-methylmorphinan-6-one hydrochloride

Chemical Formula: $C_{17}H_{19}NO_4HCl$

Introduction

Oxymorphone is a semi-synthetic opioid analgesic, which is freely soluble in water. Oxymorphone and morphine share the same benzylisoquinoline alkaloid structure with two ring closures. Oxymorphone has a molecular weight of 337.8, and differs from morphine by a ketone substitution at C6 and a saturation of the double bond at C7–C8. These structural differences make oxymorphone more lipid-soluble than morphine and may account for faster diffusion across the blood–brain barrier. Oxymorphone was first synthesized in Germany in 1914. In 1955, Dr. Ulrich Weiss synthesized and patented oxymorphone while working at ENDO Products. By January 1959, oxymorphone was introduced to the USA market as the parenteral form now available under the trade name OPANA® Injection. Oxymorphone was also made available in an immediate-release tablet and a rectal suppository; however, the oral immediate-release form of oxymorphone was withdrawn from the market in 1972. Oxymorphone ER under the trade name of OPANA® ER is a long-acting oral form of

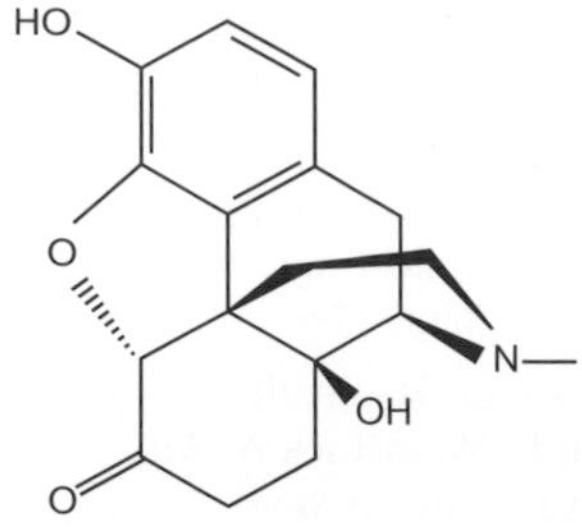

Figure 25.1.

oxymorphone that was FDA approved in June of 2006. The OPANA ER formula uses TIMERx, a controlled release delivery system, which was developed by Penwest Pharmaceuticals Co. in Danbury, Connecticut. The controlled-release technology uses an agglomerated hydrophilic matrix which releases the drug, as water penetrates the matrix, to sustain plasma levels during the 12-hour dosing interval [1].

Mode of activity

Oxymorphone is a synthetic derivative of thebane. It is an opioid agonist which has a higher specificity for the the μ opioid and δ opioid receptor when compared to the κ opioid receptor [2]. Compared to morphine, oxymorphone has a binding affinity that is logarithmically greater and has more specificity for the μ and δ opioid receptor [3]. Oxymorphone has a more rapid onset of action and several times the analgesic potency of morphine. The selective activation of the μ opioid receptor causes analgesia by activating descending inhibitory signals that modulate spinal cord pain transmission. This selective activation of the μ receptor also contributes to adverse effects such as constipation, urinary retention, hyperthermia, and respiratory depression [1]. Oxymorphone's selective activation of the δ opioid receptor potentiates the μ-mediated analgesic effects [3]. In addition, the μ opioid receptor plays a key role in the activation of reward circuitry and subsequent euphoria [4].

Metabolic pathways, drug clearance and elimination

Oxymorphone ER has an absolute bioavailability of approximately 10%. This bioavailability is thought to be primarily due to pre-systemic (first pass) metabolism in the liver [1]. Oxymorphone ER has a mean steady-state plasma concentration which linearly increases with dose [1]. The time to maximum concentration is estimated to be 25–90 minutes for all doses. Oxymorphone ER has a mean $t_{1/2}$ of 9.35–11.30 hours for doses of 5–40

mg, and if given at steady state the $t_{1/2}$ increases to 13.05 hours. Oxymorphone ER has a low fluctuation in plasma concentration when dosed at 12-hour intervals during steady state [2]. Oxymorphone ER has a maximum peak concentration that is prolonged close to 1 hour by co-administration with food. Because of the effect of food on absorption, oxymorphone ER should be taken 1 hour before or 2 hours after a meal. If ethanol is co-administered with oxymorphone ER there is a potential for increased bioavailability and a faster t_{max} [1]. In addition, there is risk from the additive effects of opiates and ethanol on CNS depression, which may lead to respiratory depression, hypotension, profound sedation, and death. Therefore co-administration of oxymorphone and ethanol should be avoided.

Absorption

Oxymorphone ER is absorbed by the gastrointestinal tract. Oxymorphone ER is a sustained-release tablet which has been developed to provide 12 hours of sustained analgesia. The mechanism of prolonged analgesia is due to the extended-release matrix, TIMERx, which delays drug dissolution and absorption of the drug from the gastrointestinal tract. The extended-release technology uses an agglomerated hydrophilic matrix which releases the drug, as water penetrates the matrix, to sustain plasma levels during the 12-hour dosing interval.

Metabolism

Oxymorphone undergoes extensive metabolism in the liver via conjugation with glucuronic acid. This produces oxymorphone's primary metabolites, oxymorphone-3-glucuronide and 6-OH-oxymorphone. 6-OH-oxymorphone and oxymorphone-3-glucuronide are both excreted in the urine and feces. In normal patients, 33–38% of the total dose of oxymorphone administered is excreted in the urine as oxymorphone-3-glucuronide and 0.25–0.62% of total dose is excreted as 6-OH-oxymorphone. The remaining 62–67% of oxymorphone ER is excreted in the feces as its metabolites oxymorphone-3-glucuronide and 6-OH-oxymorphone. Less than 1% of the oxymorphone ER is excreted as the parent compound in both feces and urine [1,5]. In patients with moderate to severe hepatic failure there is significant risk of increased bioavailability, up to 12.2-fold greater than controls, and therefore it is contraindicated in patients with moderate to severe liver impairment [1]. In patients with a creatinine clearance less than 30–50 mL/min the bioavailability of oxymorphone increased up to 65% [1]. Oxycodone, another opioid analgesic, undergoes extensive hepatic metabolism by the CYP450 system, producing the metabolite oxymorphone. Oxymorphone does not undergo significant CYP450 metabolism. The intrinsic activity of the CYP450 system is probably genetically determined and therefore a source of variation in opioid analgesic response, and can alter side-effect profiles. Up to 67% of chronic pain patients are treated with non-opiate medications which undergo CYP450 metabolism [7]. These non-opiate medications can cause either induction or inhibition of the CYP450 enzyme metabolism which can make efficacious opiate dosing more difficult when using opiates that do undergo CYP450 metabolism. Besides methadone, opiates do not induce or inhibit CYP450 metabolism directly, therefore most opioids do not directly affect the CYP450 metabolism of non-opiate medications. Oxymorphone ER does not undergo significant CYP450 metabolism, which eliminates the potential for intrinsic CYP450 enzyme activity variability and drug–drug interactions that could affect its efficacy [5].

Indications

Oxymorphone ER is indicated for the relief of moderate to severe pain in patients requiring continuous, round-the-clock opioid treatment for an extended period of time [1].

Oxymorphone ER is not intended for use as an as-needed analgesic [1].

Oxymorphone ER is not indicated for pain in the immediate post-operative period (12–24 hours following surgery) for patients not previously taking opioids because of the risk of oversedation and respiratory depression requiring reversal with opioid antagonists [1].

Oxymorphone ER is not indicated for pain in the post-operative period if the pain is mild or not expected to persist for an extended period of time [1].

Contraindications

Absolute contraindication: oxymorphone ER is contraindicated in patients with a known allergy or hypersensitivity to oxymorphone hydrochloride, morphine analogs, or other ingredients which are used in the manufacturing of oxymorphone ER [1].

Relative contraindication: oxymorphone ER is contraindicated in patients with acute or severe bronchial asthma or hypercarbia and patients with respiratory depression that is difficult to control,

monitor, or manage [1]. Oxymorphone ER is contraindicated in patients with or suspected of having a paralytic ileus [1]. Oxymorphone ER is contraindicated in patients with moderate or severe hepatic impairment [1].

Common doses and routes of administration

Adult dosing

In opioid-naive patients oxymorphone ER can be initiated in 5 mg tabs given every 12 hours. The usual titration for opioid-naive patients is to increase by 5–10 mg every 3–7 days. Oxymorphone ER should not be broken, chewed, dissolved, or crushed, because a rapid release and absorption of a potentially fatal dose of oxymorphone can occur. Oxymorphone ER should never be co-administered with alcohol because there is a risk of increased plasma levels which can lead to potentially fatal overdose [5]. Patients currently treated with opioids yet having poor analgesic response or intolerability can be converted to oxymorphone ER. A conversion table has been developed to aid dose conversion from morphine, oxycodone, and hydrocodone to oxymorphone ER [1] (Table 25.1) To convert from oxymorphone IR to oxymorphone ER, one can add the total amount of oxymorphone IR and divide that dose into two separate doses of oxymorphone ER.

Table 25.1. Conversion ratios to oxymorphone ER

Opioid analgesic	Approximate equivalent dose	Oral conversion ratio
Oxymorphone	10 mg	1
Hydrocodone	20 mg	0.5
Oxycodone	20 mg	0.5
Methadone	20 mg	0.5
Morphine	30 mg	0.333

Select opioid and multiply the dose by the conversion ratio to calculate the approximate oral oxymorphone equivalent. Sum the total daily dose for the opioid and multiply by the conversion ratio to calculate the oxymorphone total daily dose.

- For patients on a regimen of mixed opioids, calculate the approximate oral oxymorphone dose for each opioid and sum the totals to estimate the total daily oxymorphone dose.
- The dose of OPANA ER can be gradually adjusted, preferably at increments of 10 mg every 12 hours every 3–7 days, until adequate pain relief and acceptable side effects have been achieved.

125

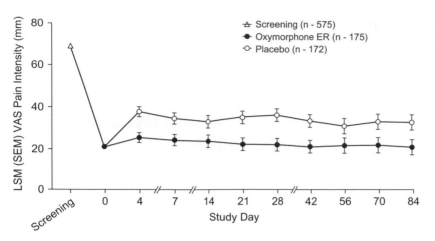

Figure 25.2. Pain Intensity as assessed with visual analog scale scores for patients with chronic low back pain during administration of oxymorphone extended-release (ER) or placebo. Screening = visit before enrollment, day 0 = baseline before randomization; *P, 0.001 versus placebo. With permission from: Peniston JH and Gould E. Oxymorphone extended-release tablets for control of chronic low back pain. *Clin Therapeutics* 2009;31:347–359.

A recent clinical trial of patients currently on chronic opioid therapy provided guidelines for dose conversion as well as information regarding oxymorphone ER's sustained and uniform analgesia effect. Oxymorphone ER was dosed every 12 hours to approximate an equianalgesic dose of their pre-study opioid medication. Patients responding to oxymorphone ER entered a 12-week double-blind treatment phase with placebo. Patients were allowed an unlimited number of oxymorphone IR 5 mg tablets, every 4–6 hours as supplemental analgesia for the first 4 days; thereafter the number was limited to two tablets per day. Seventy percent of patients treated with oxymorphone ER completed the 12-week trial. Oxymorphone ER provided superior analgesia compared to placebo (Figure 25.2). The analgesic effect of OPANA ER was maintained in 80% of patients who completed the study. A significantly higher proportion of OPANA ER patients (79.7%) had at least a 30% reduction in pain score from screening to study endpoint compared to placebo patients (34.8%).

Dosage forms

Oxymorphone ER is available as an oral medication in 5 mg, 7.5 mg, 10 mg, 15 mg, 20 mg, 30 mg and 40 mg tablets.

Potential advantages

The use of oxymorphone ER has a series of potential advantages stemming from issues relating to clinical practicality, ease of use, as well as favorable pharmacodynamic and pharmacokinetic attributes. Oxymorphone ER has high analgesic uniformity, with minimal fluctuations in plasma concentration when dosed every 12 hours during steady state [2]. Such limited variation in the oxymorphone plasma concentration

levels is likely to provide consistent pain relief and avoid the need for shortening the dosing interval as reported clinically with other long-acting agents. Less frequent dosing requirements often translate into improved compliance and oxymorphone ER is very lipid-soluble, permitting a rapid diffusion across the blood–brain barrier, and it has a greater affinity for both μ opioid and δ opioid receptors than morphine, both of which contribute to its rapid and potent analgesic effects. Oxymorphone ER provides linear pharmacokinetics which allow the physician to be confident that an increase in the dose of oxymorphone ER will have an equal and predictable increase in the plasma drug concentration. Oxymorphone ER does not undergo significant CYP450 metabolism. Oxymorphone ER is less likely to have drug–drug interactions and eliminates a potential intrinsic CYP450 enzyme activity variability that could affect its efficacy and its side-effect profile.

Potential disadvantages

Oxymorphone ER is an opioid and there is a potential for risk of abuse and both psychological and physical dependence. The development of opioid abuse is relatively rare when the drug is used for indicated medical reasons and there is no presence or history of substance abuse. Oxymorphone ER, like many other brand-name sustained-release opioids, continues to have a high cost which is a potential disadvantage to patients.

Drug-related adverse events

Patients treated with oxymorphone ER listed the following adverse events as most common (>10%): nausea, constipation, dizziness, vomiting, pruritus, somnolence, headache, sweating, and increased sedation [1]. Patients treated with oxymorphone ER listed the following adverse events as common (>1% to less than 10%): tachycardia, vomiting, constipation, dry mouth, abdominal distention, flatulence, sweating increased, dizziness, somnol-ence, headache, anxiety, confusion, disorientation, restlessness, nervousness, depression, sedation, confusion, hypoxia, pruritus, flushing, and hypertension [1].

References

1. Endo Pharmaceuticals, 2009. *Opana and Opana ER monograph*. Endo Chadds Ford.

2. Adams MP, Ahdieh H. Pharmacokinetics and dose-proportionality of oxymorphone extended release and its metabolites: results of a randomized crossover study. *Pharmacotherapy* 2004;**24**(4): 468–476.

3. Prommer E. Oxymorphone: a review. *Support Care Cancer* 2006;**14**:109–115.

4. Inturrisi CE. Clinical pharmacology of opioids for pain. *Clin J Pain* 2002;**18**(4):S3–S13.

5. Micromedex® Healthcare Series, DrugDex® Evaluations. Thompson Healthcare. Accessed August 17, 2009.

6. Adams M, Pieniazek HJ, Gammaitoni AR, Ahdieh H. Oxymorphone extended release does not affect CYP2C9 or CYP3A4 metabolic pathways. *J Clin Pharmacol* 2005;**45**:337–345.

7. National Disease Therapeutic Index (NDTI). Accessed October 25, 2007.

Oral and Parenteral Opioid Analgesics

Methadone

Keun Sam Chung

Generic Name: methadone, methadone hydrochloride injection

Trade/proprietary Name: Dolophine®

Drug class: opioid analgesic, Schedule II

Manufacturers: Roxane Laborotories Inc., 1809 Wilson Rd, Columbus, OH 43228;

Xanodyne Pharmaceutical Inc., Newport, KY 41071

Chemical Structure: see Figure 26.1

Chemical Name: 6-dimethyl amino-4,4-di phenyl-3-heptanone hydrochloride

Chemical Formula: $C_{21}H_{27}NO \cdot HCl$

Introduction

Methadone is a potent synthetic opioid analgesic, structurally unrelated to any of the opium-derived alkaloids. It is a highly lipophilic, basic drug (pKa 9.2) available as a hydrochloride powder formulation that can be reconstituted for oral, rectal, or parenteral administration. Methadone was developed in Germany in 1942 as a synthetic substitute for morphine, and has been approved and widely employed for opioid detoxification maintenance as well as acute and chronic pain management.

Mode of activity

Methadone is traditionally classified as a synthetic opioid agonist, which binds to μ, δ, and κ opioid

127

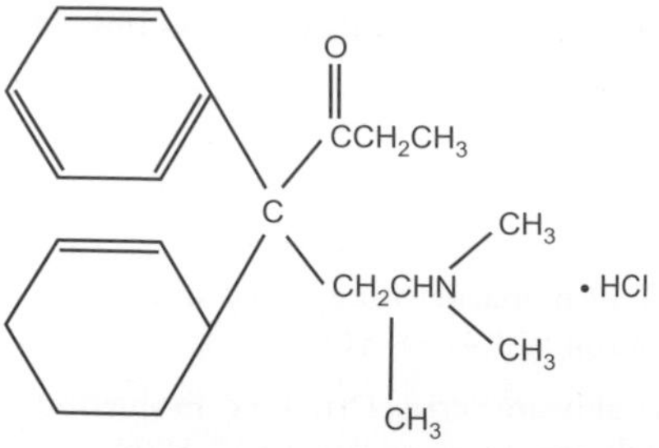

Figure 26.1.

receptors. In addition, it is also an inhibitor of serotonin and norepinephrine reuptake and a moderate antagonist at the N-methyl-D-aspartate (NMDA) receptor. It is, therefore, called a "broad-spectrum opioid". Methadone that is used clinically is a racemic mixture of equal amounts of the l-isomer and the d-isomer. The opioid-like activity of methadone is almost entirely due to l-methadone, while d-methadone has an NMDA receptor antagonist, including anti-hyperalgesic activity and the ability to prevent the development of opioid tolerance.

Unlike morphine and meperidine, methadone is well absorbed from the gastric mucosa, and has high oral bioavailability of around 75% (36–100%). It can be detected in blood 15–45 minutes after oral administration, and peak plasma concentration is achieved at 2.5–4 hours. Methadone is highly bound to plasma proteins, in particular to α1-acid glycoprotein.

Methadone is characterized by highly variable pharmacokinetics and pharmacodynamics among individuals and in an individual as well, which makes methadone one of most difficult and potentially dangerous opioids for most primary physicians to use. Its mean free fraction is around 13%, with a four-fold inter-individual variation. Methadone's volume distribution is about 4 L/kg (2–13 L/kg). Total body clearance is about 0.095 L/min with wide inter-individual variation (0.02–2 L/min). Methadone undergoes a biphasic pattern of elimination, with an alpha-elimination phase persisting 8–12 hours and a beta-elimination phase ranging from 30 to 60 hours. The alpha-elimination phase equates to the period of analgesia, which typically does not exceed 6–8 hours. This probably underscores why methadone is prescribed every 24 hours for opioid maintenance therapy and every 6–8 hours for initial analgesic titration.

Methadone undergoes hepatic metabolism and renal excretion. Because of its ionized and lipophilic properties, changes in the pH of the urinary tract can be an important determinant in the elimination of methadone. For example, at a urinary pH above 6,

renal clearance constitutes only 4% of total drug elimination. However, when urinary pH is below 6, the unchanged methadone excreted by the renal route can increase to 30% of the total administered dose.

Unlike morphine, which undergoes hepatic glucuronidation, methadone is metabolized mainly by cytochrome P450(CYP)-catalyzed hepatic N-demethylation to the pharmacologically inactive primary metabolite 2-ethyl-1,5-dimethyl-3,3-diphenylpyrrolidine (EDDP) with some urinary excretion of unchanged drug. CYP 2B6 and CYP3A4 are the main isoforms mediating N-demethylation of methadone. Interindividual variations in the genetic expression of CYP 2B6 and CYP3A4 is the main factor responsible for interindividual variability in clearance. Methadone metabolism and clearance have been attributed for over a decade to CYP3A4 on the basis of extrapolation of in vitro drug metabolism studies. Nevertheless, a recent study provided robust and unequivocal evidence against a major role for CYP3A in methadone clearance. Practitioner guidelines identifying methadone as a CYP3A substrate and warning of CYP3A-mediated drug interactions require thorough and thoughtful reevaluation.

Indications (approved/non-approved)

Maintenance for heroin addiction

Initially, methadone was limited to "detoxification treatment" or "maintenance treatment" within US Food and Drug Administration-approved narcotic addiction programs. This restriction was removed in 1976; all physicians with appropriate Drug Enforcement Agency registration now are allowed to prescribe methadone for analgesia.

Medical pain

In addition to maintenance treatment for opioid-dependent individuals, methadone is very useful as a long-acting analgesic, particularly for neuropathic pain syndromes that accompany malignancy, and chronic non-malignancy pain, or where the efficacy and side effects of commonly employed opioids are unacceptable. Pain which is poorly responsive to morphine or other opioid agonists should be identified quickly so that futile dose escalation and intolerability can be avoided.

Acute pain crisis in the emergency room

When the patient reports severe pain, uncontrolled with other potent opioids, and the pain is causing the patient and family severe distress, rotation to methadone can provide effective analgesia. When switching to methadone, the equianalgesic ratio and dose are dependent on the patient's degree of tolerance and central sensitization to the previous opioids, and they can vary over 20-fold (see Table 26.2).

Post-operative acute surgical pain

Uncontrolled post-operative acute pain, particularly in patients with a history of chronic pain and opioid dependency, can be quickly and effectively relieved by careful and slow titration of intravenous methadone. Similar results may be achieved in some opioid-naive patients who are refractory to high doses of potent opioids administered in the post-anesthesia care unit (PACU). This author uses 2.5 mg of methadone every 5–10 minutes to extinguish the "fire" associated with poorly controlled pain, and, once adequate analgesia is obtained, initiates hydromorphone intravenous PCA bolus with or without continuous infusion. It is likely that the intrinsic NMDA antagonistic property of the d-isomer of methadone blunts NMDA receptor activation and spinal sensitization induced by opioids (opioid hyperalgesia) as well as poorly controlled pain.

Intra-operative use for prolonged post-operative analgesia

Prolonged and effective post-operative analgesia (median value 25 hours) can be obtained in 40% of patients after a single intravenous dose of methadone 20 mg when it is given as an anesthetic adjunct for painful surgical procedures lasting longer than 2 hours. Supplementary PACU doses of methadone (total 2.5–10 mg in incremental doses) elevates the plasma concentration and prolongs the duration of post-operative analgesia for an additional 7 h or longer. The prolonged analgesic duration with this method appears to be related to a minimum effective analgesic concentration (MEAC) of methadone achieved and maintained by a larger loading dose followed by small incremental doses of methadone when the pain returns.

Contraindications

Absolute: patients with documented severe allergic reaction to methadone.

Relative: patients with known or suspected QT prolongation; patients taking other drugs that could prolong the QT interval; patients with known risk factors for arrhythmia, such as hypokalemia.

Common doses/uses

There is no agreement in the literature and textbooks about dosing guidelines. A safe starting dose in most opioid-naive patients is 2.5 mg every 8 hours, with dose increases occurring no more frequently than weekly. Repetitive analgesic doses of methadone lead to drug accumulation because of the discrepancy between its plasma half-life and the duration of analgesia. Sedation, confusion, and even death can occur when patients are not carefully monitored during the early accumulation period, which can last from 5 to 10 days. In older patients or those with renal or hepatic comorbidities, less frequent dosing and more cautious dose titration are recommended. Dose guidelines for methadone are provided in Table 26.1.

In opioid-tolerant patients, no single ratio is suitable for converting a specific dose of morphine into an equivalent dose of methadone and the conversion to methadone should be performed cautiously.

Table 26.1.

Injection solution: 10 mg/mL
Oral solution: 5 mg/5 mL, 10 mg/5 mL, 10 mg/mL
Oral tablet: 5 mg, 10 mg, 40 mg
Oral tablet for suspension: 40 mg

Table 26.2.

Route of administration	Pain control (q6–8h)		Maintenance for addiction (daily)
	Opioid-naive patient	Opioid-tolerant patient	
Oral	5–10 mg	0.1% to 10% morphine equivalents (lower at higher doses)	30–90 mg
Parenteral	2.5–5 mg		50–100% oral dose

Table 26.3. Conversion ratios from morphine to methadone*

Daily chronic oral morphine dose	Conversion ratio oral morphine to oral methadone
<100 mg	3:1 (90 mg to 30 mg)
100–300 mg	5:1 (300 mg to 60 mg)
300–600 mg	10:1 (600 mg to 60 mg)
600–800 mg	12:1 (800 mg to 60 mg)
800–1000 mg	15:1 (900 mg to 60 mg)
>1000 mg	>20:1 (1200 mg to 60 mg)

Note: because of incomplete cross-tolerance and the non-opioid analgesic properties of methadone, it often has greater analgesic potency than what might be expected. In general, the higher the dosage of the opioid being converted to methadone, the lower the conversion methadone dose that should be used.

Methadone guidelines for opioid-tolerant patients are provided in Table 26.2. Equianalgesic dose ratios for methadone relative to other opioids are variable and can range from 0.1% to 10% morphine equivalents (lower at higher doses). Starting methadone doses should generally not exceed 30 to 40 mg a day even in patients on high doses of other opioids. Methadone should not be used to treat breakthrough pain or as an as-needed medication. Dose conversion guidelines for methadone are provided in Table 26.3.

Intrathecal and epidural neuraxial analgesia

Intrathecal methadone, a lipophilic opioid, is rapidly cleared from the cerebrospinal fluid by absorption into the spinal cord. Consequently little, if any, is available to migrate to and activate brainstem opioid receptors. Therefore, intrathecal methadone produces analgesia by a spinal mechanism and is associated with fewer supraspinal adverse effects than highly hydrophilic morphine. Duration of analgesia is shorter than morphine but longer than highly lipophilic fentanyl because of its intermediate lipophilic and hydrophilic property.

Epidural methadone raises a dose-dependent significant plasma level and supraspinal side effects without prolongation of analgesia.

Opioid conversion

Many opioid conversion charts misrepresent the equipotency ratios of morphine to methadone, as they extrapolate a single-dose effect and are not appli-

cable to repeated therapy and its associated tissue accumulation. Adherence to new dosing guidelines could significantly diminish the risk of cumulative toxicity.

Potential advantages

Methadone has a number of clinically useful advantages:

- Once a day dosing therapy for addiction maintenance
- Highly effective analgesic for neuropathic pain, severe cancer pain, acute and chronic pain refractory to other potent opioids
- Can be administered via the oral, rectal, subcutaneous, intramuscular, intravenous and neuraxial routes
- High oral bioavailability (36–100%) and rapid mucosal absorption
- Interaction with NMDA receptors potentiates its opioid receptor-mediated analgesic effects
- No known active metabolites
- Low cost
  Availability: easily available at most hospitals

Potential disadvantages

Methadone should be adjusted frequently and increases should be based on symptoms and need for breakthrough pain.

Drug interactions

Methadone undergoes N-demethylation via the cytochrome P450 group of enzymes to such a variable extent that there can be inter-individual variability in steady-state serum levels. Thus, there are multiple potential drug interactions with medications commonly employed in pain management. While inducers of the CYP3A4 enzyme, phenytoin and carbamazepine, can potentially lead to opioid withdrawal symptoms, inhibition at CYP3A4 with serotonin reuptake inhibitors(SSRIs) can increase circulating methadone levels, amplify its effects, and possibly induce toxicity. There is also potential instability in methadone's effects related to variability in protein binding, excretion, and equianalgesic potency.

Adverse events

Methadone prolongs the QT interval. Its most severe side effect is the development of life-threatening

Torsades de pointes ventricular tachycardia and sudden cardiac-related death in the setting of a prolonged QT interval. QT prolongation is more likely to occur in patients taking high dose of methadone in the presence of contributing factors, such as cocaine abuse, other CYP450 enzyme inhibitors, and hypokalemia.

Other common/serious adverse events are similar to those described for morphine and include: respiratory depression, nausea, vomiting, dizziness, mental clouding, dysphoria, pruritus, constipation, and urinary retention.

Treatment of adverse events: naloxone is the drug of choice for reversal of respiratory depression, and sedation. Nausea and vomiting are treated with ondansetron, metaclopramide and other antiemetics. Increased QT interval and re-entry type arrhythmia should be carefully evaluated and treated with magnesium and other anti-arrhythmics.

References

1. Toombs JD, Kral LA. Methadone treatment for pain states. *Am Fam Physician* 2005;**1**(7):1353–1358.

2. Fishman SM, Wilsey B, Mahajian G, Molina P. Methadone reincarnated: novel clinical applications with related concerns. *Pain Med* 2002;**3**:339–348.

3. Eap CB, Buclin T, Baumann P. Interindividual variability of the clinical pharmacokinetics of methadone; implications for the treatment of opioid dependence. *Clin Pharmacokinet* 2002;**41**(14):1153–1193.

4. Gourlay GK, Willis RJ, Wilson PR. Post-operative pain control with methadone: influence of supplementary doses and blood concentration – response relationships. *Anesthesiology* 1984;**61**:19–26.

5. Kharasch ED, Hoffer C, Whittington D, Walker A, Bedynek PS. Methadone pharmacokinetics are independent of Cytochrome P4503A (CYP3A) activity and gastrointestinal transport. Insights from methadone interactions with ritonavir/indinavir. *Anesthesiology* 2009;**110**:660–672.

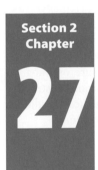

**Section 2
Chapter**

27

Oral and Parenteral Opioid Analgesics

Fentanyl oral and buccal delivery systems

Philip Levin

> **Generic Names:** fentanyl oralet, fentanyl buccal tablet
>
> **Trade/Proprietary Names:** ACTIQ™, FENTORA®
>
> **Drug Class:** opioid analgesic
>
> **Manufacturer:** Cephalon Inc., Salt Lake City, UT
>
> **Chemical Structure:** see Figure 27.1

Description

Fentanyl buccal tablet (Fentora) and fentanyl lozenge (Actiq) both contain fentanyl, an opioid agonist and a Schedule II controlled substance, with a potential abuse similar to other opioid analgesics. Fentora is formulated as a tablet meant to be placed in the oral cavity for a period sufficient to allow disintegration of the tablet and absorption of fentanyl across the oral mucosa.

Fentanyl oralet (ACTIQ) is formulated as a solid formulation of fentanyl, and is designed to be dissolved slowly in the mouth to facilitate transmucosal absorption (Figure 27.2). Fentanyl buccal tablets have a higher bioavailability of fentanyl than fentanyl oralet so they are not equivalent on a µg per µg basis.

Mode of activity

Major and minor sites of action: spinal and supraspinal opioid receptors. Fentanyl, the active ingredient in both fentora (fentanyl buccal tablets) and Actiq

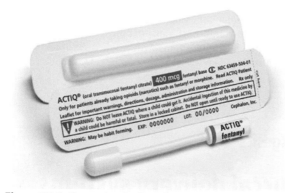

Figure 27.1.

Figure 27.2. Fentanyl oralet (Actiq™).

(fentanyl oralet), is a pure opioid agonist and it acts mostly with the μ opioid receptors which are located throughout the brain, central nervous system, and other bodily tissues. Effects include analgesia, sedation, respiratory depression, nausea and reduction in GI motility. These effects are dose-dependent and antagonized by naloxone.

Metabolic pathways: fentanyl buccal tablets have an absolute bioavailability of 65% following oral administration, compared to an absolute bioavailability of 50% following oral administration of fentanyl oralet. The difference is mainly due to the fact that 50% of the total dose administered of fentanyl buccal tablet is absorbed transmucosally vs. 25% of fentanyl oralet. The remaining half of the total dose of fentanyl buccal tablets and 75% of the total dose of fentanyl oralet is swallowed and undergoes more prolonged absorption from the gastrointestinal tract. About 1/3 of this amount (25% of the total dose) escapes hepatic and intestinal first-pass elimination and becomes systemically available. Therefore, a unit

dose of fentanyl oralet, if chewed and swallowed, might result in lower peak concentrations and lower bioavailability than when consumed as directed. Fentanyl buccal tablet has peak plasma concentrations generally attained within an hour after oral administration.

Indications (approved/non-approved)

Fentanyl buccal tablets and fentanyl oralet are both indicated for the management of breakthrough pain in patients with cancer and who are already receiving and who are tolerant to opioid therapy for their underlying continual cancer pain.

Contraindications

Absolute: fentanyl buccal tablets and fentanyl oralets are contraindicated in patients with known severe allergic reaction to fentanyl.

Relative: they are contraindicated in the management of acute or post-operative pain. They are not indicated for use in opioid non-tolerant patients. The safety and efficacy of fentanyl buccal tablets and fentanyl oralet have not been established in pediatric patients below the age of 16 years. They should be used cautiously in patients with a history of bradyarrhthymias, or with evidence of increased intracranial pressure or impaired consciousness, or with history of chronic obstructive pulmonary disease, or preexisting medical conditions predisposing them to respiratory depression.

Common doses

The initial dose of fentanyl buccal tablets should be 100 μg. Dosing can be repeated once, 30 minutes after the initial administration of fentanyl buccal tablets, if pain is not adequately relieved by one dose. Thus patients should only use a maximum of two dosages for any one breakthrough pain event. They should wait 4 hours to treat another breakthrough pain event. Patients should be closely followed and the dosage strength changed until the patient reaches a dose that provides adequate analgesia with tolerable side effects using a single fentanyl buccal tablet.

If the initial dose of 100 μg was inadequate, then the patient should be instructed to place two 100 μg tablets (one on each side of the mouth in the oral cavity) during the next breakthrough pain event, while watching for signs of over-sedation. If this dose is not acceptable, then four 100-μg tablets should be given to the patient to place two on each side of their mouth

Table 27.1. Fentora Actiq

Indications	Management of breakthrough cancer pain with Fentora (fentanyl buccal tablets)	Management of breakthrough cancer pain with Actiq (fentanyl oralet)
Initial doses	100 μg	200 μg
Dose timing	q 4 hours PRN	4 or fewer doses a per day
Adverse events	Respiratory depression, circulatory depression, nausea, vomiting, fatigue, dizziness, drowsiness, oral ulcers	Respiratory depression, circulatory depression, nausea, vomiting, fatigue, dizziness, drowsiness, dental caries

during the next breakthrough pain event. Titrate above 400 μg by 200-μg increments, never having more than four tablets in the mouth simultaneously. It is important to minimize having the patient take two different-strength tablets since there is great risk of confusion and overdose.

Once a successful dose has been established, patients should generally use only one fentanyl buccal tablet of the correct strength per breakthrough pain event. Also if the patient experiences more than four breakthrough pain episodes per day, the dose of the maintenance (round-the-clock) opioid used for persistent pain should be re-evaluated.

The fentanyl buccal tablet should not be sucked, chewed or swallowed, as this will result in lower plasma concentrations than when taken as directed. The buccal tablet should be left between the cheek and gum until it has disintegrated, which usually takes approximately 14–25 minutes. After 30 minutes, if remnants remain, then they can be swallowed with a glass of water. Fentanyl buccal comes in five different-size tablets: 100 μg, 200 μg, 400 μg, 600 μg, and 800 μg.

The initial dose of fentanyl oralet is 200 μg. During titration for unrelieved pain, patients should take only one additional dose of the same dosage strength separated by 30 minutes per breakthrough cancer pain episode. If several consecutive breakthrough pain events require more then one oralet per episode, you should increase the dosage to the next higher available strength. A single fentanyl oralet dosage unit per breakthrough pain event should be attempted. Consumption should be limited to four or fewer units per day once a successful dose is found. Fentanyl oralet comes as a solid drug matrix on handles in six different strengths: 200 μg, 400 μg, 600 μg, 800 μg, 1200 μg, and 1600 μg [3].

For patients switching from oralets to buccal tablets:

if the patient took 200–400 μg of oralet, they should start with a 100 μg buccal tablet;

if they took 600–800 μg of oralet, they should start with a 200μg buccal tablet;

if they took 1200–1600 μg of oralet, they should start with a 600 μg buccal tablet.

Potential advantages

Ease of use, tolerability: since both fentanyl buccal and oralet are oral medications they are easier to use, more portable, and require less technical expertise than medications delivered intravenously.

When comparing the two, the buccal tablets have some potential advantages over fentanyl oralets. The buccal tablet formulation is more discreet than the oralet "lollipop". Also the enhanced oral mucosal absorption allows for faster onset of pain relief (5–10 minutes) versus the oralet (10–20 minutes). Differences between the two preparations are outlined in Table 27.1.

Potential disadvantages
Toxicity

Drug interactions: since fentanyl is metabolized mainly via the human cytochrome P450 3A4 isoenzyme system (CYP3A4) possible interactions may occur when fentanyl buccal tablet or fentanyl oralet is given along with medications that affect CYP3A4 activity.

Also both fentanyl buccal tablets and fentanyl oralet should not be given to patients who have also taken an MAO inhibitor within 14 days, because MAO inhibitors have been reported to unpredictably potentiate fentanyl.

Adverse events: there is a greater risk of abuse of both fentanyl buccal tablets and fentanyl lozenges since they are both taken orally. Fentanyl oralet has been shown to have variability in fentanyl availability because of variation in patient mouth surface area, and the percentage of medication that is absorbed through oral mucosa versus the percentage swallowed.

Drug-related adverse events

The most common adverse events seen with fentanyl buccal tablets and fentanyl lozenges are typical of opioid side effects. The most serious adverse reactions with all opiods include respiratory depression, circulatory depression, hypotension, and shock. Other common opioid side effects include nausea, vomiting, fatigue, dizziness, drowsiness, constipation, and headache. Dental caries has been reported with the use of fentanyl oralet. A minor adverse event with fentanyl buccal tablets is mouth ulcer.

Treatment of adverse events

To treat the most serious adverse event, respiratory depression, ventilatory support should be implemented, intravenous access obtained, and nalaxone or other opioid antagonists should be given.

Nausea and vomiting are treated with ondansetron or metaclopramide. Constipation is treated with laxatives or stool softeners.

References

1. Actiq® Package Insert, Cephalon, Inc.; Salt Lake City, UT, 2007.

2. Fentora® Package Insert, Cephalon, Inc.; Salt Lake City, UT, Oct 2007.

3. Simpson DM, Messina J, Xie F, Hale M. Fentanyl buccal tablet for the relief of breakthrough pain in opioid-tolerant adult patients with chronic neuropathic pain: a multicenter, randomized, double-blind, placebo-controlled study. *Clin Ther* 2007;**29**(4):588–601.

4. Lecybyl R, Hanna M. Fentanyl buccal tablet: faster rescue analgesia for breakthrough pain? *Future Oncol* 2007;**3**(4):375–379.

**Section 2
Chapter
28**

Oral and Parenteral Opioid Analgesics

Fentanyl transdermal system

Hamid Nourmand

Generic Name: fentanyl transdermal system

Trade/Proprietary Name: Duragesic™

Drug Class: opioid analgesic (Schedule II)

Manufacturer: Ortho-McNeil Division of Johnson & Johnson Inc., Raritan, NJ 08869

Chemical Structure: see Figure 28.1

Chemical Name: *N*-phenyl-*N*-(1-(2-phenyl-ethyl)-4-piperidinyl) propanamide

Introduction

Fentanyl transdermal system (Duragesic™) is a rectangular transdermal patch containing a high concentration of fentanyl, a potent, short-acting Schedule II opioid agonist. Fentanyl transdermal system (FTS) provides a continuous systemic delivery of fentanyl for 72 hours, and offers additional benefits including prolonged and uniform analgesic effect as well as reduced adulteration and abuse potential. The FTS includes a drug reservoir that contains fentanyl in a gel matrix, a release membrane that allows time- and surface-limited absorption of the drug, and an adhesive backing that ensures that the preparation attaches firmly to skin (Figure 28.2).

Mode of activity

Fentanyl interacts predominantly with the mu receptors in the brain and spinal cord to produce analgesia, euphoria, and dysphoria [1,2]. Because of its low

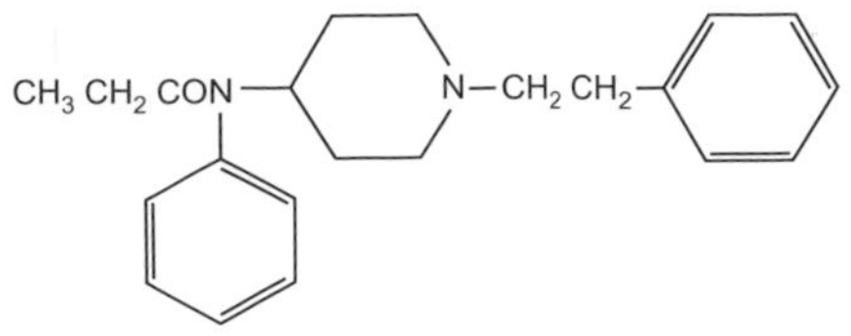

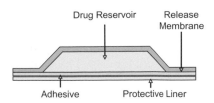

Figure 28.1.

Fentanyl Transdermal System

Drug Reservoir   Release Membrane

Adhesive   Protective Liner

Figure 28.2. Schematic representation of the fentanyl transdermal system.

molecular weight, high potency and lipid solubility, fentanyl is an ideal agent for transdermal application. Soon after application of the patch to the intact skin, a fentanyl depot concentrates in the subcutaneous fat, and it is then gradually released to the systemic circulation. Peak plasma concentration is reached between 24 and 72 hours of the treatment.

Indications (approved/non-approved)

Fentanyl transdermal system should only be used in patients who have developed tolerance to opioids. It is indicated for the treatment of chronic and long-term pain that:

- is moderate to severe in intensity, and
- is persistent, and requires continuous, round-the-clock opioid administration for an extended period of time, and
- cannot be managed by other means such as nonsteroidal analgesics, opioid combination, or immediate-release opioids.

Non-approved uses of FTS include treatment of migraine headaches, post-operative pain, or pain from an injury, and severe but short-term pain.

Contraindications

Fentanyl transdermal system is contraindicated in:

- patients with known hypersensitivity to fentanyl
- patients who are not opioid-tolerant, or in patients who are opioid-naive,
- the management of pain that is acute (such as post-operative pain), short-term, mild in intensity, or intermittent in duration
- patients who have acute or severe bronchial asthma
- patients with paralytic ileus
- patients with significant risk of respiratory depression, especially when adequate resuscitative equipment is not available.

Common doses

Fentanyl transdermal system is intended for transdermal use only. Doses should be individualized and calculated based on the PO, IM, or IV opioid requirements (see below, as published by the manufacturer). Available patch dosages are 12.5, 25, 50, 75, and 100 µg per hour. The 25 µg/h FTS patches were recalled in February 2008 due to a concern that small cuts in the gel reservoir could result in accidental exposure to fentanyl [1].

When switching to FTS, the first step is to calculate the previous 24-hour analgesic requirement and then convert it according to the dose conversion table (Table 28.1). It is important to start low and advance slowly, especially in the elderly, debilitated, cachectic, and those with impaired renal or hepatic function. The mean elimination half-life of FTS is 17 hours, and the shortest titration period is 3 days, but it takes up to 6 days to reach equilibrium on the new dose. In addition, when changing the dose, it may take 13 to 24 hours for the fentanyl to reach the new therapeutic level [1,2]. While titrating the dose, patients may require short-acting opioids for breakthrough pain.

Potential advantages

Fentanyl transdermal system provides a safe, effective, continuous, and round-the-clock delivery of fentanyl. It is ideal for the management of chronic, moderate to severe pain and in patients who are opioid-tolerant [2]. It is best reserved for patients whose opioid requirements are stable. Upon successful dose titration, and once the target analgesia is reached, the drug administration is convenient and subsequent dose titration may be safely managed in an outpatient setting. In comparison with oral opioids, FTS causes fewer gastrointestinal side effects, and, it has an obvious advantage in dysphagic patients or those that do not tolerate oral medication. FTS may result in increased quality-adjusted life-days at a nominal increased cost.

135

Table 28.1. Dose conversion guidelines

Current analgesic	Daily dose (mg/d)			
Oral morphine	60–134	135–224	225–314	315–404
IM/IV morphine	10–22	23–37	38–52	53–67
Oral oxycodone	30–67	67.5–112	112.5–157	157.5–202
IM/IV oxycodone	15–33	33.1–56	56.1–78	78.1–101
Oral codeine	150–447	448–747	748–1047	1048–1347
Oral hydromorphone	8–17	17.1–28	28.1–39	39.1–51
IV hydromorphone	1.5–3.4	3.5–5.6	5.7–7.9	8–10
IM meperidine	75–165	166–278	279–390	391–503
Oral methadone	20–44	45–74	75–104	105–134
IM methadone	10–22	23–37	38–52	53–67
Recommended Duragesic dose (µg/h)	25	50	75	100

It is important to note that the dose conversion guidelines should not be used to convert a Duragesic dose to other opioids, since it can significantly overestimate the dose of the new agent.

Potential disadvantages

Due to the delayed onset of action of FTS, and the potential for serious respiratory depression, it may take a long time to achieve adequate analgesia safely. Therefore, one main disadvantage of FTS is the slow titration process. During this period, other short-acting opioids may be administered to manage the pain. For this same reason, FTS is not suitable for the treatment of acute pain [3]. There are also reports that the effectiveness of analgesia decreases during the third day. Fentanyl transdermal system is also not ideal for end-of-life care, especially in patients with uncontrolled pain.

Drug-related adverse events

The most serious potential risk of FTS is respiratory depression due to overdose [4]. In order to minimize the risk of overdose, the recommended starting dose when converting from other opioids to FTS is probably too low for 50% of patients. Additionally, in patients receiving FTS concurrently with cytochrome P450 3A4 inhibitors (including ritonavir, fosamprenavir, amprenavir, nelfinavir, ketoconazole, fluconazole, itraconazole, troleandomycin, clarithromycin, erythromycin, nefazodone, amiodarone, aprepitant, diltiazem, verapamil, and grapefruit juice) plasma fentanyl concentration may increase and result in worsening and prolongation of the adverse events, especially fatal respiratory depression. Caution should be taken in patients who have received MAO inhibitors within 14 days of FTS use, since severe and unpredictable potentiation by MAOI has been reported. Increase in body temperature, due to fever or exercise, may hasten the absorption of fentanyl and increase the plasma concentration.

Other less serious side effects of FTS include nausea, vomiting, constipation, drowsiness, dry mouth, sweating, and pruritus.

Treatment of adverse events

Naloxone is the drug of choice for the treatment of respiratory depression. Due to the long half-life of Duragesic compared to naloxone, repeat dosing of naloxone may be necessary, and patients should be monitored for at least 24 hours following overdose.

References

1. http://www.duragesic.com/duragesic/shared/pi/duragesic.pd.

2. Payne R, Mathias SD, Pasta DJ, et al. Quality of life and cancer pain: satisfaction and side effects with transdermal fentanyl versus oral morphine. *J Clin Oncol* 1998;**16**:1588–1593.

3. Bernstein K. Inappropriate use of transdermal fentanyl for acute postoperative pain. *J Oral Maxillofac Surg* 1994;**52**: 896.

4. Horton R, Barber C. Opioid-induced respiratory depression resulting from transdermal fentanyl-clarithromycin drug interaction in a patient with advanced COPD. *J Pain Symptom Manage* 2009;**37**: 2–5.

29

Tramadol and tramadol plus acetaminophen

Julie Sramcik and Raymond S. Sinatra

Generic Names: tramadol, tramadol plus acetaminophen

Trade/Proprietary Names: Ultram®, Ultracet®, Adolonta®, Contramal®, Tramal®, Trodon®, Zydol®

Drug Class: central acting analgesic, opioid analgesic

Manufacturers: Upjohn-McNeil Division of Johnson & Johnson, Raritan, NJ; Grünenthal GmbH, Aachen, D-52099, Germany

Structural Formula: see Figure 29.1

Chemical Name: 2-[(dimethylamino)methyl]-1-(3-methoxyphenyl)-cyclohexanol]

Chemical Formula: $C_{16}H_{25}NO_2$; molecular wt 263

Introduction

Tramadol is a synthetic analgesic that has an amino-cyclohexanol structure similar to codeine [1,2–5]. It is approved to treat moderate to severe acute post-operative pain as well as chronic oncological and neuropathic pain. Tramadol was developed by Grunenthal Pharma and entered the market in West Germany in 1977 and in the USA in 1999 [1–3]. In comparison with typical opioid agonists such as morphine, tramadol rarely causes respiratory depression or physical dependence. Its analgesic efficacy is similar to codeine and propoxyphene. Tramadol is available in formulations suitable for oral, rectal, and parenteral administration. In Europe, patient-controlled analgesia (PCA) with tramadol is used and is well accepted by patients. In the US, tramadol is available only as an oral tablet (Ultram™) or combined with acetaminophen (Ultracet™). Ultracet™ was developed as a low-dose preparation (37.5 mg) which when combined with acetaminophen produced analgesia equivalent to higher doses of tramadol, but with a reduced adverse event profile [4,5].

Mode of action

Tramadol is a dual-mechanism, central-acting analgesic. It interacts weakly with μ opioid receptors and to a lesser extent at kappa and delta receptors. Interactions at these receptors provide weak opioid agonist properties. It also has effects on noradrenergic and serotonergic reuptake proteins and accentuates spinal and supraspinal monamine-based analgesia [5,6,7]. Tramadol's opioid and non-opioid sites of action appear to act additively to provide more effective pain relief. Of the two tramadol enantiomers, the (+) enantiomer acts as a μ receptor agonist and as a 5-HT reuptake inhibitor, while the (−) enantiomer is a norepinephrine reuptake inhibitor [2,5].

Tramadol behaves as a prodrug and hepatic metabolism influences its effectiveness at μ opioid receptors. Tramadol is metabolized by CYP2D6 into an active metabolite that is five times as powerful as the parent compound. This O-demethylated metabolite has 200 times greater μ receptor-affinity and 2–4 times greater potency, and a longer half-life. As with codeine, approximately 20% of individuals have CYP2D6 enzyme polymorphisms that result in poor metabolism. These patients cannot form the active metabolite and are at increased risk of analgesic failure [2,3].

Metabolism

Tramadol is metabolized in the liver by cytochrome P450 2D6 sparteine oxygenase to produce O-desmethyl tramadol (M1). As mentioned above, the desmethyl metabolite demonstrates μ receptor activity that is significantly higher than tramadol. Patients with low levels of CYP2D6 either as a result of genetics or competition by co-adminstered drugs will be unable to metabolize tramadol via this pathway. Drugs that are inducers for this enzyme may increase O-desmethyl tramadol, leading to exaggerated opioid effects. The O-desmethyl metabolite is excreted primarily through the kidneys [1,4]. Therefore, in patients with significant

137

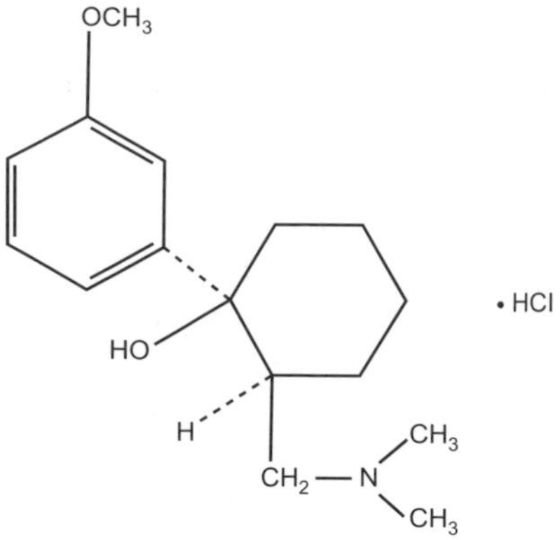

Figure 29.1.

hepatic or renal impairment, the tramadol dose should be reduced. Tramadol plasma concentrations peak 90 minutes following oral administration, and its elimination half-life is approximately 6 hours.

Indications

Chronic degenerative joint disease

Tramadol and tramadol with acetaminophen are increasingly prescribed for the treatment of osteoarthritis (OA) because unlike NSAIDs they do not produce gastrointestinal bleeding or renal problems [8]. Cepeda and coworkers [9] performed a meta-analysis of 11 RCTs with a total of 1019 participants who received tramadol or tramadol/acetaminphen and 920 participants who received placebo or active control. Patients treated with tramadol reported less pain (−8.5 units on a 0–100 scale; 95% CI −12.0 to −5.0), a 12% relative decrease in pain intensity [2], and greater global improvement in stiffness in Western Ontario Osteoarthritis Index score than patients who received placebo. In terms of adverse events, one of every five participants who received tramadol or tramadol/paracetamol experienced minor adverse events and one of every eight stopped taking the medication.

Post-operative pain

Tramadol has been shown to provide effective analgesia after both oral and intravenous administration for the treatment of post-operative pain [10]. Comparative studies have generally shown that tramadol is more effective than NSAIDs for controlling post-operative pain; however, wide individual variations exist, possibly related to low P450-2D6 metabolism in certain patients. A single 100 mg oral dose of tramadol is equivalent to 1000 mg of acetaminophen. At

doses of 100 mg, the incidence of adverse effects (headache, nausea, vomiting, dizziness, somnolence) was similar to comparator drugs. In dental trials there was increased incidence of vomiting, nausea, dizziness and somnolence compared to NSAIDs [10]. In a comparative study tramadol 50 mg was found to be a better analgesic compared to ketorolac (30 mg) for patients recovering from same-day gynecological laparoscopic procedures. Patients treated with tramadol reported lower pain scores in the post-anesthesia care unit; however, the incidence of post-operative nausea and vomiting was higher and recovery time was prolonged.

Co-administration of tramadol and NSAIDs allows the tramadol dose to be reduced and results in a lower incidence of adverse effects. Also the combination of tramadol plus acetaminophen provides superior analgesia than tramadol alone. In a randomized, double-blind, active- and placebo-controlled trial the safety and effectiveness of tramadol plus acetaminophen (APAP) were evaluated in 300 patients recovering from orthopedic or abdominal surgery [11]. Patients were randomized to receive two tablets of 37.5 mg tramadol plus 325 mg APAP ($n = 98$), codeine 30 mg plus APAP 300 mg ($n = 109$), or placebo ($n = 98$); thereafter, they received 1 or 2 tablets every 4 to 6 hours as needed for pain for 6 days. Tramadol plus APAP was superior to placebo for total pain relief, and not inferior to codeine plus APAP. For average daily pain relief, average daily pain intensity, and overall medication assessment, tramadol plus APAP was superior to placebo and codeine plus APAP. Tramadol plus APAP showed better tolerability, as the incidence of nausea, vomiting, and constipation, as well as discontinuation because of adverse events, was higher in the codeine plus APAP group.

Neuropathic pain

Because of its dual analgesic effects, tramadol may be more effective than standard opioids for neuropathic pain. The efficacy of tramadol was evaluated in patients suffering painful polyneuropathy. Forty-five patients were treated with either tramadol 200 mg/day to 400 mg/day or placebo over a period of 4 weeks. Upon study completion, ratings for pain (median 4 vs. 6), paresthesia (4 vs. 6), allodynia (0 vs. 4). and touch-evoked pain (3 vs. 5) were significantly lower with tramadol treatment than with placebo [12]. In an evaluation of safety and efficacy in painful diabetic neuropathy, patients were treated with tramadol ($n = 65$)

or placebo ($n = 66$) four times daily [13]. Tramadol, at an average dosage of 210 mg/day, was significantly ($p < 0.001$) more effective than placebo for relieving diabetic neuropathic pain. No statistically significant treatment effects on sleep were identified.

Oncology pain

Tramadol has been advocated as a safe and effective opioid analgesic for step II according to the World Health Organization guidelines for cancer pain management. Moderate cancer pain can be controlled with tramadol alone or in combination with NSAIDs and other adjuvant analgesics. Grond and colleagues [14] evaluated the efficacy and safety of high doses of oral tramadol (≥ 300 mg/d) with low doses of oral morphine (≤ 60 mg/d). Eight hundred patients received oral tramadol for a total of 23 497 days, and 848 patients received oral morphine for a total of 24 695 days. The average dose of tramadol was 428 ± 101 mg/d while the average dose of morphine was 42 ± 13 mg/d (range 10–60 mg/d). The mean pain intensity on a 0–100 scale was 27 ± 21 in the tramadol versus 26 ± 20 in the morphine group (NS). The analgesic efficacy was good in 74% and 78%, satisfactory in 10% and 7%, and inadequate in 16% and 15% of patients receiving tramadol and morphine, respectively (NS). Constipation and pruritus and the need for antiemetics were more frequent in the morphine group. The authors concluded that tramadol can be used for the treatment of moderate cancer pain, when non-opioids alone are not effective. Tramadol may be less effective in patients with severe and progressive cancer pain, and analgesic therapy may need to be advanced to a more potent opioid.

Adverse events

Tramadol is usually well tolerated; like most opioids, the main adverse reactions are gastrointestinal, and include nausea and vomiting. Other common adverse effects may include, dizziness, sedation, dry mouth, sweating, hypertension, and seizures. Although the risk of seizures is low, tramadol should be avoided in epileptics, and with concomitant use of drugs that lower seizure threshold. Like other opioids it should be avoided in patients with elevated ICP (intracranial pressure). Tramadol is contraindicated in patients taking MAO (monoamine oxidase) inhibitors as it may induce psychotic behavior. In acute pain settings, doses of tramadol should not exceed 300 mg/day. Co-administration of tramadol may increase plasma concentrations of digoxin and warfarin to toxic levels [15].

Advantages

(1) Because of its dual site of action pharmacology, tramadol is less likely to be associated with mu receptor-mediated respiratory depression, constipation, and abuse when compared to pure mu agonists. These qualities may make this drug choice more advantageous for elderly and high-risk patients with moderate pain.

(2) Although respiratory depression is unlikely following oral administration it has been observed in patients treated with intravenous tramadol. In the EU, tramadol is available for intravenous use and is used as an analgesic for childbirth and post-operative analgesia. When administered during labor, tramadol does not cause respiratory depression in neonates [3,15].

(3) Tramadol has negligible abuse potential, and is a less restricted, easily prescribed analgesic.

Disadvantages

(1) Unlike potent opioids that provide dose-dependent increases in analgesic effect, tramadol is a comparatively weak analgesic not suitable for patients with very severe pain.

(2) One of the main issues related to tramadol is the fact that it blocks serotonin reuptake and may cause serotonin syndrome in susceptible patients. Serotonin syndrome is characterized by neurological and cardiovascular stimulation, and can lead to seizures and death. Risks of developing serotonin syndrome are increased in patients treated with selective serotonin reuptake inhibitors and serotonin and norepinephrine reuptake inhibitors.

Contraindications

Absolute: tramadol should not be administered to patients with documented intolerance to the drug. It should not be administered to patients currently taking MAO inhibitors, or patients with documented histories of serotonin syndrome.

Relative: renal failure, hepatic failure, patients with seizure disorders, patients treated with SSRIs and NSRIs, patients taking coumadin or warfarin (dose reduction are required).

Preparations

Tramadol is supplied in 50 mg tablets. Tramadol extended release is supplied in 100 mg, 200 mg, and 300 mg tablets. Tramadol plus acetaminophen is available in a dose of 37.5 mg plus 325 mg of APAP. The recommended dosage is 50–100 mg orally every 4–6 hours as needed for pain. The maximum dose should not exceed

400 mg in 24 hours. In the USA, tramadol is available only in oral form and is prescribed for patients 16 years of age and older. In Europe, tramadol is used orally and parenterally in children under age 16 and adults [3,15].

References

1. Bamigbade TA, Langford RM. The clinical use of tramadol hydrochloride. *Pain Rev* 1998;**5**(3):155–182.

2. Dayer P, Desmeules J, Collart L. Pharmacology of tramadol. *Drugs* 1997;**53**(Suppl. 2):18–24.

3. Desmeules JA. The tramadol option. *Eur J Pain* 2000;**4** (Suppl. A):15–21.

4. Sinatra RS, Sramcik J. Tramadol: its use in pain management. In Hines RL, ed. *Anesthesiology Clinics of North America,* vol. 2. Philadelphia: W.B. Saunders, 1998, pp. 53–69.

5. Klotz U. Tramadol–the impact of it's pharmokinetic and pharmacodynamic properties on the management of pain. *Arzneim. Forsch./Drug Res* 2003;**53**(10):681–687.

6. Marcou TA, Marque S, Mazoit JX. The median effective dose of tramadol and morphine for post-operative patients: a study of interactions. *Anesth Analg* 2005;**100**:469–474.

7. Raffa, RB, Friderichs E, Reinann W. Opioid and nonopioid components independently contribute to the mechanism of action of tramadol, an 'atypical' opioid analgesic. *J Pharmacol Exp Ther* 1992;**260**:275–285.

8. Reig E. Tramadol in musculoskeletal pain- a survey. *Clin Rheumatol* 2002;Suppl.

9. Cepeda SM, Carmargo F, Zea C, Valencia L. Tramadol for osteoarthritis: a systematic review and metaanalysis. *J Rheumatol* 2007;**34**(3):543–555.

10. Scott LJ, Perry CM Tramadol. A review of its use in perioperative pain. *Drugs* 2000;60.

11. Smith AB, Ravikumuar T, Kamin M, et al. Combination tramadol plus acetaminophen for postsurgical pain. *Am J Surg* 2004;**187**;521–527.

12. Harati Y, Gooch D, Swenson M. Double blind randomized trial of tramadol for the treatment of diabetic neuropathy. *Neurology* 1998;**50**(6):1842–1846.

13. Sindrupab H, Andersen G, Madsen C. Tramadol relieves pain and allodynia in polyneuropathy: a randomised, double-blind, controlled trial. *Pain* 1999;**83**:85–90.

14. Grond S, Radbruch L, Meuser T, et al. High-dose tramadol in comparison to low-dose morphine for cancer pain relief. *J Pain Symptom Manage* 1999;**18**:174–179.

15. Dayer P, Desmules J, Collart L. Pharmacology of tramadol. *Drugs* 1997;**53**(Suppl 2):18–243.

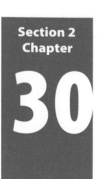

Section 2 Chapter

30

Oral and Parenteral Opioid Analgesics

Tramadol extended-release

Haruo Arita

Generic Name: tramadol ER

Trade/Proprietary Name: Ultram ER

Drug Class: central-acting analgesic

Manufacturer: PriCara, Division of Ortho-McNeil, Inc., Raritan, NJ; release technology: Biovail Corporation, Mississauga, Canada

Chemical Structure: see Figure 30.1

Chemical Name: cis-2-[(dimethylamino)methyl]-1-(3-methoxyphenyl)-cyclohexanol

Chemical Formula: $C_{16}H_{25}NO_2$; molecular wt 263.

Introduction

Tramadol ER (tramadol hydrochloride) is a centrally acting synthetic analgesic in an extended-release formulation. It offers extended duration of pain relief with potential improvements in tolerability. Tramadol

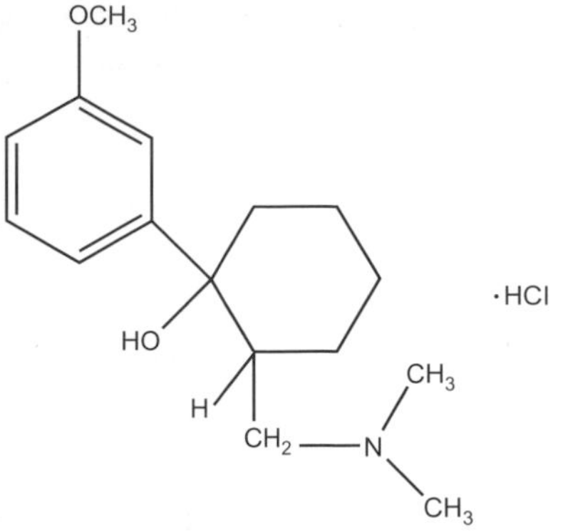

Figure 30.1.

binds to μ opioid receptors and weakly inhibits reuptake of norepinephrine and serotonin. Immediate-release tramadol has been available commercially for 15 years. An extended-release formulation of tramadol, named tramadol extended-release (ER) tablets, was formulated to be taken once daily, potentially facilitating compliance and long-term therapy [1].

Mode of activity

Tramadol is a synthetic, centrally acting analgesic with multiple mechanisms of action. The drug is a μ opioid receptor agonist, with the active metabolite (+)-O-desmethyltramadol [(+)-M1] being the major contributor to its action at μ opioid receptors. The enantiomers of tramadol also act synergistically by different mechanisms to inhibit pain transmission: the (+)-enantiomer inhibits neuronal reuptake of serotonin and the (−)-enantiomer inhibits neuronal reuptake of noradrenaline [1,2].

Tramadol ER formulation uses Biovail's Smartcoat™ diffusion-controlled tablet technology to achieve a gradual release of tramadol from the tablets, allowing for a 24-hour dosing interval. Tablets made with this technology consist of a solid tablet core, which contains tramadol and inert excipients, surrounded by a semipermeable coating that is composed of water-soluble and water-insoluble polymers and a plasticizer. Thus, the coating forms a membrane that controls the release of tramadol hydrochloride from the tablet core in vivo and is independent of pH changes as it passes through the gastrointestinal tract [1].

Indications

Tramadol ER is indicated for the management of moderate to moderately severe chronic pain in adults who require round-the-clock treatment of their pain for an extended period of time. The efficacy of tramadol ER has been investigated in two studies of patients with chronic pain caused by osteoarthritis and results from both studies confirmed the superior analgesic efficacy of tramadol ER relative to placebo [2].

Contraindications

Tramadol ER should not be administered to patients who have previously demonstrated hypersensitivity to tramadol, any other component of this product or opioids. Tramadol ER is contraindicated in any situation where opioids are contraindicated, including acute intoxication with any of the following: alcohol, hypnotics, narcotics, centrally acting analgesics, opioids, or psychotropic drugs. Tramadol ER should not be used in patients with creatinine clearance less than 30 mL/min, or severe hepatic impairment (Child-Pugh Class C).

Common doses

According to the manufacturer's prescribing information, the initial recommended dosage of tramadol ER is 100 mg once daily, with titration in 100 mg increments every 5 days (if required) up to a maximum dosage of 300 mg once daily. The drug is to be used in adults only, and may be administered without regard to food.

For patients on immediate-release (IR) tramadol, calculate the total daily IR dose and round down to the next lowest 100-mg increment. Tramadol ER tablets are supplied in 100 mg, 200 mg, and 300 mg form [1,2].

Potential advantages

Long-acting pain control; Ultram ER provides steady-state plasma concentrations sustained over 24 hours with fewer peaks and troughs. Short-acting agents dosed PRN may increase the likelihood of breakthrough pain. Night-time troughs may lead to breakthrough pain and interrupt sleep, for which patients are forced to re-dose during the night [3]. Poor sleep results in an increased pain intensity.

Ease of use, tolerability: tramadol ER was well tolerated in controlled clinical trials, with a safety profile similar to short-acting tramadol, which has been used for over 10 years in the USA and 30 years worldwide. Tramadol ER appears to be better tolerated than narcotic preparations with fewer adverse events for the level of analgesia achieved. Tramadol ER does not contain acetaminophen or NSAIDs. Tramadol has low potential for induction of respiratory depression and dependence. Unlike NSAIDs and COX-2 inhibitors, tramadol does not have black-box warnings regarding cardiovascular or gastrointestinal risk or lower-level warnings for renal toxicity with long-term use. Ultram® ER had a low incidence of cognitive side effects. For example, cognitive disorders, impaired balance, disturbance in attention, and sedation also occured at low rates.

NSAID dose-sparing potential: combination of tramadol with NSAIDs for the management of chronic pain has the potential to reduce NSAID requirements, while providing more effective pain relief.

Availability: tramadol ER is widely available at most pharmacies and is not a federally scheduled drug.

Less abuse potential: the use of opioid analgesics is accompanied by concerns regarding the potential for abuse, dependence, diversion, misuse, addiction, tolerance, and withdrawal. In contrast, short-acting tramadol has been shown to have a low potential for abuse, probably even less with tramadol ER.

Potential disadvantages

Tramadol ER must be swallowed whole and must not be chewed, crushed, or split. Chewing, crushing, or splitting the tablet will result in the uncontrolled delivery of the opioid and could result in overdose and death. This risk is increased with concurrent abuse of alcohol and other substances. Tramadol, like other opioids used in analgesia, can be abused [1,2].

Seizures have been reported in patients receiving tramadol. The risk of seizure is increased with doses of tramadol above the recommended range. Concomitant use of tramadol increases the seizure risk in patients taking tricyclic antidepressants, selective serotonin reuptake inhibitors, or other opioids. Tramadol may enhance the seizure risk in patients taking MAO inhibitors, neuroleptics, or other drugs that reduce the seizure threshold. Risk of convulsions may also increase in patients with epilepsy, those with a history of seizures, or in patients with a recognized risk for seizure (such as head trauma, metabolic disorders, alcohol and drug withdrawal, CNS infections).

Tramadol ER should be used with caution and in reduced dosages when administered to patients receiving CNS depressants such as alcohol, opioids, anesthetic agents, narcotics, phenothiazines, tranquilizers, antidepressants, or sedative hypnotics. Tramadol ER increases the risk of CNS and respiratory depression in these patients.

The development of a potentially life-threatening serotonin syndrome may occur with tramadol, particularly when combined with serotonergic drugs such as SSRIs, SNRIs, TCAs, MAOIs, triptans, drugs that alter metabolism of serotonin, and drugs that alter metabolism of tramadol (CYP2D6 and CYP3A4 inhibitors) [1,2]. When combined treatment with these drugs is clinically warranted, patients should be closely observed for signs and symptoms of serotonin

Table 30.1. Incidence (%) of patients with adverse event rates ≥ 5% from two 12-week placebo-controlled studies in patients with moderate to moderately severe chronic pain by dose

MedDRA preferred term	Ultram ER				Placebo
	100 mg (n = 403) n (%)	200 mg (n = 400) n (%)	300 mg (n = 400) n (%)	400 mg (n = 202) n (%)	(n = 406) n (%)
Dizziness (not vertigo)	64 (15.9)	81 (20.3)	90 (22.5)	57 (28.2)	28 (6.9)
Nausea	61 (15.1)	90 (22.5)	102 (25.5)	53 (26.2)	32 (7.9)
Constipation	49 (12.2)	68 (17.0)	85 (21.3)	60 (29.7)	17 (4.2)
Somnolence	33 (8.2)	45 (11.3)	29 (7.3)	41 (20.3)	7 (1.7)
Flushing	31 (7.7)	40 (10.0)	35 (8.8)	32 (15.8)	18 (4.4)
Pruritus	25 (6.2)	34 (8.5)	30 (7.5)	24 (11.9)	4 (1.0)
Vomiting	20 (5.0)	29 (7.3)	34 (8.5)	19 (9.4)	11 (2.7)
Insomnia	26 (6.5)	32 (8.0)	36 (9.0)	22 (10.9)	13 (3.2)
Asthenia	14 (3.5)	24 (6.0)	26 (6.5)	13 (6.4)	7 (1.7)
Postural hypotension	7 (1.7)	17 (4.3)	8 (2.0)	11 (5.4)	9 (2.2)

syndrome such as mental status changes, autonomic instability, neuromuscular aberrations, and/or gastrointestinal symptoms, especially during treatment initiation and dosage escalation. Patients with serotonin syndrome require immediate medical attention.

Drug-related adverse events

Tramadol ER was administered to a total of 3108 patients during studies conducted in the USA. These included four double-blind studies in patients with osteoarthritis and/or chronic low back pain and one open-label study in patients with chronic non-malignant pain. A total of 901 patients were 65 years or older. Adverse events increased with dose from 100 mg to 400 mg in the two pooled, 12-week, randomized, double-blind, placebo-controlled studies in patients with chronic non-malignant pain [4] (see Table 30.1)

There are no specific drugs for reversal of adverse effects; however, naloxone may be used to treat respiratory depression.

References

1. Hair PI, Curran MP, Keam SJ. Tramadol extended-release tablets. *Drugs* 2006;**66**(15):2017–2027.

2. Ultram ER. Prescribing information. www.ultram-er.com.

3. Barking RL. "Extended-release tramadol (ULTRAM ER): a pharmacotherapeutic, pharmacokinetic, and pharmacodynamic focus on effectiveness and safety in patients with chronic/persistent pain. *Am J Ther* 2008;**15**:157–166.

4. Ganal T, Pascual MG. Extended-release tramadol in the treatment of osteoarthritis: a multicenter, randomized, double-blind, placebo-controlled clinical trial. *Curr Med Res Opin* 2006;**22**: 1391–1401.

Section 2 Chapter

Oral and Parenteral Opioid Analgesics

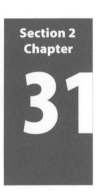

Tapentadol

Dan Froicu and Raymond S. Sinatra

Generic Name: tapentadol hydrochloride

Trade Name: Nucynta™

Drug Class: opioid analgesic, Class II, central-acting analgesic

Manufacturer: PriCara, Division of Johnson & Johnson Inc., Raritan, NJ 08869

Chemical Name: 3-[(1*R*,2*R*)-3-(dimethylamino)-1-ethyl-2-methylpropyl]phenol monohydrochloride

Chemical Structure: see Figure 31.1

Chemical Formula: $C_{14}H_{23}NO\cdot HCl$; molecular wt:257.8

Introduction

Tapentadol is the first new analgesic for moderate to severe acute pain in more than 25 years [1]. Grunenthal GbmH and Johnson & Johnson Research signed a licensing agreement for tapentadol in 2003, and have shared development responsibilities. Grunenthal licensed marketing rights to tapentadol to Ortho-McNeil-Janssen Pharmaceuticals, Inc. for the USA, Canada, and Japan. Grunenthal maintains marketing rights in Europe and other parts of the world.

In November 2008, the FDA approved tapentadol for marketing in the USA as a drug for moderate-to-severe acute pain. Tapentadol was licensed and approved for distribution as a schedule II (strong

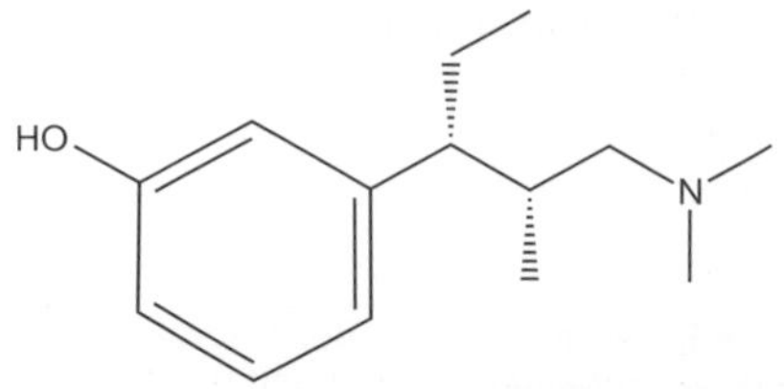

Figure 31.1.

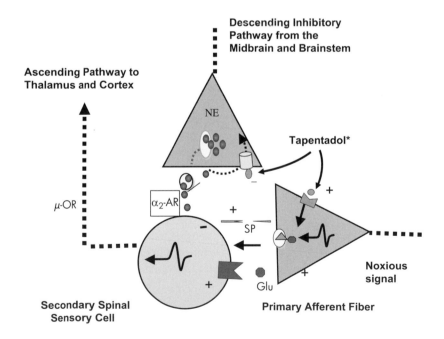

opioid) in June 2009. Tapentadol is marketed as Nucynta™ (possibly derived from "new central acting analgesic") and is available as 50, 75 and 100 mg immediate-release tablets. Immediate-release tablets are film-coated to facilitate oral administration and should not be broken or crushed. Sustained-release tablets are in development for chronic pain management (refer to Chapter 115).

Mode of activity

Tapentadol is a centrally acting analgesic. While its action mechanism is unknown it is presumed that tapentadol has dual effects in suppressing pain transmission, combining μ opioid receptor (MOR) agonism with monoamine reuptake inhibition (Figure 31.2) [1–3]. Tapentadol has an 18-fold lower affinity for the human μ opioid receptor compared with morphine but is only 2–3-fold less potent than morphine, which is probably due to its norepinephrine reuptake inhibition activity [2,3]. In animal trials tapentadol had only minor effects on serotonin reuptake. Tapentadol exists as a single active enantiomer [3] and is metabolized mainly by O-glucuronidation; its principal metabolite is inactive, having no affinity for MOR or the NE transporter. As the analgesic activity of tapentadol is limited to the primary molecule, no enzymes are needed to convert it to an active metabolite (such as tramadol, or codeine). This implies fewer if any individual variations in its action compared to drugs that require polymorphic enzymes.

Tapentadol provides high analgesic efficacy that is comparable to classic opioids, but is associated with unexpectedly improved gastrointestinal tolerability [4,5,6,7]. Its two mechanisms of action appear to be additive and provide an opioid-sparing effect while maintaining effective analgesia. The efficacy and safety of various doses of tapentadol IR compared

Figure 31.2. Diagram demonstrating sites of tapentadol activity in the pain transmission pathway. Tapentadol binds to and activates mu opioid receptors and also blocks norepinephrine reuptake by inhibiting the NE transporter protein. NE = norepinephrine; α_2-AR = alpha$_2$-adrenoceptor; μ-OR = μ opioid receptor; SP = substance P; Glu = glutamate. Cylinder represents the NE reuptake transporter protein. After (1) Tzschentke TM et al. *J Pharmacol Exp Ther* 2007;**323**(1):265–276; (2) American Pain Society.

with oxycodone HCl IR have been evaluated in several placebo-controlled acute post-operative pain trials [4,5]. A large phase III study ($n = 901$) demonstrated that tapentadol IR 50 and 75 mg provided efficacy that was non-inferior to oxycodone HCl IR 10 mg for the management of moderate to severe pain after bunionectomy [5]. Prespecified tolerability comparisons showed that a significantly lower percentage of patients in the tapentadol IR 50 mg group reported composite nausea and/or vomiting than patients treated with oxycodone HCl IR 10 mg (35% vs. 59%; $P < 0.001$). The percentage of patients who experienced nausea and/or vomiting in the tapentadol IR |75 mg group was also lower (51%) than the oxycodone HCl IR 10 mg group (59%), but the difference marginally failed to reach statistical

Table 31.1. Percentages of patients experiencing nausea and vomiting in randomized, double-blind, placebo-controlled, studies of tapentadol IR

Phase 3 study	Adverse event	Placebo	Tapentadol IR 50 mg	Tapentadol IR 75 mg	Tapentadol IR 100 mg	Oxycodone HCl IR (10 or 15 mg)
Bunionectomy 1 trial	Nausea	13	35	38	49	67
	Vomiting	3	18	21	32	42
	Nausea and/or vomiting	–	–	41[a]	53[b]	70
Bunionectomy 2 trial	Nausea	17	34	46	–	57
	Vomiting	0	12	28	–	26
	Nausea and/or vomiting	–	35[c]	51[d]	–	59
End-stage joint disease	Nausea	5	18	21	–	41
	Vomiting	4	7	14	–	34
	Nausea and/or vomiting	–	22[c]	30[c]	–	57

Data taken from references 4, 5, and 6.
[a]IR, immediate release.
[b]$P = 0.007$ vs oxycodone HCl IR 15 mg.
[c]$P < 0.001$ vs oxycodone HCl IR 10 mg.
[d]$P = 0.057$ vs oxycodone HCl IR 10 mg.

Table 31.2. Percentage of patients reporting adverse events in a 90-day safety trial

System/organ class	Tapentadol IR 50 mg or 100 mg ($n = 679$), % of subjects	Oxycodone IR 10 mg or 15 mg ($n = 170$), % of subjects
Gastrointestinal disorders	44.2	63.5
Nausea	18.4	29.4
Vomiting	16.9	30.0
Constipation	12.8	27.1
Diarrhea	6.6	5.9
Dry mouth	5.3	2.9
Dizziness	18.1	17.1
Headache	11.5	10.0
Somnolence	10.2	9.4
Pruritus	4.3	11.8

significance ($P = 0.057$). A similar reduction in the incidence of nausea and vomiting with tapentadol IR compared with oxycodone IR was demonstrated in a separate phase III study of tapentadol IR in patients with moderate to severe osteoarthritis pain from end-stage joint disease [6] (Table 31.1). Analgesic onset with tapentadol 5–100 mg is fairly rapid and comparable to other immediate-release opioid agonists. Data taken from 602 patients enrolled in the post-operative bunionectomy pain trials indicated that tapentadol provided perceptible pain relief as early as 32 to 46 minutes following administration [4,5].

The FDA required a safety study of 90 days duration in at least 300 patients where tapentadol was compared to another immediate-release opioid [7]. For the 849 adult subjects enrolled in this study, the average baseline pain intensity score was 7.1. About half the patients were opioid-experienced. Supplemental analgesics (acetaminophen 2 g per day or ibuprofen 400 mg per day) were allowed in this study. The treatment groups were tapentadol IR 50 mg or 100 mg every 4 to 6 hours PRN versus oxycodone IR 10 mg or 15 mg every 4 to 6 hours PRN. Adverse events were monitored as part of the tolerability evaluation. Tapentadol was well tolerated, and had a lower incidence of GI adverse events than in patients treated with the comparator (refer to Table 31.2). Other tolerability evaluations included findings from the Clinical Opioid Withdrawal Scale (COWS) which indicated that 83% of patients abruptly discontinued from therapy did not experience withdrawal symptoms within 2 to 4 days of treatment cessation.

Indications

Tapentadol is FDA approved for moderate to severe acute pain management in patients age 18 or older.

Contraindications

Significant respiratory depression in unmonitored settings or the absence of resuscitative equipment. Nucynta™ is also contraindicated in patients with acute or severe bronchial asthma or hypercapnia in unmonitored settings or the absence of resuscitative equipment.

Paralytic ileus (proven or suspected).

Patients who are receiving monoamine oxidase (MAO) inhibitors or who have taken them within the last 14 days due to potential additive effects on norepinephrine levels which may result in adverse cardiovascular events.

Relative contraindications

Patients at risk of developing serotonin syndrome: the development of a potentially life-threatening serotonin syndrome may occur with use of SNRI products, including tapentadol, particularly with concomitant use of serotonergic drugs such as SSRIs, SNRIs, TCAs, MAOIs, and triptans, and with drugs which impair metabolism of serotonin (including MAOIs). Serotonin syndrome may include mental-status changes (e.g. agitation, hallucinations, coma), autonomic instability (e.g. tachycardia, labile blood pressure, hyperthermia), and neuromuscular aberrations (e.g. hyperreflexia, incoordination).

Common doses

Tapentadol can be given in doses of one tablet of 50 mg, 75 mg, or 100 mg every 4 to 6 hours depending on the pain intensity. The maximum daily dose of tapentadol is 700 mg (for the first day of treatment) and 600 mg (day 2 and after). Doses higher than 700 mg per day have not been studied. No dosage adjustment is needed in mild or moderate renal impairment. Little information exists regarding tapentadol dosing in opioid-dependent patients. Data taken from the 90-day safety trial in which some patients had been taking opioids prior to enrollment suggest that tapentadol doses of 100 mg every 4 hours may be appropriate. Although tapentadol IR has only been approved for acute pain management there is no limitation with regards to duration of therapy listed in the package insert.

Potential advantages

Unlike tramadol, tapentadol is an active molecule, it is not a prodrug and does not have to be converted into an active form.

Metabolized by glucoronidation: less individual variability due to the fact that there is no interaction with CYP-450 or CYP-2AD-6.

Better gastrointestinal tolerability than hydrocodone, less nausea, vomiting, and constipation in an end-term osteoarthritis efficacy trial and 90-day safety trial.

Nephrotoxicity or hepatotoxicity have not been reported.

Potential disadvantages

Risk of opioid-induced respiratory depression, nausea, vomiting and constipation. Tapentadol should not be used during breast feeding.

Drug-related adverse events

Tapentadol has an abuse potential similar to other opioids and is subject to criminal diversion. After 90 days of continuous administration, abrupt discontinuation of tapentadol was associated with mild to moderate withdrawal symptoms in 17% of patients

References

1. Micromedex® Healthcare Series, DrugDex® Evaluations, Thompson Healthcare. 2009.

2. Vanderah TW. Pathophysiology of pain. *Med Clin North Am* 2007;**91**(1):1–12.

3. Tzschentke TM et al. *J Pharmacol Exp Ther* 2007;**323**(1):265–276.

4. Daniels SE, Upmalis D, Okamoto A, Lange C, Häeussler J. A randomized, double-blind, phase III study comparing multiple doses of tapentadol IR, oxycodone IR, and placebo for postoperative (bunionectomy) pain. *Curr Med Res Opin* 2009;**25**(3):765–776.

5. Daniels S, Casson E, Stegmann J-U, et al. A randomized, double-blind, placebo-controlled phase 3 study of the relative efficacy and tolerability of tapentadol IR and oxycodone IR for acute pain. *Curr Med Res Opin* 2009;**25**(6):1551–1561.

6. Hartrick C, Van Hove I, Stegmann J-U, Oh C, Upmalis D. Efficacy and tolerability of tapentadol immediate release and oxycodone HCl immediate release in patients awaiting primary joint replacement surgery for end-stage joint disease: a 10-day, phase III, randomized, double-blind, active- and placebo-controlled study. *Clin Ther* 2009;**31**(2):1–12.

7. Hale M, Upmalis D, Okamoto A, Lange C, Rauschkolb C. Tolerability of tapentadol immediate release in patients with lower back pain or osteoarthritis of the hip or knee over 90 days: a randomized, double-blind study. *Curr Med Res Opin* 2009;**25**(5):1095–1104.

8. Nucynta™(Tapentadol) Package insert 2008, PriCara®, Division of Ortho-McNeil-Janssen Pharmaceuticals, Inc. Raritan, NJ 08869.

Section 2 Chapter

Oral and Parenteral Opioid Analgesics

32 Remifentanil

Marjorie Podraza Stiegler

Generic Name: remifentanil hydrochloride

Trade Name: Ultiva®

Drug Class: opioid analgesic

Manufacturer: GlaxoSmithKline, GSK House, Brentford, London, UK; Abbott Laboratories, Abbott Park, IL

Chemical Structure: see Figure 32.1

Chemical Name: 1-(2-methoxycarbonyl-ethyl)-4-(phenylpropionyl-amino)-piperidine-4-carboxylic acid methyl ester hydrochloride

Chemical Formula: $C_{20}H_{28}N_2O_5 \cdot HCl$

Introduction

Remifentanil is a unique μ opioid agonist that has a rapid blood–brain equilibration half-time of 1 ± 1

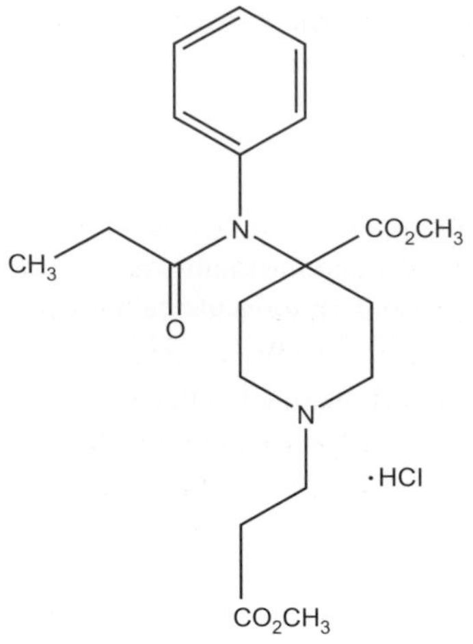

Figure 32.1.

minutes, and very rapid onset and offset of analgesic effects. It is a 4-anilidopiperidine fentanyl analog with dose-dependent adverse effects similar to other μ opioids [1,2].

Mode of activity

Remifentanil binds to and activates μ receptors in the brain and spinal cord. It is generally administered as an intravenous bolus or continuous infusion. The average clearance of remifentanil in young healthy adults generally correlates with total body weight; in severely obese patients it correlates with ideal body weight. Blood concentration decreases 50% in 3 to 6 minutes after cessation of infusion and clinical recovery from the effects occurs rapidly, within 5 to 10 minutes. The terminal half-life is 10 to 20 minutes. Distinct from other opioids in its class, the duration of action does not increase with prolonged administration [1,2].

Remifentanil is rapidly and extensively metabolized by nonspecific blood and tissue esterases (but not plasma cholinesterase) to a carboxylic acid derivative that is 4600 times less active than the parent compound [2]. Approximately 95% of remifentanil is excreted in the urine as this metabolite. It follows that the pharmacokinetics of remifentanil are not significantly changed in patients with renal impairment. The clearance of the carboxylic acid metabolite is reduced with renal dysfunction; however, there is no demonstrated clinical relevance of the accumulated metabolite. The pharmacokinetics are also unchanged in patients with severe hepatic impairment (even those awaiting liver transplant,

or during the anhepatic phase of liver transplant surgery).

Remifentanil crosses the placenta, resulting in fetal blood concentrations approximately half that of maternal blood. Additionally, remifentanyl may be transferred to breastmilk. Neonates can metabolize remifentanil. The half-life of remifentanil is not significantly different in neonates or pediatric patients as compared to adults.

Among patients >65 years of age, the EC_{50} for delta-wave formation on EEG is 50% lower; thus, the initial dose should be reduced accordingly, with careful titration to effect.

Indications
Adjunct with induction of anesthesia

Remifentanil can be used as an adjunct, and only when intubation and mechanical ventilation are intended. Remifentanil is inadequate as a sole induction agent, as loss of consciousness cannot be ensured [2,3].

Intra-operative analgesia during anesthesia maintenance

Because remifentanil can be rapidly titrated, it is useful for analgesia intra-operatively without prolonging recovery. It is particularly useful in procedures that are generally associated with little post-operative pain but significant intra-operative stimulation. If post-operative pain is anticipated, long-acting narcotics should be administered prior to discontinuing remifentanil. Even after prolonged infusion, recovery from respiratory depression adequate for extubation can be expected within 5 to 10 minutes of discontinuation. Remifentanil is inadequate as a sole agent for maintenance of anesthesia.

Post-operative analgesia

Due to its potential for respiratory depression, remifentanil is not recommended for post-operative analgesia, except in mechanically ventilated patients in a properly supervised environment.

ICU sedation

Infusion rates of 0.1–0.15 μg/kg per min are effective for establishing and maintaining analgesia and sedation in a wide range of ICU patients, including those with severe renal or hepatic impairment.

Hemodynamic effects are similar to those of morphine or fentanyl.

Procedural sedation

With proper monitoring and personnel skilled in airway rescue procedures, remifentanil may be used safely for analgesia and sedation during procedures.

Off-label indications

Rapid-sequence intubation: remifentanil has been reported for use in lieu of neuromuscular blockade during rapid sequence intubations and is reported to provide good to excellent intubating conditions with doses of 3–4 µg/kg given as a slow IV push. Notably, studies do not indicate chest wall rigidity or hypotension as problematic with this technique.

Labor analgesia: remifentanil has also been reported for PCA use in obstetric analgesia during the first stage of labor.

Contraindications

Absolute: contraindicated for epidural and intrathecal use, due to glycine in the formulation; unsuitable as the sole agent for induction or maintenance of general anesthesia.

Relative: not recommended for use in spontaneous ventilation anesthesia; not recommended as an analgesic in the immediate post-operative period except in ventilated patients.

Common doses

Remifentanil is only available for parenteral administration, either as a bolus or infusion.

Manufacturer-recommended doses range from 0.1 µg/kg per min to 0.5 µg/kg per min, and as high as 1.0 µg/kg per min in children. These doses are much higher than those used in actual clinical practice, which generally range from 0.025–0.1 µg/kg per min for sedation and up to 0.1–1 µg/kg per min for anesthesia, titrated to effect. Remifentanil may also be used in a process called target controlled infusion, in which computer-controlled infusion pumps maintain desired plasma concentrations.

For induction of anesthesia, the dose of 1 µg/kg should be administered over 60 seconds. As a replacement for neuromuscular blocker, a higher dose of 3–4 µg/kg is suggested, again over 60 seconds. A hypnotic agent is still required, though the dose may be reduced by as much as 75%, as remifentanil is synergistic with thiopental and propofol.

Potential advantages

The primary advantage to remifentanil remains its rapid onset, offset, and ease of titration, even when using a prolonged infusion. This may result in faster time to extubation both in the OR and in the ICU [2,3].

"Fast-track" cardiac anesthesia.

High-dose infusion (starting doses 1–3 mg/kg per min) effectively attenuates response to major surgical stress, such as sternal spread, and is still associated with a rapid recovery profile. However, remifentanil may be associated with a higher incidence of intra-operative hypotension.

Neuroanesthesia

Remifentanil may be particularly advantageous for procedures in which a crisp post-operative neurological exam is desired.

Potential disadvantages

Side effects: remifentanil may cause adverse effects characteristic of µ opioids, such as respiratory depression, bradycardia, hypotension, pruritus, and skeletal muscle rigidity.

Incompatibilities: nonspecific esterases in blood products may lead to the hydrolysis of remifentanil to its carboxylic acid metabolite. Therefore, administration of ULTIVA into the same IV tubing with blood is not recommended.

Hyperalgesia: infusions of remifentanil have been associated with acute tolerance development and opioid-induced hyperalgesia. Both factors can increase post-operative opioid dose requirements and increase pain intensity scores [4].

Schedule II with potential for abuse.

Pregnancy Category C, although no animal studies have demonstrated tetratogenic effects, even at doses 400 times the maximum recommended human dose.

Cost: remifentanil costs about ten times as much as fentanyl. If operating-room time or ICU stay is reduced, this cost may be offset. This has not been demonstrated conclusively.

Drug-related adverse events

Adverse events including respiratory depression, bradycardia, hypotension, pruritus, and skeletal muscle rigidity will dissipate within minutes of discontinuing or decreasing the infusion rate; they can also be reversed promptly with naloxone.

Remifentanil is known to cause nausea and vomiting.

Hypotension and bradycardia are vagally mediated and unrelated to histamine release.

Diaphoresis, post-operative shivering, dizziness, and agitation have also been reported.

References

1. Servin FS, Billard V. Remifentanil and other opioids. *Handb Exp Pharmacol* 2008;(**182**):283–311.

2. Komatsu R, Turan AM, Orhan-Sungur M, McGuire J, Radke OC, Apfel CC. Remifentanil for general anaesthesia: a systematic review. *Anaesthesia* 2007;**62**(12):1266–1280.

3. Beers R, Camporesi E. Remifentanil update: clinical science and utility. *CNS Drugs* 2004;**18**(15):1085–1104.

4. Joly V, Richebe P, Guignard B, et al. Remifentanil-induced postoperative hyperalgesia and its prevention with small-dose ketamine. *Anesthesiology* 2005;**103**(1):147–155.

| Section 2 Chapter **33** | **Oral and Parenteral Opioid Analgesics** |

Nalbuphine

Ana M. Lobo

Generic Name: nalbuphine

Brand Names: Nubain™, Nubain™ Injectable (USA), Nalbufina™ (Argentina)

Class: opioid agonist–antagonist analgesic

Manufacturer: Hospira Inc., 275 North Field Drive, Lake Forest, IL 60045. Also: Astra-Zeneca Pharmaceuticals, Moore, H.L. Drug Exchange Inc., Southwood Pharmaceuticals Inc.

Chemical Structure: see Figure 33.1

Chemical Name: (−)-17-(cyclobutylmethyl)-4,5α-epoxymorphinan-3,6α,14-triol hydrochloride

Chemical Formula: $C_{21}H_{27}NO_4$; molecular wt: 393.91

Introduction

Nalbuphine is a semi-synthetic agonist–antagonist opioid of the phenanthrene series. It is structurally similar to, and chemically related to, both the potent opioid agonist oxymorphone, and the narcotic antagonist naloxone [1]. Nalbuphine is a moderately potent analgesic that simultaneously exhibits opioid antagonist activity. It is primarily a kappa receptor agonist and partial mu receptor antagonist. Analgesic potency is equivalent to that of morphine, milligram to milligram for doses up to 10 mg. At higher doses morphine provides progressively improved analgesic efficacy. Typically, at normal dosages, pulmonary artery pressure, myocardial work load, and systemic vascular resistance do not increase. The same degree of respiratory depression may occur with nalbuphine as with equianalgesic doses of morphine. However, in the absence of other central nervous system depressants which are compromising respiration, nalbuphine shows a ceiling effect on further respiratory compromise, in doses in excess of 30 mg. Similarly, at this juncture, there is a ceiling effect on analgesia. Naloxone is 25 times more potent than nalbuphine with respect to its antagonistic effects [1,2]. Nalbuphine's antagonist effect occurs at doses equal to, or lower than, those which produce analgesia. Indeed, respiratory depression

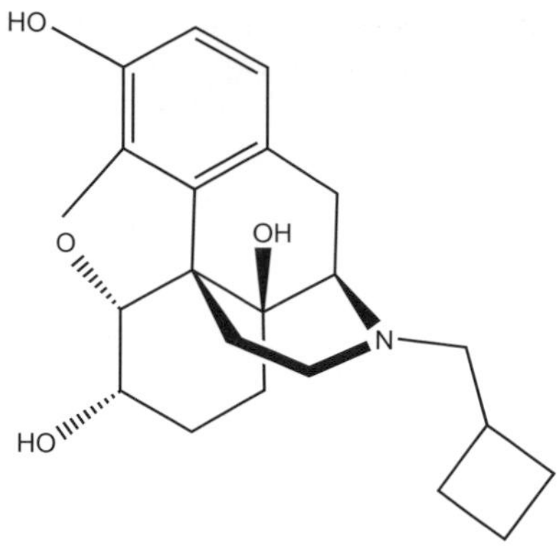

Figure 33.1.

caused by other concomitantly administered mu agonists may be blocked or partially reversed by nalbuphine. If given orally, this drug may be 80% less potent than when it is administered intramuscularly [2].

Pharmacokinetics

Nalbuphine loses much of its potency, when given orally, due to first-pass metabolism in the liver. In terms of distribution, it is not bound to plasma proteins, and crosses the placenta. Metabolism, to pharmacologically inactive conjugates, occurs in the liver. Conjugates and unchanged drug are secreted into bile [1–3]. Elimination is predominantly fecal. Seven percent is excreted in the urine unchanged. The plasma elimination half-life is 2–3 hours in healthy adults and children over the age of eight, only 1 hour in children between the ages of 1.5 and 8 years, and 4 hours in neonates. Clinical effect is maintained for approximately 3–6 hours [1–3].

Indications

Nalbuphine is indicated for the treatment of moderate to severe somatic and visceral pain. Additional indications include its use as a component of balanced anesthesia, treatment of pain associated with labor

and delivery, and for the treatment of pre-operative and post-operative pain. Unlabeled uses include treatment pf pruritus secondary to intrathecal morphine in patients recovering from cesarean section. Intrathecal and epidural dosing have also been studied [1,3].

Dosage

The recommended adult dose is 10 mg SQ/IM/IV per 70 kg every 3–6 hours [1–3]. Dosing should be adjusted based on severity of pain, the patient's medical and overall condition, and the presence or absence of concommitent narcotic use and/or dependency. In non-dependent patients, no more than 20 mg/dose should be administered, or 160 mg/day. Activation of kappa opioid receptors can attenuate visceral pain in animals, and like other mixed agonist–antagonist opioids nalbuphine is effective for controlling abdominal and pelvic visceral pain [3]. Doses of 0.1–0.2 mg/kg may be administered to control pain associated with gall stones, renal stones, and discomfort following laparoscopic pelvic surgery. There is evidence to suggest that nalbuphine is more effective in female patients [4].

When used as part of a balanced anesthetic, induction doses range from 0.3 mg/kg to 3 mg/kg IV over 10–15 minutes [1,3]. Maintenance doses of 0.25 to 0.5 mg/kg may be utilized, as required, in single intravenous boluses. The advantage in general anesthesia is that patients will exibit less respiratory depression upon emergence, and in PACU, than patients treated with morphine or fentanyl. In our experience, these patients may be moderately to very sedated in PACU, resulting in delays in discharge. Over-sedation may be treated with low doses of naloxone (40–80 μg as required).

Nalbuphine has been evaluated for use with intravenous patient-controlled analgesia. In a double-blind trial of 48 patients, nalbuphine, morphine, and pethidine (meperidine) administered with IV-PCA were compared in the first 24 hours after cholecystectomy.

Table 33.1. Self-administered nalbuphine following cholecystectomy

PCA drug	Mean VAS pain score (24 h)	Mean pain score with movement	24 h self-administered dose
Nalbuphine	50 mm	70 mm (2)	70 mg
Morphine	44 mm	52 mm (5)[a]	46 mg
Meperidine	53 mm	67 mm (7)	614 mg

mm = millimetres; 0 = no pain, 100 = worst pain.
[a]Significant reduction vs. nalbuphine (P > 0.05).
From: Bahar M, Rosen M, Vickers MD. Self administered nalbuphine, morphine, and pethidine. *Anaesthesia* 2007;**40**:529–532.

Using this mode of administration nalbuphine 15 mg was approximately equivalent to morphine 10 mg or meperidine 120 mg; however, nalbuphine's ability to reduce pain with movement was inferior to that provided by morphine [5] (Table 33.1).

The safety and efficacy of nalbuphine, with respect to the treatment of pediatric pain, have not been fully established. For patients older than 1 year of age, doses of 0.1–0.2 mg/kg SQ/IM/IV every 3–4 hours are utilized, and individualized, as above [6]. The maximum dose is 20 mg/administration and the daily total dose should not exceed 160 mg. Nalbuphine, in doses of 0.05–0.1 mg/kg SQ/IM/IV, has been used to facilitate weaning from mechanical ventilation in the pediatric intensive care unit setting. Nalbuphine is also used to relieve pruritus, caused by narcotic administration, in this population as well as in adults.

The efficacy and adverse effects of intrathecal nalbuphine were evaluated in patients recovering from cesarean delivery. Doses of 0.8 mg added to bupivacaine provided the longest duration of effective pain relief. Increasing the nalbuphine dose to 1.6 mg did not further improve analgesia. Intrathecal nalbuphine provided a significantly faster onset of pain relief than the comparator, intrathecal morphine (0.2 mg), probably because of its lipophilic properties. Analgesic duration was significantly less than morphine (240 min vs. 600 min). Unlike the comparator pruritus and PONV were not observed with nalbuphine 0.2 and 0.8 mg [7].

Nalbuphine 5–10 mg IV has been used to reduce the incidence and severity of pruritus in patients treated with intrathecal morphine and other neuraxially administered opioids. The efficacy of nalbuphine and propofol for treating intrathecal morphine-induced pruritus was evaluated in a randomized, double-blinded study [8]. One-hundred and eighty-one patients recovering from cesarean section who developed moderate to severe pruritus after the administration of intrathecal morphine were treated with either 3 mg IV nalbuphine (n = 91) or 20 mg IV propofol (n = 90). The treatment success rate was higher in the nalbuphine group than in the propofol group (83% vs. 61%; P < 0.001). Recurrence rates of moderate to severe pruritus within 4 h were not significantly different (nalbuphine 9% versus propofol 7%; P = 0.76). Sedation with both drugs and pain on injection with propofol were the two most common side effects, and had no clinical consequences.

Administration of naloxone (0.2–0.4 mg) is indicated to treat an overdosage of, or adverse reaction to, nalbuphine. Additional supportive measures such as oxygen administration, respiratory support, intravenous fluids, and vasopressors may also be indicated [1,2].

Drug interactions

Nalbuphine may cause psychological or physical dependence. Abrupt discontinuation after prolonged use can cause signs and symptoms of opioid withdrawal. Increased CNS and respiratory depression may be observed when nalbuphine is used with other CNS depressants and barbiturates. If such medications are currently being administered, decreasing the dose of nalbuphine, or lengthening the time interval between dosing, should be considered. In opioid-naive patients, doses of nalbuphine should be decreased. Nalbuphine does not consistently antagonize other narcotics in opioid-naive patients, and may potentiate analgesic effects when given in close proximity. Nalbuphine is ten times more potent than pentazocine as an antagonist and will precipitate withdrawal in opiate-tolerant individuals. Nalbuphine-induced withdrawal has been observed in patients chronically treated with opioid agonists as well as those abusing narcotics. It should not be used to control post-operative pain or labor and delivery pain in patients treated with methadone or those abusing heroin. Concomitant use of drugs which potentially depress liver function should be taken in consideration when nalbuphine will be administered for more than 24 h [1,9].

Adverse reactions

The most common adverse reaction noted with nalbuphine is sedation, occurring in 30% of patients receiving this drug. Other side effects which occur with a frequency of < 10% include the following: nausea/vomiting, sweaty/clammy feeling, vertigo/dizziness, headache, and dry mouth. Other side effects, occurring with a frequency of < 1%, include the following [1,2,9]:

CNS: confusion, faintness, dysphoria, hallucinations, unusual dreams, restlessness

cardiovascular: hypotension, bradycardia, hypertension, tachycardia

gastrointestinal: dyspepsia, cramps, nausea, vomiting, biliary tract sphincter spasm

respiratory: depression

dermatological: flushing, itching, burning

obstetric: fetal bradycardia, pseudo-sinusoidal heart rhythm, decrease in fetal heart rate variability

Contraindications: nalbuphine should not be used in patients with known major or minor hypersensitivity reactions to any of the ingredients in the injectable preparation.

Use during labor and delivery: nalbuphine readily and rapidly crosses the placenta. Documented fetal adverse effects include bradycardia, apnea and/or respiratory depression at birth, hypotonia, and cyanosis. These adverse effects have resulted in permanent neurological damage to the fetus. If nalbuphine has been administered to a pregnant or laboring female, it is prudent to monitor the fetus, after birth, for any of the above. In addition, nalbuphine is frequently administered in combination with vistaril or benadryl, to potentiate its perceived effect. Both may add to maternal sedation with concomitant fetal compromise. Nalbuphine is a Pregnancy Category B drug [1,9].

Nursing mothers: nalbuphine is excreted in maternal milk, but in small amounts (<1% of administered dose). The effect on the fetus is clinically insignificant. Administer to a lactating female with caution.

Abuse liability: caregivers must recognize that as an injectable formulation, nalbuphine may be liable to abuse; however, it is less attractive to heroin addicts or highly tolerant opioid abusers due to its potent antagonist effects. A limited number of anecdotal reports suggest that nalbuphine is abused by healthcare professionals and by body-builders (anabolic steroid users). Nalbuphine is rarely encountered by law enforcement personnel or submitted to forensic laboratories for analysis. This may, in part, be due to its non-controlled status.

Routes of administration: intravenous, intramuscular and subcutaneous; intrathecal and epidural (off-label use).

Formulation: sterile, non-pyrogenic injectable solution in water containing sodium citrate hydrous, citric acid anhydrous, sodium metabisulfite, methyl-paraben and propylparaben. pH is adjusted with hydrochloric acid or sodium hydroxide. Supplied as ampoules or bottles, concentration10 mg/mL, 20 mg/mL.

References

1. Gutstein HB, Akil H. Opioid analgesics. In Hardman JG, Limbird LE, Gilman AG, eds. *Goodman & Gilman's The Pharmacological Basis of Therapeutics*, 10th ed. New York: McGraw-Hill, 2002, pp. 569–619.

2. The Merck Manual. www.merck.com/mmpe/index.htm

3. www.drugs.com/pro/Nalbuphine.html: Use of the mixed agonist–antagonist nalbuphine in opioid based analgesia.

4. Gear RW, Miaskowski C, Gordon NC, Paul SM, Heller PH, Levine JD. The kappa opioid nalbuphine produces gender- and dose-dependent analgesia and antianalgesia in patients with post-operative pain. *Pain* 1999;**83**;339–345.

5. Bahar M, Rosen M, Vickers MD. Self administered Nalbuphine, morphine, and pethidine. *Anaesthesia* 2007;**40**:529–532.

6. Yaster M, Deshpande JK. Management of pediatric pain with opioid analgesics. *J Pediatrics* 1988;**113**(3):421–429.

7. Culebras X, Gaggero G, Zatloukal J, et al. Advantages of intrathecal nalbuphine compared to intrathecal morphine after cesarean section. *Anesth Analg* 2000;**91**:601–605.

8. Charuluxananan S, Kyokong O, Somboonviboon W, et al. Nalbuphine versus propofol for treatment of intrathecal morphine-induced pruritus after cesarean delivery. *Anesth Analg* 2001;**93**:162–165.

9. Gunion MW, Marchionne AM, Andersons CTM, Seifert S. Opioid medications. In Dart RC, ed. *Medical Toxicology*, 3rd ed. Philadelphia: Lippincott Williams and Wilkins, 2003, pp. 756–782.

Oral and Parenteral Opioid Analgesics

Butorphanol

J. Michael Watkins-Pitchford

Generic Name: butorphanol, butorphanol tartrate, butorphanol tartrate injection, USP, butorphanol tartrate nasal spray

Trade/Proprietary Names: Nasal Stadol™; Moradol™ and Beforal™ (the brand name Injectable Stadol™ is no longer available in the USA)

Manufacturers: Roxane Laboratories, 1809 Wilson Rd, Columbus, OH; Barr Laboratories, 223 Quaker Road, Pomona, NY

Structure: see Figure 34.1

Chemical Name: (−)-17-(cyclobutylmethyl)morphinan-3,14-diol D-(−)-tartrate(1:1)(salt)

Chemical Formula: $C_{21}H_{29}NO_2 \cdot C_4H_6O_6$; molecular wt 477.6

Introduction

Butorphanol tartrate is a synthetically derived opioid agonist–antagonist analgesic of the phenanthrene series, structurally similar to levorphanol. In the USA, butorphanol is used as a substitute for meperidine for patients complaining of moderate pain. Butorphanol and other mixed agonist–antagonists appear to be more effective in female patients and are primarily prescribed for visceral pain and headache [1,2]. It is used to control pain associated with ureteral and gall stones and is also employed for labor and delivery analgesia.

General pharmacology and mechanism of action

Butorphanol has antagonistic activity at μ opioid receptors. It is an agonist at κ opioid receptors, effecting visceral and spinal analgesia. With this set of differential effects, it can provide pain relief, while blocking μ-mediated respiratory depression.

Butorphanol increases cardiac work and can cause pulmonary hypertension. At super-therapeutic doses, it can incite dysphoria. Other CNS effects include depression of spontaneous respiratory activity and cough, stimulation of the emetic center, miosis, and sedation. Effects possibly mediated by non-CNS mechanisms include alteration in cardiovascular resistance and capacitance, bronchomotor tone, gastrointestinal secretory and motor activity, and bladder sphincter activity. Butorphanol metabolites have minor analgesic activity [2,3].

Uptake and elimination

Butorphanol is extensively metabolized in the liver. Metabolism is qualitatively and quantitatively similar following intravenous or intramuscular administration. Oral bioavailability is only 5 to 17% because of extensive first-pass metabolism of butorphanol [2,3].

The major metabolite of butorphanol is hydroxybutorphanol, while norbutorphanol is produced in small amounts. Both have been detected in plasma following administration of butorphanol, with norbutorphanol present at trace levels at most time points. The elimination half-life of hydroxybutorphanol is about 18 hours and, as a consequence, considerable accumulation (~5-fold) occurs when butorphanol is dosed to steady state [2–4].

Elimination occurs by urine and fecal excretion. When ³H-labeled butorphanol is administered to normal subjects, most (70 to 80%) of the dose is recovered in the urine, while approximately 15% is recovered in the feces.

About 5% of the dose is recovered in the urine as butorphanol. Forty-nine percent is eliminated in the urine as hydroxybutorphanol. Less than 5% is excreted in the urine as norbutorphanol [3,4].

Butorphanol pharmacokinetics in the elderly differ from younger patients.

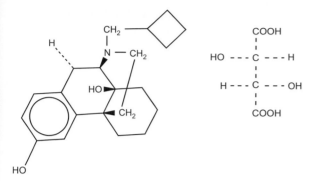

Figure 34.1.

In renally impaired patients with creatinine clearances <30 mL/min, the elimination half-life was approximately doubled and the total body clearance was approximately one-half of that in healthy subjects.

After intravenous administration to patients with hepatic impairment, the elimination half-life of butorphanol was approximately triple and total body clearance was approximately one-half compared to healthy subjects.

Indications

Parenteral: management of moderate-to-severe pain; pre-operative medication, a supplement to balanced anesthesia, management of pain during labor, anesthesia.

Nasal spray: management of moderate-to-severe pain, including migraine headache pain [4].

Dose guide

IV for pain: 1 mg repeated every 3 to 4 hours, as necessary. However, depending on the severity of pain, dosing can range from 0.5 mg to 2 mg repeated every 3 to 4 hours [3,4].

IM: 2 mg repeated every 3 to 4 hours as necessary. A dose range is 1 mg to 4 mg repeated every 3 to 4 hours. There are insufficient clinical data to recommend single doses above 4 mg. Higher doses are associated with increased drowsiness and somnolence, so bed rest is advised.

Use as pre-operative/preanesthetic medication

The usual adult dose is 2 mg IM, 60 to 90 minutes before surgery, roughly similar to the sedative effect of 10 mg morphine or 80 mg meperidine.

Use in balanced anesthesia

The usual dose is 2 mg IV shortly before induction and/or 0.5 mg to 1 mg IV in increments during anesthesia. Larger increments may be used, up to 0.06 mg/kg (4 mg/70 kg), depending on other drugs administered. The total dose ranges between 4 mg and more than 12.5 mg (approximately 0.06 to 0.18 mg/kg) [2–4].

Labor

For parturients in early labor, a 1 to 2 mg IV or IM may be repeated 4 hourly, but other analgesia should be employed if delivery is expected within 4 hours.

Contraindications

Hypersensitivity to butorphanol or any component of the formulation. Opiate-dependent patients may experience acute opiate withdrawal.

Butorphanol tartrate injection is contraindicated in patients hypersensitive to butorphanol tartrate or the preservative benzethonium chloride in the multiple-dose vial.

Precautions and relative contraindications

Head injury and increased intracranial pressure

Butorphanol use in patients with head injury may be associated with carbon dioxide retention and secondary elevation of cerebrospinal fluid pressure, drug-induced miosis, and alterations in mental state. As with other opioids, such use may obscure important clinical signs in patients with head injuries.

Disorders of respiratory function or control

Butorphanol may produce respiratory depression, with other medications with significant CNS action and in patients with CNS or respiratory diseases.

Hepatic and renal disease

Hepatic or renal impairment may indicate a half-dose initially (0.5 mg IV and 1 mg IM). Repeat doses in these patients should be determined by the patient's response. As a guide, the interval should not be less than 6 hours.

Cardiovascular effects

Butorphanol may increase the work of the heart, and is associated with pulmonary hypertension, so butorphanol use with acute myocardial infarction, ventricular dysfunction, or coronary insufficiency should only be used if the benefits clearly outweigh the risk. Severe hypertension has been reported rarely. Naloxone and anti-hypertensive drugs have been found effective.

Use in ambulatory patients

Car driving or operating machinery can be impaired by drowsiness or dizziness as with other opioids. These effects may persist for varying periods of time but are common in the first hour. Patients should not drive or operate dangerous machinery until the effects of the drug are no longer present [4].

Alcohol is associated with increased drowsiness and impairment of mental functions; it should be avoided.

Butorphanol has abuse potential, particularly the nasal spray. Patients and prescribers need to be aware of the danger.

Drug interactions

Concurrent use of butorphanol with central nervous system depressants (e.g. alcohol, barbiturates, tranquilizers, and antihistamines) may result in increased central nervous system depressant effects. When used concurrently with such drugs, the dose of butorphanol should be the smallest effective dose and the frequency of dosing reduced as much as possible when administered concomitantly with drugs that potentiate the action of opioids.

It is not known whether the effects of butorphanol are altered by concomitant medications that affect hepatic metabolism of drugs (erythromycin, theophylline, etc.), but physicians should be alert to the possibility that a smaller initial dose and longer intervals between doses may be needed.

Caution should be used if butorphanol treatment is considered with MAO inhibitors.

Mixed opioid agonist–antagonist analgesics such as buprenorphine, butorphanol, nalbuphine, and pentazocine may theoretically decrease the analgesic effects of tramadol or cause withdrawal symptoms in patients who have been taking tramadol and other opioids [1,2,4].

Cost

US$100–200/month, depending on source and product.

Adverse events

Many adverse events have been reported, though it is unclear in many instances whether butorphanol was to blame. The following is a list of common events reported in trials at a frequency of 1% or more, and probably related to the use of butorphanol:

Body as a whole: asthenia/lethargy, headache, sensation of heat.

Cardiovascular: vasodilatation, palpitations.

Digestive: anorexia, constipation, dry mouth, nausea and/or vomiting, stomach pain.

Nervous: anxiety, confusion, dizziness, euphoria, floating feeling, insomnia, nervousness, paresthesia, somnolence, tremor.

Respiratory: bronchitis, cough, dyspnea, epistaxis, nasal congestion, nasal irritation, pharyngitis, rhinitis, sinus congestion, sinusitis, upper respiratory infection.

Skin and appendages: sweating/clammy, pruritus.

Special senses: blurred vision, ear pain, tinnitus, unpleasant taste.

References

1. http://dailymed.nlm.nih.gov/dailymed/drugInfo.cfm?id=4752 #nlm34089–3 Butorphanol, description by NIH-NLM-H&HS, "DailyMed".

2. https://online.epocrates.com/noFrame/showPage.do?method=drugs&MonographId=1685 Butorphanol on Epocrates.

3. Brunton LL, ed. Opioid analgesics (Chapter 21). In *Goodman & Gilman's The Pharmacological Basis of Therapeutics*,11th ed. New York: McGraw Hill, 2006.

4. http://www.drugs.com/pro/butorphanol.html Butorphanaol on Drugs.com.

35 Buprenorphine: intravenous neuraxial and transdermal applications

Nalini Vadivelu

Generic Name: buprenorphine, buprenorphine hydrochoride

Trade/Proprietary Names: Anorfin™; Buprenex™; Buprex™; Buprine™

Chemical Class: opioid analgesic

Manufacturers: Spectrum Chemical Mfg Corp., 202 E Laurel Street, Bellingham, WA 98225, USA; Archimedes Pharma Ltd (United Kingdom), 250 South Oak Way, Green Park, Reading,RG2 6UG; Reckitt Benckiser Pharmaceuticals Inc., 10710 Midlothian Turnpike, Richmond, VA 23235; Otsuka Pharmaceuticals Co. Limited (Japan), 2–27, Otedori, 3-Chome, Chuoku, Osaka 5400021

Chemical Structure: see Figure 35.1

Chemical Name: 17-(cyclopropylmethyl)-α-(1,1-dimethylethyl)-4,5-epoxy-18,19-dihydro-3-hydroxy-6-methoxy-α-methyl-6,14-ethenomorphinan-7-methanol, [5α,7α(S)]

Chemical Formula: $C_{29}H_{41}NO_4$; molecular wt: 467

Introduction

Buprenorphine was first synthesized in 1966 as a semisynthetic opioid alkaloid derivative of thebain. Its unique mixed agonist–antagonist properties combined with its long-acting lipid solubility make it a useful analgesic with a lower abuse liability in humans. Its high affinity to mu opioid receptors along with a slow dissociation rate has led to its use as an analgesic for patients with opioid dependence as well. Buprenorphine has been widely used as an analgesic in the peri-operative setting and as an analgesic for moderate to severe acute pain as well as for chronic pain.

Pharmacodynamics and pharmacokinetics of buprenorphine

Buprenorphine binds to mu, kappa, and delta opioid receptor subtypes. It has a partial agonist activity at mu receptors and an antagonist activity at kappa receptors. Less is known about the activity of buprenorphine at delta receptors. Buprenorphine is more lipophilic than morphine and penetrates the blood–brain barrier more easily and has a rapid onset of effect.

The onset of action of buprenorphine is 5–15 minutes for intravenous of intramuscular injection and 15–45 minutes for sublingual buprenorphine. Buprenorphine has been seen to have a antinociceptive potency about 20–70 times greater than that of morphine [1].

Buprenorphine is metabolized to an active N-dealkylated metabolite, norbuprenorphine. Norbuprenorphine has one-fourth the potency of buprenorphine. It is metabolized in the liver and the gut. It is seen that the excretion of buprenorphine is not affected by the presence of end-stage renal failure.

Side effects

Its high affinity to the mu receptors and slow dissociation could lead to a lower incidence of side effects of sedation, nausea, pruritus, respiratory depression, and urinary retention. Being an agonist and antagonist it has side effects seen with this group of drugs such as dry mouth, lightheadedness, confusion, and blurred vision [2].

Buprenorphine for acute pain relief

Initial studies performed in animals demonstrated the analgesic efficacy of buprenorphine. These were followed by human analgesic trials evaluating different routes of administration. Buprenorphine does not have

157

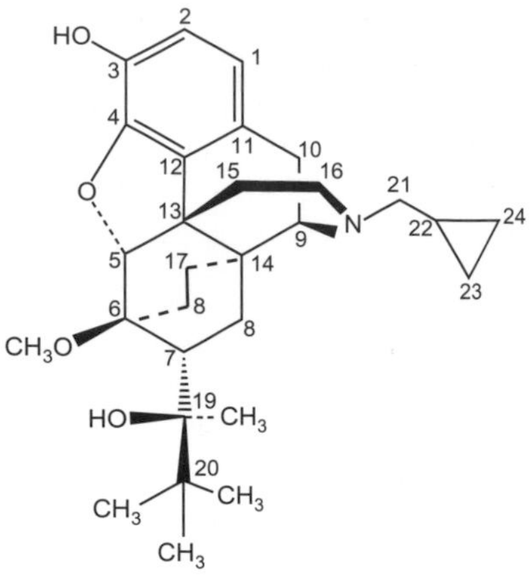

Figure 35.1.

Table 35.1. Commonly used routes and doses of buprenorphine for analgesia

Route	Dose
Intravenous	4–14 µg/kg
Subcutaneous	30 µg/h
Sublingual	0.5–2 mg single dose
Intramuscular	0.3–0.4 mg single dose
Epidural	15 µg/h
Caudal in pediatrics	3–4 µg/kg
Transdermal buprenorphine	35, 52.5, and 70 µg/h
Intrathecal	0.2 mg single dose

significant therapeutic value when given orally because of its poor absorption and oral bioavailability; however, multiple clinical trials have demonstrated its analgesic efficacy following administration via epidural, intrathecal, sublingual, intramuscular, intra-articular, and transdermal routes (Table 35.1).

Epidural buprenorphine

Epidural buprenorphine has been used to provide analgesia after a wide range of surgeries. Mehta et al. [3] found that post-operative analgesia produced by buprenorphine administered at lumbar epidural sites was comparable to that provided at thoracic sites in patients recovering from CABG surgery. Epidural buprenorphine can produce spinal segmental analgesia, which develops 2 to 6 hours after administration. This property is useful for control of pain after rib fractures [4]. A study by Miwa et al. [5] showed that epidurally administered buprenorphine in a dose of 4 or 8 µg/kg provided post-operative analgesia as effec-

tive as morphine in doses of 80 µg per hour. Buprenorphine can also be used as a continuous epidural infusion. A dose of 15 µg per hour can produce satisfactory post-operative pain relief after lower abdominal surgery [6]. Buprenorphine has also been used caudally in children to safely and reliably produce post-operative pain relief. Kamal and Khan. [7] compared caudal buprenorphine with caudal bupivacaine in children aged 1–11 years undergoing genitourinary surgery looking at quality and duration of analgesia. They found that patients with caudal buprenorphine had better immediate post-operative relief as well as delayed post-operative relief after 20–24 hours with fewer side effects as compared with caudal bupivacaine.

Epidural buprenorphine has been shown to produce good post-operative pain control for patients recovering from gynecological surgery [5]. Epidural doses of 4 or 8 µg/kg provided good post-operative analgesia. Buprenorphine has also been used epidurally in the management of pain associated with multiple rib fractures [8]. It is interesting to note that there was no urinary retention or hypotension in these patients. Nausea, vomiting, and pruritus were the only complications [4].

Intrathecal buprenorphine

Intrathecal administration of buprenorphine provides potent and effective analgesia with fewer adverse effects than the epidural route since the dose of buprenorphine is significantly less [10–12]. Intrathecal buprenorphine has been used effectively to control pain after cesarean section. The doses of intrathecal buprenorphine in this study were between 0.03 mg and 0.045 mg buprenorphine with the higher dose of intrathecal buprenorphine producing a longer duration of analgesia [11].

Intravenous buprenorphine

Intravenous buprenorphine has been used in doses in the range of 5–15 µg/kg body weight with good pain relief. The high (15 µg/kg) dose produced analgesia lasting up to 13 hours [13].

In a study of patients recovering from gynecological surgery, buprenorphine was noted to have an intravenous analgesic potency 24 times greater than morphine [14]. Intravenous buprenorphine was compared with thoracic epidural buprenorphine/bupivacaine mixture for treatment of post-thoracotomy pain. Surprisingly, it was shown that patients in the intravenous buprenorphine group required significantly less rescue analgesics as compared to the epidural buprenorphine/bupivacaine group [15]. Subcutaneous administration of buprenorphine offers advantages in palliative care settings where intravenous access may be a problem. Matsumoto et al. [16] found that an effective dose of subcutaneous buprenorphine is 30 μg an hour for early post-operative pain relief.

Sublingual buprenorphine

The great lipophilicity of buprenorphine allows it to be a suitable sublingual agent [17]. Sublingual buprenorphine in doses of 0.2 mg has been used as a premedication for extracorporeal kidney lithotripsy [18] and prostatectomy [19], providing effective analgesia with few side effects. Witjes et al. [20] evaluated sublingual buprenorphine in patients recovering from cholecystectomy. They reported that there was a need for supplemental analgesics for some of the patients. The authors recommended intravenous PCA for such cases.

Buprenorphine via other routes

Buprenorphine can also be used intramuscularly where it provides an analgesic onset at 15 minutes, peak effect at 1 hour and a duration of 6 hours. The development and use of transdermal buprenorphine for the treatment of chronic pain is ongoing and is discussed in Chapter 121. Buprenorphine in conjunction with local anesthetic has been used intra-articularly for control of pain after knee arthroscopy [21] and for perivascular axillary brachial plexus block [22]. It was seen that buprenorphine in conjunction with local anesthetic produced analgesia that was three times longer than the analgesia produced by the use of bupivacaine alone. Buprenorphine added to the local anesthetic for axillary brachial plexus block prolongs post-operative analgesia [23].

Finally, buprenorphine has been found to be effective and safe for the treatment of chronic pain that is refractory to treatment with long-term opioids [24]. In another study treating chronic pain it was shown that sublingual and intravenous buprenorphine produced longer antihyperalgesic effects than pure mu agonists [25].

Conclusion

Recent studies have revealed that buprenorphine has a great potential as an analgesic and it has been used as an effective analgesic for the treatment of acute pain as well as for the treatment of chronic pain. Its advantages over the commonly used mu agonists include effectiveness via many different routes of administration, greater potency, smaller molecular weight, longer duration of action and less respiratory depression.

References

1. Capogna G, Celleno D, Tagariello V, Loffreda-Mancinelli C. Intrathecal buprenorphine for post-operative analgesia in the elderly patient. *Anaesthesia* 1988;**43**(2):128–130.

2. Harcus A, Ward A, Smith D. Buprenorphine in post-operative pain: results in 7500 patients. *Anaesthesia* 1980;**35**(4):382–386.

3. Mehta Y, Juneja R, Madhok H, Trehan N. Lumbar versus thoracic epidural buprenorphine for post-operative analgesia following coronary artery bypass graft surgery. *Acta Anaesthesiol Scand* 1999;**43**(4):388–393.

4. Govindarajan R, Bakalova T, Michael R, Abadir A. Epidural buprenorphine in management of pain in multiple rib fractures. *Acta Anaesthesiol Scand* 2002;**46**(6):660–665.

5. Miwa Y, Yonemura E, Fukushima K. Epidural administered buprenorphine in the perioperative period. *Can J Anaesth* 1996;**43**(9):907–913.

6. Hirabayashi Y, Mitsuhata H, Shimizu R, Saitoh J, Saitoh K, Fukuda H. [Continuous epidural buprenorphine for post-operative pain relief in patients after lower abdominal surgery]. *Masui* 1993;**42**(11):1618–1622.

7. Kamal R, Khan F. Caudal analgesia with buprenorphine for post-operative pain relief in children. *Paediatr Anaesth* 1995;**5**(2):101–106.

8. Govindarajan R, Bakalova T, Michael R, Abadir AR. Epidural buprenorphine in management of pain in multiple rib fractures. *Acta Anaesthesiol Scand* 2002;**46**(6):660–665.

9. Girotra S, Kumar S, Rajendran K. Comparison of caudal morphine and buprenorphine for post-operative analgesia in children. *Eur J Anaesthesiol* 1993;**10**(4):309–312.

10. Tejwani G, Rattan A. The role of spinal opioid receptors in antinociceptive effects produced by intrathecal administration of hydromorphone and buprenorphine in the rat. *Anesth Analg* 2002;**94**(6):1542–1546.

11. Celleno D, Capogna G. Spinal buprenorphine for post-operative analgesia after caesarean section. *Acta Anaesthesiol Scand* 1989;**33**(3):236–238.

12. Dahm P, Lundborg C, Janson M, Olegård C, Nitescu P. Comparison of 0.5% intrathecal bupivacaine with 0.5% intrathecal ropivacaine in the treatment of refractory cancer and noncancer pain conditions: results from a prospective, crossover, double-blind, randomized study. *Reg Anesth Pain Med* 2000;**25**(5):480–487.

13. Abrahamsson J, Niemand D, Olsson A, Törnebrandt K. [Buprenorphine (Temgesic) as a peroperative analgesic. A multicenter study]. *Anaesthesist* 1983;**32**(2):75–79.

14. Ho S, Wang J, Liu H, Tzeng J, Liaw W. The analgesic effect of PCA buprenorphine in Taiwan's gynecologic patients. *Acta Anaesthesiol Sin* 1997;**35**(4):195–199.

15. Satoh M, Hirabayashi Y, Seo N. [Intravenous patient controlled analgesia combined with continuous thoracic epidural analgesia for post-thoracotomy pain]. *Masui* 2000;**49**(11):1222–1225.

16. Matsumoto S, Mitsuhata H, Akiyama H, Terada H, Matsumoto H. [The effect of subcutaneous administration of buprenorphine with patient controlled analgesia system for post-operative pain relief]. *Masui* 1994;**43**(11):1709–1713.

17. Bullingham R, McQuay H, Dwyer D, Allen M, Moore R. Sublingual buprenorphine used post-operatively: clinical observations and preliminary pharmacokinetic analysis. *Br J Clin Pharmacol* 1981;**12**(2):117–122.

18. Tauzin-Fin P, Saumtally S, Houdek M, Muscagorry J. [Analgesia by sublingual buprenorphine in extracorporeal kidney lithotripsy]. *Ann Fr Anesth Reanim* 1993;**12**(3):260–264.

19. Gaitini L, Moskovitz B, Katz E, Vaisberg A, Vaida S, Nativ O. Sublingual buprenorphine compared to morphine delivered by a patient-controlled analgesia system as post-operative analgesia after prostatectomy. *Urol Int* 1996;**57**(4):227–229.

20. Witjes W, Crul B, Vollaard E, Joosten H, von Egmond J. Application of sublingual buprenorphine in combination with naproxen or paracetamol for post-operative pain relief in cholecystectomy patients in a double-blind study. *Acta Anaesthesiol Scand* 1992;**36**(4):323–327.

21. Rodriguez N, Cooper D, Risdahl J. Antinociceptive activity of and clinical experience with buprenorphine in swine. *Contemp Top Lab Anim Sci* 2001;**40**(3):17–20.

22. Varrassi G, Marinangeli F, Ciccozzi A, Iovinelli G, Facchetti G, Ciccone A. Intra-articular buprenorphine after knee arthroscopy. A randomised, prospective, double-blind study. *Acta Anaesthesiol Scand* 1999;**43**(1):51–55.

23. Candido K, Winnie A, Ghaleb A, Fattouh M, Franco C. Buprenorphine added to the local anesthetic for axillary brachial plexus block prolongs postoperative analgesia. *Reg Anesth Pain Med* 2002;**27**(2):162–167.

24. Malinoff H, Barkin R, Wilson G. Sublingual buprenorphine is effective in the treatment of chronic pain syndrome. *Am J Ther* 2005 Sep-Oct;**12**(5):379–384.

25. Koppert W, Ihmsen H, Körber N, Wehrfritz A, Sittl R, Schmelz M, Schüttler J. Different profiles of buprenorphine-induced analgesia and antihyperalgesia in a human pain model. *Pain* 2005;**118**(1–2):15–22.

36

Opioid dosing in pediatric patients

Debra E. Morrison, Abraham Rosenbaum, Co T. Truong and Zeev N. Kain

General principles of opioid dosing and pain management in pediatric patients

Opioids are usually used for acute and chronic pain management in pediatric practice, as described below. However, an opioid may be used as an anesthetic in a critical premature or newborn infant who either cannot tolerate a conventional ventilator or cannot tolerate a volatile anesthetic: this will be addressed at the end of the chapter.

There are size and developmental considerations to consider when prescribing opiates to pediatric patients in addition to the setting in which opiates are prescribed.

Pediatric patients from birth through adolescence can be classified into six groups:

(1) Premature infants (less than 38 weeks gestation)
(2) Newborn/neonate (term birth to 1 month or 40–44 weeks gestational age)
(3) Infant (1 month or 44 weeks to 24 months)
    (a) term infant less than 6 months of age
    (b) term infant more than 6 months of age
(4) Young child (2 to 4 years)
(5) Older child (6 to12 years)
(6) Adolescent (13 to 18 years)

All pediatric drug orders and prescriptions should include weight.

A comparative oral and parenteral dosage table and initial approximate oral and parental dosage tables are included below.

Dosing for pediatric patients who weigh less than 50 kg is in mg or µg per kg.

Dosing for pediatric patients who weigh 50 kg or greater is similar to adult dosing.

Dosing for pediatric patients in the 50–70 kg range can be more closely titrated by using a ratio to determine dose/kg: $1/70 \times$ adult dose = dose/1 kg.

Weight may not be proportional to developmental age.

Ideal body weight should be considered when patient's weight is out of proportion to height and age, especially in dosing water-soluble opiates. Older children and adolescents who are developmentally appropriate can tolerate patient-controlled analgesia (PCA). PCA by proxy for younger children is not recommended, except with certain parents who have experience with and understanding of their child's pain management.

Opiates are indicated when adjunct medications (local anesthetics, acetaminophen, NSAIDS) are inadequate, but these medications should not be abandoned when opiates are added to the regimen: drugs should be layered as pain management escalates.

Parents as well as all members of the healthcare team caring for pediatric patients should be educated about pediatric pain and pain management with a goal of achieving optimal pain management.

It is easier to use non-combination opiates in order to avoid confusion leading to acetaminophen toxicity, and to prescribe acetaminophen separately, despite the ease and familiarity (for the prescriber) of prescribing combination drugs.

Dosing should start low and titrate upward, but pain management should be aggressive.

Codeine, a weak opiate with many side effects, including nausea, is generally not a good drug for pediatric patients. In addition, many people, especially many African-Americans and Asians, do not metabolize codeine.

Pain management should not be limited in end of life care.

Doses for breakthrough pain should always be available.

Doses for treatment of side effects should be calculated in advance.

Even young children and their parents who have past experience with opiates will be able to give credible histories of dysphoria but inadequate pain relief with one opiate but not another: please listen.

Issues of tolerance and withdrawal are relevant to pediatric pain management.

Initial opiate dosage guide for patients over 6 months of age

For children too young to swallow pills, an oral elixir is the best option (awake children often find suppositories undignified, but suppositories may be necessary in patients who find swallowing even liquid painful). Opiates available in liquid form include:

Morphine

Oral regular release 10 mg/5mL, 20 mg/mL, 20 mg/5mL

(Roxanol®) 20 mg/mL

Hydromorphone (Dilaudid®) 1 mg/mL

Codeine 15 mg/5 mL

Codeine phosphate/acetaminophen elixir

(Tylenol® #2) 15 mg codeine/300 mg acetaminophen

(Tylenol® #3) 30 mg codeine/300 mg acetaminophen

(Tylenol® #4) 60 mg codeine/300 mg acetaminophen

Hydrocodone elixir (Lortab®) 2.5 mg hydrocodone/167 mg acetaminophen/5 mL

Methadone oral solution 5 mg/mL (5, 500 mL), 10 mg/5mL (500 mL)

Oxycodone

(Roxicodone®) solution 5 mg/5 mL

(Roxicet®) 5 mg oxycodone/325 mg acetaminophen/5 mL

Remember that not all neighborhood pharmacies have liquid opiates available.

For patients whose pain will be short-term in nature, oxycodone (in appropriate formulation) can be given around the clock. For patients whose pain is anticipated to be longer-term in nature, oxycodone HCl CR (Oxycontin) or MS Contin can be given.

Oral opioid dose recommendations are presented in Table 36.1.

IV equivalent doses

Morphine, with a half-life of 3 hours, is the basic unit of comparison: other drugs are compared to morphine. Morphine 1 mg : hydromorphone 0.2 mg : fentanyl 50 μg : meperidine 10 mg.

Table 36.1. Initial approximate oral doses and intervals

Codeine	0.5–1 mg/kg every 3–4 h	30–60 mg every 3–4 h
Morphine	Immed. release	Immed. release
	0.3 mg/kg	15–30 mg
	every 3–4 h	every 3–4 h
		Sustained release
		30–45 mg
		every 3–4 h
Oxycodone	0.1–0.2 mg/kg	5–10 mg
	every 3–4 h	every 3–4 h
Methadone	0.1 mg/kg	10 mg
	every 4–8 h	every 4–8 h
Hydromorphone	0.04–0.08	2–4 mg
	every 3–4 h	every 3–4 h
Meperidine[a]	2–3 mg/kg	100–150 mg
	every 3–4 h	every 3–4 h

[a]Avoid if other drugs available, avoid chronic use since metabolite causes seizures.

The average morphine loading dose is 100 µg/kg. The average morphine infusion is 20 µg/kg per h. Drugs appropriate for PCA include morphine and hydromorphone.

PCA morphine dose should start at a bolus dose of 0.03 mg/kg, with or without a continuous infusion of 0.03 mg/kg per h, with a 6–10 min lockout. If pain is not controlled, increase bolus by 10–20%, increase infusion by 20–40%, decrease interval, and check to see that patient is not reaching the 4 h maximum dose. Refer to Table 36.2 for IV-PCA dosing.

If the patient is experiencing side effects, such as itching, nausea and vomiting, hallucinations, dysphoria, constipation, urinary retention: consider switching opioids and/or treating treatable side effects (itching, nausea and vomiting, constipation) individually.

Table 36.2. Approximate PCA doses and dose intervals

Drug	Child <50 kg	Child > 50 kg
Morphine	Bolus:	Bolus:
	0.1–0.3 mg/kg	5–8 mg
	every 2–4 h	every 2–4 h
	Infusion:	Infusion:
	0.2.–0.3	1.5 mg/h
	mg/kg per h	
Methadone	0.1 mg/kg	5–8 mg every 4–8 h
	(see sliding scale)	
Fentanyl	Bolus:	Bolus:
	0.5–1.0 µg/kg	25–50 µg
	every 1–2 h	every 1–2 h
	Infusion:	Infusion:
	0.5–2.0 µg/kg per h	25–100 µg/h
Hydromorphone	Bolus:	Bolus:
	0.01–0.02 mg/kg	1 mg
	every 2–4 h	every 2–4 h
	Infusion:	Infusion:
	0.006 mg/kg per h	0.3 mg/h
	(6 µg/kg/ per h)	
Meperidine[a]	Bolus:	Bolus:
	0.8–1.0 mg/kg	50–75 mg
	every 2–3 h	every 2–3 h
	(No infusion)	(No infusion)

[a]Avoid if other drugs available, avoid chronic use since metabolite causes seizures
Methadone sliding scale: The methadone sliding scale or "reverse PRN" method is useful for patients for whom PCA is not appropriate. The patient is assessed every 4 hours for the first 24 hours, then every 6 hours subsequently. Methadone is titrated to pain intensity at the time of assessment. The drug is given around the clock and held only for significant side effects.

Pain score	Dose
Zero–mild pain	25 µg/kg
Mild–moderate pain	50 µg/kg
Moderate–severe pain	75 µg/kg

Diphenhydramine (Benadryl®) 5 mg/kg per 24 h, given every 6–8 h (not recommended for <1 yr old because of its sedative side effect)

Naloxone (Narcan®)

Respiratory depression 10 µg/kg IV push every 3 minutes

Apnea or impending apnea 100 µg/kg, maximum 2 mg/dose

Antiemetics (see appropriate chapter)

Stool softeners and laxatives

Neuraxial opiates will not be addressed, since in pediatric patients, opiates may be given enterally or parentally as adjuncts to regional or neuraxial analgesia.

Transdermal fentanyl (Duragesic®) can be used in older and larger children (>50 kg).

Fentanyl Oralet (Actiq®) can be a useful adjunct in children with cancer pain or other chronic pain. Don't call it a lollipop.

Other sedating agents are held for 1 hour before and after the methadone dose to avoid respiratory depression.

Accumulation of methadone occurs after several days, so a decrease in dosing frequency and/or dose is necessary with prolonged administration.

For tolerance, in patients with chronic or escalating pain, the sliding-scale dose can be increased by 25 µg/kg.

Breakthrough pain can be treated first with adjunct agents, and second with immediate release oral morphine or IV morphine every 1–2 h PRN.

Dosing conversion from oral to iV opioids are presented in Table 36.3.

Initial opioid dosage guide for patients under 6 months of age

For term infants under 6 months of age, if non-opiate pain medications are inadequate, use dosing tables above, but limit drugs to morphine and fentanyl.

If the patient is naive to opioids, start with a smaller than recommended dose per kg, and titrate up.

If the patient has received prior opioids, use past history as a guideline to determine starting doses.

Consider leaving patients intubated post-operatively after major/painful surgery in order to allow safe and effective pain relief.

Consider regional and continuous neuraxial analgesia (without opiates) with low-dose opiates for breakthrough pain.

Opioids as anesthetics

An opiate may be used as an anesthetic in a critical premature or newborn infant who either cannot tolerate a conventional ventilator or cannot tolerate a volatile anesthetic.

Premature infants who require ligation of a patent ductus arteriosus (PDA) or who present with necrotizing enterocolitis (NEC) often weigh less than 1 kg and are not on conventional ventilators, thus often cannot be moved from the neonatal intensive care unit and cannot tolerate an anesthesia machine or a volatile anesthetic.

Other larger but very critical infants who are able to be transported to the operating room may be too unstable to tolerate a volatile anesthetic.

Fentanyl, in high doses, can be used as the sole anesthetic, with a nondepolarizing muscle relaxant. Doses used in our practice are 50–150 µg/kg (or higher,

Table 36.3. Comparing oral and parenteral doses

Drug	Equianalgesic doses parenteral	Oral	Parenteral/oral dose ratio
Codeine	120 mg	200 mg	1:2
Morphine	10 mg	30 mg (long-term)	1:3
Oxycodone	N/A	15–20 mg	N/A
Methadone	10 mg	10–20 mg	1:2
Fentanyl	100 µg (0.1 mg)	N/A	N/A
Hydromorphone	1.5–2 mg	6–8 mg	1:4
Meperidine[a]	75–100 mg	300 mg	1:4

[a]Avoid if other drugs available, avoid chronic use since metabolite causes seizures.

depending on the length of operation, the degree of surgical stimulation, and whether or not local anesthetics can be used as adjuncts). The goal is to block pain such that any rise in heart rate is attributable only to hypovolemia. These patients are not extubatable for other reasons, thus respiratory depression is not an issue here. Although remifentanil might seem like a candidate as an anesthetic in this setting, it is not FDA-approved for this population, and it is much more likely to cause hypotension than is fentanyl, which allows these patients to remain surprisingly stable.

Clinical pearls

For routine post-operative analgesia, we rely on acetaminophen, local anesthetics, NSAIDS if not contraindicated, and, finally, opiates. Even if pain control is adequate without opiates, small doses of fentanyl may be used at the time of emergence to ease a patient through emergence delirium and the first moments in PACU when even parental presence is not a comfort.

References

1. Anand KJS, Stevens BJ, McGrath PJ. *Pain in Neonates and Infants*, 3rd ed. Philadelphia: Elsevier, 2007.

2. Bartolome SM, Cid JL-H, Freddi N. Analgesia and sedation in children: practical approach for the most frequent situations. *J Pediatr (Rio J)* 2007;**83**(2 Suppl):S71–82.

3. Fortier MA, MacLaren JE, Martin SR, Perret-Karimi D, Kain ZN. Pediatric pain after ambulatory surgery: where's the medication? *Pediatrics* 2009;**124**;e588-e595; originally published online Sep 7 2009; DOI: 10.1542/peds.2008–3529.

4. Kraemer FW, Rose JB. Pharmacologic management of acute pediatric pain. *Anesthesiology Clin* 2009;**27**: 241–268.

5. Tobias JD, Desphande JK. *Pediatric Pain Management for Primary Care*, 2nd ed. American Academy of Pediatrics, 2005.

6. Tollison CD, Satterthwaite JR, Tollison JW, eds. *Practical Pain Management*, 3rd ed. Philadelphia: Lippincott, Williams & Wilkins, 2002.

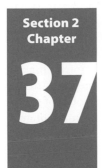

Section 2
Chapter

37

Oral and Parenteral Opioid Analgesics

Opioid tolerance and dependence

Sukanya Mitra

Introduction

Anesthesiologists, surgeons, pharmacists and nursing staff are increasingly asked to care for a variety of opioid-tolerant patients in peri-operative and pain management settings. The majority are those suffering from chronic pain conditions, who have been taking opioid analgesics for a prolonged period (months to years). A less common but important second group exhibiting tolerance includes the opioid abuser or addicted patient. Former addicts enrolled in long-term methadone or buprenorphine maintenance programs constitute an increasing third group. A final subset of opioid-dependent patients comprises those who suffer well-documented chronic pain who, superficially, resemble opioid abusers by virtue of their often obsessive drug-seeking behavior. These patients are usually found to have visited numerous physicians and have filled multiple prescriptions for opioids. In actuality these individuals are not addicted but undermedicated and are only seeking adequate pain relief. This phenomenon was not recognized until recently and has been termed pseudo-addiction.

Opioid tolerance

Opioid tolerance is a normal and predictable pharmacological adaptation of the body to continued opioid administration. Continued opioid exposure results in a rightward shift in the dose-response curve and patients require increasing amounts of drug to maintain the baseline pharmacological effects. The phenomenon of tolerance develops to analgesic, euphoric, sedative, respiratory depressant, and nauseating effects of opioids, but very little to their effects on miosis and constipation. Further, tolerance develops to some drug effects much more rapidly than to other effects of the same drug. For example, tolerance develops rapidly to the euphoria produced by opioids such as heroin. In contrast, tolerance to the gastrointestinal effects of opiates develops more slowly. The discrepancy between the rapid development of tolerance to euphorigenic effects and slow development of tolerance to effects on respiration and blood pressure can lead to potentially fatal accidents in opioid addicts.

The degree or gradation of opioid tolerance is generally related to duration of exposure, daily dose requirement, and receptor association/disassociation kinetics. While there are no clear gradation guidelines, individuals requiring the equivalent of 1 mg or more intravenous or 3 mg or more of oral morphine per hour for a period greater than 1 month may be considered clinically to have high-grade opioid tolerance.

Tolerance is observed in patients legitimately prescribed opioids for pain management as well as in those abusing this class of drug. In general, the higher the daily dose requirement the greater the degree of tolerance development. This is of importance for many patients and caregivers who perceive an increasing opioid dose requirement as reflecting harmful addiction rather than normal pharmacological adaptation.

Types of opioid tolerance

Several types of opioid tolerance including innate (genetic) tolerance, pharmacokinetic tolerance, learned tolerance and pharmacodynamic tolerance may be observed. Innate tolerance refers to genetically determined lack of sensitivity to a drug that is observed the first time that the drug is administered (and hence it is not true tolerance according to the definition of tolerance, which requires repeated or continuous opioid administration). Recent research has identified certain genetic variations of the mu opioid receptor gene (particularly the A118G single nucleotide polymorphism), beta-2-adrenergic receptor gene and the abcb1b gene of the P glycoprotein drug transporter to be associated with innate opioid tolerance.

The other three types of tolerance (pharmacokinetic, pharmacodynamic, and learned) are clubbed as acquired tolerance. In contrast to innate tolerance, this type of tolerance develops with continued opioid administration, and thus represents true tolerance rather than genetically mediated lack of sensitivity to opioids.

Learned tolerance refers to a moderation of the effects of a drug (usually behavioral) because of learning mechanisms that are acquired by past experiences. An example of learned behavioral tolerance is continuing the complex psychomotor act of driving despite high blood alcohol levels and the motor impairment produced by alcohol intoxication. This probably involves both acquisition of motor skills and the learned awareness of one's deficit. At higher levels of intoxication, of course, behavioral tolerance is overcome and the deficits are unmasked.

Pharmacokinetic tolerance refers to changes in distribution or metabolism of the drug, usually by enzyme induction and subsequent acceleration in metabolism. Opioids are biotransformed in the liver by two types of metabolic processes. Phase I reactions include oxidative and reductive reactions, such as those catalyzed by the cytochrome P450 (CYP) enzyme system, and hydrolytic reactions. Phase II reactions involve conjugation of a drug or its metabolite to an endogenous substrate, such as D-glucuronic acid, generating highly hydrophilic chemicals that are then excreted primarily by the kidneys. With the exceptions of the N-dealkylated metabolite of meperidine and the 6- and possibly 3-glucuronides of morphine, opioid metabolites are generally inactive. Since the P450 enzyme system is inducible by a host of compounds including opioids, barbiturates and antiepileptics, patients chronically exposed to these drugs can metabolize some opioids faster, thus producing pharmacokinetic tolerance. The CYP2D6 oxidation system has been particularly implicated in the hypoalgesic effect of opioids.

Perhaps the most important form of tolerance relevant to opioids is pharmacodynamic tolerance. Pharmacodynamic tolerance has been related to neuroadaptive changes that take place following chronic exposure to the drug. These include changes at various levels: receptor properties, receptor coupling to G proteins, signal transduction pathways, genetic expression profiles of several enzymes, receptors and other molecules, neural and glial networks, etc.

Mechanisms of pharmacodynamic tolerance

Basic animal research has provided a better though yet incomplete understanding of the cellular and molecular mechanisms mediating pharmacodynamic opioid tolerance. These mechanisms occur at three levels and have been termed receptor-level tolerance, cellular-level tolerance and system-level tolerance.

Receptor tolerance occurs at the level of the opioid receptor and involves receptor desensitization upon chronic or repeated exposure to opioids. The concept of receptor desensitization underlies acute-onset opioid tolerance. Receptor desensitization means loss in the coupling of mu opioid receptor to its cellular effectors, particularly its major cellular effector – the G-protein-regulated inwardly rectifying potassium channel. Several potential mechanisms could account for tolerance at this level of organization, but changes in coupling to G protein and perhaps expression of the receptors on the cell surface appear to be most important.

Earlier, removal of opioid receptors from the cell surface by beta-arrestin mediated endocytosis (a process termed "internalization") was also thought to be important in producing receptor tolerance. However, the observation that morphine, while causing very poor receptor internalization, nonetheless produces severe tolerance has led to a recent re-thinking on this mechanism. Internalized μ opioid receptors are not degraded but predominantly dephosphorylated and recycled to the cell surface in a reactivated state. In fact, it has been demonstrated that agonist induced μ receptor internalization plays an important role in actually reducing the development of opioid tolerance after chronic agonist treatment. The tentative explanation for this apparently paradoxical phenomenon is that internalized receptors quickly resurface in an activated state, whereas morphine-bound receptors remaining at cell surface remain desensitized (i.e., uncoupled to K^+ channel and other intracellular effectors) and thus produce tolerance.

Receptor-level tolerance represents the early (minutes to hours) and often short-lived adaptations to opioid administration. The slower-onset (hours to days) and longer-lasting adaptation to chronic opioid administration is better explained by cellular-level and system-level tolerance. Cellular tolerance refers to the second-messenger and further downstream changes induced by opioids that eventually counter-act opioids' own action. There are many different pathways, involving several enzymes (e.g., adenylyl cyclase, protein kinase A, protein kinase C, calcium/calmodulin-dependent kinase type 2, G protein-coupled receptor kinase, mitogen-activated protein kinase, other protein kinases, monoxide signaling systems heme oxygenase and nitric oxide synthase, phospholipase C) and their signaling cascades. Perhaps the best-established pathway involves up-regulation of the cyclic adenosine monophosphate (cAMP). Acutely, opiates inhibit the functional activity of the cAMP pathway by blocking adenylyl cyclase (AC), the enzyme that catalyzes the synthesis of cAMP. However, with chronic opiate exposure, the cAMP pathway gradually recovers, and tolerance develops. Up-regulation of cAMP may be responsible for physical dependence and physiological changes associated with withdrawal. In this regard, the activity of the cAMP pathway increases far above baseline levels following abrupt discontinuance of opioid binding. Although up-regulation of cAMP has been most clearly demonstrated in the locus coeruleus of the brain, up-regulation within the spinal cord dorsal horn appears to be responsible for tolerance to opioid-induced analgesia. Up-regulation of calcium ion channels is another mechanism of cellular-level tolerance.

Prolonged or long-term tolerance may represent a persistent neural adaptation, and is best explained by evoking the concept of system-level tolerance that involves altered sensitivity, functionality or even microstructure of not only opioid but related non-opioid neural and neural-glial networks. This phenomenon may be observed in patients who discontinued prescribed or illicit opioid use many months or years ago yet continue to exhibit diminished responsiveness or opioid insensitivity. Long-term adaptations at the molecular and cellular level involve, amongst others: (1) induction of transcription factors, such as delta Fos B, which regulate the function of several genes in a stable fashion, thus initiating neuronal plasticity; (2) activation of the central glutamate system and NMDA receptor activation as the "pronociceptive system". Prolonged exposure to morphine indirectly activates NMDA receptors via second-messenger mechanisms, and also down-regulates spinal glutamate transporters. The resultant high synaptic concentration of glutamate and NMDA activation contribute to opioid tolerance and abnormal pain sensitivity.

Opioid dependence

Physical dependence is a *state* that develops as a result of the adaptation of the body to repeated opioid use because of resetting of various homeostatic processes to a different set point (a process known as *allostasis*). Opioids affect numerous systems that previously were in equilibrium; these systems find a new balance in the presence of chronic inhibition by opioids. A person in this adapted or physically dependent state requires continued administration of the drug to maintain normal function. However, if and when administration of the drug is stopped abruptly, there is another imbalance (because the allostatic set points are different from the original ones), and the affected systems again must go through a process of readjusting to a new equilibrium without the drug. This readjustment process is often clinically manifest as a set of characteristic symptoms and signs known as the *withdrawal syndrome*. The appearance of a withdrawal syndrome when administration of the drug is terminated is the only actual evidence of physical dependence. Withdrawal signs and symptoms occur when drug administration in a physically dependent person is terminated abruptly. Thus, abrupt termination of a

Table 37.1. Substance use disorder: related definitions

Addiction	Commonly used term meaning the aberrant use of a specific psychoactive substance in a manner characterized by loss of control, compulsive use, preoccupation, and continued use despite harm; pejorative term, replaced in the DSM-IV-TR in a non-pejorative way by the term "substance use disorder (SUD)" with psychological and physical dependence
Dependence	1. Psychological dependence: need for a specific psychoactive substance either for its positive effects or to avoid negative psychological or physical effects associated with its withdrawal
	2. Physical dependence: a physiological state of adaptation to a specific psychoactive substance characterized by the emergence of a withdrawal syndrome during abstinence, which may be relieved in total or in part by readministration of the substance
	3. One category of psychoactive substance use disorder
Chemical dependence	A generic term relating to psychological and/or physical dependence when one or more psychoactive substances or classes of psychoactive substances are abused (alcohol; sedatives, hypnotics and anxiolytics; cannabis; opioids; cocaine; amphetamine and other sympathomimetics; hallucinogens; caffeine; nicotine; phencyclidine)
Substance use disorders	Term of DSM-IV-TR[19] comprising two main groups:
	1. Substance dependence disorder and substance abuse disorder
	2. Substance-induced disorders (e.g., intoxication, withdrawal, delirium, psychotic disorders)
Tolerance	Normal neurobiological event; a state in which an increased dosage of a psychoactive substance is needed to produce the original effect. Cross-tolerance: induced by repeated administration of one psychoactive substance that is manifested toward another substance to which the individual has not been recently exposed
Withdrawal syndrome	The onset of a predictable constellation of signs and symptoms following the abrupt discontinuation of or a rapid decrease in dosage of a psychoactive substance
Polydrug dependence	Concomitant use of two or more psychoactive substances in quantities and frequencies that cause individually significant physiological, psychological, and/or sociological distress or impairment (polysubstance abuser)
Recovery	A process of overcoming both physical and psychological dependence on a psychoactive substance with a commitment to sobriety
Abstinence	In recovery, non-use of any psychoactive substance
Maintenance	Prevention of craving behavior and withdrawal symptoms of opioids by permanently acting opioid (e.g., methadone, buprenorphine)
Substance abuse	Use of a psychoactive substance in a manner outside sociocultural conventions; according to this, any use of illicit and licit drugs in a manner not dictated by convention (e.g., according to physicians' order) is abuse
Pseudo-addiction	Behavioral changes in patients that seem similar to those in patients with opioid dependence or addiction but are secondary to inadequate pain control
Drug-seeking behaviors	Directed or concerted efforts on the part of the patient to obtain opioid medication or to ensure an adequate medication supply: may be an appropriate response to inadequately treated pain
Opioid-induced hyperalgesia	A neuroplastic change in pain perception resulting in an increase in pain sensitivity to painful stimuli, thereby decreasing the analgesic effects of opioids.

drug (such as an opioid agonist) that produces miotic (constricted) pupils and slow heart rate will produce a withdrawal syndrome including dilated pupils and tachycardia. Tolerance, physical dependence, and withdrawal are all biological phenomena. They are the natural consequences of drug use and can be produced in experimental animals and in any human being who takes certain medications repeatedly. These symptoms in themselves do not imply that the individual is involved in abuse or addiction. Patients who take medicine for appropriate medical indications and in correct dosages still may show tolerance, physical dependence, and withdrawal symptoms if the drug is stopped abruptly rather than gradually.

In contrast, some persons repeatedly taking opioids develop a psycho-behavioral syndrome characterized by a compulsive, irresistible quality in their drug-taking behavior, which persists despite drug-induced harm and which continues at the cost of neglecting other interests and responsibilities of life. These persons "crave" the drug (even in the absence of pain or other obvious physical reasons), cannot control the initiation, quantity, or termination of the drug intake, and spend a lot of time arranging for the drug, using it, or recovering from its effects. The diagnostic system of the American Psychiatric Association uses the term substance dependence instead of "addiction" for this behavioral syndrome. It also applies the same general criteria to all types of drugs regardless of their pharmacological class.

Thus, the word "opioid dependence" can mean two different things: one, a biological state produced in all receiving chronic opioid administration, primarily characterized by appearance of withdrawal phenomena when the opioid is abruptly stopped; and two, a clinical syndrome seen in some opioid consumers, characteristics of which may include tolerance and

Table 37.2. Guidelines for peri-operative pain management in opioid-tolerant patients

Pre-operative	
1.	Evaluation: should include early recognition and high index of suspicion
2.	Identification: identify factors such as total opioid dose requirement, previous surgery/trauma resulting in undermedication, inadequate analgesia or relapse episodes
3.	Consultation: meet with addiction specialists and pain specialists with regard to peri-operative planning
4.	Reassurance: discuss patient concerns related to pain control, anxiety, and risk of relapse
5.	Medication: calculate opioid dose requirement and mode(s) of administration, provide anxiolytics or other medications: as clinically indicated
Intra-operative	
1.	Maintain baseline opioids (oral, transdermal, intravenous)
2.	Increase intra-operative and post-operative opioid dose to compensate for tolerance
3.	Provide peripheral neural or plexus blockade, consider neuraxial analgesic techniques when clinically indicated
4.	Utilize non-opioids as analgesic adjuncts
Post-operative	
1.	Plan pre-operatively for post-operative analgesia; formulate primary strategy as well as suitable alternatives
2.	Maintain baseline opioids
3.	Employ multimodal analgesic techniques.
4.	Patient-controlled analgesia: as primary therapy or as supplementation for epidural or regional techniques
5.	Continue neuraxial opioids: intrathecal or epidural analgesia
6.	Continue continuous neural blockade
Post-discharge	
1.	If surgery provides complete pain relief, opioids should be slowly tapered, rather than abruptly discontinued
2.	Develop a pain management plan prior to hospital discharge; provide adequate doses of opioid and non-opioid analgesics
3.	Arrange for a timely outpatient pain clinic follow-up or a visit with the patient's addictionologist

withdrawal, but which is essentially characterized by an overpowering sense of compulsion to take the drug and the range of behaviors associated with it. Failure to appreciate this difference can lead to inappropriate undermedication of biologically opioid-dependent people who need opioids for the control of their pain conditions. Table 37.1 provides the definitions of some of these and related terms.

Patient management

Detailed pain management of patients displaying opioid tolerance or dependence is beyond the scope of this brief chapter (see the references below for detailed reviews). However, the broad goals of pain management in the opioid-dependent patients are:

1. Identification of the populations at risk: patients on long-term opioid therapy for various chronic pain situations (musculoskeletal, neuropathic, sickle cell disease, HIV-related disease, and palliative care), drug abusers, recovering addicts in opioid maintenance programs.
2. Prevention of withdrawal symptoms and complications.
3. Symptomatic treatment of psychological affective disorders such as anxiety.
4. Effective analgesic treatment in acute phase.
5. Rehabilitation to an acceptable and suitable maintenance opioid therapy.

Peri-operative management of these patients can present unique challenges. Table 37.2 provides an overview of the peri-operative management of opioid-tolerant and dependent patients. There are several general principles that help guide the anesthesiologist and pain specialist with peri-operative pain management. First and foremost is to uncover the fact that

their patient is an opioid user or an abuser and to recognize that issues related to physical and psychological dependence and opioid tolerance could profoundly influence the post-operative course. The importance of patient assessment and early recognition cannot be overemphasized, because failing this essential first step, principles that follow becomes less relevant.

References

1. Mitra S, Sinatra RS. Perioperative management of acute pain in the opioid-dependent patient. *Anesthesiology* 2004;**101**:212–227.

2. Gutstein HB, Akil H. Opioid analgesics. In Brunton LL, Lazo JS, Parker KL, eds. *Goodman and Gilman's The Pharmacological Basis of Therapeutics*, 11th ed. New York: McGraw-Hill, 2006, pp. 569–619.

3. O'Brien CP. Drug addiction and drug abuse. In Brunton LL, Lazo JS, Parker KL, eds. *Goodman and Gilman's The Pharmacological Basis of Therapeutics*, 11th ed. New York: McGraw-Hill, 2006, pp. 621–642.

4. Mehta V, Langford RM. Acute pain management for opioid dependent patients. *Anaesthesia* 2006;**61** : 269–276.

5. Christie MJ. Cellular neuroadaptations to chronic opioids: tolerance, withdrawal, and addiction. *Br J Pharmacol* 2008;**154**:384–396.

6. Ueda H, Ueda M. Mechanisms underlying morphine analgesic tolerance and dependence. *Front Biosci* 2009;**14**:5260–5272.

7. Chu LF, Clark D, Angst MS. Molecular basis and clinical implications of opioid tolerance and opioid-induced hyperalgesia. In Sinatra RS, de Leon-Casasola OA, Ginsberg B, Viscusi ER, eds. *Acute Pain Management*. New York: Cambridge University Press, 2009, pp. 114–146.

38

Opioid-induced hyperalgesia

Sukanya Mitra

Introduction

In recent years it has become increasingly clear that opioids can produce paradoxical pain and hyperalgesia under many circumstances, and that such an effect might contribute to the drawbacks of acute and chronic administration of opioids. This phenomenon (opioid-induced lowering of pain threshold) has been described as opioid-induced hyperalgesia (also termed opioid-induced abnormal pain sensitivity, opioid hyperalgesia, opioid-induced paradoxical pain, or opioid-induced abnormal pain). The recognition of opioid-induced hyperalgesia (OIH) has important clinical implications. A major issue confronting the clinician dealing with patients on opioids is to disentangle apparent opioid tolerance from true tolerance vis-à-vis OIH. The differential diagnosis of a patient not responding to, or even complaining of increased pain in response to, high doses of opioids necessitates a rational and scientific clinical approach to the problem. Further management will necessarily depend on such clarification.

Characteristics of OIH

The common underlying clinical theme of OIH is the worsening of pain in patients receiving high, escalating doses of opioids, and, more importantly, appearance of pain with characteristics *different* from those of the original pain syndrome for which the opioid treatment was instituted, e.g., pain arising in a different location, becoming more diffuse in nature, often spreading beyond the original disease location, even giving rise to whole-body hyperesthesia, and allodynia (pain elicited by normally innocuous stimulation such as touch). This may be accompanied or followed by generalized neuro-excitatory features such as agitation, multifocal myoclonic jerks, seizures, and even delirium. Thus, although there is an apparent tolerance to the analgesic action of opioids in these patients, opioid-induced hyperalgesic syndrome is more than

simply an opioid tolerance phenomenon. Table 38.1 gives a comparison between true opioid tolerance and opioid-induced hyperalgesia.

Pathophysiology

The pathophysiology of OIH is poorly understood. Various non-opioid chemicals, neurotransmitters, and receptors have been implicated, e.g., cholecystokinin (CCK), N-methyl D-aspartate (NMDA) receptor, neurokinin, etc. One mechanism for opioid-induced enhanced pain sensitivity may be the neuroplastic changes that result in part from the activation of descending pain facilitation mechanisms arising from the rostral ventromedial medulla (RVM) by increasing the activity of CCK in the RVM. These activated descending neural tracts facilitate nociceptive processing in the spinal cord.

A conceptual model of OIH implicates a state of disturbed balance between the anti-nociceptive and pro-nociceptive systems. Under normal states, there is an assumed balance between [1] the activity produced by endogenous opioids (the "anti-nociceptive" system) and [2] the "anti-opioid" system involving the NMDA receptor and CCK (the "pro-nociceptive" system). Immediately after morphine administration, increased release of excitatory peptides such as substance P by morphine produces transient hyperalgesia. With time, the inhibitory effect of morphine grows, resulting in analgesia. However, along with its usual expected analgesic effects due to its action on the opioid receptors, morphine itself also paradoxically somehow activates the pro-nociceptive system. This is manifested as a transient period of delayed hyperalgesia when the opioid-induced inhibition is diminished and the activity of anti-opioid mechanisms is increased. Then the system oscillates back to equilibrium as before.

In the opioid-tolerant state, however, due to chronic opioid exposure the anti-opioid system is upregulated, resulting in an increased pro-nociceptive

Table 38.1. Opioid tolerance versus opioid-induced hyperalgesia (OIH)

		Opioid tolerance	OIH
Background factors	Duration of opioid exposure	Long (chronic exposure)	May be long (chronic exposure) or short (acute exposure)
	Opioid dose escalation	Slow (over weeks to months)	May be slow, but typically rapid escalation (days to weeks)
Clinical characteristics	Nature of pain	Unaltered from the original pain condition	Altered from the original pain condition (usually more diffuse in nature)
	Location of pain	Unaltered from the original pain condition	Altered from the original pain condition (usually extends to other locations, even whole body hyperalgesia)
	Quality of pain	Unaltered from the original pain condition	Altered from the original pain condition (e.g., allodynia)
	Pain sensitivity	Unchanged	Increased
	Pain threshold	Unchanged	Decreased
	Additional clinical features	Usually absent	May be present as generalized neuro-excitatory features (agitation, mutifocal myoclonus, seizures, even delirium)
Basic postulated mechanism		Attenuation of anti-nociceptive system (primarily involving opioid receptors and cells)	Enhancement of pro-nociceptive system (involving non-opioids e.g., NMDA, CCK, and other system e.g., RVM)
Management implications	Effect of additional opioids	At least temporarily relieves pain	Pain is typically increased further, especially with rapid escalation of opioid doses
	Effect of adjunct non-opioid agents (especially NMDA-blockers, e.g., ketamine)	May be useful	Often useful
	Essential focus during clinical management	Ensure adequate (often very high) doses of opioids to overcome tolerance temporarily. Additional methadone or opioid rotation often useful. Non-opioid adjuncts may be useful	Avoid escalation of opioid doses. May substitute with methadone (because of its additional NMDA-blocking properties). Use of ketamine seems promising

Source: reprinted with permission from: Mitra S. Opioid-induced hyperalgesia: pathophysiology and clinical implications. *J Opioid Manage* 2008;**4**:123–130.

activity under basal conditions. Further repeated opioid administration actually helps even more up-regulation of the anti-opioid system, possibly through CCK-mediated descending pain facilitation at the RVM as described above. The net result is the clinical phenomenon of opioid hyperalgesia. Although attractive as a conceptual model, this awaits experimental verification.

Clinical and management implications of OIH

Recognition of the phenomenon of opioid-induced hyperalgesia in the clinical setting is the foremost challenge for the clinician. When a patient receiving opioids starts complaining of worsening pain, often demanding more opioids, the clinician is immediately confronted with a dilemma. The increasing pain complaints, despite the opioids that the patient is already on, could be because of several distinct reasons, each meriting a different response: (a) the original underlying pain-producing pathology; (b) true opioid tolerance; (c) opioid addiction, or severe psychological problems such as anxiety or depression; and (d) opioid-induced hyperalgesia. In contrast to all the three clinical scenarios mentioned above, even a short-term further escalation of opioid doses in OIH would lead to further worsening of pain, allodynia,

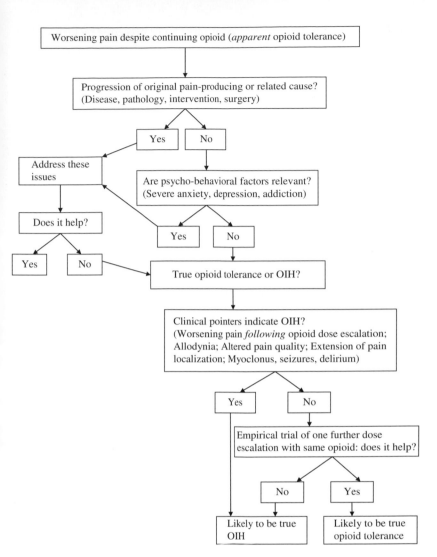

Figure 38.1. Clinical algorithm for differentiating worsening pain states despite continuation of opioid therapy. (Reprinted with permission from: Mitra S. Opioid-induced hyperalgesia: pathophysiology and clinical implications. *J Opioid Manage* 2008;**4**:123–130.)

Table 38.2. Some therapeutic options available for empirical trial in OIH, after reduction in doses of the primary opioid

Methods/Agents	Specific drugs	Comments/Cautions
Opioid rotation	Buprenorphine; methadone; other mu receptor agonists	Some of these drugs, including methadone, might themselves cause or add to OIH
NMDA receptor antagonists	Ketamine (low dose); dextromethorphan	Many case reports available. S-ketamine, if available, may be used at even lower doses, though risk of adverse effects remains
NSAIDs and COX-2 inhibitors	Indirect evidence for NSAID	
Direct evidence for IV parecoxib	Timing of parecoxib administration important for preventing OIH	
Others	Clonidine; magnesium sulfate; ultra-low-dose opioid antagonists; ultra-rapid opioid detoxification	Anecdotal or single case-report-based evidence: not recommended for use currently
Change of route of opioid	From IV to spinal	Single case report of two cases

extension of pain from the original pain site, etc. Hence, however counterintuitive it may sound, further opioid dose escalation is clearly contraindicated in this situation.

It may be difficult to differentiate the two phenomena of true tolerance and OIH purely on clinical grounds. At this point, it has been suggested the best practical step would be to go for a trial of another opioid dose escalation, using the same opioid as before. If the patient's pain improves, the cause of the pain is more likely to be tolerance. However, if the patient's pain worsens or changes character, it is likely to be due to opioid-induced hyperalgesia. This approach has been schematically shown as a clinical algorithm for differentiating worsening pain states despite continuation of opioid therapy (Figure 38.1).

After this crucial distinction is clinched by this empirical dose escalation trial and OIH is suspected, the immediate next step should be reduction of the opioid dose. Along with this vital step, several other options are potentially available (Table 38.2), though these are based on case reports and empirical trials rather than controlled trials preceded by formal diagnosis of OIH.

References

1. Chu LF, Clark D, Angst MS. Molecular basis and clinical implications of opioid tolerance and opioid-induced hyperalgesia. In Sinatra RS, de Leon-Casasola OA, Ginsberg B, Viscusi ER, eds. *Acute Pain Management*. New York: Cambridge University Press, 2009, pp. 114–146.

2. Mitra S. Opioid-induced hyperalgesia: pathophysiology and clinical implications. *J Opioid Manage* 2008;**4**:123–130.

3. Chang G, Chen L, Mao J. Opioid tolerance and hyperalgesia. *Med Clin N Am* 2007;**91**: 199–211.

4. Koppert W, Schmelz M. The impact of opioid-induced hyperalgesia for postoperative pain. *Best Pract Res Clin Anaesthesiol* 2007;**21**:65–83.

5. Angst MS, Clark JD. Opioid-induced hyperalgesia. A qualitative systematic review. *Anesthesiology* 2006;**104**:570–587.

Section 2
Chapter

39

Oral and Parenteral Opioid Analgesics

Opioid rotation

Raymond S. Sinatra

Introduction

The overall effectiveness of analgesic therapy is determined by the efficacy and tolerability of the drug(s) administered. Opioid analgesics remain the foundation of acute and chronic pain management; however, their associated adverse effects often result in intolerability, poor dosing compliance, and inadequate analgesia [1–3]. In a systematic review that analyzed post-operative opioid-associated adverse events, 31% of patients experienced troubling gastrointestinal events, including nausea, vomiting, ileus, or constipation. Other common adverse events included excessive sedation, (30.4%), pruritus (18.3%), and urinary retention (17.5%) [1]. In a different post-operative study the severity of opioid-related side effects was considered more important than the quality of pain relief, suggesting that many patients were willing to "trade" analgesic efficacy for a reduction in side-effect severity [2].

Patients with chronic pain also experience opioid-induced nausea, sedation, cognitive dysfunction, and constipation that can be so troublesome that many choose to cope with pain rather than continue taking their medication. Such adversity not only prevents opioids from being dosed to maximal efficacy, but is also responsible for premature discontinuation of therapy. Studies of patients with chronic pain have shown that patients often switch opioid medications at least once, and sometimes as many as three or four times, before achieving effective analgesia with tolerable AEs [3,4].

Most patients requiring long-term opioid therapy experience moderate to high-grade tolerance development. Tolerance, or diminishing response to a given dose, develops rapidly to the analgesic and euphoric effects of opioids, more slowly to their sedative and nauseating effects, and rarely to their inhibition of bowel function and constipatory effects [5,6]. Tolerance occurs most rapidly with immediate-release short-duration opioids which achieve rapid and high peak plasma levels (C_{max}) followed by rapid decline (C_{min}). Tolerance development has been related to up-regulation of metabolic enzymes, enhanced drug elimination, down-regulation of receptors, and receptor endocytotic activity [6]. The major clinical issue associated with tolerance development is that moderate to very large escalations in opioid dose may be required in order to maintain baseline analgesic effects. Opioid dose escalation often results in a progressive increase in sedation, loss of appetite, and constipation that may become intolerable and limit further dose augmentation.

Another troubling clinical alteration that can lead to treatment failures in patients receiving long-term opioid therapy is termed "opioid-induced hyperalgesia". This phenomenon is characterized by paradoxical increases in pain intensity (hyperesthesia), the development of new pain complaints, and alterations in pain characteristics (allodynia) in response to continued administration or increased dosing of opioid analgesics [7]. Treatment of OIH includes discontinuation or dose reduction of the offending opioid/metabolite, switching (or rotation) to a different opioid including methadone, and use of analgesic adjuvants including ketamine.

Variabilities in opioid response

A therapeutic failure with one opioid agonist does not necessarily mean that the patient will fail to respond to others. Pharmacokinetic and pharmacodynamic variabilities as well as genetic polymorphisms in mu opioid receptors are known to influence opioid dose response. These inter-individual variations are respon-

sible for clinically measurable differences in analgesic efficacy, adverse effect profile and tolerance development between opioid agonists [8,9]. The concept of incomplete cross-tolerance describes the unexpectedly improved effectiveness or tolerability of newly prescribed agonists when compared to equivalent doses of others the patient has found unacceptable. This concept must be appreciated in order to understand the rationale underlying opioid rotation. Incomplete cross-tolerance may be related to a variety of factors including differences in CNS penetration, CSF transport, and receptor affinity of one agonist such as fentanyl over another such as morphine. In addition, variability in the phenotypic expression of mu opioid receptors may allow one agonist to achieve greater binding affinity and intrisic efficacy than another. Alterations in metabolic enzymes may result in greater or lesser amounts of free drug in plasma and CNS. Finally, some agonists such as methadone and tapentadol may provide additional non-opioid receptor mediated analgesic effects.

Historically, leaders in pharmacology believed that there were more similarities than differences between opioid agonists used in clinical practice [10]. However, observed inter-individual variations in opioid dose response and side-effect profile as well as incomplete cross-tolerance underscored the inaccuracy of this statement. We now recognize that "one size does not fit all" and that patients responding poorly to one agonist may do well with another. In recent years, pharmacogenomic research has uncovered significant mu receptor polymorphisms with over 10 different genetic variants detected [11–13]. Differences in mu opioid receptor gene (OPRM1) expression appear to influence subsequent activation of associated proteins and second messengers [12,13] and may affect pain intensity and morphine requirements. In the first "bench-to-bedside" evaluation of mu opioid receptor polymorphism, OPRM1 genotypes of patients undergoing total knee arthroplasty were analyzed preoperatively [14]. The authors found that patients homozygous for allele G118 self-administered significantly more morphine during the first 48 hours following surgery (homozygous AA, 25 mg; heterozygous AG, 26 mg; homozygous GG, 40 mg). Similar variability was observed in cancer pain management, with homozygous GG patients requiring an average morphine dose that was 93% higher than that needed by homozygous AA patients [15].

Box 39.1. Patient variability in opioid response

A variety of genetic, pharmacological, and pathophysiological factors influence patient response to opioid analgesics

(1) Genetic polymorphisms
  (a) OPRM1 encoding mu-opioid receptor
  (b) Enzymes responsible for opioid metabolism (CYP2D6 and others)
  (c) Genes modifying receptor activation (transporter P-glycoprotein COMT)
(2) Receptor endocytotic efficacy
(3) Incomplete cross-tolerance
(4) Extremes in patient age
(5) Exposure to drugs that compete for metabolic enzymes
(6) Exposure to drugs that increase CNS depression
(7) Patient comorbidity (hepatic failure, CNS lesions, renal failure)

Genetic variability of the catechol-*O*-methyltransferase (COMT) gene also influences morphine dose requirements. Patients homozygous for the Val:Val genetic variant required 63% more drug than Met:Met variants [16]. Heterozygous Val:Met variants required 23% more. When the two genes are taken into account the Met/Met genotype required the least amount of morphine to maintain equivalent analgesia. The transporter P-glycoprotein (ABCB1) system influences opioid clearance from cerebrospinal fluid. In a recent article, Park and coworkers reported that genetic polymorphism in this enzyme system significantly influenced respiratory rate in patients exposed to 2.5 µg/kg of fentanyl [17]. Genetic variations of this enzyme system affect the clearance of morphine, methadone, and fentanyl but not meperidine.

Genetic variations in hepatic enzyme cytochrome P450 2D6 are also associated with important metabolic consequences [18]. Cytochrome 2D6 metabolizes a number of opioid agonists and its activity ranges from complete deficiency to ultrafast metabolism, depending on at least 16 different known allele polymorphisms. Codeine, substituted derivatives of codeine (oxycodone, hydrocodone), and tramadol are *O*-demethylated into active compounds by CYP-2D6. Loss of CYP2D6 function alleles with poor to absent drug metabolism is noted in 10% of Caucasians. These patients gain superior analgesic effects with equianalgesic doses of morphine, hydromorphone, and oxymorphone, which are primarily metabolized by glucoronyl transferase [19].

The above-mentioned receptor polymorphisms and genetic variations in enzymes involved in metabolism and clearance contribute to the wide range of patient responses to opioid analgesics. If the clinician has been unable to achieve adequate pain control with acceptable adverse effects, an alternative opioid should be considered. At the present time, opioid rotation is the only method available to determine which patient will respond best to a particular drug [19–21]. Patient variabilities that influence opioid response are summarized in Box 39.1.

Opioid rotation

Pain specialists often discontinue an offending opioid analgesic and switch patients to an alternative agonist (rotation) in order to identify a derivative that produces the most favorable ratio of analgesia to adverse effects [19–21]. Opioid rotation has been shown to be an effective strategy for managing increasing adverse events associated with dose escalation. The availability of multiple opioid analgesics is crucial to achieving clinically satisfactory outcomes, and the development of new opioids or new formulations such as oxymorphone ER and IR, and tapentadol IR, as well as existing preparations such as oxycodone ER, fentanyl transdermal patch, and morphine ER provide useful options. Opioid rotation guidelines can facilitate discontinuation and introduction of a new prescription, and are intended to reduce the risk of relative overdosing or underdosing.

The first and perhaps most important rotation guideline is the assumption that caregivers will utilize standardized opioid equianalgesic dosing tables and become thoroughly familiar with their use and limitations. Tables provide evidence-based values for the relative potencies of different opioid agonists and var-

Table 39.1. Opioid dosing guidelines

Opioid	Route	Dose	Potency	Metabolism	Comments
Morphine	IV	10 mg	1.0	Glucoronidation	The standard of comparison for opioid analgesia
Morphine	PO	30 mg	0.3	Glucoronidation	Poor oral effect, active metabolite
Meperidine	PO	200 mg	0.02	Demethylation	Toxic metabolite, not for chronic pain
Hydrocodone	PO	15 mg	0.5	CYP450	Good oral analgesic, Schedule III
Oxycodone	PO	15 mg	0.5	CYP2D6	Good oral bioavailability
Codeine	PO	200 mg	0.01	Demethylation	Prolonged elimination
Hydromorphone	PO	10 mg	1.0	Glucoronidation	Well tolerated
Oxymorphone	PO	10 mg	1.0	Demethylation	Low oral bioavailability, stable release kinetics
Methadone	PO	10 mg	1.0	Demethylation	Difficult to titrate, may accumulate in tissues
Tramadol	PO	200 mg	0.02	CYP2D6	*O*-demethylated to an active compound
Tapentadol	PO	100 mg	0.5	Glucoronidation	No active metabolites, Dual acting analgesic
Fentanyl (TDS)	TDS	25 µg	40.0	Demethylation	12 h latency to peak effect

Equianalgesic dosing table. Values listed represent approximations based on single dose calculations. According to this conversion scheme, IV morphine 10 mg is assigned a potency of "1" while oral morphine is considered 0.3 due to its poor bioavailability and higher dose requirement. Methadone values represent single-dose effects; accumulation of drug and duration of action will increase with continued dosing. To calculate oral to oral dose conversions, determine the prior 24 h opioid dose (both scheduled and rescue doses) then utilize opioids according to the PO equianalgesic dose and potency listed above. Utilize the following proportion: potency of current opioid /24 h dose of current opioid = potency of new opioid / X. X equals the 24 h dose of the new opioid. Solve for X by cross multiplying. Divide the 24 h dose and administer into increments according to the duration of action of the new drug. For patient safety the recommended "conservative dose" should be 25 to 50% less than the amount calculated. Subsequent dosing may be increased or decreased as necessary. Dose conversions to and from fentanyl TDS are complicated. Please refer to the prescriber guidelines, product information. Adapted from references 22,23,24.

ying routes of administration [22–24] (Table 39.1). Equianalgesic dosing tables simplify opioid rotation by listing agonist potencies relative to a standard of comparison, which is parenteral morphine 10 mg. It is important to note that doses recommended in many equianalgesic dose tables represent comparisons following single-dose administration and that opioid dose response is associated with wide inter-patient variability. These values may not be accurate in patients who have developed tolerance or have been taking

opioids for long periods of time. Based on clinical experience, the starting "conservative" dose for opioid rotation should always be less than the calculated equianalgesic dose. There are several reasons to err on the side of caution with the first and several follow-up doses of the new agonist. First, there is a potential for incomplete cross-tolerance whereby the analgesic potency and adverse effects may be greater than expected. Also, because of clinically significant inter-individual pharmacokinetic and pharmacodynamic

Box 39.2 Opioid rotation: a clinical example

Over the past 24 hours a patient has received 60 mg sustained release (SR) morphine (30 mg, PO, q12h), as well as six 10 mg PO doses of immediate-release (IR) morphine for breakthrough pain and is complaining of excessive nausea and sedation. You wish to rotate the patient to oxymorphone.

First step: calculate total opioid dose over 24 hours
Baseline (SR morphine) doses: 30 mg × 2 doses = *morphine 60 mg (PO)*
Breakthrough doses: 10 mg × 6 doses = *morphine 60 mg (PO)*
Total: morphine 120 mg (PO) per 24 hours

Second step: conversion to an equivalent dose of oral oxymorphone
Oral morphine potency (= 0.03) to oral oxymorphone potency (= 1.0); ratio ~ 3:1
Thus, 120 mg morphine (PO)/24 h is equivalent to 40 mg oxymorphone (PO)/24 h.

Third step: divide equianalgesic dose by 2
Split calculated oxymorphone dose into two divided doses; (i.e. 20 mg SR oxymorphone BID)

Fourth step: convert the equianalgesic dose to a conservative dose
To compensate for incomplete cross tolerance – round down 24 h oxymorphone dose by 25 to 50% (i.e. 10–15 mg SR oxymorphone BID)

Fifth step: breakthrough analgesia
This may or may not be required. If the patient complains of moderate to severe breakthrough pain, provide immediate release oxymorphone 2.5–5 mg every 6 h as required. If frequent breakthrough doses are required, increase the SR oxymorphone dose to 20 mg BID, and assess the quality of analgesia and incidence of adverse events. If, on the other hand, the patient notices improved pain relief, does not require breakthrough doses, but still complains of sedation, nausea or vomiting, consider reducing the SR oxymorphone dose to 7.5 mg BID.

variabilities, opioid potency ratios listed in the equianalgesic table may over- or underestimate the effectiveness of the new agonist. Finally, the caregiver should always exercise caution when rotating agonists in patients with comorbidities that increase opioid risk, including COPD, sleep apnea, obesity, polydrug dependency, hepatic or renal disease, and advanced age [22–24]. A clinical example of opioid rotation is presented in Box 39.2.

The following dosing guidelines provide a reasonable starting point. For patients reporting good pain control but unacceptable adverse events the starting dose of the agonist being rotated to can usually be reduced to 40–60% of the calculated equianalgesic dose of poorly tolerated opioid [20,21]. For patients with poor pain control and unacceptable AEs, the starting dose of the new agonist should probably be lowered to 25–50% of the calculated equianalgesic dose. On the other hand, patients reporting severe pain after receiving several conservative doses of the new agonist should have the dosage increased to the calculated equianalgesic dosage without delay [19–22].

Exceptions to these guidelines exist for conversions to and from transdermal fentanyl and oral methadone. Opioid rotation to a TDS fentanyl patch offers dosing convenience and uniform plasma concentrations, and appears to cause significantly less constipation than oral doses of morphine [25]. Fentanyl has high affinity at mu opioid receptors, can accumulate in fatty tissue, and has no active metabolites. Dosing equivalency between transdermal and orally administered opioids is complicated and referral to the TDS fentanyl package insert is recommended [26]. In general, 25 µg/h of TDS fentanyl is equipotent to 1–3 mg oral morphine/h. Since there is a latency to peak effect of 10–12 h with this preparation, the patient may notice a period of less effective pain control followed by progressive increases in efficacy as well as diminished safety. For this reason, initial doses should be reduced significantly (40–50% of the equipotent calculation) and analgesia supplemented as needed with rapid-acting short-duration opioids.

Caution should be provided when rotating patients to methadone. Based on clinical findings of greater than expected potency gain when switching to methadone from morphine, a significant 75% to 90% reduction in the calculated equianalgesic dose may be warranted [20,27]. The increase in analgesic effect is greater when converting patients on very high daily doses of morphine than for patients on low to moderate doses [21,27]. The greater analgesic effectiveness of methadone may be related to its *d*-isomer, which blocks the *N*-methyl-D-aspartate receptor, providing independent analgesic effects and partial reversal of opioid tolerance.

Patients participating in opioid rotation and dose conversion should be monitored closely to assess the adequacy of pain relief as well as the incidence and severity of therapy-related AEs. As with any opioid regimen, subsequent dose adjustments, gradual upwards or downwards dose titration, will probably be necessary. In some individuals rotation will be unsuccessful and a second rotation and possibly conversion to methadone may be required. If tolerability and efficacy improve following rotation, the new treatment plan may be maintained; however, if moderate symptoms remain, other options may be considered. Many patients may accept the new opioid if residual adverse effects such as excessive sedation are treated with CNS stimulants and constipation is controlled with peripheral opioid antagonists [28]. Others may experience reductions in pain intensity and greater tolerability by reducing the daily dose of the new opioid and providing multimodal non-opioid analgesic supplementation [29,30].

References

1. Wheeler M, Oderda GM, Ashburn MA, Lipman AG. Adverse events associated with post-operative opioid analgesia: a systematic review. *J Pain* 2002;3:159–180.

2. Eberhart LH, Morin AM, Wulf H, Geldner G. Patient preferences for immediate post-operative recovery. *Br J Anaesth* 2002;89:760–761.

3. Moore RA, McQuay HJ. Prevalence of opioid adverse events in chronic non-malignant pain: systematic review of randomised trials of oral opioids. *Arthritis Res Ther* 2005;7:R1046–1051.

4. Quang-Cantergrel, et al. Opioid rotation in non cancer pain. *Anesthesia Analg* 2000;90:933–937.

5. Cherny N, Ripamonti C, Pereira J, et al. Strategies to manage the adverse effects of oral morphine: an evidence-based report. *J Clin Oncol* 2001;19:2542–2554.

6. Zastrow M, Svingos A, Haberstock H, et al. Regulatory endocytosis of opioid receptors: cellular mechanisms and proposed role in physiological adaptation to opiate drugs. *Curr Opin Neurobiol* 2003;13:348–353.

7. Angst MS, Clark JD. Opioid-induced hyperalgesia: a qualitative systematic review. *Anesthesiology* 2006;104:570–587.

8. Trescot AM, Boswell MV, Atluri SL, et al. Opioid guidelines in the management of chronic non-cancer pain. *Pain Physician* 2006;9:1–40.

9. Mercadante S, et al. *J Clin Oncol* 1999;17:3307–3312.

10. Bonica JJ. Biochemistry and modulation of nociception and pain. In Bonica JJ, ed. *The Management of Pain*, 2nd ed. Philadelphia: Lea and Febiger, 1990, pp. 94–121.

11. Galer BS, Coyle N, Pasternak GW, Portenoy RK. Individual variability in the response to different opioids: report of five cases. *Pain* 1992;49:87–91.

12. Pan YX, Xu J, Bolan E, Moskowitz HS Pasternak GW. Identification of four novel exon 5 splice variants of the mouse mu opioid receptor gene. *Mol Pharmacol Fast Forward* 2005;68:866–875.

13. Uhl GR, Sora I, Wang Z. The mu opiate receptor as a candidate gene for pain: polymorphisms, variations in expression, nociception, and opiate responses. *Proc Natl Acad Sci U S A* 1999;96:7752–7755.

14. Chou WY et al. *Acta Anaesthesiol Scand* 2006;50(7):787–792.

15. Klepstad P, et al. *Acta Anaesthesiol Scand* 2004;48(10):1232–1239.

16. Reyes Gibby CC, Shete S, et al. Exploring joint effects of genes and the clinical efficacy of morphine for cancer pain; OPRM1 and COMT gene. *Pain* 2007;130:25–30.

17. Park HJ, Shinn HK, Lee HS, et al. Genetic polymorphism in the ABCB1 gene and the effects of fentanyl in Koreans. *Clin Pharm Ther* 2007;81:539–546.

18. Lovlie R, et al. *Pharmacogenetics* 2001;11(1):45–55.

19. American Academy of Pain Medicine; American Pain Society. The use of opioids for the treatment of chronic pain. A consensus statement from the American Academy of Pain Medicine and the American Pain Society. *Clin J Pain* 1997;13:6–8.

20. Indelicato RA, Portenoy RK. Opioid rotation in the management of refractory cancer pain. *J Clin Oncol* 2002;20:348–352.

21. Mercadante S, Portenoy RK. Opioid poorly-responsive cancer pain. part 1: clinical considerations. *J Pain Symptom Manage* 2001;21:144–150.

22. Anderson A, Saiers JH, Abram S, Schlicht C. Accuracy in equianalgesic dosing conversion dilemmas. *J Pain Sympt Management* 2001;21:397–406.

23. Gordon D, Stevenson K, Griffie J, et al. Opioid equianalgesic calculations. *J Palliat Med* 1999;2:209–218.

24. Sinatra RS. Oral and parenteral opioids. In Sinatra RS, Viscusi G, de Leon-Cassasola O, Ginsberg B, eds. *Acute Pain Management*. London: Cambridge Press, 2009.

25. Peng PW, Sandler AN. Fentanyl for postoperative analgesia: a review. *Anesthesiology* 1999;**90**: 576–599.

26. Duragesic™ Transdermal Delivery System, Johnson & Johnson Pharmaceuticals, Princeton NJ. Full prescribing information, 2008.

27. Moryl N, Santiago-Palma J, Kornick C, et al. Pitfalls of opioid rotation: substituting another opioid for methadone in patients with cancer pain. *Pain* 2002;**96**:325–328.

28. Thomas J, Karver S, Austin Cooney G, et al. Methylnaltrexone for opioid-induced constipation in advanced illness. *NEJM* 2008;**358**:2332–2343.

29. Martin TJ, Eisenach JC. Pharmacology of opioid and nonopioid analgesics in chronic pain states. *J Pharmacol Exp Ther* 2001;**299**:811–817.

30. Cherny N, Ripamonti C, Pereira J, et al. Strategies to manage the adverse effects of oral morphine: an evidence-based report. *J Clin Oncol* 2001;**19**: 2542–2554.

40

Epidural morphine

Siamak Rahman

Name of Analgesic Agent: Duramorph, Infumorph

Generic Name: morphine sulfate, preservative-free

Chemical Name: $(C_{17}H_{19}NO_3)_2 \cdot H_2SO_4 \cdot 5H_2O$

Manufacturer: Baxter Healthcare, Round Lake, IL 60073

Class of Drug: opioids

Chemical Structure: see Figure 40.1

Mode of activity

Epidural morphine must redistribute to the spinal cord to produce analgesia, although it is not clear how exactly epidural morphine reaches the spinal cord. Injection of morphine, the prototypic hydrophilic opioid with octanol:water partition coefficients of 1.42, results in slow onset and a wide band of analgesia surrounding the site of injection in epidural space. Transfer to the systemic circulation is slow and concentrations within the CSF decline more slowly than similar doses of lipophilic opioids, accounting for the greater degree of rostral spread, and delayed respiratory depression. Analgesic contribution from systemic redistribution is minimal after the first 30–60 minutes of epidural administration.

Historical development

The discovery of opioid receptors within the brain and spinal cord followed direct application of morphine at the spinal cord level for patients with severe pain associated with advanced cancer.

Major and minor sites of action

Opiate receptors in the substantia gelatinosa of the spinal cord appear to be the main site of drug action after epidural drug administration. However, an additional systemic effect for this selective spinal analgesia cannot be excluded.

Receptor interactions: binds to various opioid receptors, producing analgesia and sedation (opioid agonist).

Metabolic pathways/drug clearance and elimination: morphine is metabolized primarily in the liver and approximately 87% of a dose of morphine is excreted in the urine within 72 hours of administration. Morphine is primarily metabolized into morphine-3-glucuronide (M3G) and morphine-6-glucuronide (M6G) via glucuronidation by the phase II metabolism enzyme UDP-glucuronosyl transferase-2B7. About 60% of morphine is converted to M3G, and 6–10% is converted to M6G. The cytochrome P450 (CYP) 2D6 family of enzymes involved in phase I metabolism plays a lesser role. Not only does the metabolism occur in the liver but it may also take place in the brain and the kidneys. M3G does not undergo opioid receptor binding and has no analgesic effect. M6G binds to mu receptors and is a more potent analgesic than morphine.

Indications (approved/non-approved)

Preservative-free morphine is the same medication as for systemic opioid analgesia, but used for epidural administration. It is used for the management of pain not responsive to non-narcotic analgesics. Preservative-free morphine administered epidurally provides selective dermatomal pain relief for extended periods without attendant loss of motor, sensory or sympathetic function.

Labor analgesia: in isolation, the efficacy of epidural (up to 7.5 mg) morphine for labor analgesia is limited by a long latency (15–60 min), incomplete analgesia, and maternal side effects. It needs to be used in combination with local anesthetic and/or lipophilic opioids, to prolong or improve labor analgesia.

Cesarean delivery: morphine is currently the "gold-standard" neuraxial opioid for post-cesarean analgesia. It provides effective post-operative analgesia for 12–24 h.

181

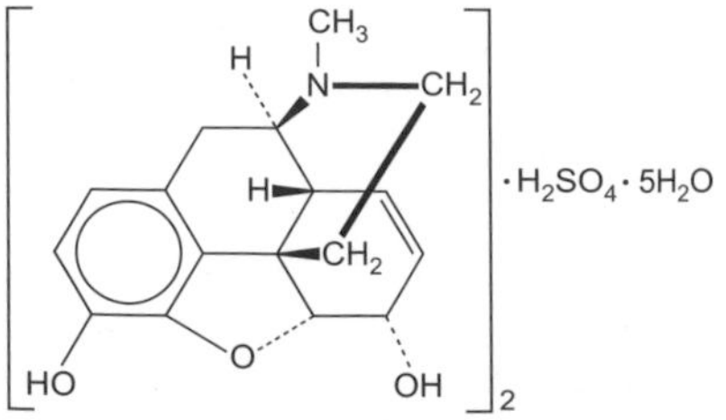

Figure 40.1.

Surgical acute pain: in patients undergoing abdominal surgery, pelvic and lower extremity surgery, epidural morphine with or without added local anesthetic provides better analgesia than parenteral opioids.

Medical pain: has been successfully used for advanced peripheral vascular disease.

Chronic nonmalignancy pain: has been used widely with help of an externalized, tunnelled epidural catheter. Since an externalized catheter may only be maintained for a few months, an intrathecal catheter plus an internal delivery system is prefered.

Cancer pain: it has been used widely with help of an externalized, tunnelled epidural catheter.

Somatic, visceral, or neuropathic pain: epidural morphine is capable of relieving visceral as well as somatic and neuropathic pain.

Contraindications

Preservative-free morphine is contraindicated in those medical conditions which would preclude the administration of opioids by the intravenous route – allergy to morphine or other opiates, acute bronchial asthma, upper airway obstruction.

Preservative-free morphine, like all opioid analgesics, may cause severe hypotension in an individual whose ability to maintain blood pressure has already been compromised by a depleted blood volume or a concurrent administration of drugs, such as phenothiazines or general anesthetics.

Absolute: allergy to morphine.

Relative: use in patients with increased intracranial pressure or head injury. Preservative-free morphine should be used with extreme caution in patients with head injury or increased intracranial pressure. Pupillary changes (miosis) from morphine may obscure the existence, extent, and course of intracranial pathology

Use in chronic pulmonary disease: care is urged in using this drug in patients who have a decreased respiratory reserve (e.g. emphysema, severe obesity, kyphoscoliosis, or paralysis of the phrenic nerve).

Preservative-free morphine should not be given in cases of chronic asthma, upper airway obstruction or in any other chronic pulmonary disorder without due consideration of the known risk of acute respiratory failure following morphine administration in such patients.

Use in hepatic or renal disease: the elimination half-life of morphine may be prolonged in patients with reduced metabolic rates and with hepatic and/or renal dysfunction. Hence, care should be exercised in administering preservative-free morphine epidurally to patients with these conditions, since high blood morphine levels, due to reduced clearance, may take several days to develop.

Use in biliary surgery or disorders of the biliary tract: as significant morphine is released into the systemic circulation from neuraxial administration, the ensuing smooth muscle hypertonicity may result in biliary colic.

Use with disorders of the urinary system: initiation of neuraxial opiate analgesia is frequently associated with disturbances of micturition, especially in males with prostatic enlargement. Early recognition of difficulty in urination and prompt intervention in cases of urinary retention is indicated.

Use in ambulatory patients: patients with reduced circulating blood volume, impaired myocardial function or on sympatholytic drugs should be monitored for the possible occurrence of orthostatic hypotension, a frequent complication in single-dose neuraxial morphine analgesia. Epidural morphine should not be given to outpatient surgical patients.

Use with other central nervous system depressants: the depressant effects of morphine are potentiated by the presence of other CNS depressants such as alcohol, sedatives, antihistaminics or psychotropic drugs. Use of neuroleptics in conjunction with neuraxial morphine may increase the risk of respiratory depression.

Common doses

Usual single epidural dose for post-operative pain is initial injection of 2–5 mg in the lumbar region. If adequate pain relief is not achieved within 1 hour, careful administration of incremental doses of 1 to 2 mg at intervals sufficient to assess effectiveness may be given. No more than 10 mg/24 h should be administered. For continuous infusion, an initial dose of 2 to 4 mg/24 h is recommended. Doses need to be selected according to history of sleep apnea, coexisting diseases or conditions (e.g. diabetes, obesity), current medications (including pre-operative opioids), and adverse effects after opioid administration. The lowest efficacious dose of neuraxial opioids should be administered to minimize the risk of respiratory depression. No information is available regarding the use of preservative-free morphine in patients under the age of 18.

Potential advantages

Preservative-free Duramorph (morphine sulfate injection, USP) is a sterile, nonpyrogenic, isobaric solution of morphine sulfate, free of antioxidants, preservatives or other potentially neurotoxic additives. Selective blockade of pain sensation is possible by neuraxial application of morphine and duration of analgesia may be much longer by this route compared to systemic administration.

Ease of use: preservative-free morphine should be administered by or under the direction of a physician experienced in the techniques and familiar with the patient management problems associated with epidural or intrathecal drug administration.

Potential disadvantages

Preservative-free morphine contains no preservative or antioxidant, so it has to be protected from light and kept in controlled room temperature 20–25°C (68–77°F). Most of the potential side effects associated with systemic administration of opioids such as CNS effects, respiratory depression, sedation, nausea and vomiting, pruritus, and urinary retention are still seen with epidural administration.

Drug interactions

Epidural chlorprocaine: the efficacy and duration of epidural morphine analgesia is diminished when administered after 2-chloroprocaine compared with lidocaine. The mechanism of the interaction between 2-chloroprocaine and morphine is unknown. The observed interaction between epidural morphine and 2-chloroprocaine may be a result of differences in onset and duration of action of the two drugs.

Adverse events

Observational studies report a range in the occurrence of respiratory depression from 0.01% to 3.0% of patients who are given single-injection neuraxial opioids. When single-injection neuraxial opioids are compared with parenteral (i.e. intravenous, intramuscular, or intravenous patient-controlled) opioids, meta-analysis indicates no difference in the frequency of respiratory depression and less somnolence or sedation. Although respiratory depression risk is dose-related and larger doses are more likely to cause respiratory depression, small doses can also cause respiratory depression. Neuraxial opioids depress the respiratory centers in the brainstem via direct and/or indirect mechanisms. Respiratory depression after neuraxial morphine is biphasic; it can occur early (30–90 min) after epidural administration of hydrophilic morphine due to systemic vascular absorption, or it can occur late (6–18 h) after epidural or intrathecal morphine due to rostral spread in cerebrospinal fluid and slow penetration into the brainstem.

Delays gastric emptying: gastric emptying is delayed and orocecal transit time prolonged after epidural morphine.

Post-operative delirium and cognitive decline: the available studies suggest that IV or epidural techniques do not influence cognitive function differently.

Pruritus: mild to severe genralized pruritus is the only side effect that is seen more frequently following neuraxial dosing than with systemic administration.

Prevention of respiratory depression: opioid effects on respiration include decreased minute ventilation (decreased respiratory rate, tidal volume, or both), decreased response to hypoxia, and a rightward shift and depression of the CO_2 response. So, all these patients receiving epidural morphine need appropriate methods of respiratory monitoring (e.g. respiratory rate, depth of respiration [assessed without disturbing a sleeping patient]), oxygenation (e.g. pulse oximetry when appropriate), and level of consciousness. Monitoring should be performed for a minimum of 24 h after administration, at least once per hour for the first 12 h after administration, followed at least once every 2 h for the next 12 h. In the case of continuous infusion or PCEA with morphine, monitoring should be performed the same as above for the first 24 h. After 24 h monitoring should be performed at least once every 4 h.

Less common adverse events: recurrence of oral herpes simplex virus (HSV) infections involving the third division of the trigeminal nerve with epidural morphine.

Treatment of adverse events: supplemental oxygen should be administered to patients with altered level of consciousness, respiratory depression, or hypoxemia and continued until the patient is alert and no respiratory depression or hypoxemia is present. In the presence of severe respiratory depression, reversal agent (naloxone), single-dose or continous infusion, should be given and appropriate resuscitation should be initiated. Consider non-invasive positive-pressure ventilation if frequent or severe airway obstruction or hypoxemia occurs during post-operative monitoring.

Availability

Available in the USA as a schedule II drug.

Pearls

Intravenous access should be maintained for 24 h after administration of epidural morphine. Whether the addition of parenteral opioids or hypnotics to neuraxial opioids is associated with increased occurrence of respiratory depression or hypoxemia is unclear.

Parenteral opioids or hypnotics should be cautiously administered in the presence of neuraxial opioids. The concomitant administration of neuraxial opioids and parenteral opioids, sedatives, hypnotics, or magnesium requires increased level of monitoring.

References

1. Practice guidelines for the prevention, detection, and management of respiratory depression associated with neuraxial opioid administration. An updated report by the American Society of Anesthesiologists Task Force on Neuraxial Opioids. *Anesthesiology* 2009;**110**:218–230.

2. Carvalho B. Respiratory depression after neuraxial opioids in the obstetric setting. *Anesth Analg* 2008;**107**:956–961.

3. Epocrates®.

4. Micromedex® Healthcare Series, DrugDex® Evaluations.

5. *Goodman and Gilmans Pharmacological basis of therapeutics.* New York: McGraw-Hill.

Section 3 Chapter	Neuraxial Opioid Analgesics
41	# Epidural fentanyl

Bita H. Zadeh

Generic Name: fentanyl

Chemical Name: fentanyl citrate

Trade Name: Sublimaze™

Manufacturer: multiple, including Hospira, Inc., Lake Forest, IL 60045; Baxter Healthcare Corporation, Deerfield, IL 60015

Class: analgesic, opioid, schedule II drug

Chemical Structure: see Figure 41.1

Description

Fentanyl was first created in 1959 by a chemist named Dr. Paul Jannsen. It was released for human use in 1963. Fentanyl citrate is a sterile, nonpyrogenic solution of fentanyl citrate in water.

Fentanyl citrate has a molecular weight of 528.6. Each milliliter contains fentanyl (as the citrate) 50 µg (0.05 mg). May contain sodium hydroxide and/or hydrochloric acid for pH adjustments. pH is 4–7.5 and pKa 7.3–8.4.

It is freely soluble in organic solvents and sparingly soluble in water. It has a relative lipid solubility of 580.

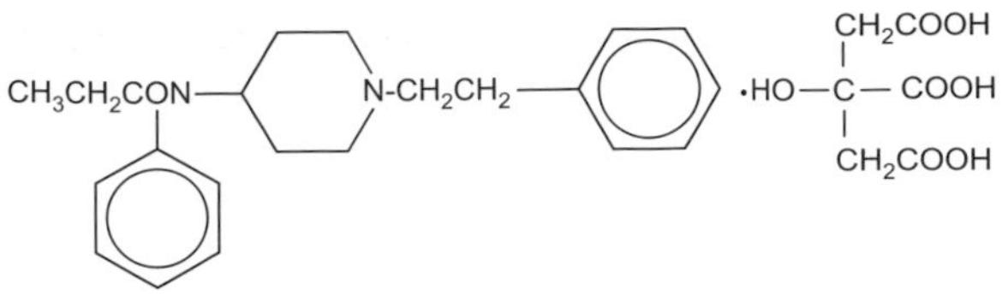

Figure 41.1.

Mode of activity

Epidural fentanyl has been used in practice since 1975. When fentanyl is placed in the epidural space, it must first cross the dura mater before it can reach the spinal cord. Epidural fentanyl binds to opioid receptors located throughout the spinal cord and nerve roots, and provides analgesia. The epidural space is highly vascularized, and some redistribution of drug to the systemic circulation occurs. The epidural space also contains fat, connective tissues, a lymphatic network, and the dorsal and ventral roots of the spinal nerves, all of which can serve as repositories for lipophilic agents.

Epidural fentanyl, given as a bolus, will redistribute to the lipophilic sites found in the epidural space and limit rostral spread. However, given as a continuous infusion, those sites will become saturated and serum levels 24 hours after a continuous-rate infusion are similar to those obtained from a similar IV infusion.

Depending on whether epidural administration of fentanyl is as a bolus or a continuous infusion, analgesic effects are predominantly mediated by spinal or supraspinal mechanisms, respectively.

Fentanyl is metabolized primarily in the liver via the cytochrome P450 3A4 isoenzyme system. It is metabolized primarily by *N*-dealkylation to norfentanyl and other inactive metabolites that do not contribute materially to the observed activity of the drug.

Fentanyl is excreted primarily by the kidneys, 90% as metabolites, 10% as unchanged drug.

Indications

The benefits of giving fentanyl in the epidural space for improving intra-operative and post-operative analgesia are very clear. The analysis of current literature shows that the addition of fentanyl to local anesthetics for intra-operative and post-operative epidural analgesia is safe and advantageous. The reduction in the incidence of pain is quantitatively high, and adverse effects are mild.

Epidural fentanyl has been approved for a variety of circumstances including surgical acute pain. Fentanyl given in thoracic epidurals (thoracotomy, bowel cases, etc.) works extremely well; due to its lipopholic quality, it will give more segmental analgesia and have less rostral spread. It is also used in lumbar epidurals for labor and any surgery in the pelvic region or lower extremity. Fentanyl can be used as the sole analgesic in epidurals. This can be very useful in laboring patients who require minimal or no motor blockade, "walking epidural".

It can be used in thoracic or lumbar epidurals, to treat other pains such as medical pain, chronic non-malignancy pain, and cancer pain within those dermatomes.

Contraindications

The only absolute contraindication to epidural fentanyl is in patients with known intolerance to the drug.

The use of cervical epidural administration of fentanyl is questionable. In a study of patient-controlled cervical epidural fentanyl infusion, compared with patient-controlled IV fentanyl infusion for pain relief after pharyngolarynx surgery, results show that cervical epidural fentanyl analgesia provides marginally better pain relief at rest with no decrease in fentanyl consumption. Also, administration of fentanyl in the cervical epidural space is questionable because of the possible complications of the technique.

Common doses/uses

The dose of epidural fentanyl should be appropriately reduced in elderly, debilitated, pregnant, or pediatric patients as well as in patients with obstructive sleep apnea.

Epidural fentanyl can be given as a single bolus, a continuous infusion, or a combination of both.

Fentanyl can be given as a one-time bolus during initiation of epidural analgesia. The dose range is 50–200 µg, with an average onset time of 10–15 minutes, and duration of 2–3 hours. Based on review of current literature, 100 µg fentanyl, administered as a single bolus into the epidural space appears to be the optimal safe dose for most patients. Dose must be appropriately reduced for patients at an increased risk of respiratory depression.

For continuous infusion techniques, fentanyl 0.5–1.0 µg/kg per h, after initial bolus administration, provides effective analgesia both alone and in combination with low concentrations of local anesthetic.

Lumbar epidural analgesia for labor requires effective analgesia with significantly less motor block. In these patients, a continuous infusion of fentanyl (1–2 µg/mL) in combination with low concentrations of a local anesthetic at a rate of 6–8 ml/h is effective.

Epidural fentanyl 5–20 µg/h at an infusion rate of 3–10 mL/h used as solo anesthetic can provide near total analgesia with minimal side effects, while allowing the patient to ambulate safely and more comfortably.

Potential advantages

Epidural fentanyl markedly improves the analgesic effect of epidural infused local anesthetic. It works synergistically with and helps prevent tachyphylaxis to local anesthetics. In addition to better analgesia, one can reduce the local anesthetic concentration to avoid motor block. Because of its greater lipophilicity, fentanyl offers a number of advantages over morphine for epidural analgesia, including a lower incidence of side effects and reduced risk of delayed-onset respiratory depression. The greater lipid solubility of epidural fentanyl results in rapid-onset analgesia and rapid clearance from cerebrospinal fluid, resulting in a relatively short duration of action. Fentanyl's relatively short duration of action makes it more ideally suited for continuous infusion or PCEA (patient-controlled epidural analgesia). Epidural fentanyl lacks spread through the cerebrospinal fluid, and therefore achieves a segmental nature to the analgesia. Hence the location of epidural catheter placement is most important when fentanyl is used. Rapid clearance from cerebrospinal fluid allows for less cephalad spread, causing fentanyl to be associated with fewer and less severe adverse effects.

Potential disadvantages

Prolonged infusion of epidural fentanyl may result in systemic concentrations not dissimilar to IV infusion, and therefore it is more efficacious to combine it with a low concentration of local anesthetic to get a synergistic effect. Although the addition of fentanyl to local anesthetic in the epidural space has been shown to reduce the incidence of pain in adults, this may not be true for pediatric patients. In fact, the addition of 0.2 µg/kg per h fentanyl to 1.5 mg/mL ropivacaine increased the incidence of side effects without improvement of analgesia in infants and children undergoing urological surgery.

Another disadvantage of epidural fentanyl is that it reduces the shivering threshold when combined with epidural local anesthetic. Epidural local anesthetics and IV opioids both decrease the core temperature, which triggers shivering. Fentanyl is often added to local anesthetic to improve the quality of epidural blockade and to reduce side effects. However, it has been shown that patients are at increased risk of hypothermia when fentanyl is added to local anesthetics.

Epidural fentanyl analgesia is commonly used as a therapeutic modality in the management of pain during labor. Healthcare providers have a general perception that drugs administered in the maternal epidural space remain there and do not compromise the respiratory status of newborns. There have been case reports of newborns developing respiratory depression following epidural fentanyl analgesia. Respiratory depression in the newborn related to fentanyl is more related to the amount of drug received within 2 to 4 hours preceding delivery than used during the entire course of labor.

There are variations in fentanyl maternal-placental-fetal kinetics, and hence it is not easy to pinpoint with complete certainty which baby will have respiratory depression following birth. However, the case reports suggest that babies delivered after mothers have received >300 µg fentanyl (approx 5 µg/kg) during the last 4 hours of labor may be at greater risk.

Drug-related adverse events

One great advantage of epidural fentanyl administration compared to morphine is its lower incidence and severity of adverse effects.

Adverse reactions include pruritus (most common in 10–35%); nausea and/or vomiting (5–30%), and urinary retention (0–5%). Mild to moderate sedation can occur early on and is brief. Early respiratory depression is rare and there is no delayed respiratory depression. Shivering has been reported. There are a few case reports of respiratory depression of newborn and decreased apgar scores (if >5 µg/kg are given within the last 4 hours of labor). Reactivation of oral herpes simplex virus, which has been reported with epidural morphine, has not been reported with fentanyl.

References

1. Micromedex® Healthcare Series.

2. Ginosar Y, Riley E, Angst M. The site of action of epidural fentanyl in humans: the difference between infusion and bolus administration. *Anesth Analg* 2003;**97**:1428–1438.

3. Curatolo M, Petersen-Felix S, Scaramozzino Z, Binden A. Epidural fentanyl, adrenaline and clonidine as adjuvants to local anesthetics for surgical analgesia: meta-analyses of analgesia and side-effects. *Acta Anaesthesiol Scand* 1998;**42**: 910–920.

4. Grass JA. Fentanyl: clinical use as postoperative analgesic-epidural/intrathecal route. *J Pain Symptom Manage* 1992;7:419–430.

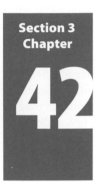

Section 3
Chapter

42

Neuraxial Opioid Analgesics

Epidural hydromorphone

Susan Dabu-Bondoc and Greg Albert

Generic Name: hydromorphone (dihydromorphinone-HCl)

Proprietary Name: Dilaudid™ (preservative-free)

Drug Class: opioid analgesic

Manufacturer: Abbott Laboratories, 8401 Trans-Canada Highway, Saint-Laurent, Québec, Canada H4S 1Z1

Chemical Name: 4,5a-epoxy-3-hydroxy-17-methylmorphinan-6-one hydrochloride

Chemical Structure: see Figure 42.1

Description

Hydromorphone is a semisynthetic opioid agonist prescribed for control of moderate to severe pain. It was first synthesized in 1924 and introduced by Knoll pharmaceuticals under the brand name Dilaudid™. Intravenous hydromorphone is about 5–6 times more potent than morphine; however, when administered epidurally, morphine provides greater spinal selectivity and 2–3 times greater analgesic potency than hydromorphone. Hydromophone is available as a preservative-free solution which has been advocated for neuraxial administration. While not formally FDA-approved, hydromorphone was one of the first opioids administered via the epidural route, and its safety and analgesic efficacy have been evaluated in a number of clinical trials [1–3].

Major and minor sites of action

Epidural hydromorphone's primary site of action is at endogenous opioid receptors located on neurons in lamina I–II (substantia gelatinosa) and lamina V of the spinal dorsal horn. Following epidural administration, hydromorphone enters the spinal cord and activates pre- and postsynaptic mu receptors and suppresses pain transmission. Systemic absorption and activation of central opioid receptors may provide additional analgesia. Hydromorphone is not particularly hydrophilic, and rostral migration in CSF is of lower magnitude than that observed with morphine. Rostral spread of hydromorphone may result in undesirable side effects such as pruritus, nausea and vomiting, and sedation. Epidural hydromorphone is associated with dose-dependent reductions in respiratory rate and minute ventilation; however, unlike morphine, delayed-onset respiratory depression is less likely to occur [3,4].

187

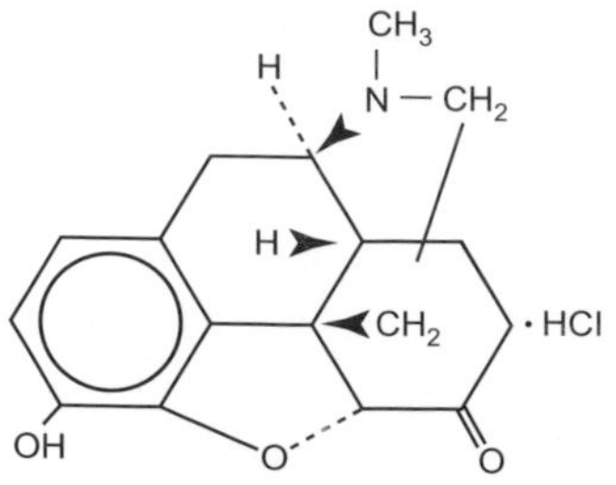

Figure 42.1.

Metabolic pathways, drug clearance and elimination

Epidural hydromorphone has a short metabolic and elimination half-life: typically 2–4 hours (2–3 hours with IV hydromorphone), with peak plasma levels achieved in 2–14 minutes (5–10 min with IV hydromorphone, 30–60 min with oral dosing), and peak CSF levels achieved in 60 min after epidural administration. In those with renal impairment, the half-life of hydromorphone can increase to as much as 40 hours, hence caution must be exercised when dosing hydromorphone in patients with kidney problems which can result in drug accumulation. Fortunately the glucoronated metabolite has minimal clinical activity. Single-dose epidural hydromorphone (1 mg) has an average clinical analgesic duration of 6–7 h, only one-third as long as morphine.

Indications

Surgical acute pain: epidural hydromorphone alone or in combination with dilute local anesthetics can effectively relieve moderate to severe surgical pain.

Chronic pain: infusions of intrathecal and epidural hydromorphone may be employed for control of chronic benign and malignancy-related pain.

Contraindications

Contraindications to epidural hydromorphone infusions include documented severe allergic reaction or hypersensitivity, patient refusal, infection or tumor at the insertion site, septicemia, vertebral fractures/instability, neural deficit, coagulopathy, and treatment with low molecular weight heparinoids. As with other epidural opioids, the American Society of Regional Anesthesia (ASRA) issued guidelines with respect to the safe use of anticoagulants when considering neuraxial anesthesia/analgesia.

Epidural doses

Intermittent bolus dosing

Chestnut and colleagues [5] were first to evaluate single doses of epidural hydromorphone (1 mg in 10 mL saline) or placebo for pain control following cesarean delivery. Patients assigned to the epidural hydromorphone group benefited from superior pain control, with 92% reporting good or excellent pain relief versus 56% in the control group. Time to first request for supplemental analgesia (IV hydromorphone) was extended (13 vs. 3.1 h), and 24 hour requirement was reduced (4.7 vs. 10.2 mg). Patients undergoing lower extremity orthopedic and vascular procedures with epidural anesthesia plus conscious sedation may be given an intra-operative epidural dose of 0.5–1.5 mg hydromorphone with appropriate doses of 0.5–0.75% bupivacaine or ropivacaine to achieve surgical anesthesia. Supplemental boluses of local anesthetic may be administered as required during the procedure. Epidural hydromorphone may be administered for relief of post-operative pain following arthroscopic and less invasive pelvic/perineal surgery.

Continuous epidural infusion

Patients undergoing orthopedic, abdominal, and thoracic surgeries with general anesthesia plus epidural anesthesia/analgesia may be given an intra-operative loading dose of 0.5–1.5 mg hydromorphone alone or in combination with 0.125–0.25% bupivacaine or 0.2–0.5% ropivacaine depending on patient age and comorbidities. Supplemental boluses of local anesthetic are administered as required during the case. In extremely prolonged procedures, an additional bolus of hydromorphone (25–50% of loading dose) is given 6 hours into the procedure. Alternatively, for elderly debilitated patients, a light general anesthesia may be combined with epidural infusion using a reduced hydromorphone loading dose of 0.25–0.75 mg with 8–10 mL 0.125% bupivacaine or 0.2% ropivacaine followed by an intra-operative infusion of dilute hydromorphone (10–20 µg/mL) plus 0.1–0.031% bupivacaine at a rate of 8–16 mL/h. Infusions are maintained during the course of a light sevoflurane, desflurane, or propofol-based general anesthetic. On near completion of the surgical procedure or following arrival in the PACU, the intra-operative basal infusion may be maintained for 24–72 h. Infusion rates are reduced by one-third to one-half in patients greater than 70 yrs or when administered via thoracic catheters.

Epidural patient-controlled analgesia

Guidelines for loading doses and continuous infusion rates are similar or slightly less than those described for the continuous infusion technique. When patients become alert and oriented in the post-anesthesia care unit, the patient is given a PCA button. PCA bolus doses (1–4 mL of solution) with a 6–8-minute lockout interval are added to supplement the epidural infusion. To further improve the overall quality of analgesia, non-opioid analgesics such as IV ketorolac (7.5–15 mg every 6 hours), and oral Celecoxib™ (200 mg twice a day) may be prescribed to augment hydromorphone-based epidural analgesia. A standardized order set for epidural PCA (EPCA) with hydromorphone is presented in Table 42.1.

Epidural PCA is maintained for 2–4 days, depending upon the procedure and potential benefit to the patient. Most patients make a smooth transition to oral opioids such as oxycodone or oxycodone-acetaminophen compounds, or to low-dose IV-PCA therapy for some who remain nil per os (NPO) for extended periods. For opioid-dependent or chronic pain patients the loading dose of epidural hydromorphone is increased by 50–100% and the infusion concentration increased by 100% or more to compensate for opioid tolerance and down-regulation of spinal opioid receptors. Judicious use of adjuvants such as epidural clonidine, or IV ketamine infusions, or methadone may be administered to further augment pain relief in opioid-dependent patients. These patients should always receive their baseline opioids either orally or parenterally (IV-PCA) in addition to the epidural infusion, to prevent opioid withdrawal and provide supraspinal analgesic potentiation [2]. Dosing guidelines for epidural hydromophine are summarized in Table 42.2.

At Yale New Haven Hospital, epidural solutions are prepared by hospital pharmacy services by adding 5 mg (0.5 mL) preservative-free hydromorphone (taken from a mutidose vial of Dilaudid-HP 10 µg/mL) to a 500 mL normal saline solution. Calculated volumes of 0.75% bupivacaine (without epinephrine) are added to achieve infusate concentrations of 0.0625–0.031%, kept sterile and refrigerated at 40°F [2,4].

Table 42.1. Hydromorphone EPCA order set

1.	Patient has an epidural catheter for post-operative pain control and will be managed by the anesthesiology pain management service, beeper _____
2.	Catheter is placed at _____ interspace. and is _____cm at the skin
3.	Please check the insertion site per shift. Notify the pain service if any of the following is observed: leaking of infusate, redness, bleeding
4.	Epidural analgesic: hydromorphone 10 µg/mL plus bupivacaine 0.031%
	Hydromorphone 10 µg/mL plus bupivacaine 0.0625%
	Hydromorphone 20 µg/mL plus bupivacaine 0.625%
	Hydromorphone_____µg/mL
	Hydromorphone _____µg/mL plus ropivacaine 0.1%
5.	Epidural continuous infusion rate_____mL/h
6.	Epidural bolus dose_____mL, per_____min
7.	Four hour dose limit_____mL
8.	Adjunctive analgesia: ketorolac_____mq, _____h
	Celecoxib_____mg, _____h
9.	Treatment of adverse events:
	_____ (Pruritus) naloxone infusion (400 µg/L, infuse at _____mL/h)
	_____ (Nausea) ondansetron _____mg, _____h
	_____ (Nausea) droperidol _____mg, _____h
	_____ (Respiratory depression) naloxone_____ µg
10.	Notify the anesthesiology pain service if the patient has a respiratory rate of 10 or less, oxygen saturation 90% or less, is troubled by pain intensity greater than 5, or is troubled by nausea, vomiting and pruritus unresponsive to standard therapy

Table 42.2. Dosing guidelines for epidural hydromorphone

1.	Single bolus technique: administer 0.5–1.5mg[a] in 10 mL preservative free saline, or dilute local anesthetic every 6–8 h
2.	Continuous infusion technique: administer 0.5–1 mg bolus[a] followed by infusion (hydromorphone 10–20 μg/mL) alone or with local anesthetic (bupivacaine 0.1–0.031% or ropivacaine 0.1–0.2%) at a rate of 8–16 mL/h
3.	Patient-controlled technique: administer 0.5–1 mg bolus[a] followed by infusion (hydromorphone 10–20 μg/mL) alone or with local anesthetic (bupivacaine 0.1–0.031% or ropivacaine 0.1–0.2%) at rate of 8–12 mL/h, Provide PCA boluses of 2–4 mL of solution with lockout of 6–8 min
4.	Adjunctive therapy[b]: ketorolac IV (7.5–15 mg every 6 h), celecoxib PO (200 mg every 12 h)

[a]Dependent on age, physical status, height, extent of surgical dissection, degree of opioid tolerance and so on, reduce dose by 25–33% with thoracic epidural placement.
[b]Unless contraindicated.

Potential advantages

Being moderately lipid-soluble, vascular uptake of epidural hydromorphone is lower than that of fentanyl, although its ability to remain in CSF and spread rostrally is greater. This property provides important clinical advantages: (1) like morphine, doses administered via high lumbar and low thoracic catheters can control pain at higher dermatomal segments, and (2) epidural administration is associated with three times greater potency than similar amounts given IV. Unlike morphine, which is more hydrophilic, rostral spread to brainstem respiratory centers and delayed respiratory depression is less likely to occur. The short latency and long duration of analgesia in spinal cord regions far distant from the site of hydromorphone injection are desirable characteristics. Epidural hydromorphone has a more rapid onset, and a less troublesome side-effect profile compared to morphine. Its safety and side-effect profile is superior to morphine as equianalgesic doses are associated with less risk of excess sedation and delayed respiratory depression. In our experience, epidural hydromorphone is associated with less nausea and vomiting, less sedation, and fewer histamine-related side effects such as itching and skin erythema, than that observed with morphine. Preservative-free hydromorphone is relatively inexpensive and is widely available. Cost: 4 mg/mL (20 cartridges, 1 mL): $35.00.

Potential disadvantages

Like other epidural opioids, invasiveness and placement/follow-up expenses are greater compared to parenteral administration.

Like most other neuraxial opioids, it may increase risk of respiratory compromise in patients who are morbidly obese or have chronic obstructive pulmonary disease and those with chronic sleep apnea.

Hydromorphone may compete with other drugs for hepatic glucoronidation.

Drug-related adverse events and treatments

Common adverse events: sedation, respiratory depression, pruritus, nausea/vomiting, constipation, and urinary retention, which are treated with a naloxone 40–80 μg IV bolus followed by an infusion of 50–100 μg/h. However, these adverse events are relatively less commonly observed with epidural hydromorphone than with neuraxial morphine regimens. Pruritus is treated with a naloxone infusion of 50–100 μg/h, diphenhydramine 12.5–50 mg or propofol infusion of 10 mg/h. Nausea and vomiting is best treated with either ondansetron (4–8 mg IV), low-dose droperidol (0.625–1.25 mg IV), metoclopramide (10 mg IV every 4–6 h), or transdermal scopolamine patch during the first 10 hours following administration.

References

1. Brose WG, Tanelian DL, et al. CSF & blood pharmacokinetics of hydromorphone and morphine following lumbar epidural administration. *Pain* 1991;**45**:11–15.

2. Dabu-Bondoc S, Franco S, Sinatra R. Neuraxial analgesia with hydromorphone, morphine, and fentanyl: dosing and safety guidelines. In Sinatra RS, de Leon-Casasola OA, Ginsberg B, Viscusi ER, eds. *Acute Pain Management.* New York: Cambridge University Press, 2009, pp. 230–244.

3. Wong C, et al. *Spinal and Epidural Anesthesia.* New York: McGraw-Hill, 2007, pp. 75–110.

4. Ayoub C, Sinatra RS. Postoperative analgesia: epidural and spinal techniques. In Chestnut DH, ed. *Obstetric Anesthesia: Principles and Practice*, vol. III. St Louis: Mosby, 2004.

5. Chestnut DH, Choi WW, Isbell TJ. Epidural hydromorphone for postcesarean analgesia. *Obstet Gynecol* 1986;**68**(1):65–69.

43

Epidural sufentanil

Jill Zafar, Anthony T. Yarussi and Laura Mechtler

Generic Name: sufentanil

Trade Name: Sufenta

Chemical Name: N-{4-(methoxymethyl)-1-(2-thiophen-2-ylethyl)piperidin-4-yl}-N-phenyl-propanamide

Manufacturer: Claris Lifesciences Inc., 542 Industrial Way West, Eastontown, NJ 07724

Class: opioid analgesic

Chemical Structure: see Figure 43.1

Description

Sufentanil is a potent opioid analgesic that is primarily administered intravenously as an adjunct in anesthesia during surgery or as an epidural analgesic during labor and vaginal delivery. Sufentanil is a synthetic anilinopiperidine that binds to and activates the mu opioid receptors on neuronal cell membranes which are present in large quantities in the periaqueductal gray matter (human brain) and the substantia gelatinosa (spinal cord). Activation of mu receptors predominantly causes analgesia and sedation along with other side effects. Sufentanil is the thienyl analog of fentanyl and is approximately 5–10 times more potent than fentanyl.

Mode of activity

Sufentanil (as other opioids) given epidurally can produce analgesia one of three ways. It can spread cephalad in the CSF to supraspinal centers, be absorbed systemically and transfer to supraspinal centers, or act directly in the dorsal horn of the spinal cord on the spinal opioid receptors. It is felt that the main site of action of epidural sufentanil is pre-synaptic modulation of the nociceptive signal in the lamina of Rexed in the spinal cord. Sufentanil has a fast onset of action when it selectively binds to the spinal mu receptors. Mu opioid receptors are coupled to G proteins and are thus able to activate the intracellular secondary messenger system when the opioid agonist binds to its receptor in the CSF. Subsequently, activated G protein subunits alter the ion channel conductance of the neuron by inhibiting Ca influx and enhancing the outward movement of K from the cell. Presynaptically this inhibits the release of neurotransmitters such as substance P and glutamate.

Duration of action of epidural sufentanil is between that of fentanyl and morphine, usually between 2 and 4 hours. Once systemically absorbed it is metabolized by the liver and excreted by the kidney.

Indications

In the 1970s sufentanil was first introduced as a new potent opioid for use in anesthesia. The use of this drug was originally recommended for intravenous peri-operative analgesia. In the following years other uses for this opioid were explored, such as intrathecal and epidural use for peri-operative analgesia, labor and delivery, and chronic pain. Although epidural sufentanil is only FDA-approved for use in labor and delivery, studies have found it to be an acceptable option in other clinical situations.

Labor and delivery

The addition of epidural sufentanil to local anesthetics significantly potentiates their analgesic effects. They also provide for safe and effective analgesia at a lower concentration and dose of local anesthetics. As a result this decreases the incidence of side effects such as motor blockade and hypotension.

Post-operative pain management

Sufentanil is an effective analgesic when used in continuous epidural infusions. It has been used for

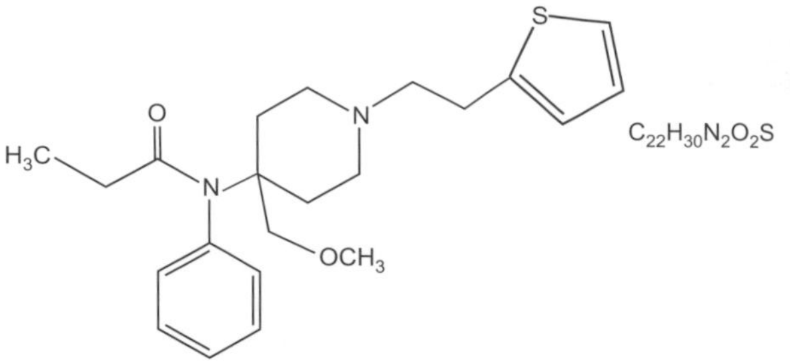

Figure 43.1.

post-operative pain control in general surgery, orthopedic, thoracic, and cesarean section procedures. When sufentanil is combined with bupivacaine epidurally, the dose requirement for post-operative analgesia has been shown to be 50% less than intravenous requirements.

Chronic pain

Epidural sufentanil is beneficial in chronic pain patients tolerant to morphine. Recent evidence has shown that tolerance occurs from a progressive loss of receptor site action due to prolonged agonist exposure. With prolonged opioid use there is an eventual loss of receptors on the cell surface and fewer binding sites, resulting in higher dose requirements. When this occurs, sufentanil can be used as it is a more effective opioid. It has a higher intrinsic efficacy than morphine, and an analgesic effect will occur with less receptor binding.

Epidural sufentanil is not typically used for neuropathic pain.

Contraindications

Absolute: patients with known hypersensitivity to sufentanil or known intolerance to other opioid agonists.

Relative: patients with chonic obstructive pulmonary disease and head injuries. In addition, patients with hepatic or renal impairment are at risk due to the importance of these organs in the metabolism and excretion of sufentanil.

Common doses/uses

Epidural opioids are frequently used for the management of pain. Sufentanil, which is five times more potent than fentanyl, has been studied for its analgesic effects epidurally. It can be administered by either bolus dose or continuous infusion technique. Bolus

dosing can range from 10 to 50 µg with a duration of action of approximately 2–4 hours. Continuous infusion techniques can also be used. Rates of 0.3 µg/kg per h have been shown to provide rapid onset and sustained analgesia in abdominal surgery. In addition rates of 4–8 mL h of a 1–2 µg/mL solution have been used with good success. These techniques may be safer as they take advantage of the drug's shorter duration of action and can reduce the respiratory risks that are present with bolus use. Patient-controlled epidural anesthesia can be used as well at a dose of 2.5 µg every 10 min as needed. During labor and vaginal delivery 10 to 15 µg doses can be given epidurally mixed with 10 mL of 0.125% bupivacaine. This dose can be repeated two times at intervals of not less than 1 hour until delivery.

Potential advantages

Sufentanil is a sterile, preservative-free, aqueous solution that is readily available in the majority of hospitals and pain clinics in the USA. Due to its lipophilicity and high affinity for the mu opioid receptors, sufentanil has a more rapid onset of action (5 to 15 minutes) and shorter duration of action as an analgesic than morphine. Sufentanil is effective in epidural PCA and provides a good quality of analgesia. It is primarily used as a multimodal agent combined with local anesthetics epidurally for post-operative pain control. A combination of analgesic drugs provides more effective pain control at lower doses than relying on one drug alone. In addition, the drug combination reduces the risk of adverse effects from any one drug.

It produces less respiratory depression due to its lipophilic properties so less drug accumulates in the CSF.

Potential disadvantages

There is no known toxicity even at epidural doses as high as 600–800 µg/day. Patients on high doses should be monitored with neurological exams for myoclonic movements or changes in behavior.

Epidural spread of lipophilic drugs is limited in the epidural space as a result of their high lipid solubility. As a result, these opioids are more dermatomally restricted than hydrophilic ones so that epidural catheters need to be placed at the center of the dermatomes involved in the surgical procedure to achieve a good quality of analgesia.

Table 43.1. Drug-related adverse events

Body system	Common/serious adverse side effects	Less common adverse effects
Central nervous system	Sedation	Spinal cord damage from toxic preservatives rare, tonic skeletal muscle rigidity
Respiratory	Regulatory depression within 2 hours from systemic absorption	
Gastrointestinal	Nausea, vomiting	Delayed gastric emptying
Genitourinary	Urinary rentention	
Dermatological	Pruritus – most common side effect from neuraxial opioids, most cases are mild; due to cephalad migration of opioid in CSF	Cold sores from viral reactivation

Drug interactions: barbiturates, tranquilizers, other narcotics, antihistamines, antidepressants, MAO inhibitors, and alcohol can all increase CNS depression. The risk of bradycardia and hypotension increases for patients on beta blockers and calcium channel blockers. Cimetidine, used to treat peptic ulcers, interacts with sufentanil and increases the risk of respiratory depression.

Cost: sufentanil provides a faster onset and a more rapid recovery than morphine or fentanyl. However, morphine and fentanyl are chosen as the cost effective alternatives.

Drug-related adverse events

See Table 43.1 for the main adverse effects.

Other infrequent side effects include ocular dysfunction with miosis and nystagmus. Inhibition of shivering from loss of thermoregulatory function and oliguria with water retention from ADH stimulation can occur.

Naloxone, an opioid antagonist, is used clinically to reverse respiratory depression, sedation, or opioid overdose caused by sufentanil. Naloxone has a high mu receptor affinity and therefore competes with the opioid from the same receptor sites. Intravenous doses of naloxone (0.1–0.4 mg) repeated every 2 to 3 minutes are administered until the patient is breathing or responds.

References

1. Ballantyne J, Fishman S, Salahadin A, eds. *The Massachusetts General Hospital Handbook of Pain Management*, 2nd ed. Philadelphia: Lippincott Williams & Wilkins, 2002.

2. Joris JL, Jacob EA, Sessler DI. Spinal mechanisms contribute to analgesia proceduced by epidural sufentanil combined with bupivacaine for postoperative analgesia. *Anesth Analg* 2003;**97**(5):1446–1451.

3. *Sufenta*. Janssen-Ortho Inc., 26 July 1985. http://www.janssen-ortho.com/JOI/pdf_files/sufenta_E.pdf. Accessed August 4, 2009.

4. de Leon-Casasola OA, Lema MJ. Epidural bupivacaine/sufentanil therapy for postoperative pain control in patients tolerant to opioid and unresponsive to epidural bupivacaine/morphine. *Anesthesiology* 1994;**80**:303–309.

Extended-release epidural morphine

Akta Patel, Eugene R. Viscusi and Leslie Schechter

Generic Name: morphine extended-release liposome injection

Trade/Proprietary Name: DepoDur®

Drug Class: opioid analgesic

Manufacturer: Pacira Pharmaceuticals Inc., San Diego, CA 92121; distributed by EKR Therapeutics Inc., Cedar Knolls, NJ 07927

Chemical Structure: see Figure 44.1

Chemical Name: 7,8-didehydro-4,5α-epoxy-17-methylmorphinan-3,6α-diol sulfate (2:1) (salt) pentahydratemax

---

Introduction

DepoDur® is a sterile, non-pyrogenic, white to off-white, preservative-free suspension of multi-vesicular lipid-based particles containing morphine sulfate, USP. The lipid carrier is a proprietary drug delivery system known as DepoFoam®. After the administration of DepoDur® into the epidural space, morphine sulfate is released from the multivesicular liposomes over a period of time [1–3] (Figures 44.2 and 44.3).

Mode of activity

Major and minor sites of action

It is absorbed both neuraxially and systemically. Depo-Dur® has a principal effect on opioid receptors in the dorsal horn of the spinal cord as well as in other regions of the central nervous system (CNS). Additionally, it works in the gastrointestinal (GI) tract and other smooth muscles. However, it does not have a major effect on the cardiovascular system at therapeutic doses.

Effects on the CNS: principal therapeutic action of morphine is analgesia; other effects include euphoria, anxiolysis, and feelings of relaxation.

Effects on the GI tract and other smooth muscles: decreases gastric, biliary, and pancreatic secretions; causes a reduction in motility.

Effects on the cardiovascular system: no major effects; may result in orthostatic hypotension and fainting.

Receptor interactions: morphine is a pure opioid agonist relatively selective for the μ receptor, although it can interact with other opiate receptors at higher doses.

Metabolic pathways/drug clearance and elimination: the major metabolic pathway is conjugation, either with D-glucuronic acid in the liver to produce glucuronides or with sulfuric acid to give morphine-3-etheral sulfate. Approximately 10% of morphine dose is excreted unchanged in the urine. Most of the dose is excreted as glucuronide metabolites, including morphine-3-glucuronide (M3G; about 50%) and morphine-6-glucuronide (M6G; about 5 to 15%). M3G has no significant analgesic activity. M6G has been shown to have opiate agonist and analgesic activity in humans. Seven to ten percent is excreted in the feces. The mean adult plasma clearance is about 20–30 mL/min per kg. The terminal half-life of morphine is approximately 2 hours.

Indications

DepoDur® is approved for the treatment of pain following major surgery or after clamping the umbilical cord during cesarean section by a single-dose administration into the lumbar epidural space.

It is not intended for intrathecal, intravenous, or intramuscular administration. Administration of Depo-Dur® into the thoracic epidural space or higher has not been evaluated and therefore is not recommended.

Contraindications

Absolute: patients with known hypersensitivity to morphine, morphine salts, or any components of the product.

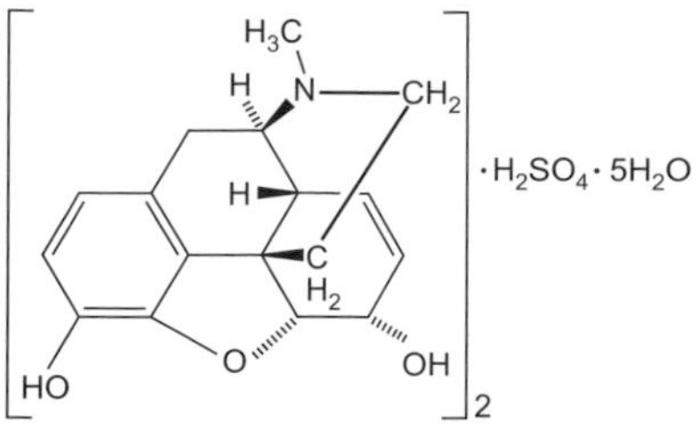

Figure 44.1.

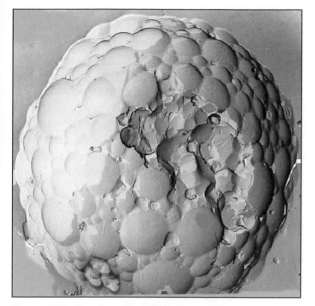

Figure 44.2. DepoFoam® Particle.

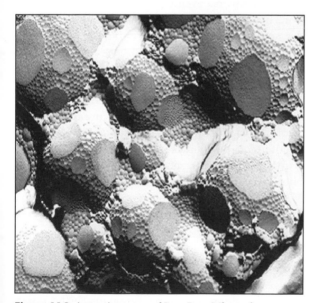

Figure 44.3. Internal structure of DepoFoam® (freeze fracture electron microscope image).

Relative: patients with respiratory depression, acute or severe bronchial asthma, and upper airway obstruction; any patient who has or is suspected of having paralytic ileus; patients with suspected or known head injury or increased intracranial pressure. It is contraindicated in circulatory shock as it causes vasodilatation, which may exacerbate hypotension and hypoperfusion.

Approved doses (based on FDA pivotal trials)

Major orthopedic surgery of the lower extremity – 15 mg

Lower abdominal or pelvic surgery – 10 to 15 mg

Some patients may benefit from a 20-mg dose of DepoDur®

Cesarean section – 10 mg

Clinically useful dosing (based on the authors' clinical experience)

In most circumstances and particularly with multimodal analgesia, patients may benefit from doses of EREM lower than those in the label. Lower dosing may reduce opioid-related side effects.

Total hip arthroplasty – 7.5 – 10 mg

Total knee arthroplasty – 10 – 12.5 mg

Lower abdominal surgery– 7.5 – 10 mg

Cesarean section 7.5 – 10 mg

How supplied

Preservative-free DepoDur® – 10 mg/mL single-use, amber vials for epidural administration

10 mg/1 mL vial packaged in cartons of 5

15 mg/1.5 mL vial packaged in cartons of 5

Potential advantages

Ease of use: the potential of providing extended analgesia without an epidural catheter and epidural pump or IV-PCA pump is very desirable. External pump technology is cumbersome for the patient, time-consuming for the nursing staff, and is associated with medication errors and pump programming errors. In many surgical settings, anticoagulation to prevent venous thromboembolism is now standard care. Consequently, indwelling epidural catheters may increase the risk of epidural hematoma formation. DepoDur® may provide extended analgesia without the need for indwelling epidural catheters and without the difficulties associated with current epidural and IV-PCA pumps.

Tolerability: DepoDur® is intended for single-dose administration; therefore accumulation of morphine or its metabolites is not expected even in patients with impaired hepatic or renal function [3].

In a pilot study including 37 patients, the opioid-sparing effect of DepoDur® on subsequent fentanyl PCA requirements was assessed. DepoDur® use resulted in reduced total fentanyl requirements, increased time-to-rescue, and lower pain ratings over 48 hours [4].

In a double-blind, double-dummy, sham-controlled study including 168 total knee arthroplasty patients, subjects were assigned to receive DepoDur® 30 mg, DepoDur® 20 mg, or sham epidural injection, to compare DepoDur® with morphine PCA. DepoDur® patients experienced less pain and required less opioid rescue as compared to morphine PCA patients [5].

Hartrick and Hartrick [1] conducted a study assessing the safety of DepoDur® by combining and analyzing the adverse effects from previous trials. This study showed that patients in the high-dose DepoDur® group experienced a higher incidence of pruritus as compared to standard epidural morphine. There were no differences between low-dose DepoDur® and standard epidural morphine. In general, opioid-related adverse effects were seen in all groups, which is not surprising, as multimodal analgesia was not used to reduce DepoDur® dose in many of these studies.

Availability: widely available at most hospitals.

Cost : although the cost of DepoDur® ($327–$491/dose) is significantly greater than morphine sulfate injection (~$1/syringe), there are many cost advantages for DepoDur®, which include the following:

(1) decreased post-operative IV-PCA use and therefore costs and potential for pump programming errors;
(2) decreased use of sciatic nerve blocks, which can last up to 24 hours and delay time to ambulation and physical therapy and may impact length of stay;
(3) ability to initiate anticoagulation (heparin, LMWH) after surgery without the risk of spinal hematomas associated with epidural catheters.

Potential disadvantages

Toxicity: prolonged and serious respiratory depression or apnea has occurred when administration of epidural DepoDur® was associated with subarachnoid puncture.

Drug interactions: administration of DepoDur® after an analgesic dose of bupivacaine (0.25% – 20 mL) increases peak serum concentrations of morphine. Increasing the interval between the analgesic dose and DepoDur® administration to greater than 30 minutes minimizes this pharmacokinetic interaction.

Warnings: epidural local anesthetics should not be used before or after DepoDur® except: (1) in the form of a 3 mL test dose with lidocaine 1.5% and epinephrine 1:200,000, or (2) a therapeutic dose of bupivacaine 0.25% – 20 mL.

Do not mix or co-administer DepoDur® with any other medications, including local anesthetics. Once DepoDur® has been administered, no other medication should be administered into the epidural space for at least 48 hours [2,3].

Drug-related adverse events

Common adverse events (>10%): decreased oxygen saturation, hypotension, urinary retention, vomiting, constipation, nausea, pruritus, pyrexia, anemia, headache, and dizziness.

Adverse events (5–10%): hypoxia, tachycardia, insomnia, and flatulence.

Other adverse events (2–5%): respiratory depression, hypercapnia, paralytic ileus, somnolence, bladder spasm, abdominal distension, dyspepsia, rigors, dyspnea, hypokalemia, paresthesia, and decreased hematocrit.

The concurrent use of other CNS depressants, including sedatives, hypnotics, general anesthetics, droperidol, phenothiazines or other tranquilizers, or alcohol, increases the risk of respiratory depression, hypotension, profound sedation, or coma.

MAOIs markedly potentiate the action of morphine. DepoDur® should not be used in patients taking MAOIs or within 14 days of stopping such treatment.

Treatment of adverse events

Respiratory depression: naloxone – slow titration to achieve adequate ventilation without reversing all analgesia is recommended. An initial dose of 0.1 mg IV may be administered; an infusion may be necessary to treat ongoing respiratory depression. In situations of severe respiratory depression, assisted or controlled ventilation may be necessary.

Nausea: ondansetron 4 mg IV every 6 h; metoclopramide 10 mg PO/IVP every 6 h; promethazine 6.25 mg IV every 8 h. Preventive treatment is recommended.

Pruritus: diphenhydramine 25–50 mg PO/IVP every 6 hours. Non-sedating antihistamines are also effective. Low-dose opioid antagonists may be effective when antihistamines are ineffective.

References

1. Hartrick CT, Hartrick KA. Extended-release epidural morphine (DepoDur®): review and safety analysis. *Expert Rev Neurother* 2008;**8**(11):1641–1648.

2. DepoDur® (package insert). Cedar Knolls, NJ: EKR Therapeutics, Inc., 2007

3. DepoDur® (updated package insert). Bedminster, NJ: EKR Therapeutics, Inc., 2008

4. Gambling D, Hughes T, Martin G, et al. A comparison of DepoDur, a novel, single-dose extended-release epidural morphine, with standard epidural morphine for pain relief after lower abdominal surgery. *Anesth Analg* 2005;**100**(4):1065–1074.

5. Viscusi ER, Martin G, Hartrick CT, et al. Forty-eight hours of postoperative pain relief after total hip arthroplasty with a novel, extended-release epidural morphine formulation. *Anesthesiology* 2005;**102**(5):1014–1022.

6. Viscusi ER. Liposomal drug delivery for postoperative pain management (translational vignette). *Reg Anesth Pain Med* 2005;**30**(5):491–496.

7. Viscusi E, Gambling D, Hughes T, Manvelian G. The serum pharmacokinetics of extended-release epidural morphine sulfate (DepoDur®): a pooled analysis of 6 clinical studies. *Am J Health-Syst Pharm* 2009;**66**:1020–1030.

8. Viscusi ER, Manvelian G. A randomized controlled study of the serum pharmacokinetics, effectiveness, and safety of thoracic extended-release epidural morphine (Depodur®) after lidocaine-epinephrine test dose administration in patients undergoing upper abdominal surgery. *Int J Pharmacol Ther* 2009;**47**:659–670.

Section 3 Chapter

Neuraxial Opioid Analgesics

Intrathecal morphine

James M. Moore

Class: analgesic agent

Generic Name: morphine, intrathecal

Chemical Structure: see Figure 45.1

Structural Formula: 5α,6α-7,8-didehydro-4,5-epoxy-17-methylmorphinan-3,6-diol; molecular wt 285.34; for intrathecal use, morphine is available as the sulfate salt with the following formula: $(C_{17}H_{19}NO_3)_2 \cdot H_2SO_4 \cdot 5H_2O$; molecular wt 758.83

Description

Morphine is the principal active alkaloid of opium and a phenanthrene derivative. Morphine sulfate for intrathecal administration is available in the USA under the brand names Astramorph/PF and Duramorph for use in acute pain and Infumorph for chronic intrathecal use. These preparations are all isobaric and preservative-free aqueous solutions.

Mode of activity

Intrathecal morphine binds opioid receptors within the neurons of the gray matter of the dorsal horn of the

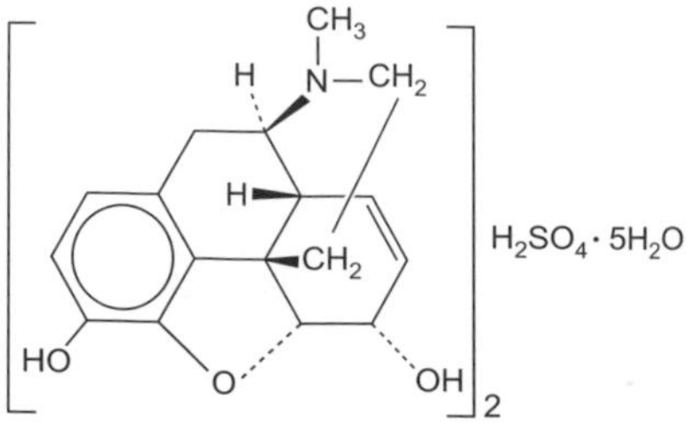

Figure 45.1.

spinal cord, including but not limited to the substantia gelatinosa. Opioid receptor activation blocks release of substance P and other excitatory neurotransmitters, causing inhibition of ascending nociceptive pathways and altering the perception of and response to pain.

Due to morphine's hydrophilic nature, the spinal cord's exposure over time to intrathecal morphine greatly exceeds that of other spinal opioids, leading to a prolonged analgesic effect but also greater rostral spread and the potential for delayed respiratory depression and sedation. Compared to less hydrophilic opioids, morphine has a lower spinal cord distribution volume, slower clearance from the spinal cord into the plasma, and higher bioavailability in the extracellular fluid space of the spinal cord [1].

Drugs injected into the cerebrospinal fluid may redistribute into the epidural space and fat, and morphine does so to a significant extent. However, doses of intrathecal morphine used clinically are so small that substantial plasma levels are not seen. The propensity for intrathecal morphine to penetrate the spinal cord to enter the gray matter of the dorsal horn is greater than for other less hydrophilic opioids. Although pulsation of the cerebrospinal vasculature produces motion of cerebrospinal fluid, such motion is complex and less pronounced in the lumbar region than in the cervical region. Other factors that may influence the spread of intrathecal morphine include the baricity and volume of injectate as well as the force of injection.

Indications (approved/non-approved)

Intrathecal morphine is indicated for the management of pain not responsive to non-narcotic analgesics, but it should be administered in a fully equipped and staffed environment. Naloxone injection should be immediately available. Patients receiving intrathecal morphine should remain in this environment for at least 24 hours following the initial dose. Repeated intrathecal injections of morphine for acute pain are not recommended.

Single-dose intrathecal morphine may be effective for patients at risk for severe post-operative pain from a variety of major surgical procedures, including lower extremity orthopedic surgery, abdominal surgery, and operations of the lumbar and thoracic spine. It is commonly given for analgesia for patients undergoing cesarean section.

In some cases usually amenable to continuous epidural analgesia, the use of an indwelling epidural catheter at an optimal spinal level is not feasible, such as when epidural catheter placement is unsuccessful or is precluded by planned post-operative anticoagulation. In such circumstances, intrathecal morphine may be given instead.

Non-approved uses include administration of intrathecal morphine to pediatric patients, and use in pediatric patients undergoing scoliosis repair is common.

Contraindications

Intrathecal morphine is contraindicated in the presence of a true allergy to morphine and in patients with preexisting severe respiratory depression or sedation. It should be avoided in patients with elevated intracranial pressure and used with caution in patients with or at risk for upper airway obstruction. Systemic morphine administration can exacerbate bronchospasm in patients with acute asthma, and systemic absorption of intrathecally administered morphine might have a similar effect, although the amount of morphine entering the systemic circulation is small.

Like all opioid analgesics, intrathecal morphine may cause severe hypotension in a patient whose ability to maintain blood pressure is already compromised by hypovolemia or concurrent drug administration.

Common doses

Intrathecal morphine may be given alone for analgesia or as part of a surgical spinal anesthetic. Limited information is available on which to base rational dosing choices. It is unclear whether any anthropometric patient characteristics such as height and weight relate to intrathecal morphine dose requirement for analgesia. Elderly patients are more at risk for respiratory depression and sedation and should receive lower doses than other patients. The more cephalad the site of spinal innervation of the surgical site, the greater the dose requirement may be. On the other hand, dosing is constrained by potential side effects, especially respiratory depression and sedation, and in some models escalating intrathecal morphine dose does not confer further analgesia over low doses.

In many patients, intrathecal morphine at a dose of 0.1–0.2 mg produces effective analgesia for at least 12 hours and acceptable side effects. Higher doses may be used, but increasing dose can increase the risk of pruritus and especially respiratory depression.

For hip arthroplasty in elderly patients, a dose of 0.2 mg confers analgesia with a favorable side-effect profile [2]. For major abdominal surgery a dose of 0.2–0.4 mg has been reported. Much higher doses are sometimes used in cardiac surgery in patients who will initially have post-operative ventilation. Effectiveness limits the use of intrathecal morphine in patients undergoing thoracotomy. Adult patients undergoing major spine surgery receive effective analgesia and a low risk of respiratory depression with an intrathecal morphine dose of 0.3 mg [3].

For cesarean section, intrathecal morphine is often given as part of the surgical spinal anesthetic. Most commonly doses of 0.1–0.2 mg morphine are given, and a dose of 0.1 mg may be as effective as higher doses with less risk of pruritus [4].

For pediatric patients undergoing posterior spinal fusion and segmental spinal administration for idiopathic scoliosis, a dose of pre-operative intrathecal morphine ranging from 9 to 19 µg/kg with a mean of 14 µg/kg provided effective analgesia with a low frequency of respiratory depression and intensive care unit admission [5]. Another report of pediatric spinal fusion patients showed no advantage of 15 µg/kg intrathecal morphine over a dose of 5 µg/kg [6].

Potential advantages

Compared to epidural and intravenous use, intrathecal morphine administration produces profound analgesia at a low dose and leads to minimal systemic absorption and low plasma levels. Intrathecal needle placement is often technically easier and less traumatic than epidural needle placement.

A single dose of intrathecal morphine may produce analgesia for 12 to 33 hours.

Potential disadvantages

For post-operative analgesia, intrathecal morphine is usually given as a one-time injection, thus limiting the duration of effect and obviating the ability to titrate the dose to effect as can be done with opioids administered by other routes.

Information on appropriate dosing is limited. Generally, effective dosing must be tempered to avoid side effects, especially respiratory depression.

Drug-related adverse events

Opioid side effects may occur with intrathecal morphine just as with any opioid administration.

The most concerning and least common opioid side effect with intrathecal morphine is the combination of respiratory depression and sedation, often occurring approximately 8 hours after intrathecal morphine administration with a steady, gradual onset. Monitoring patients on an hourly basis for changes in respiratory rate and sedation level for at least 12 hours after intrathecal morphine dosing should detect clinically significant episodes of respiratory depression and sedation. The need for and duration of such monitoring may depend on the dose of morphine. A traditional dose of intrathecal morphine is at least 0.1 mg, but much lower doses have not been well studied and may be associated with very low risk of respiratory depression. Intrathecal morphine dose of <0.3 mg may be less likely to produce respiratory depression than higher doses [7].

Pruritus is the most common opioid side effect of intrathecal morphine. It may occur even with small doses and can be effectively treated with either intermittent intravenous nalbuphine or an infusion of low-dose intravenous naloxone. Pruritus due to intrathecal morphine does not respond well to diphenhydramine.

Urinary retention may occur and may be due to reduced parasympathetic output causing detrusor muscle relaxation and inhibition of sphincter relaxation. Some patients have urinary catheters prophylactically inserted out of concern for this side effect.

Nausea and vomiting may occur, possibly due to direct stimulation of the medullary vomiting center [8].

References

1. Umenhofer WC, et al. Comparative spinal distribution and clearance kinetics of intrathecally administered morphine, fentanyl, alfentanil, and sufentanil. *Anesthesiology* 2000;**92**:739–753.

2. Rathmell JP, et al. Intrathecal morphine for post-operative analgesia: a randomized, controlled, dose-ranging study after hip and knee arthroplasty. *Anesth Analg* 2003;**97**:1452–1457.

3. Boezaart AP, et al. Intrathecal morphine: double-blind evaluation of optimal dosage for analgesia after major lumbar spinal surgery. *Spine* 1999;**24**: 1131–1137.

4. Gurgin NK, et al. Intrathecal morphine in anesthesia for cesarean delivery: dose-response relationship for combinations of low-dose intrathecal morphine and spinal bupivacaine. *J Clin Anesth* 2008;**20**: 180–185.

5. Tripi PA, et al. Intrathecal morphine for postoperative analgesia in patients with idiopathic scoliosis undergoing posterior spinal fusion. *Spine* 2008;**33**:2248–2251.

6. Eschertzhuber S, et al. Comparison of high- and low-dose intrathecal morphine for spinal fusion in children. *Br J Anaesth* 2008;**100**:538–543.

7. Gehling M, Tryba M. Risks and side-effects of intrathecal morphine combined with spinal anaesthesia: a meta-analysis. *Anaesthesia* 2009;**64**:643–651.

8. Gwirtz KH. Intrathecal analgesia. *Problems Anesth* 1998;**10**:71–79.

Section 3
Chapter

46

Neuraxial Opioid Analgesics

Evaluating epidural catheters

Anna Clebone and Raymond S. Sinatra

General considerations

First! Gather all relevant information from the anesthesia team and record to determine where the catheter is and its functionality.

Always remember: continuous monitoring of BP, HR, and SaO_2 is required before, during, and after epidural test or bolus dosing in all patients.

Before dosing any medication:

a. *Who placed the epidural?* A senior experienced attending (probably placed correctly) or a very junior resident (catheter could be anywhere!).

b. *How sure is the team of the catheter's placement?* If the team states "we think it's in" or "it was difficult but we think it's in", it is probably not placed correctly!

c. *How many attempts were required?* If multiple attempts were required, or the team may have caused a dural puncture, be very cautious giving a test dose and use only dilute 1/8% bupivacaine (see "Dosing" box below).

d. *How deep is the catheter placed?* How many cm is the catheter from the skin and into the epidural space? The OR team will have recorded this in the anesthesia record. Ideally it should be 3 cm into the epidural space. If too deep and not working

well, consider pulling the catheter out to 3 cm. If the catheter is only 1.5 cm or less in the epidural space, it may not be usable, but consider retesting before discontinuing completely (see "Dosing" box below).

e. *How much supplemental anesthesia was needed?* If the team states "the blood pressure dropped following boluses of local anesthesia", or "the patient required minimal general anesthesia", it may be positioned correctly in the epidural space!

How to determine initial dosing

a. *Was the catheter bolused intra-operatively with fentanyl or hydromorphone?* If not, consider bolusing with 50 µg fentanyl, 0.5–1 mg hydromorphone.

b. *When was the catheter dosed?* If more than 6 hours ago, the patient may a need a rebolus of hydromorphone 0.5–1 mg.

c. *Is the patient opioid-dependent/tolerant?* Consider rebolus with 1.5–2 times the standard hydromorphone dose (up to 2 additional mg). Then consider a double strength epidural infusion (hydromorphone 20–30 µg/mL and bupivacaine 1/16%).

d. *Where was the catheter placed?* If the patient has a low lumbar catheter for an upper abdominal/thoracic incision, you may need to bolus large volumes (15–20 mL) of dilute local anesthetic (bupivacaine 1/16–1/8%) to cover the affected dermatomes. If the patient has a thoracic (T6–7–8) epidural for an upper abdominal/thoracic incision, consider reducing the bolus dose and infusion rate by one third.

Before dosing medications: ensure that the epidural infusion or test dose will not destabilize the patient

First, evaluate for adequate respiration and oxygenation, hemodynamic stability, and absence of oversedation. Special care should be exercised in elderly, frail, or post-pneumonectomy patients who are at increased risk of epidural complications.

How to manage

Continuous monitoring of BP, HR, and SaO_2 is required before, during, and after dosing in all patients.

If the patient is hypovolemic, anemic, or hypotensive, avoid testing the catheter with local anesthetic until the patient is volume-repleted. Infusions containing only an opioid will decrease blood pressure less than those containing both an opioid and a local anesthetic.

Ensure that the epidural catheter is not placed intravascularly or intrathecally

Always aspirate the epinephrine catheter in the PACU before starting an infusion or giving a test dose.

How to manage

If a small quantity of free-flowing blood or any CSF is aspirated, the catheter will need to be repositioned or removed. Pulling out the catheter by 1/2 cm at a time and re-aspirating can occasionally reposition the catheter into the epidural space.

Give a test dose: if no blood or CSF is detected on aspiration, test the catheter with a small quantity of local anesthetic containing epinephrine (see "Dosing" box):

Evaluate for hemodynamic changes: increases in heart rate or blood pressure immediately after dosing signify that the catheter is in the intravascular space. Reposition, re-aspirate, and re-dose, or remove.

Evaluate for toxicity due to intravascular placement: symptoms such as lightheadedness, dizziness, a metallic taste, ringing in the ears, or perioral numbness signify potential intravascular injection and risk for toxicity. Local anesthetic toxicity can also cause late symptoms such as hypotension, blurry vision, seizures, and cardiac arrhythmias. Stay with the patient for the first 10 minutes after a test dose or bolus.

Always remember: continuous monitoring of BP, HR, and SaO_2 is required before, during, and after epidural test or bolus dosing in all patients.

Before dosing any epidural, aspirate the catheter and rule out the presence of blood or cerebrospinal fluid.

Never bolus more than 3 mL of local anesthetic at any time; additional boluses may be given incrementally every 2–3 min after watching the hemodynamic response. The minimum dose of epidural to achieve a reliable hemodynamic reponse is 15 µg.

Evaluate for intrathecal placement: results that are "too good" from the test dose (such as dense sensory or motor block) can indicate intrathecal placement of the catheter.

Evaluate for equivocal results: if you are unsure of the catheter's placement after a test dose, you may rebolus another 3 mL. With attending supervision/approval, you may bolus up to 10 mL 1/8% bupivicaine with epinephrine or 20 mL 1/16% bupivacaine with epinephrine (3 mL at a time).

Dosing

Typical test dose:
   3 mL of 0.5% lidocaine with 1:200 000 epinephrine (5 µg/mL) or 3 mL of 0.5–0.25% bupivacaine with 1:200 000 epinephrine (5 µg/mL) or a combination of the two.
   Typical infusion solution:
   10 µg/mL Dilaudid with 0.031% bupivicaine at 8–14 mL/h, with patient-controlled bolus of 3 mL every 6 minutes.

Troubleshooting: how to manage a patient with an epidural who complains of pain in the post-operative care unit (PACU)

Patients with mild to moderate incisional pain

(Most likely a well-placed functional catheter, in a non-opioid-dependent patient.)

Ensure continuous HR, BP and O$_2$ Sat monitoring. Aspirate catheter, attach to the infusion pump, and bolus 10–20 mL of infusion solution. Infusion solutions: 0.031% bupivacaine with hydromorphone (10µg/mL) or fentanyl (2–4µg/mL)

- If pain is unchanged or worsening after 10 minutes, and blood pressure has not declined, consider the catheter to be suboptimal, and test with local anesthetic (refer to dosing box below).
- If pain intensity and blood pressure have declined, consider the catheter to be functional, and either start a standard infusion rate (10–12 mL per hour) or slightly increase the infusion rate (14–16 mL per hour).

Patients with moderate to severe incisional pain

(Possibly a well placed functional catheter, in a non-opioid-dependent patient.)

Ensure continuous HR, BP and O$_2$ Sat monitoring. Aspirate catheter, test with local anesthetic (see "dosing" box).

- Evaluate for significant increases in HR or symptoms of local anesthetic toxicity (which could signify intravascular catheter placement, signifying the need to reposition and re-test, or remove).
- If pain is unchanged or worsening after 10 minutes, and the blood pressure has not declined, the catheter is probably non-functional. However,

before discontinuing, consider retesting with a more concentrated local anesthetic (6–8 mL lidocaine 2% with epi, or 6–8 mL of lidocaine 1% with epi combined with bupivacaine 0.25% with epi, given 3 mL at a time). If no improvement, discontinue catheter, consider placing another epidural immediately. If the patient notices some relief and blood pressure drops slightly, consider the catheter to be functional, and start infusion.

- If the pain remains at a point higher than the level of the catheter, with good pain relief lower than the level of the catheter, consider infusing larger volumes of solution (14–16 mL/h). To further optimize pain relief, consider giving an additional loading dose of 0.5 mg hydromorphone. Alternatively consider an additional loading dose of 10–20 mL of infusion solution via the epidural pump.

Patients with severe incisional pain (crying-screaming!)

(Most likely a non functional catheter! but also assess placement, intra-operative dosing, and opioid dependency variables.)

Ensure continuous HR, BP and O$_2$ Sat monitoring. Aspirate catheter, test with concentrated local anesthetic (6–10 mL lidocaine 2% with epi or 6–10 mL lidocaine 1% with epi combined with bupivacaine 0.25% with epi).

- If pain relief or a drop in BP is not observed within 10 minutes, pull epidural catheter, administer IV opioids and consider immediate replacement of the epidural.
- If partial pain relief is noted but analgesia is better on one side than the other, the catheter could be in too far or off midline. If the catheter is in greater than 3 cm, pull it out one or two cm then rebolus with 10–20 mL of infusate solution.
- If the pain remains at a point higher than the level of the catheter, consider infusing larger volumes of solution (14–16 mL/h). As above, consider giving an additional loading dose of 0.5 mg hydromorphone

Dosing

Typical test dose:

    3 mL of 0.5% lidocaine with 1:200 000 epinephrine (5 µg/mL) or 3 mL of 0.5–0.25% bupivacaine with 1:200 000 epinephrine (5 µg/mL) or a combination of the two.

    Typical infusion solution:

    10 µg/mL Dilaudid with 0.031% bupivicaine at 8–14 mL/h, with patient-controlled bolus of 3 mL every 6 minutes.

epidurally, or up to 2 mg hydromorphone if the patient is opioid-dependent. Also consider a more concentrated epidural infusion. Finally, patients with very high incisions often benefit from small parenteral (IV) doses of morphine (2–4 mg) or hydromorphone (0.5–1 mg). After consulting with the surgical team, a judicious dose of ketorolac (15–30 mg) may also be administered to control upper abdominal and thoracic pain.

Always remember: continuous monitoring of BP, HR, and SaO_2 is required before, during, and after epidural test or bolus dosing in all patients.

Before dosing any epidural, aspirate the catheter and rule out the presence of blood or cerebrospinal fluid.

Troubleshooting: how to manage a patient with an epidural who complains of pain or in the intensive care unit

Patients with moderate incisional pain

(Patients may have finished ambulating or physical therapy, or were more comfortable earlier.)

- Check epidural site for leakage, catheter withdrawal, or catheter obstruction. Aspirate catheter to rule out intravascular migration. Consider surgical complications.
- Assess epidural PCA use. If minimal, educate the patient to press the bolus button every 6 minutes as needed. If approaching the maximum, consider increasing the bolus dose by 25–33%. Also consider an epidural loading dose of 10 mL of infusion solution, which may be repeated 15 minutes later.
- Consider supplementing with parenteral opioids, taking into consideration the patient's hemodynamic, respiratory, and sedation status.

Patients with moderate to severe incisional pain

(Patients may have finished ambulating or physical therapy, or were more comfortable earlier.)

- Check epidural site for leakage, catheter withdrawal, or catheter obstruction. Aspirate catheter to rule out intravascular migration. Consider surgical complications such as compartment syndrome.
- Treat similarly as above instructions for "In the PACU"; however, dose with a maximum of 3 mL of local anesthetic on the floor as an inpatient.

Patients with severe pain (crying-screaming!)

(Most likely a non-functional catheter! But also assess placement, intraop dosing, and opioid-dependency variables.)

- Ensure continuous HR, BP and O_2 Sat monitoring. Also ensure that a senior-level resident or attending is immediately available.
- Prescribe small doses of parenteral hydromorphone (1–2 mg), less if opioid-naive.
- Check epidural site for leakage, catheter withdrawal, or catheter obstruction. Aspirate catheter to rule out intravascular migration. Consider surgical complications such as compartment syndrome.
- Aspirate the catheter, and test with local anesthetic (4–6 mL lidocaine 1% with epi, or lidocaine 1% with epi combined with bupivacaine 0.25% with epi). The patient must be closely observed for the next 20 minutes. If pain relief or a drop in BP is not observed within 10 minutes, pull out the epidural catheter, administer IV opioids and consider immediate replacement of the epidural. If the catheter cannot be replaced,

Dosing

Typical test dose:

3 mL of 0.5% lidocaine with 1:200 000 epinephrine (5 µg/mL) or 3 mL of 0.5–0.25% bupivacaine with 1:200 000 epinephrine (5 µg/mL) or a combination of the two.

Typical infusion solution:

10 µg/mL Dilaudid with 0.031% bupivicaine at 8–14 mL/h, with patient-controlled bolus of 3 mL every 6 minutes.

initiate IV-PCA hydromorphone and follow the patient overnight.

- If you have relief over only part of the incisional site, consider infusing larger volumes of solution (14–16 mL/h). As above, consider giving an additional loading dose of 0.5 mg hydromorphone epidurally, or up to 2 mg hydromorphone if the patient is opioid-dependent. Also consider a more concentrated epidural infusion.
- If the patient is highly opioid-dependent, consider administering a more concentrated epidural infusion (hydromorphone 20–30 µg/mL plus bupivacaine 1/16th%). In addition, opioid-dependent patients will almost always require oral or IV opioid supplementation. They may benefit from combined IV-PCA hydromorphone (0.4–1 mg q 6 min) plus a continuous epidural infusion of more concentrated solution. Alternatively, parenteral doses of morphine

(4–10 mg) or hydromorphone (1–3 mg) or baseline doses of oral oxycontin may be provided. Opioid-dependent patients also exhibit polydrug dependence and may require benzodiazepines for anxiolysis, sleep, and muscle spasm.

Symptom management

An epidural catheter that is working very well but causing hypotension, excessive pruritus, and muscle weakness could be in the intrathecal space. Alternatively, the catheter could be in the epidural space but the infusate could be leaking into the intrathecal space through a dural puncture made inadvertently during placement of the epidural. Decrease the infusate solution rate to 1–2 mL/h, and use a dilute naloxone solution of 400–800 µg/L of the IVF already prescribed by the primary team (at a rate of 75–150 mL/h dependent on patient's fluid requirements).

Section 3
Chapter

47

Neuraxial Opioid Analgesics

Anticoagulants and regional anesthesia

Gregory Cain, Michael Seneca and Ashley Vaughn

Introduction

Neuraxial and peripheral anesthetic techniques provide several unique advantages when used in lieu of or in combination with systemic analgesics and anesthetic agents. Regional techniques have been demonstrated to offer reductions in post-operative morbidity and mortality, although the extent of this reduction and applicability to all patient populations remain controversial. Specific benefits offered by regional techniques include decreased intra-operative blood loss, earlier ambulation, improved post-operative pain control, and a decreased incidence of post-operative nausea and vomiting. However, these

techniques also have a unique set of risks that warrant consideration when planning the anesthetic management of patients.

One factor that has been particularly controversial is how to adjust neuraxial and peripheral techniques and timing for the anticoagulated patient. The relationship between anticoagulants and the development of bleeding complications remains complex and multifactorial. Many patients receiving systemic anticoagulants have safely undergone neuraxial techniques without sequelae. Conversely, there are documented cases of patients spontaneously developing severe bleeding complications such as epidural hematoma without having previously received exogenous anticoagulants. Nevertheless, assessment of coagulation status remains a central component when considering regional anesthetic techniques. Establishment of standards for venous thromboembolic prophylaxis as well as development of more efficacious anticoagulant agents have made the management of regional anesthetic techniques increasingly challenging and complex. Additionally, a paucity of data regarding certain facets of patient management, such as timing, in the face of newer or even multiple anticoagulants has been a continual source of controversy. The American Society of Regional Anesthesia and Pain Medicine (ASRA) released a set of guidelines based upon available data that aimed to simplify management for patients undergoing neuraxial anesthetic techniques. However, minimal data exist and significant controversy remains with regard to peripheral techniques. This chapter will summarize and highlight the most current ASRA guidelines as well as some additional research data that may provide some direction to practitioners managing these patients.

Potential complications

Recent advancements in regional anesthesia are often paralleled by the introduction of new thromboprophylaxis guidelines and therapeutic agents. Complications including bleeding, infection, hematoma, and transient or permanent neurological injury from peripheral and neuraxial anesthesia can be particularly devastating to the patient. Although sources vary, the incidence of hematoma is estimated to be 1:150 000 for epidural techniques and 1:220 000 for spinal techniques. The introduction of low molecular weight heparin (LMWH) in 1993 was implicated in over 40 spinal hematomas over a 5-year period. The widespread use of antithrombotic agents continues to pose a significant challenge to practitioners considering regional techniques. Guidelines were introduced in 1998 and subsequently revised in 2002 and 2010 [1] by ASRA to help simplify management of these patients based upon available data. However, it is important to note that adverse clinical events have been reported even when procedures were performed within the guidelines. Tam et al. [2] presented a case study in which the patient developed an epidural hematoma after a combined spinal-epidural anesthetic while concomitantly taking clopidogrel and dalteparin for thromboprophylaxis. An epidural hematoma developed despite following standard guidelines concerning administration of LMWH peri-operatively and discontinuing the clopidogrel 7 days prior to the scheduled anesthetic.

Even low-risk patients treated with antiplatelet agents that currently have no specific recommendations undergoing epidural anesthesia are at risk for developing complications such as epidural hematoma. Gilbert et al. [3] published a case report in which an epidural hematoma developed post-operatively in a 35-year-old healthy patient who underwent an outpatient knee arthroscopy under epidural anesthesia. An atraumatic L3–L4 epidural catheter was placed. Thirty milligrams of ketorolac was administered intravenously 45 minutes after epidural placement. The operation was uneventful, the catheter was removed in the recovery room, and the patient was discharged home. The patient developed severe back pain and was advised to return to the surgery center immediately, where she was administered multiple intravenous doses of fentanyl in addition to a repeat dose of ketorolac. The patient developed lower extremity weakness and was subsequently diagnosed with an L1–L3 epidural hematoma via magnetic resonance imaging (MRI). An emergency decompressive laminectomy with hematoma evacuation was performed. The patient had full return of motor function in the following weeks with some persistent sensory deficit over the right soleus area. This case raised the issue of the use of nonsteroidal anti-inflammatory (NSAIDS) drugs during the immediate and post-operative course.

Anticoagulated patients are considered at an increased risk for epidural hematoma. The removal of an intrathecal or epidural catheter is as important as its placement when considering the risk involved. The coagulation status must be evaluated prior to discontinuing these catheters as noted in the case report presented by Rosen et al. [4]. An 18-year-old patient presented for aortic valve replacement secondary to aortic stenosis. A thoracic T9–T10 epidural was placed after an inhalation induction of general anesthesia. Three hours later, the patient received 21 000 units of heparin in preparation for cardiopulmonary bypass (CPB). After CPB the heparin was reversed with protamine. Forty-nine hours post-operatively, intravenous heparin was started for thrombophylaxis of the prosthetic aortic valve. Fifty-three hours post-operatively, the PICC line became clotted and 2 mg of alteplase was administered. Intense back pain and blood in the epidural catheter and around the epidural puncture site were noted. The pediatric team removed

205

the epidural catheter with the onset of the intense back pain. The patient's activated partial thromboplastin time (aPTT) at that time was found to be 87.4 seconds. With removal of the catheter, sudden onset of numbness and weakness distal to T9 was observed. An MRI revealed a T9–T10 epidural hematoma with cord displacement and compression. An urgent decompressive laminectomy was performed. Six weeks following the laminectomy, the patient's neurological status had returned to baseline. The authors postulated that the blood loss through the epidural catheter helped to decrease the pressure effects of the developing hematoma. Removal of the epidural catheter in the presence of impaired coagulation may have increased the bleeding and compounded the problem.

Epidural anesthesia has been demonstrated to be an effective and acceptable alternative to opioid patient-controlled analgesia in many patients. However, the increased risks of hematoma in patients receiving anticoagulants have limited its use beyond the recovery period in these patients.

The following guidelines are adapted from The 2010 Third ASRA Consensus Conference on Neuraxial Anesthesia and Anticoagulation, with additional information provided when available from current literature.

Heparin

Heparin is frequently used in the intra-operative period and may be associated with increased risk when combined with spinal or epidural anesthesia. Three main risk factors have been identified: traumatic needle placement, less than 1 hour between needle placement and heparin administration, and concomitant use of other anticoagulants.

Subcutaneous (SC) heparin use for prophylaxis of venous thromboembolism, typically 5000 units every 12 hours, has been used extensively and is not a contraindication for neuraxial techniques. Withholding heparin until the block is placed and assessing platelet count in patients who have received heparin for more than 4 days may reduce the risk of complications.

Intra-operative systemic anticoagulation with heparin is generally compatible with neuraxial anesthesia and has been used safely in vascular and cardiopulmonary bypass surgery. Most of the published case studies regarding CPB and systemic heparinization have observed the following recommendations: avoid neuraxial blocks in patients with existing coagulopathies of any origin, a minimum of 24 hour delay in the

event of traumatic needle placement, time from instrumentation to systemic heparinization should be greater than 1 hour, heparin effect and its reversal should be tightly controlled, epidural catheters should be removed only when normal coagulation is restored, and patients should be monitored closely for a minimum of 24 hours for signs and symptoms of hematoma formation.

The following recommendations are advised for combining spinal or epidural anesthesia with heparin during vascular anesthesia: delay heparin administration for a minimum of 1 hour following block or catheter placement, avoid in patients with existing coagulopathies, indwelling catheters should be removed 2–4 hours after the last dose of heparin and assessment of the patient's coagulation status, and reheparinization should occur a minimum of 1 hour after catheter removal.

Low molecular weight heparin (LMWH)

Underestimating the pharmacological differences between LMWH and standard heparin led to over 40 reported cases of spinal hematoma within 5 years of its introduction into the US market. New indications and labeling for LMWH warrant additional discussion and research regarding the anesthetic management of patients on these medications.

Patients presenting for surgery on LMWH thromboprophylaxis should have needle placement delayed until at least 10–12 hours after the LMWH dose. These patients can be assumed to have altered coagulation states. Patients on higher treatment doses of LMWH will require delays of at least 24 hours to return to normal coagulation states prior to needle placement.

Management of post-operative thromboprophylaxis and neuraxial anesthesia may be done safely and is based on total daily dosing, timing of dosing, and dosing schedule. Twice-daily dosing of LMWH may be associated with an increased risk of spinal hematoma and the first dose should be administered no earlier than 24 hours post-operatively. If a catheter is left in place for a continuous technique, it should be removed at least 2 hours prior to the first dose of LMWH.

Single daily dosing, which more closely approximates the European dosing regime and its associated lower incidence of neuraxial complications, should be administered 6–8 hours post-operatively, with the second dose no sooner than 24 hours after the initial dose. Indwelling catheters may be maintained safely, although the catheter should not be removed until 10–12 hours after the last dose. Subsequent LMWH doses should be held until at least 2 hours following catheter removal.

Fondaparinux (Arixtra)

Fondaparinux is a newer, unique anticoagulant utilized for thromboembolic prophylaxis. It is a synthetic Factor Xa inhibitor. Data with this drug in patients receiving regional anesthesia are limited. Current recommendations suggest avoiding indwelling catheters and utilizing neuraxial techniques with extreme caution. However, a study by Singelyn et al. in 2007 [5] suggested that both neuraxial techniques and indwelling catheters may be safe. The Singelyn study had a sample of 5704 patients who received 2.5 mg SC injections of fondaparinux once daily. Of this sample, 1553 patients had indwelling neuraxial or peripheral nerve catheters. The incidence of venous thromboembolism in this study was the same (about 1%) for patients with and without indwelling catheters. There were no reports in this study of neuraxial or peripheral hematoma. Singelyn recommended discontinuing fondaparinux for 48 hours before discontinuing an indwelling catheter.

Oral anticoagulants (warfarin)

Warfarin exerts its anticoagulant effects indirectly by inhibiting the synthesis of vitamin K-dependent clotting factors. The effects of warfarin are not clinically apparent until a significant amount of inactive factors are synthesized and the remaining active factors are consumed. Individual patient variability, a narrow therapeutic range, a lack of data regarding complications, risks in the patient who recently discontinued warfarin, and a long list of drugs that potentiate warfarin are just some of the challenges presented to practitioners managing this patient population. Peri-operative management of these patients remains controversial.

Caution should be used when considering neuraxial techniques in patients who have recently discontinued warfarin therapy, and prothrombin time (PT/INR) should be assessed prior to needle placement. Therapy should be withheld 4–5 days prior to the operation. It is important to note that concomitant use of other medications that affect the clotting mechanism, such as aspirin or heparin, may interact synergistically with warfarin without any demonstrated prolongation of the PT/INR. Other medications that may potentiate warfarin include NSAIDs, clopidogrel, LMWH, and ticlopidine.

If a patient has received an initial oral dose of warfarin greater than 24 hours prior to surgery the PT/INR should be checked. The PT/INR should also be checked if the patient has received more than one oral dose, even if less than 24 hours has gone by.

Patients receiving continuous epidural anesthesia and low-dose warfarin therapy should have their PT/INR monitored daily and assessed prior to catheter removal. Most studies evaluating low-dose warfarin therapy have observed 5 mg dosing of warfarin. Higher doses may require more frequent assessment. When initiating thromboprophylaxis with warfarin, the catheter should be removed when the INR is less than 1.5, as this is associated with clotting factor activity levels of more than 40%. Neurological, sensory and motor function assessment should be performed on all patients receiving warfarin therapy and epidural anesthesia. It is preferable to choose an anesthetic technique that minimizes the degree of sensory and motor blockade. These assessments should be continued for a minimum of 24 hours following catheter removal and longer if the INR was greater than 1.5 at the time it was removed.

An INR greater than 3 may require the next dose of warfarin to be held or reduced in patients with an indwelling catheter. There are no recommendations or consensus views regarding the removal of neuraxial catheters in patients with therapeutic levels of anticoagulation. Reduced doses of warfarin should be considered in patients who may have an enhanced or exaggerated response to the drug.

Antiplatelet agents

The safety of neuraxial blockade in combination with NSAIDs has been demonstrated in several large studies and is also supported by both the rarity of case reports and the widespread usage in the general population. There are no restrictions at this time with regard to NSAID administration and timing of neuraxial anesthesia. There are few data, however, regarding neuraxial anesthesia in the presence of thienopyridine derivatives or GP IIb/IIIa platelet receptor antagonists. Surgical and radiology recommendations include delay of elective surgery for 24 to 48 hours following abciximab and 4 to 8 hours after eptifibatide and tirofiban. Concomitant therapy with other anticoagulants and antiplatelet medications has been shown to increase the risk of hemorrhagic complications.

Direct thrombin inhibitors (DTIs)

Numerous DTIs have been studied clinically, although only a few are in routine clinical use. In particular, argatroban is often used for anticoagulation in patients with or at risk for heparin-induced thrombocytopenia. The effects of these drugs can be monitored using the aPTT, similar to heparin. Few data exist establishing the safety of these agents alongside neuraxial anesthesia, so caution is recommended.

Herbal therapies

Herbal medications, including garlic, ginko, and ginseng, alone do not appear to represent any additional risk in patients having epidural or spinal anesthesia. However, combination therapy with herbal medications and other forms of anticoagulation may increase the risk of bleeding complications and there is not yet an accepted test to measure hemostasis in this patient population. Some sources recommend discontinuing herbal agents 5–7 days to surgery. However, the 2010 recommendations by ASRA are to allow patients to continue any herbal remedies without interruption. Additionally, the current ASRA recommendations provide no restrictions to neuraxial or peripheral techniques on patients taking herbal medications (Table 47.1).

Complications in peripheral nerve blocks

A lack of data available to the first two ASRA conferences limited the ability to offer specific guidelines on continuous peripheral nerve blocks (CPNB) in anticoagulated patients. Case reports suggest that significant blood loss, not neurological deficits, may be the most common and serious complication of peripheral anesthesia in the anticoagulated patient. Prior conferences also noted that applying the same neuraxial guidelines to CPNB could be overly restrictive. However, the 2010 ASRA guidelines recommend using the same guidelines for neuraxial techniques in deep plexus and peripheral blocks. The development of guidelines regarding peripheral nerve blocks in anticoagulated patients by ASRA has not been done within the same environment of urgency in which the neuraxial guidelines were developed. As stated, the most common serious complications related to CPNB are from bleeding rather than neurological damage. Anecdotal evidence suggests that CPNB is safe in anticoagulated patients. However, the decision to proceed with CPNB should be made considering the risks and benefits for individual patients. Additionally, the availability of qualified personnel for performance and follow-up as well as resources at the institution where blocks are performed should be considered.

Recent data, presented by Buckenmaier et al. [6], described the use of CPNB in polytrauma combat casualty patients at Walter Reed Army Medical Center. The high risk of thromboembolism in this patient population necessitated the use of twice-daily dosing of LMWH and, according to the ASRA guidelines, would have precluded the use of CPNBs as well as requiring waiting 24 hours before the first dose of LMWH. The study, noting ASRA's lack of available data, the round-the-clock availability of an acute pain service, and twice-daily visits by an anesthesia provider, elected for a more liberal approach. Ten to 12 hours after the last dose of prophylactic enoxaparin, patients could receive an indwelling catheter or single injection block, as well as have a catheter discontinued. Patients on therapeutic enoxaparin differed slightly, allowing for a single injection block at staff discretion and requiring a 24-hour wait between the last dose and CPNB placement, which was not to be placed if therapeutic anticoagulation was to be continued. If a CPNB catheter was in place and the dose of enoxaparin increased to therapeutic dosage, with the exception of lumbar plexus blocks, CPNB was recommended to be continued. Lumbar plexus catheters were to be removed 24 hours after the last dose due to the relatively higher risk of bleeding complications. No bleeding complications were reported in any of the 187 patients included in the study. The patient population was primarily composed of young, otherwise healthy, male military personnel and may not be applicable to other patient populations.

A retrospective case study was conducted by Chelly et al. [7] that examined patients receiving warfarin therapy and continuous lumbar plexus block following total hip replacemnt. At the time of lumbar plexus catheter removal, 36.2% of patients had an INR >1.4, 24% had an INR between 1.5 and 1.9, while 12% had an INR above 2.0. Six hundred and seventy patients were included in this study. There was one reported case of bleeding at the catheter site after removal in which the INR was 3.0 at the time of removal. The bleeding was managed with direct pressure and vitamin K. The preliminary findings of this study suggested that the removal of a deep perineural catheter

Table 47.1. Guidelines for neuraxial techniques in patients receiving anticoagulants

	Guidelines	Additional Notes
Heparin	Subcutaneous heparin: delay dosing until after neuraxial technique, if possible	Evaluate platelet count in patients receiving heparin for >4 days
	Intravenous heparin: discontinue 1 hour before and after needle placement	
	Discontinue infusion 2–4 hours prior to catheter removal	
	Avoid resuming infusion for minimum of 1 hour after catheter removal	
	Monitor for 24 hours after removal	
LMWH	Avoid administration for minimum of 10–12 hours before or after needle placement: patients on higher dosing regimens may require 24 hours for normal coagulation	
Fondaparinux (Arixtra)	Avoid indwelling catheters	Utilize neuraxial techniques with extreme caution
	Avoid traumatic needle placement	
Warfarin (Coumadin)	Discontinue 4–5 days prior to needle placement	Monitor PT/INR, ensure INR <1.5 prior to needle placement or catheter removal
	Monitor for 24 hours after epidural or spinal techniques	
Antiplatelet agents	Aspirin/NSAIDs (no restrictions)	
	Clopidogrel (Plavix) discontinue 5–7 days prior to needle placement;	
	Ticlopidine (Ticlid), discontinue 14 days prior to needle placement	
	Eptifibatide (Integrilin) and Tirofiban (Aggrastat), avoid neuraxial anesthesia	
Direct thrombin inhibitors (DTIs)	Hirudin-based, bivalent DTIs including bivalirudin (Angiomax), lepirudin (Refludan), and desirudin (Iprivask), risk of bleeding complications unknown	Monitor aPTT
	Univalent DTIs including argatroban and dabigatran (Pradaxa), risk of bleeding complications unknown	
Herbal medications	No restrictions	Agents of concern: ginger, ginkgo, ginseng, garlic, feverfew, and vitamin E. Prior recommendations were to discontinue 5–7 days prior

Where available, based upon 2010 ASRA Guidelines. When inconsistencies were observed in literature, more conservative guidelines are utilized

The 2010 ASRA guidelines are the first to provide recommendations regarding deep plexus and peripheral blocks in patients receiving anticoagulants. Current ASRA recommendations are to apply the same guidelines for neuraxial blockade to deep plexus and peripheral blocks.

may be safely performed with an INR >1.4 in patients receiving warfarin for thromboprophylaxis.

Conclusion

For a variety of reasons, recommendations in the current literature can be inconsistent regarding the management of anticoagulated patients receiving regional anesthesia. Pharmacological therapies for thromboembolic prophylaxis are continually evolving and dosing regimens for anticoagulants can vary by patient population, indications, and even by region. Numerous case studies demonstrate inconsistent results with current recommendations, which focus on neuraxial anesthesia and may be overly restrictive when applied to peripheral nerve blocks. However, current ASRA guidelines are conservative in this regard and recommend using the same guidelines whether performing neuraxial, deep plexus, or peripheral techniques.

References

1. Horlocker TT, Wedel DJ, Denise J, et al. Regional anesthesia in the patient receiving antithrombotic or thrombolytic therapy: American Society of Regional Anesthesia and Pain Medicine Evidence-Based Guidelines (Third Edition). *Reg Anesth Pain Med* 2010;**35**(1):64–101.

2. Tam NLK, Pac-Soo C, Pretorius PM. Epidural haematoma after a combined spinal-epidural anaesthetic in a patient treated with clopidogrel and dalteparin. *Br J Anaesth* 2006;**96**(2):262–265.

3. Gilbert AG, Owens BD, Mulroy MF. Epidural hematoma after outpatient epidural anesthesia. *Anesth Analg* 2002:**94**(1):77–78.

4. Rosen DA, Hawkinberry DW, Rosen KR, et al. *Anesth Analg* 2004;**98**(4):966–969.

5. Singelyn FJ, Verheyen C, Piovella F, Van Aken HK, Rosencher N. The safety and efficacy of extended thromboprophylaxis with fondaparinux after major orthopedic surgery of the lower limb with or without a neuraxial or deep peripheral nerve catheter: The EXPERT Study. *Anesth Analg* 2007;**105**(6):1540–1547.

6. Buckenmaier CC, Shields CH, Auton AA, et al. Continuous peripheral nerve block in combat casualties receiving low molecular weight heparin. *Br J Anaesth* 2006;**97**(6):874–877.

7. Chelly JE, Szczodry DM, Neumann KJ. International normalized ratio and prothrombin time values before the removal of a lumbar plexus catheter in patients receiving warfarin after total hip replacement. *Br J Anaesth* 2008;**101**(2):250–254.

48

Nonselective nonsteroidal anti-inflammatory drugs, COX-2 inhibitors, and acetaminophen

Jonathan S. Jahr and Vivian K. Lee

Analgesics, such as nonselective nonsteroidal anti-inflammatory drugs (NSAIDs), COX-2 inhibitors, and acetaminophen, are amongst the most commonly used medications in the USA and worldwide. An estimated 70 million NSAID prescriptions are written every year in the USA alone. Moreover, non-presciption strength NSAIDs and oral acetaminophen are readily accessible over-the-counter. In the peri-operative setting, these analgesics are gaining recognition as an important alternative and/or adjunct to the historically mostly opioid-based analgesia.

The appeal of NSAIDs, COX-2 inhibitors, and acetaminophen is that the unfavorable opioid-related side effects may be mitigated. Although opioids are potent and effective drugs for pain control, they are well known for adverse side effects such as excessive sedation, dose-dependent respiratory depression, pruritus, nausea, vomiting, biliary spasm, hypotension, constipation, and urinary retention. Minimizing these effects has the advantage of earlier ambulation post-operatively and consequently a shorter hospitalization, as well as higher patient satisfaction and quality of recovery.

The multimodal analgesic approach aims to reduce opioid-related adverse effects peri-operatively. Multimodal analgesia combines different classes of analgesics and methods of pain management to provide superior pain relief than any one class or method alone. The basic principle is that using various classes of medications will simultaneously and synergistically inhibit the different pain receptor pathways. The combination reduces the dose of each analgesic and thereby decreases the incidence of side effects of any particular medication used. The American Society of Anesthesiologists Task Force on Acute Pain Management currently advocates this approach. In fact, guidelines suggest all patients receive NSAIDs, COX-2 inhibitors, or acetaminophen for acute pain management peri-operatively, unless contraindicated. This is consistent with the World Health Organization

(WHO) "pain ladder" method of controlling pain (see Figure 48.1). The WHO "pain ladder" was initially created for treating cancer pain but is now commonly used as a paradigm for treating all types of pain. The bottom rung of the ladder consists of non-opioids such as NSAIDs, COX-2 inhibitors, and acetaminophen. If pain persists, medications of escalating strength are recommended.

No medication is without adverse effects, and NSAIDs, COX-2 inhibitors, and acetaminophen are no exception. These adverse effects may or may not be less significant compared to the adverse effects of opioids. Nonselective NSAIDs, for example, invariably affect platelet aggregation and it remains controversial whether administration peri-operatively increases the risk of bleeding. Clinicians must weigh the risk of bleeding with the reduction in opioid consumption if the NSAID is administered preemptively prior to emergence. On the other hand, the anti-platelet effects of the nonselective NSAID aspirin are beneficial when used for venous thromboembolism prophylaxis. Without prophylaxis, the reported incidence of deep venous thrombosis and pulmonary embolism following total hip arthroplasty and total knee arthroplasty has been reported to be as high as 50–60% and 7–11%, respectively. Studies have demonstrated that aspirin can be used for venous thromboembolism prophylaxis in low-risk patients being discharged home following orthopedic surgery.

Aside from their important role in multimodal analgesic therapy, they have also been extensively studied in preemptive analgesia. Preemptive analgesia is an anticipatory anesthetic approach that intends to prevent the pain and inflammatory response initiated by surgical incision and manipulation, and prevent the "wind-up phenomenon". NSAIDs, COX-2 inhibitors, and acetaminophen have all demonstrated efficacy in the management of mild to moderate post-operative pain. Additionally, they are

The Essence of Analgesia and Analgesics, ed. Raymond S. Sinatra, Jonathan S. Jahr and J. Michael Watkins-Pitchford. Published by Cambridge University Press. © Cambridge University Press 2011.

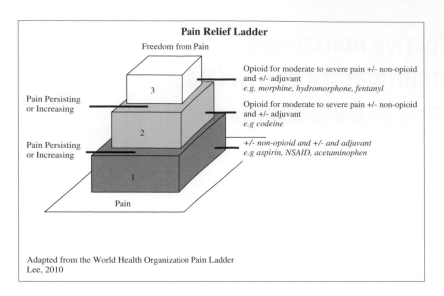

Pain Relief Ladder

Freedom from Pain

3

Opioid for moderate to severe pain +/- non-opioid
and +/- adjuvant
e.g. morphine, hydromorphone, fentanyl

Pain Persisting
or Increasing

2

Opioid for moderate to severe pain +/- non-opioid
and +/- adjuvant
e.g codeine

Pain Persisting
or Increasing

1

+/- non-opioid and +/- and adjuvant
e.g aspirin, NSAID, acetaminophen

Pain

Adapted from the World Health Organization Pain Ladder
Lee, 2010

Figure 48.1. WHO pain ladder (adapted from http://www.abpi.org.uk).

important analgesic adjuncts in moderate to severe post-operative pain.

Nonselective nonsteroidal anti-inflammatory drugs

The nonselective nonsteroidal anti-inflammatory drugs (NSAIDs) are mostly derived from carboxylic and enolic acids. They possess analgesic, anti-inflammatory, as well as antipyretic properties, and have proven efficacy in the treatment of headache, rheumatoid arthritis, dysmenorrhea, gout, osteoarthritis, among many other clinical disorders. Because of these properties, they have also proven to be useful in the pre-operative and post-operative period. There are more than 20 different NSAIDs currently available. There are oral, rectal, and parenteral forms, although the only intravenous NSAIDs that are approved for clinical use in the USA are ketorolac and ibuprofen. Many studies have demonstrated no major difference in analgesic efficacy among the various NSAIDs. However, the doses leading to toxicity can be highly variable. When selecting which NSAID to use, it is therefore important to consider toxicity, bioavailability, duration of analgesia, cost, and route of administration. For example, the bioavailability of orally administered NSAIDs has been shown to be higher than after rectal administration. In post-operative patients who are unable to tolerate oral medications, it may be a more prudent choice to administer the drug parentally rather than rectally even though the intravenous form may be more expensive.

The mechanism of action of NSAIDs involves the inhibition of prostaglandin synthesis in response to tissue injury. Lipases release arachidonic acids from membrane phospholipids when cells are faced with insult. The arachidonic acids are normally oxidized to eicosanoids, fatty-acid-derived signaling molecules that have been implicated in pathways affecting the cardiovascular system, nervous system, reproductive system, coagulation, gastrointestinal system, among others. Prostaglandins are among the four known families of eicosanoids and are synthesized by the cyclooxygenase (COX) enzymes. The COX enzymes are required for both prostaglandin and thromboxane synthesis. The NSAIDs are reversible inhibitors of the COX enzymes with the exception of aspirin, which irreversibly inactivates cyclooxygenase.

At least two cyclooxygenase isoenzymes exist – COX-1 and COX-2 – which are differentially expressed in the tissues of the human body (see Figure 48.2). COX-1 is expressed constitutively and functions in platelet aggregation, renal blood flow, and gastric protection. In contrast, COX-2 expression is induced by factors mediating the inflammatory cascade. The COX-2 enzyme is therefore responsible for inflammation and pain. Aspirin and nonselective NSAIDs inhibit both COX-1 and COX-2. Common adverse effects of this class of drugs are related to the nonspecific inhibition of prostaglandin and thromboxane synthesis, and include an increased risk of significant gastrointestinal bleeding, compromised platelet function, and renal dysfunction.

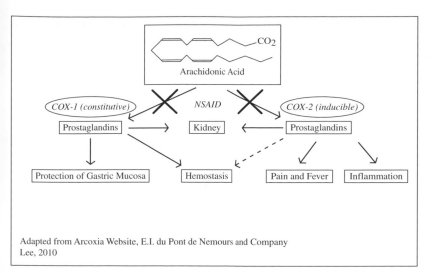

Figure 48.2. NSAIDs mechanism of action (adapted from http://www.arcoxia.ae).

COX-2 inhibitors

COX-2 inhibitors are a subclass of NSAIDs that are relatively more specific inhibitors of the cyclooxygenase-2 enzyme. Research and development of this subclass was initially driven by the potential to improve the gastrointestinal safety profile of traditional NSAIDs while providing similar analgesic relief. The mechanisms by which NSAIDs cause gastrointestinal damage include disruption of the gastric mucosal layer, vasoconstriction, and decreased bicarbonate secretion. Selective inhibition of the COX-2 enzyme provides the anti-inflammatory and analgesic effects without compromising COX-1 expression and causing gastrointestinal insult. The adverse effects on the gastrointestinal tract affect an estimated 60% of patients taking NSAIDs.

COX-2 inhibitors are not absolutely selective for the COX-2 enzyme. Rather, all NSAIDs have some COX-1 and COX-2 inhibition, but along this continuum, the COX-2 inhibitors are much more selective for the COX-2 enzyme. Increasing COX-2 selectivity does not necessarily correlate with increased therapeutic efficacy.

The first COX-2 inhibitor approved by the US Food and Drug Administration (FDA) in 1998 was celecoxib (Celebrex). This was soon followed by the approval of rofecoxib (Vioxx) and valdecoxib (Bextra). Since then, valdecoxib and rofecoxib have both been voluntarily withdrawn from the US market because of an increased stroke and cardiovascular risk, especially that of thrombosis. Currently, celecoxib is the only COX-2 inhibitor available in the US market and and has a FDA-mandated black-box warning regarding cardiovascular risk. Its FDA-approved indications include treatment of osteoarthritis, rheumatoid arthritis, ankylosing spondylitis, primary dysmenorrhea, familial adenomatous polyposis, as well as acute pain management. Other COX-2 inhibitors used in Europe but not yet approved for use in the USA include parecoxib, etoricoxib, and lumiracoxib.

Additional use of the COX-2 inhibitors in the perioperative setting helps avoid the adverse effects of opioids. Given the increased cardiovascular risk and FDA-mandated black-box warning, however, the COX-2 inhibitors seem to have fallen out of favor in the management of post-operative pain. Regardless, it is important to be aware of the general guidelines for using COX-2 inhibitors.

Studies have suggested a dose-dependent increase in cardiovascular risk, and the lowest effective dose for the shortest duration possible should be used when COX-2 inhibitors are indicated. According to current American Heart Association recommendations, naproxen is the safest alternative to COX-2 inhibitors in patients at increased risk of major thrombotic events. There is, however, no clear data that traditional NSAIDS are without the cardiovascular risk of COX-2 inhibitors. In patients who have a history of gastrointestinal bleeding, current guidelines suggest pairing a COX-2 inhibitor with a proton pump inhibitor. Additionally, eradication of *Helicobacter pylori* in the GI tract seems to reduce the risk of gastrointestinal complications caused by NSAIDS. COX-2 inhibitors alone have been shown to more effectively protect

213

the gastrointestinal tract than a traditional NSAID along with a gastroprotective agent such as a proton pump inhibitor, an H2 receptor antagonist, or prostaglandin analogs.

Acetaminophen

In patients who may be highly susceptible to the adverse effects of traditional NSAIDs and COX-inhibitors, acetaminophen is a favorable alternative. Acetaminophen is a commonly used analgesic and antipyretic that is readily available in its oral form as an over-the-counter drug. It is also known as para-cetamol or *N*-acetyl-para-aminophenol (APAP), and is supplied in oral, rectal, and parenteral forms. Although the intravenous form has been available in various countries worldwide since 2002, it is currently still undergoing approval by the US Food and Drug Administration at the time of writing of this chapter.

Acetaminophen exerts weaker inhibition of peripheral prostaglandin synthesis than NSAIDs. Its mechanism of action is not clearly understood but involves central inhibition of cyclooxygenases. Some studies have suggested that NSAIDs seem to be a more effective analgesic than acetaminophen, but it may also depend on the type of surgery being performed. Regardless, acetaminophen is a useful drug for the monotherapy management of mild to moderate peri-operative pain, and as an adjunct to other analgesics for the management of moderate to severe peri-operative pain.

Although acetaminophen has a narrow therapeutic index, when used within the recommended dosage ranges it has been shown to have an extremely low incidence of adverse effects. It can be used as an adjunct to the NSAIDs to decrease the incidence of NSAID-related adverse effects, and similarly as an adjunct to opioids to decrease the incidence of opioid-related adverse effects.

In day-to-day practice, clinicians must weigh the risk/benefit ratio for each medication they prescribe to patients. Given their widespread usage peri-operatively as well as non-peri-operatively, a basic understanding of NSAIDs, COX-2 inhibitors, and acetaminophen is certainly imperative. The following chapters provide an overview of key points regarding specific agents within these classes, such as their recommended doses, indications, advantages, disadvantages, and both common and serious adverse reactions. With this information, clinicians can choose the optimal agent from their armamentarium to treat patients in the acute peri-operative setting.

References

1. Jahr JS, Donkor KN, Sinatra RS. Non-selective non-steroidal anti-inflammatory drugs (NSAIDs), cyclooxygenase-2 inhibitors (COX-2Is), and acetaminophen in acute perioperative pain: analgesic efficacy, opiate-sparing effects, and adverse effects. In Sinatra R, de Leon-Casasola O, Ginsberg B, Viscusi ER, eds. *Acute Pain Management*, 2nd ed. New York: Cambridge University Press 2009, pp. 332–365.

2. Ong CKS, et al. An evidence-based update on nonsteroidal anti-inflammatory drugs. *Clin Med Res* 2007;**5**(1):19–34.

3. Hyllested M, et al. Comparative effect of paracetamol, NSAIDs or their combination in post-operative pain Management: a qualitative review. *Br J Anaesth* 2002;**88**(2):199–214.

4. Scheiman JM. Balancing risks and benefits of cyclooxygenase-2 selective nonsteroidal anti-inflammatory drugs. *Gastroenterol Clin N Am* 2009;**38**:305–314.

5. Jones R, et al. Gastrointestinal and cardiovascular risks of nonsteroidal anti-inflammatory drugs. *Am J Med* 2008;**121**(6):464–474.

6. Sinatra RS, Jahr JS, Reynolds LW, Viscusi ER, Groudine SB, Payen-Champenois C. The analgesic efficacy and safety of single and repeated administration of intravenous paracetamol (acetaminophen) 1 g for the treatment of postoperative pain following orthopedic surgery. *Anesthesiology* 2005;**102**:822–831.

7. Sinatra RS, Boice JA, Loeys TL, Ko AT, Kashuba MM, Jahr JS, Rhondeau S, Singla N, Cavanaugh PF. Evaluation of the effect of perioperative rofecoxib treatment on pain control and clinical outcomes in patients recovering from gynecologic abdominal surgery: a randomized, double-blind, placebo-controlled clinical study. *Reg Anesth Pain Med* 2006;**31**(2):134–142.

8. Buvanendran A, Kroin JS. Multimodal analgesia for controlling acute postoperative pain. *Curr Opin Anaesthesiol* 2009; [Epub ahead of print].

9. Snyder BK. Venous thromboembolic prophylaxis: the use of aspirin. *Orthop Nurs* 2008;**27**(4):225–230.

Ibuprofen

Eric C. Lin and Shu-ming Wang

Generic Name: ibuprofen

Trade/Proprietary Names: Advil™, Motrin™

Chemical Structure: see Figure 49.1

Chemical Name: D2-(4-isobutylphenyl)propanoic acid

Description

Ibuprofen (2-arylpropionate derivatives) contains a stereocenter in the α-position of the propinate moiety. Ibuprofen is also known as Advil, Genpril, Ibu, Midol, Motrin, and Nuprin. Ibuprofen was developed during the 1960s by the research arm of Boots Group in the UK. Stewart Adams, John Nicholson, and Collin Burrows discovered this compound and patented it in 1961. In 1969, this drug was launched as a treatment for rheumatoid arthritis in the UK and later on was launched in the USA in 1974. The clinical outcomes of ibuprofen as a treatment for pain, inflammation, and fever won Boots Group the Queen's Award for Technical Achievement in 1987.

Mode of activity

Major sites of action: ibuprofen produces reversible cyclooxygenase inhibition by competing with the substrate, arachidonic acid, for the active site of enzyme. This leads to the inhibition of prostaglandin synthesis. The inhibition of prostaglandin synthesis by ibuprofen has been demonstrated in a wide variety of cell types and tissues.

Receptor interactions: ibuprofen interacts nonselectively with cyclooxygenase 1 (COX-1) and 2 (COX-2). Effects of ibuprofen include analgesia and antipyretic and anti-inflammatory properties through the COX-2 inhibition. Unwanted effects, such as preventing platelet aggregation and ulcerating gastrointestinal mucosa, are mediated through COX-1 inhibition. In contrast to other NSAIDs, ibuprofen shows non-time-dependent inhibition, but retains its initial ratio of activity against COX-1/COX-2.

Metabolic pathways: ibuprofen is absorbed from the gastrointestinal tract and peak plasma concentrations are reached within about 1 to 2 hours after ingestion. Bioavailability is greater than or equal to 80%, 99% of ibuprofen is bound to plasma proteins, and 90% is transformed to two inactive metabolites. Following a single dose ingestion, the plasma half-life is about 2 ± 0.5 hours. However, as the dosage increases, the half-life ranges between 4 and 8 hours. Ibuprofen is rapidly excreted in the urine, mainly as metabolites and their conjugates. The majority of the dose is recovered in the urine within 24 hours as the hydroxy (25%) and carboxypropyl (37%) phenylpropionic acid metabolites. The percentages of free and conjugated ibuprofen found in urine are about 1% and 14% respectively. The remainder of the drug is found in the stool as both metabolites and an unabsorbed drug.

Indications (approved/non-approved)

Oral suspension

Fever: ibuprofen is indicated for the reduction of fever in patients aged 6 months and older.

Medical pain: ibuprofen is commonly used to relieve mild to moderate pain and primary dysmenorrhea.

Cancer pain: a small randomized clinical trial indicated that ibuprofen combined with methadone has significantly increased analgesia in patients suffering from moderate to severe cancer-related pain.

Chronic non-malignancy pain: ibuprofen frequently is used to assist in the management of various chronic pain syndromes such as osteoarthritis, rheumatoid arthritis, low back pain, fibromyalgia, and peripheral neuropathy.

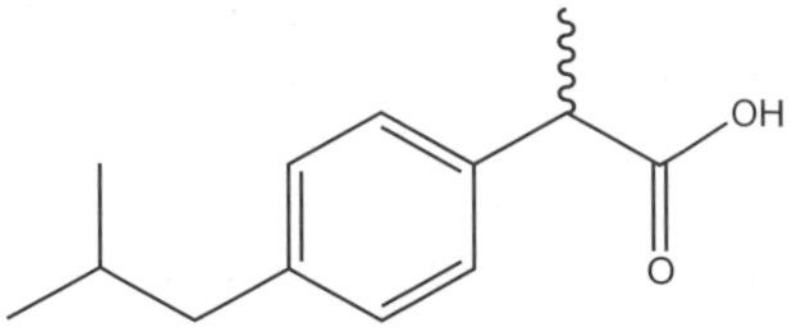

Figure 49.1.

Topical cream and gel

Medical pain: 5% ibuprofen cream is found to be useful in treating acute ankle sprains and knee osteoarthritis.

Acne treatment: 5% ibuprofen cream is found to be effective in treating patients with mild acne.

Contraindications

Absolute: patients with documented hypersensitivity to ibuprofen, individuals with a history of allergic manifestations to aspirin or other NSAIDs, and severe anaphylactic-like reaction to ibuprofen.

Relative: (1) patients with serious gastrointestinal events and other risk factors known to be associated with peptic ulcer disease such as alcoholism, smoking, etc. (2) Elderly and debilitated patients who cannot tolerate ulceration or bleeding well. (3) Patients with bronchospastic reactivity (e.g. asthma), nasal polyps, or those with a history of angioedema can have an anaphylactoid reaction after ibuprofen. (4) Patients with advanced renal disease should be monitored closely during the treatment of ibuprofen.

Common doses

Oral: the recommended dosage is based upon body mass and indications. Generally, the oral dosage is 200–400 mg for adults or 5–10 mg/kg for children every 4–6 hours. The usual dose in adults is 400–800 mg daily for analgesia and up to 1600 to 2400 mg for its anti-inflammatory action. The maximum daily ibuprofen dose for over-the-counter use is 1200 mg. Under the medical direction of physicians, the daily allowable dose can be up to 3200 mg.

Drug preparation

Tablets – 200 mg, 400 mg, 600 mg and 800 mg

Chewable tablets – 50–100 mg

Capsule – 200 mg

Suspension – 100 mg/2.5 mL and 100 mg/5 mL

Oral drops – 40 mg/mL

Topical – 5% cream

Suppository – 60 mg

Potential advantages

Ease of use, tolerability: for most patients, ibuprofen is well tolerated and has less toxicity as compared to other analgesic treatments.

Cost: relatively inexpensive when generic versions are available.

Availability: widely available in every hospital and pharmacy.

As monotherapy: ibuprofen has been used to treat fever and relieve mild to moderate pain.

As used for multimodal analgesia: study has shown that ibuprofen can be used as an adjunct for narcotics in managing cancer pain.

Potential disadvantages

Toxicity: ibuprofen has become very common ever since it was licensed as an over-the-counter medication. Although there are many ibuprofen overdose experiences in the medical literature, the frequency of life-threatening complications from the overdose is low. The toxic effect is unlikely at doses below 100 mg/kg, but the toxic effect can be severe when ibuprofen is above 400 mg/kg. The lethal dose may vary with age, weight, and concomitant diseases of the individual patient. Therapy for the overdose of ibuprofen is largely symptomatically. In cases presented early, gastric decontamination is recommended (by using active charcoal to absorb the ibuprofen before it enters the systemic circulation).

Drug interactions: ibuprofen affects the antihypertensive effect of ACE inhibitors, reduces the natriuretic effects of furosemide and thiazides, elevates the plasma lithium level by reducing renal lithium clearance, enhances the toxicity of methotrexate, and affects prothrombin time.

Drug-related adverse events

Common adverse events

(1) Serious gastrointestinal toxicity such as ulceration, bleeding, and perforation can occur at any time, with or without warning symptoms in patients receiving chronic ibuprofen treatment. In patients

treated with ibuprofen for 3–6 months, 1% of patients can present with symptomatic upper GI ulcers, gross bleeding or perforation. When the duration of ibuprofen treatment increases to 1 year, 2–4% of patients will have gastrointestinal toxicity.

(2) Ibuprofen can increase the risk of life-threatening cardiovascular events, including heart attack or stroke.

(3) Fluid retention can occur in association with ibuprofen usage. Therefore, the drug should be used with caution in patients with a history of cardiac decompensation or hypertension.

(4) Ibuprofen can inhibit platelet aggregation. But unlike aspirin, its effect on platelet function is reversible, quantitatively less, and of shorter duration. Thus, in patients with underlying hemostatic defects, ibuprofen should be used with caution.

(5) Elevation of one or more liver function tests (LFTs) may occur in up to 15% of patients who receive ibuprofen treatment. The changes of LFTs can be transient or may progress with continued treatment.

(6) Blurred and diminished visions, scotomata, and changes in color vision have been reported with ibuprofen treatment.

(7) Dizziness, headache, and nervousness can occur.

(8) Rashes and pruritus can be present.

Rare adverse events

(1) Anaphylactoid reactions may occur in patients with bronchospastic reactivities and angioedema.

(2) Aseptic meningitis with fever and coma has been observed on rare occasions in patients on ibuprofen therapy. It is probably more likely to occur in patients with systemic lupus erythematosus and related connective tissue diseases.

Treatment of adverse events

The treatment will have to be based on the adverse events. Physicians should discuss with their patients the potential adverse events associated with ibuprofen treatment. They should also advise patients to report to their physicians about signs and symptoms of chest pain, weakness, shortness of breath, slurred speech, gastrointestinal ulceration, bleeding, blurred vision or other eye symptoms, skin rash, weight gain, or edema.

References

1. Vane JR, Botting RM. Mechanism of action of anti-inflammatory drugs. *Scand J Rheumatol* 1996;**25** (suppl 102):9–12.

2. Frölich JC, Fricker RM. Pain therapy and analgesics-antipyretics (nonsteroidal antirheumatic drugs-NSAR). In Frölich JC, Kirch W, eds. *Praktiche Arzneitherpie*, 4th ed. Heidelberg: Springer, 2006, pp. 675–706.

3. Vale JA, Meredith TJ. Acute poisoning due to non-steroidal anti-inflammatory drugs. Clinical features and management. *Med Toxicol* 1996;**1**:12–31.

50 Injectable ibuprofen

James H. Shull

Generic Name: injectable ibuprofen

Trade Name: Caldolor™

Chemical Class: nonsteroidal anti-inflammatory drug

Manufacturer: Cumberland Pharmaceuticals, Nashville, TN

Chemical Name: D2-(4-isobutylphenyl)propanoic acid

Chemical Structure: see Figure 50.1

Description

Ibuprofen is a nonsteroidal anti-inflammatory drug with a long history that has found a broad range of uses in a wide variety of clinical settings. Initially released in oral form in the UK in 1969 (and later in the USA in 1974) as a treatment for rheumatoid arthritis, ibuprofen is now used to treat acute and chronic pain, fever, inflammation and as an anti-platelet agent. Although originally released as an oral agent, later an injectable form became available in Europe, Australia, and New Zealand and has been used as an alternative to indomethacin in the treatment of patent ductus arteriosus. Injectable ibuprofen was recently studied, FDA-approved and introduced to the US market by Cumberland Pharmaceuticals under the trade name Caldolor®. Injectable ibuprofen in the USA is marketed both as an analgesic for use in mild to moderate pain and as an adjunct to opiods in the treatment of moderate to severe pain. In addition to its use as an analgesic, injectable ibuprofen may also be useful as an antipyretic in patients, for whom oral ibuprofen is not an option, although it is not FDA-approved for this indication.

Mode of activity

Injectable ibuprofen is thought to act through the inhibition of cyclooxygenase-mediated prostanoid (prostaglandin, prostacyclin, and thromboxane) formation through nonselective inhibition of both COX-1 and COX-2 isoenzymes. COX-2 is an inducible enzyme found at sites of inflammation. Inhibition of COX-2 activity at sites of inflammation is chiefly responsible for the analgesic, anti-inflammatory, and antipyretic actions of injectable ibuprofen (and NSAIDs in general). In contrast, the COX-1 isoenzyme is a constitutive enzyme found in a wide variety of sites throughout the body and is responsible for many of the untoward effects of ibuprofen administration, including the formation of gastric ulcers and anti-platelet activity.

Indications

Injectable ibuprofen is FDA-approved for the treatment of mild to moderate pain and the treatment of moderate to severe pain as an adjunct to opiod analgesics.

Contraindications and precautions

(1) Patients with known hypersensitivity to ibuprofen or previous hypersensitivity reactions to other NSAIDS.

(2) Injectable ibuprofen is contraindicated in the peri-operative period in patients undergoing coronary artery bypass graft (CABG) surgery secondary to an increased risk of thrombotic events and myocardial infarction.

(3) Patients who have previously had asthma, urticaria, or allergic-type reactions after taking NSAIDS.

(4) Injectable ibuprofen should not be used in pregnant women after 30 weeks of gestation because of the potential for premature closure of the fetal ductus arteriosis. Prior to 30 weeks gestation ibuprofen is Pregnancy Class C.

(5) The safety and effectiveness of injectable ibuprofen in the pediatric population has not been established.

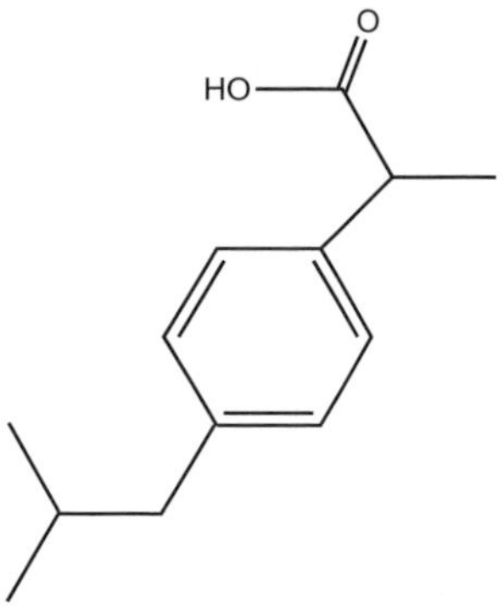

Figure 50.1.

Potential advantages

The chief advantage of injectable ibuprofen is as a means to provide non-opioid analgesia in patients with mild to moderate pain in whom the oral route is not possible or not preferred. Injectable ibuprofen is also useful in the setting of moderate to severe pain when an intravenous route is preferred for an adjunct to opioid analgesia to reduce opioid requirement and thus unwanted opioid side effects such as respiratory depression, pruritus, and nausea. Injectable ibuprofen has not been compared directly with injectable ketorolac; however, efficacy and overall safety of equivalent doses would be expected to be comparable. Like IV ketorolac, injectable ibuprofen may play a role in post-operative multimodal analgesia. In several clinical trials in gynecological and orthopedic surgery, the combination of IV ibuprofen and PCA morphine was superior to IV-PCA morphine alone (Table 50.1).

The analgesic effect of IV ibuprofen was evaluated in two large double-blind, placebo-controlled studies in post-surgical patients, all with access to IV or IV-PCA morphine (Table 50.1) [3–5]. The first was a dose-ranging study in patients recovering from abdominal and orthopedic surgery. Patients randomized to receive 800 mg IV ibuprofen had a 22% reduction in median morphine use while patients receiving 400 mg had a 3% reduction, compared with those receiving placebo. Patients receiving 800 mg IV ibuprofen reported reductions in rest and movement associated VAS pain intensity scores over the 24 hours following surgery (P = 0.001) Patients receiving 400 mg reported a 7% reduction in pain intensity over the 24 hours following surgery (P = 0.057) (Table 50.2) [4]. These data formed the basis for the dosing in the second study, the Abdominal Hysterectomy Pain Study. In this second study, patients undergoing abdominal surgery had a 19.5% reduction in median morphine usage with IV

(6) Like any NSAID, injectable ibuprofen should be avoided in patients with renal dysfunction.

(7) Injectable ibuprofen may cause toxic epidermal necrolysis, exfoliative dermatitis, or Stevens–Johnson syndrome. The drug should be discontinued if a local skin reaction occurs.

(8) Patients taking ACE inhibitors should closely monitor their blood pressure as NSAIDs may reduce ACE inhibitors' antihypertensive effect.

Common doses

Injectable ibuprofen is administered for analgesia in doses of 400 mg to 800 mg every 6 hours as needed, with the total 24 hour dose not to exceed 3200 mg. Injectable ibuprofen is available in single-dose vials of 400 mg/4 mL and 800 mg/8 mL. The 400 mg dose should be diluted in no less than 100 mL of diluent (normal saline, lactated Ringer's, or D5W), while the 800 mg dose should be diluted in no less than 200 mL of diluent. Both the 400 mg and 800 mg doses should be infused in no less than 30 minutes. Rapid IV boluses may cause pain and adverse events (phlebitis, venous injury) and are not recommended [1].

Table 50.1. Reduction in pain intensity: effect of Caldolor, 24 hours post-surgery

	400 mg	800 mg
Medium decreases[a] at hour 24 at rest	0%	33%
P value[b]	P = 0.419	P = 0.009
Medium decreases[a] at hour 24 with movement	−2%	18%
P value[b]	P = 0.894	P = 0.005

[a]In those receiving ibuprofen multimodal therapy compared with those receiving standard, morphine-only therapy.
[b]The analysis is based on a linear 4-way ANOVA model with fixed effects for age group, weight group, randomization center, and treatment group. The P values are based on the difference in LS means from the final ANOVA model.
Source: Key IV Ibuprofen (Caldolor™) Clinical Trials. From: http://www.caldolor.com/.

ibuprofen 800 mg as compared with placebo ($P < 0.001$) (Table 50.2). In addition to using less morphine, patients receiving 800 mg IV ibuprofen reported a 21% median reduction in pain intensity following surgery from post-op through study hour 24 ($P = 0.011$) (Table 50.3) [3–5]. Based on these findings and subsequent approval of IV ibuprofen, physicians comfortable with the use of oral ibuprofen have been given an alternative therapy for pain and fever in the hospital setting where an injectable medicine is often needed [3–5].

Another advantage of injectable ibuprofen is the lack of black-box warning for pre-operative dosing. Unlike ketorolac, injectable ibuprofen is approved for administration prior to tissue injury where it can inhibit traumatic synthesis of prostaglandin and more effectively attenuate the intra-operative inflammatory response.

A final advantage is that ibuprofen and the proprietary preparation Motrin™ are well-recognized and respected analgesics that are widely accepted by patients and caregivers alike. Patients may be treated with injectable doses to initiate analgesia and anti-inflammatory effects, and then converted to and maintained on oral ibuprofen, which is inexpensive and widely available as an over-the-counter analgesic.

Table 50.2. Injectable ibuprofen dose ranging study: pain at rest and with movement and incidence of gastrointestinal adverse events

	IV ibuprofen 400 mg + PCA morphine	IV ibuprofen 800 mg + PCA morphine	IV placebo + PCA morphine
	(n = 111)	(n = 116)	(n = 115)
Pain at rest (VAS[a]- AUC mm-h) 1–24 h, Mean (SD)	81.9 (44.6)	76.9 (41.0)	90.2 (45.5)
Pain with movement (VAS[a]- AUC mm-h) 1–24 h, mean (SD)	111.8 (44.1)	108.5 (45.0)	122.1 (47.3)
PCA morphine requirement (mg) mean (SD)	44.7 (27.0)	42.1 (32.0)	48.8 (28.3)
Incidence of nausea, number (%)	77 (57)[b]	82 (59)	94 (70)
Incidence of vomiting, number (%)	30 (22)	31 (22)	38 (28)
Incidence of constipation, number (%)	23 (17)	25 (18)	28 (21)

[a]As measured using a visual analog scale (VAS scale, 0 = no pain, 100 = intense pain), area under the curve.
[b]Significant difference $P = 0.042$ vs. placebo.
Source: Southworth S, Peters J, Ludbrook G, et al: A multicenter, randomized, double-blind, placebo-controlled trial of intravenous ibuprofen for the management of post-operative pain in adults. *Clin Ther* 2009;**31**:1–13.

Table 50.3. Injectable ibuprofen: analgesic effects observed during the immediate 24 hours following abdominal hysterectomy

Variable	IV-PCA morphine + IV placebo	IV-PCA morphine + IV ibuprofen (800 mg)
Number of patients	153	166
Mean morphine dose (mg) (SD)	56.0 (20.6)	47.3 (25.6)*
Median morphine dose (mg)	54.0	43.5*
Percentage reduction in median morphine dose	–	19.5%*
Pain intensity (rest)	–	Significant Reduction
Pain intensity (movement)	–	Significant Reduction
Incidence of nausea	56%	48%
Incidence of vomiting	8%	9%

[a]Significant reduction $P < 0.05$.

Source: Kroll, P., et al. Randomized double blind, placebo-controlled trial of ibuprofen injection for treatment of pain in post-operative adult patients. Poster #50, 20th Annual AAPM Meeting, Oct 10, 2009.

Potential disadvantages

Injectable ibuprofen shares disadvantages in common with oral ibuprofen and other NSAID analgesics including gastrointestinal irritation and ulceration, increased bleeding secondary to antiplatelet effects, renal toxicity, and cardiovascular complications including stroke and myocardial infarction. IV ibuprofen is contraindicated for patients recovering from coronary artery bypass surgery. As a new entry to the market in the USA, injectable ibuprofen suffers a price disadvantage when compared to the other widely available injectable NSAID, ketorolac, which is available in generic form. Nevertheless it is a drug that is well-recognized and proven safe and efficacious in over 40 years of use. It also offers the caregiver ease of dosing transition from an IV preparation to an inexpensive oral preparation which can be easily purchased and continued upon hospital discharge. Further comparative studies of both effectiveness and the relative side-effect profiles of the respective drugs are needed to determine whether the higher cost for brand-name injectable ibuprofen is justified.

Drug-related adverse reactions

The most common adverse reactions reported with injectable ibuprofen are nausea, flatulence, vomiting, headache, dizziness, and hemorrhage. The most common reaction that leads to discontinuation of the drug is pruritus, which occurs in less than 1% of patients.

References

1. Caldolor® product monograph: available from Cumberland Pharmaceuticals, Nashville, TN.

2. Vane JR, Botting RM. Mechanism of action of anti-inflammatory drugs. *Scand J Rheumatol* 1996;**25**(suppl 102): 9–12.

3. Data on file and Cumberland Pharmaceuticals Inc.

4. Kroll P, Meadows L, Rock A, et al. Randomized double blind, placebo-controlled trial of ibuprofen injection for treatment of pain in postoperative adult patients. *Poster #50, 20th Annual AAPM Meeting*, October 10, 2009

5. Southworth S, Peters J, Ludbrook G, et al. A multicenter, randomized, double- blind, placebo-controlled trial of intravenous ibuprofen for the management of postoperative pain in adults. *Clin Ther* 2009;**31**:1–13.

Section 4 Chapter

51

NSAIDs

Naproxen

Dorothea Hall, Tyson Bolinske and Elizabeth Sinatra

Generic Name: naproxen, naproxen sodium
Trade/Proprietay Names: Naprosyn™, Anaprox™, EC-Naprosyn™, Alleve™, Naprelan™, numerous generics
Drug Class: nonsteroidal anti-inflammatory drug
Manufacturer: Roche Laboratories USA, Nutley, NJ 07110; Bayer Health Care, 100 Bayer Road, Pittsburgh, PA 15205–9741; Pfizer-Wyeth Pharmaceuticals, 235 East 42nd Street, New York, NY 10017
Chemical Name: sodium 2-(6-methoxynaphthalen-2-yl)propanoate
Chemical Structure (salt form): see Figure 51.1
Chemical Formula: $C_{14}H_{14}O_3$

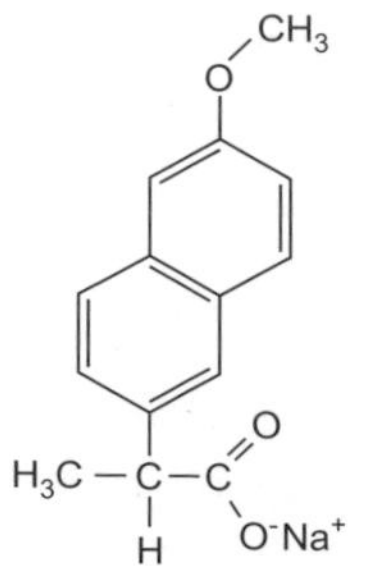

Figure 51.1.

Description

Naproxen is one of many drugs in the group classified as nonsteroidal anti-inflammatory drugs (NSAIDs). Naproxen is in the chemical class of propionic acid derivatives and possesses analgesic, antipyretic, and anti-inflammatory properties. It was first introduced in 1976 under the trade name Naprosyn™ by Roche Pharmaceuticals. Both the acid and salt formulations are currently used, with the salt form having a slightly more rapid absorption rate. Reduced-dose naproxen sodium was approved as an over-the-counter (OTC) pain reliever in the USA in 1994 and entered the market under the trade name of Alleve™ [1,2].

Mechanism of action

In a manner similar to other NSAIDs, naproxen decreases pain by inhibiting inflammation and nociception at the cellular level. Naproxen reversibly inhibits cyclooxygenase (COX). Cyclooxygenase converts arachidonic acid to endoperoxides, and blocks the COX-1-mediated production of thromboxane A2 as well as the COX-2-mediated production of prostaglandin E2. Whereas COX-1 is constitutive and synthesizes prostaglandins for normal renal and gastrointestinal function, COX-2 is inducible and primarily responsible for synthesis of prostaglandins involved in inflammatory reactions. Prostaglandins have direct effects on peripheral terminals of nociceptor sensory neurons, sensitizing pain receptors to histamine and bradykinin and thus reducing their threshold to peripheral noxious stimuli [1].

Pharmacodynamics and pharmacokinetics

Although the exact mechanism of action is not fully understood, it is known that by blocking synthesis of prostaglandins and suppressing the peripheral inflammatory response, activation and amplification of nociceptive inputs and sensitization of nociceptive receptors are diminished.

Both naproxen and its sodium salt are rapidly absorbed in the gastrointestinal tract and are generally fully absorbed when taken orally. Peak plasma levels are obtained in 2–4 hours after ingestion of naproxen, and 1–2 hours after ingestion of the sodium salt form (Anaprox™). The latter has significantly increased aqueous solubility. The enteric coated form of naproxen dissolves in the small intestine as opposed to the stomach; therefore its absorption is delayed.

Distribution: naproxen has a volume of distribution of 0.16 L/kg. The elimination half-life of naproxen is approximately 15 hours following normal therapeutic doses. Naproxen is almost completely (99%) bound to albumin and other plasma proteins. It crosses the placenta and appears in the milk of lactating women at approximately 1% of the plasma level concentration. Substantial amounts are found in the spinal fluid [1–3].

Metabolism: naproxen undergoes various forms of hepatic metabolism (95%) with about 30% of the drug being subjected to 6-demethylation. Most of this metabolite, along with naproxen itself, is excreted as the glucuronide or other conjugate. After liver conjugation, 95% of the drug is excreted by the kidneys, primarily in the metabolite form. Decreased kidney function as seen in the elderly or patients with end-stage liver disease may increase drug elimination half-life two-fold or greater. The combination of decreased protein binding and delayed excretion put the elderly at increased risk of drug toxicity [2,3].

Indications

Acute surgical pain: depending upon the extent of surgery and intensity of post-operative pain, naproxen may be administered as monotherapy or combined with opioid analgesics such as morphine, oxycodone, hydrocodone, or hydromorphone. Oral doses of naproxen 500 mg and naproxen sodium 400 mg provide effective analgesia in adults with moderate to severe acute post-operative pain following dental surgery and bunionectomy. Concomitant use of naproxen in a multimodal analgesic regimen has been shown to reduce pain intensity and the amount of narcotic medications patients require for effective post-operative analgesia. In a recent review of 1509 patients, 400 to 500 mg of oral naproxen provided effective analgesia in adults with moderate to severe acute post-operative pain [4]. In randomized double-blinded trial, pre-operative doses of oral naproxen (550 mg) were compared to placebo in 44 patients recovering from laparoscopic tubal ligation [5]. Patients treated with naproxen benefited from lower VAS pain intensity scores (0.9 vs. 2.3 cm, $P > 0.05$), reduced need for opioids in the PACU (0% vs. 34%), and reduced day surgery stay (168 vs. 188 min, $P > 0.05$) (Table 51.1). Except for one patient in the naproxen group who developed gastric discomfort, there were no other adverse events [5].

Although opioid dose requirements are reduced with short-term use of NSAIDs including naproxen, it remains unclear whether reductions in dose are associated with a decrease in opioid-related adverse events such as nausea, vomiting, and constipation. Like other nonselective NSAIDs, naproxen is often withheld in the peri-operative period for fear of surgical site and GI bleeding. It should be appreciated that unlike aspirin, inhibition of platelet aggregation with naproxen is reversible, and temporally related to serum drug concentration.

Medical pain and non-malignancy chronic pain: naproxen can be used to treat mild to moderate pain. Enteric coated naproxen, however, is not indicated for the treatment of acute pain. Common indications for enteric coated preparations include general somatic pain, acute gout, osteoarthritis, rheumatoid diseases, juvenile arthritis, tendonitis, bursitis, ankylosing, spondylitis, and dysmenorrhea. Recommended dosing for these conditions is 250–500 mg PO q12h with daily dosage caps set between 1250 and 1500 mg/day. These levels should be maintained no longer than 6 months to limit adverse reactions and potential CV and GI morbidity. Naproxen is also used to treat acute gout. It is generally recommended to have a dosing scheme of 250 mg PO q8h with divided doses reaching no higher than 750 mg per day.

Cancer pain: naproxen and other NSAIDs are used for the treatment of cancer pain, often in combination with an opioid. NSAIDs alone have been shown to be efficacious in treating cancer pain in the short term. Naproxen dosage schemes have not been formulated specifically for cancer pain; however, patients experiencing mild to moderate pain may be treated with 250–500 mg PO q12h for acute use with a 1250 mg/day maximum. Maximum dose should be reduced to 1000 mg/day if used for long-term maintenance analgesia. When using naproxen as an adjunct to opioid analgesics for management of moderate to severe cancer pain, dosage must be tailored to the patient's coagulation status to limit hemostatic side effects.

Contraindications

Absolute: hypersensitivity to naproxen, aspirin, other NSAIDs, or a component of their formulations. Post-coronary artery bypass graft (CABG) surgery.

Relative: history of renal insufficiency, peptic ulcer disease, gastrointestinal (GI) bleeds.

Concomitant use of corticosteroids: increased risk of gastroduodenal ulcers. Patients undergoing anticoagulation therapy with products such as warfarin or heparin.

Patients with a bleeding disorder including hemophilia, von Willebrand disease, various factor deficiencies, disseminated intravascular coagulation (DIC), idiopathic thrombocytopenia purpura (ITP), antithrombin III deficiency, or protein C or S deficiency.

Third trimester of pregnancy, Pregnancy Category D, meaning the drug has been found to be unsafe but its use in certain circumstances may be justified. The use of acetaminophen is recommended instead.

The drug is extensively bound to albumin, therefore use with caution in patients with liver disease.

May increase levels of methotrexate, lithium, phenytoin, digoxin, and cyclosporine.

Fluid retention from an inhibition of renal prostaglandins may exacerbate heart failure.

Caution if patient is under sodium restriction or if using a diuretic.

Naproxen increases intravascular fluid volume and blunts the effects of antihypertensive medications.

Table 51.1. Visual analog pain scores following tubal ligation

	Naproxen group	Control group	P
	(n = 23)	(n = 21)	
Pain Intensity (1 h)	0.9 + 0.2	3.5 + 0.6	<0.05
Pain Intensity (2 h)	1.1 + 0.2	2.4 + 0.5	<0.05
Pain Score (Next Day)	0.2 + 0.1	0.6 + 0.2	NS

With permission from Comfort KV, Code WE, Rooney ME et al. *Can J Anesthesia* 1992;**39**:349–392.

Naproxen should not be used in patients with creatinine clearance of less than 30 mL/min, in patients at risk for surgical bleeding and gastrointestinal bleeding and those treated with anticoagulants.

Cigarette smoking and alcohol consumption may increase the risk of ulcers.

Common doses/uses

Dosing is generally based on naproxen content; 200, 500 mg naproxen = 220, 550 mg naproxen sodium.

Naproxen tablets or suspension at 250, 375 or 500 mg q12 hours

EC-naproxen delayed-release enteric coated tablets at 375 or 500 mg q12 hours

Naproxen sodium at 220 mg, 275 mg, 550 mg, and 825 mg q12 hours

The maximum daily dose of naproxen is 1500 mg/day and is the point where increased doses are no longer efficacious and produce significant side-effect risks.

Naproxen is administered orally (PO). To start treatment, the lowest dose likely to be effective for a given patient is prescribed twice daily. The dose is then adjusted by observing benefit and possible adverse effects.

For post-operative pain, 500 mg of oral naproxen or 550 mg of oral naproxen sodium have been shown to provide effective analgesia [3].

Adverse events

Common side effects: these occur in approximately 3–10% of patients treated and are seen at higher frequencies in patients on higher doses and who undergo treatment for longer periods of time. Naproxen is observed to primarily affect the gastrointestinal tract; heartburn, abdominal pain, nausea, constipation, diarrhea, dyspepsia, and stomatitis. More severe gastrointestinal side effects include stomach ulcers and GI bleeds. Elderly patients are at greater risk for suffering from gastrointestinal side effects, edema, visual disturbances, hearing disturbances, headache, dizziness, drowsiness, lightheadedness, and pruritus. Gastrointestinal side effects and the potential for developing ulcers and GI bleeding remain the limiting factor in the widespread use of naproxen for analgesia.

Less common adverse events include cardiovascular palpitation, lightheadedness, vertigo, purpura, rash, diarrhea, dyspepsia, stomatitis, gross bleeding/perforation, indigestion, ulcers, vomiting, abnormal renal function, anemia, increased bleeding time, diaphoresis, thirst, and increased hepatic enzymes (LFTs) [1–3].

Treatment of non-acute adverse events is directed toward utilizing the lowest effective dose for the shortest duration of time. Patients at a high risk for adverse effects should be evaluated for the use of alternative therapies.

Cardiovascular risk: increasing evidence is surfacing that NSAID use, but particularly the use of COX-2 selective NSAIDS, elevates the risk of cardiovascular morbidity and mortality. This is especially true in patients with preexisting cardiovascular disease. Thrombotic cardiovascular events are related to a relative increase in thromboxane and a relative diminution in prostacycline. Since most selective as well as nonselective NSAIDS affect this relative imbalance of thromboxane over prostacycline they are all implicated in increasing the risk for thrombotic cardiovascular events [6]. However, naproxen appears to be risk-neutral with regard to cardiovascular events and may in fact be somewhat cardioprotective due to its nonselectivity [7].

Potential advantages

Easy to use and administer

Over-the-counter formulations available

Little risk of side effects with a low-dose non-chronic dosing schedule

Opioid-sparing when employed as multimodal analgesia

Unlike opioids, naproxen does not cause physical or psychological dependency, severe cognitive dysfunction, excessive nausea, vomiting, or constipation

Regular administration of naproxen 500 mg BID can produce an antiplatelet COX-1 effect similar to that of low-dose aspirin

Potential disadvantages

Naproxen toxicity can occur at very high doses (150–500 mg/kg). Naproxen toxicity is relatively uncommon compared to other NSAIDs such as aspirin and ibuprofen. See below for description of signs and symptoms of naproxen toxicity.

Drug interactions occur with many commonly prescribed medications and are mostly due to naproxen's effects on renal prostaglandins and the associated changes in kidney filtration rate, although many other mechanisms exist. Many drug interactions exist, with examples being ACE inhibitors, beta blockers, methotrexate, lithium, probenecid, antiplatelet agents, diuretics, and vancomycin.

The ceiling effect of naproxen limits the amount of pain relief that can be expected. It may increase risk of gastrointestinal irritation, inflammation, ulceration, bleeding, and perforation. Enteric coated formulations are available to help reduce the risk of such complications.

Toxicity

Toxicity most commonly begins within 4 hours of ingestion with symptoms such as headache, tinnitus, drowsiness, abdominal pain, nausea, and vomiting. Severe toxicity is reported mainly in children. Severe toxicity occurs with ingestions of 400 mg/kg or more of naproxen with symptoms including seizures, apnea, hypertension, and renal and hepatic dysfunction.

References

1. Capone M, Tacconelli S, Sciulli M, et al. Clinical pharmacology of platelet, monocyte and vascular cyclooxygenase inhibition by naproxen and low-dose aspirin in healthy subjects. *Circulation* 2004;**109**: 1468–1471.

2. Hamilton RJ, ed. *Tarascon Pocket Pharmacopoeia 2009 Deluxe Edition.* Sudbury, MA: Jones and Bartlett, pp. 7–9.

3. MICROMEDEX® Healthcare Series: DRUGDEX® Drug Point.

4. Derry C, Derry S, Moore RA, McQuay HJ. Single dose oral naproxen and naproxen sodium for acute post-operative pain in adults. *Cochrane Database Syst Rev* 2009;**1**:CD004234.

5. Comfort KV, Code WE, Rooney ME, et al. Naproxen premedication reduces postoperative tubal ligation pain. *Can J Anesthesia* 1992;**39**:349–392.

6. Hennekens CH, Borzak S. Cyclooxygenase-2 inhibitors and most traditional nonsteroidal anti-inflammatory drugs cause similar moderately increased risk of cardiovascular disease. *J Cardiovasc Pharmacol Ther* 2008;**13**(1):41–45.

7. Bing RJ, Lomnicka M. Why do cyclo-oxygenase-2 inhibitors cause cardiovascular events? *J Am Coll Cardiol* 2002;**39**:521–522.

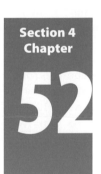

Section 4
Chapter

52

NSAIDs

Diclofenac gel and diclofenac patch

Neil Singla

Generic Names: diclofenac sodium topical gel; diclofenac epolamine topical patch

Trade/Proprietary Names: Voltaren® Gel; Flector® Patch

Drug Class: nonsteroidal anti-inflammatory drug (NSAID)

Manufacturer: Novartis Pharma Produktions GmbH, Oflinger Strasse 44, D-79644 Wehr/Baden, Germany; King Pharmaceuticals, Inc., 501 Fifth Street, Bristol, TN 37620

Chemical Names: 2-[(2,6-dichlorophynyl)amino]benzeneacetic acid, monosodium salt; 2-[(2,6-dichlorophenyl)amino]benzeneacetic acid, 2-(pyrrolidin-1yl)ethanol salt

Chemical Structures: diclofenac sodium topical gel (Figure 52.1); molecular formula: $C_{14}H_{10}Cl_2NNaO_2$; diclofenac epolamine patch (Figure 52.2); molecular formula; $C_{20}H_{24}Cl_2N_2O_3$

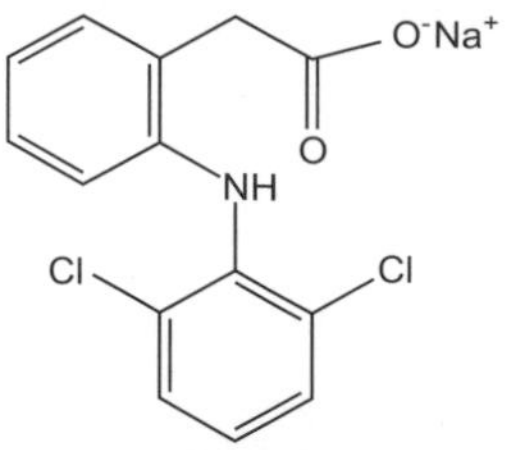

Figure 52.1.

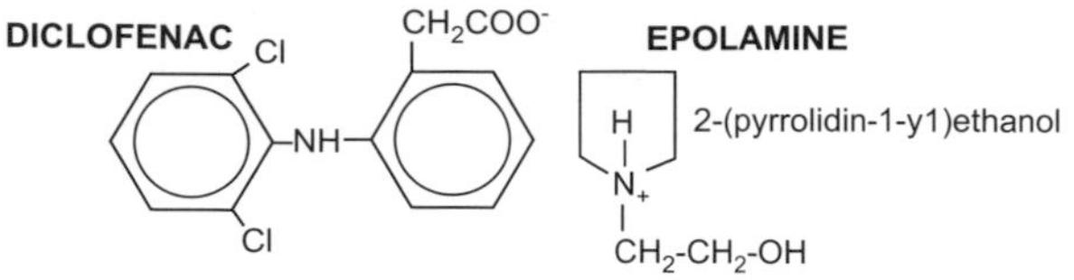

DICLOFENAC   EPOLAMINE

2-(pyrrolidin-1-y1)ethanol

Figure 52.2.

Introduction

Diclofenac is a nonsteroidal anti-inflammatory drug (NSAID) and is the active ingredient in both the gel and patch formulations described in this chapter. Diclofenac inhibits the enzyme cyclooxygenase (COX), an early component of the arachidonic acid cascade, resulting in reduced formation of prostaglandins, thromboxane, and prostacyclin. It is not completely understood how reduced synthesis of these compounds results in therapeutic efficacy. The chief therapeutic effects of diclofenac are anti-inflammatory activity, anti-nociception and antipyresis. When applied topically (via gel or patch), diclofenac is absorbed into the epidermis. However, the amount of topical diclofenac absorbed and the ultimate systemic exposure is substantially less than that seen after oral administration of the compound.

After application of 4 grams of the 1% gel to the knee four times daily (total daily dose of 160 mg of diclofenac sodium) for 7 days, the mean C_{max} was 15 ± 7.3 ng/mL, the time to the maximum concentration was 14 hours (range 0–24 hours), and the AUC over 24 hours was 233 ± 128 ng/h per mL. The C_{max} was 0.6%, and the AUC was 5.8% of the values obtained after administration of oral diclofenac sodium 50 mg three times daily.

Ten to 20 hours after a single application of the diclofenac patch to the upper inner arm, peak plasma diclofenac concentrations of 0.7–6 ng/mL were recorded. Diclofenac plasma concentrations of 1.3–8.8 ng/mL were noted after 5 days of twice-daily patch application.

Diclofenac appears to be widely distributed, with significant amounts in synovial fluid. Protein binding is roughly 99%, primarily to albumin. It is unknown whether diclofenac crosses the placenta. Significant distribution into breast milk does not occur. Metabolism of diclofenac via hepatic cytochrome P450 2C9 and 3A4 involves conjugation at the carboxyl group of the side chain or single or multiple hydroxylations resulting in several phenolic metabolites, most of which are converted to glucuronide conjugates. The elimination half-life of diclofenac is about 1.2–2 hours after oral administration. After application of the diclofenac patch, the elimination half-life is approximately 12 hours. Metabolites are subsequently excreted through urinary and biliary pathways. About 65% of a dose is excreted in the urine and about 3.5% in the bile [1].

Indications

Diclofenac gel is indicated for the relief of the pain of osteoarthritis of the joints amenable to topical treatments such as the knees and those of the hands. Diclofenac patch is indicated for the topical treatment of acute pain due to minor strains, sprains and contusions [2,3]. In controlled trials during the pre-marketing development approximately 600 patients with minor sprains, strains, and contusions were treated safely with diclofenac patch for up to 2 weeks [4]. A randomized, double-blind, placebo-controlled, trial evaluated the efficacy and tolerability of diclofenac patch, self-administered every 12 h to injury site, in 384 patients aged 18–65 years with minor soft tissue injury and moderate to severe pain intensity ≥ 5 (0–10 scale). The most common injuries were contusion (42.6%), strain (31.1%), and sprain (24.4%); most common sites were ankle, shoulder, knee, and foot (67.3%). Patients treated with diclofenac patch experienced improved mean pain scores (40.4% of baseline score) vs. patients using placebo (47.4%, $P < 0.05$); with an overall pain reduction of 14.8% (Figure 52.3). Patients treated with the patch reached pain resolution 3 days sooner than those in the placebo group (median 10.0 vs. 13.5 days, $P = 0.01$). Patient response to treatment was rated good to excellent 57.8% for the diclofenac patch vs. 48.4% placebo ($P < 0.01$).

Diclofenac patch and gel preparations have not been evaluated for use in labor and delivery, in pregnant and nursing women or in pediatrics. The Flector® diclofenac patch is supplied in resealable envelopes,

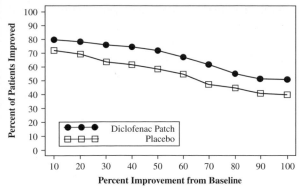

Figure 52.3. Patients achieving various levels of pain relief at end of study; 14-day study percent improvement from baseline. With permission from Carr W, Beks P, Jones C, et al: (Poster Presentation American Pain Society Annual meeting 2008) *The Journal of Pain* Volume 9, Issue 4, Supplement 2, 45; April 2008.

each containing 5 patches (10 cm × 14 cm), with six envelopes per box. Each patch contains 180 mg of diclofenac epolamine in an aqueous base (13 mg of active drug per gram of adhesive or 1.3%). The patch is intended for topical use only. The envelopes should be sealed at all times when not in use.

Contraindications

The absolute and relative contraindications for diclofenac, both the topical and gel formulations, are described below:

Absolute

- Known hypersensitivity to diclofenac, aspirin, or other NSAIDs.
- History of asthma, urticaria, or other allergic-type reactions after taking aspirin or other NSAIDs.
- Use during the peri-operative period in the setting of coronary artery bypass graft (CABG) surgery.

Relative

- Serious and potentially fatal cardiovascular (CV) thrombotic events, myocardial infarction, and stroke can occur with NSAID treatment. Diclofenac should be used with caution in patients with known CV disease or risk factors for CV disease.
- Diclofenac can cause serious GI adverse events including inflammation, bleeding, ulceration and perforation. Patients with a prior history of ulcer disease or GI bleeding should be treated with caution.
- Long-term administration of NSAIDs can result in renal papillary necrosis and other renal injury. Diclofenac should be used with caution in patients at greatest risk, including the elderly, those with impaired renal function, heart failure, liver dysfunction, and those taking diuretics and ACE inhibitors.
- Fluid retention and edema have been observed in some patients taking NSAIDs and therefore diclofenac should be used with caution in patients with a history of fluid retention or heart failure.

Common doses/uses

Diclofenac gel is available in tubes, each containing 100 g of gel. One gram of the gel base contains 10 mg of the active ingredient, diclofenac sodium. Dosing information is considered in terms of grams of gel, not in terms of milligrams of diclofenac. Total daily dose should not exceed 32 g of gel per day over all affected joints. When prescribed, a dosing card is dispensed to the patient so they can appropriately measure 2 and 4 g aliquots of the gel. Specific dosing information is as follows:

- Lower extremities; the gel (4 g) is applied to the affected area four times daily. More than 16 g daily should not be applied to any one of the affected joints of the lower extremity.
- Upper extremities; 2 g of gel should be applied to the affected area up to four times daily. More than 8 g daily should not be applied to any one of the affected joints of the upper extremity.

The diclofenac patch measures 10 cm × 14 cm and is composed of an adhesive material containing 1.3% diclofenac epolamine. There is a total of 180 mg of diclofenac epolamine distributed throughout each patch (13 mg of diclofenac per gram of adhesive). The recommended dose of the diclofenac patch is one patch to the most painful area of the body applied up to twice daily.

Potential advantages

Both diclofenac gel and the diclofenac patch have been designed with the idea of providing local analgesia while reducing systemic NSAID exposure. The local analgesic effects of both the gel and patch formulations have been fairly well established in the literature. PK data (as described above) seem to indicate that systemic exposure after application of either formulation is relatively limited when compared to routine oral dosing. In this regard, systemic exposure (AUC) and maximum plasma concentrations of diclofenac, after repeated dosing for 4 days with diclofenac patch, were lower (<1%) than after a single oral 50 mg diclofenac sodium tablet [5].

A literature review suggests that the clinical adverse event data may demonstrate a lower potential for systemic toxicities than oral diclofenac [6].

Potential disadvantages

The active ingredient, diclofenac, has a side-effect profile similar to most NSAIDs. The main clinical concerns with this class of agents are GI bleeding and renal insufficiency. A more complete description of the side-effect profile can be gleaned from the contraindications mentioned above. When using NSAIDs over long periods of time to treat chronic conditions such as osteoarthritis, the risk of serious side effects becomes more significant. In the controlled trials, 3% of patients in both the diclofenac patch and placebo patch groups discontinued treatment due to an adverse event. The most common adverse events leading to discontinuation were application site reactions, occurring in 2% of both the diclofenac patch and placebo patch groups. Application site reactions leading to dropout included pruritus, dermatitis, and burning. Rare toxicities associated with diclofenac are: Stevens–Johnson syndrome, toxic epidermal necrolysis, anaphalactoid reactions, and hepatic insufficiency.

Drug-related adverse events

For both the gel and patch preparations of diclofenac, by far the most common drug-related adverse events were site-specific reactions such as itching and irritation.

References

1. Rainsford KD. Review of the pharmaceutical properties and clinical effects of the topical NSAID formulation, diclofenac epolamine. *J Curr Med Res Opin* 2008;**24**(10): 2967–2992.

2. Petersen B. Diclofenac epolamine (Flector) patch: evidence for topical activity. *J Clin Drug Investig* 2009;**29**:1–9.

3. *Flector® Patch* (diclofenac epolamine topical patch 1.3%). Prescribing information; September 2007, Alpharma, Inc., Bridgewater, NJ.

4. Carr W, Beks P, Jones C, et al. Efficacy and tolerability of FLECTOR Patch (diclofenac epolamine topical patch) in the treatment of minor soft tissue injury pain (Poster Presentation American Pain Society Annual meeting 2008). *J Pain* 2008;**9**(4, Suppl. 2):45.

5. Voltaren® Gel (diclofenac sodium topical gel) Prescribing information. October 2007, Novartis Consumer Health, Inc. Parsippany, NJ.

6. Gold Standard Inc. 2009: Diclofenac. Drug Monograph. MD Consult Web site, Core Collection. Available at http://www.mdconsult.com/das/pharm/body/162078605–3/892674727/full/183. Accessed September 22, 2009.

53

Diclofenac oral and diclofenac plus PPI

Nehal Gatha

Generic Name: diclofenac sodium, diclofenac potassium, diclofenac with misoprostol

Proprietary Names: Voltaren™, Cataflam™, Voltaren-XR™, Solaraze™, Arthrotec™

Manufacturers: Novartis Pharmaceuticals, Basel, Switzerland; Pfizer, New York City, NY; Kowa Pharmaceuticals Inc, Montgomery, AL

Drug Class: nonsteroidal anti-inflammatory drug

Chemistry: diclofenac is a phenylacetic acid derivative; its chemical name is 2-(2-(2,6-dichlorophenylamino)phenyl)acetic acid

Chemical Structure: see Figure 53.1

Molecular Formula: $C_{14}H_{11}Cl_2NO_2$

Introduction

Diclofenac sodium was introduced with the aim of developing a nonsteroidal anti-inflammatory drug (NSAID) with high activity and improved tolerability. Three older and highly effective NSAIDS, indomethacin, phenylbutazone, and mefenamic acid, all have favorable acidity constants, pKa, between 4 and 5, a similar degree of lipophilicity, and two aromatic rings that are twisted in relation to each other. The diclofenac molecule includes these favorable characteristics. It has a pKa of 4.0, a partition coefficient of 13.4, and includes a phenylacetic acid group, an amino group, and a phenyl ring containing chlorine, which results in maximal twisting of the ring. Arthrotec is a combination of diclofenac and misoprostol. It was developed to create a combination drug with protective effects against the major gastrointestinal side effects of NSAIDS.

Major and minor sites of action, receptor interactions

Diclofenac acts primarily by inhibiting prostaglandin synthesis via inhibition of cyclooxygenase (COX-1 and 2). This provides its anti-inflammatory, antipyretic, and analgesic actions. Inhibition of COX receptors also decreases prostaglandins in the epithelium of the stomach. Diclofenac has a moderate preference to block the COX-2 receptor, but is not as selective as celecoxib. The exact mechanism of diclofenac, as with other NSAIDS, is not completely known. There is also some evidence that diclofenac inhibits the lipoxygenase pathways, reducing inflammation by decreasing production of leukotrienes. There has been suggestion that diclofenac also inhibits phospolipase A2. Diclofenac also may work by inhibiting reactivation of volatage-dependent sodium channels, blocking acid-sending ion channels, as well as modulation of KCNQ- and BK-potassium channels.

Misoprostol is a synthetic prostaglandin E1 analog with gastric mucosal protective properties. There are specific prostaglandin receptors in the gastric mucosa which have a high affinity for misoprostol and its metabolites. Receptor affinity for misoprostol has been shown to correlate with antisecretory activity of gastric acid. Misoprostol also produces a decrease in pepsin concentrations. Deficiency of prostaglandins such as misoprostol in the gastric and duodenal mucosa may lead to diminishing mucus and bicarbonate secretion, which are protective in these mucosa.

Metabolic pathways, drug clearance and elimination

Diclofenac oral is absorbed directly from the GI tract. The pharmaceutical preparations of diclofenac commonly available are not as soluble in gastric fluid (lower pH), but allow a more rapid release of drug in the duodenum, which has a slightly higher pH. Approximately

229

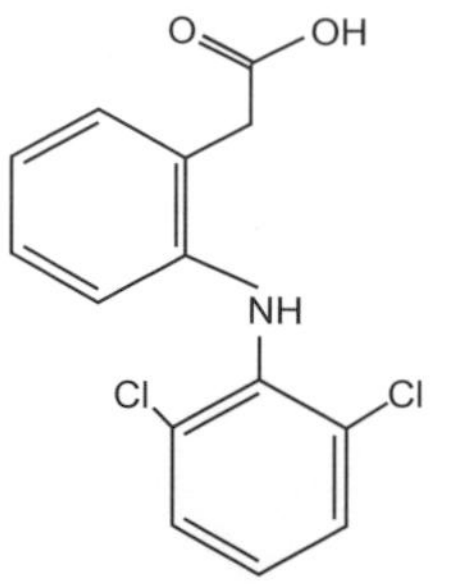

Figure 53.1.

50% of the absorbed dose is available due to first-pass metabolism. Peak plasma levels of the drug are achieved within 1–4 hours, with plasma levels declining in a bio-exponential fashion, with the terminal phase having a half-life of approximately 2 hours. Clearance is 350 mL/min with a volume of distribution of approximately 550 mL/kg. Diclofenac sodium is more than 99% reversibly bound to plasma albumin. Diclofenac is metabolized and broken down into its glucuronide and sulfate conjugates, with elimination occurring through metabolism and also subsequent urinary and biliary excretion of these conjugates. Sixty-five percent is excreted through the urine, with the remaining 35% in bile. Conjugates of unchanged diclofenac account for 7% of the dose excreted in the urine, and for less than 5% in the bile. Less than 1% of the drug is excreted unchanged or unconjugated. Conjugates of the major metabolite account for 20–30% of the drug excreted in the urine and 10–20% of the dose in the bile. The accumulation and activity of diclofenac metabolites are unknown. The action of a dose of diclofenac sodium is 6–8 hours, much longer than the aforementioned short half-life. This could be due to high concentration levels in the synovial fluids.

The misoprostol in diclofenac + misoprostol is extensively absorbed, and is metabolized rapidly to its active metabolite, misoprostol acid. Misoprostol acid reaches peak plasma concentration within 20 minutes and has an elimination half-life of 30 minutes. No accumulation of misoprostol acid has been found. The serum protein binding of this metabolite is less than 90%. Approximately 70% of misoprostol is excreted in the urine. Activity of misoprostol is evident within 30 minutes of administration and lasts for 3 hours. Administration of diclofenac and misoprostol together as diclofenac + misoprostol leads to similar absorption and elimination as when the two are administered alone.

Indications

Diclofenac oral, as in many NSAIDS, has a wide application of use in acute, subacute, and chronic pain. It is approved to use, and most commonly used, for conditions relating to chronic musculoskeletal type pain. These include osteoarthritis, rheumatoid arthritis, ankylosing spondylitis, spondylarthritis, and gout. It is also indicated in the treatment of acute visceral and somatic pain related to nephrolithiasis, cholelithiasis, and abdominal pain. An additional use is for the treatment of acute migraines. Diclofenac is commonly used to treat mild to moderate surgical pain post-operatively or post-traumatically, once the patient is taking oral medications; however, it is less useful as a sole agent in a patient with moderate to severe pain acutely post-operatively. Diclofenac has also been shown to be effective against menstrualtype pain.

Arthrotec is indicated for these patients who will be on NSAIDS long-term, or those at high risk for GI bleed or gastric irritation, as long-term use can predispose to peptic ulcer.

Diclofenac is also used off-label or for investigational trials in chronic pain patients with cancer, especially when inflammation is present. Examples include patients with breast or prostate cancer with bony metastases.

It has also showed limited effectiveness in reducing fever in patients with malignant lymphogranulomatosis.

Contraindications

Black-box warning: cardiovascular risk – may increase risk of cardiovascular thrombotic events, MI, stroke. GI risk – may increase risk of serious GI adverse events such as bleeding, ulceration, or perforation. Arthrotec also carries these black-box warnings, but with additional black-box warnings for pregnant patients as well as in women of child-bearing age as misoprostol increases the chance of miscarriage and can induce labor.

Absolute: hypersensitivity to drug class, third-trimester pregnancy, patients with active stomach or duodenal ulceration or gastrointestinal bleeding; patients with angioedema or bronchospastic reactions to NSAIDs.

Relative: use caution in patients with cardiovascular disease or status post cardiac surgery, patients with history of allergic reactions following the use of aspirin or other NSAIDS, HTN, CHF, peptic ulcer disease, inflammatory intestinal disorders such as Crohn's or ulcerative colitis, patients using corticosteroids, patients using anticoagulants or with history of coagulopathy, history of alcohol use or smoking, elderly patients, patients with hepatic or renal insufficiency, patients taking ACEI or ARBs, patients with preexisting hepatic porphyria. Use extreme caution in patients with severe, active bleeding such as cerebral hemorrhage.

Common doses/uses

Diclofenac sodium: 25, 50, 75 mg tablets, 100 mg extended-release tablets. Common doses include 25–75 mg PO BID-TID with a maximum dose of 150 mg/day. Alternative dose includes 100 mg ER daily.

Arthrotec: 50/0.2, 75/0.2 diclofenac/misoprostol. Common doses include 1 tab PO TID-QID, with a maximum dose of 225 mg/day diclofenac.

Potential advantages

As an NSAID, diclofenac is easy to use, and has been shown to be efficacious in arthritic syndromes, as well as for acute treatment of migraines, and small procedures. A major advantage of diclofenac, as with other NSAIDs, is its use in multimodal analgesia. In patients who are post-operative or with certain chronic pain syndromes, diclofenac can be used to provide additive analgesia and an opioid-sparing effect. Diclofenac has decreased side effects when compared to opioids in terms of nausea, respiratory depression, sedation, and constipation.

A major advantage of diclofenac as compared to other NSAIDs is that it has an approximately 10-fold preference to block the COX-2 isoenzyme, which leads to reduced incidence of GI upset, peptic ulcers, and GI bleeding compared with other NSAIDs. In patients at increased risk of GI complications, diclofenac with misoprostol is available to protect from diclofenac's effects.

Cost is also a potential advantage as there are now generic forms available relatively inexpensively, and can reduce cost as part of a multimodal approach to pain.

Potential disadvantages

NSAIDs can lead to gastric complications, including GI upset, peptic ulcers, and GI hemorrhage. This risk is increased with long-term use, use in the elderly, and use with anticoagulants or steroids. These complications are exceedingly rare when diclofenac is used in the short term, and even less when used in the combination form of diclofenac with misoprostol. Diclofenac,

as with other NSAIDS, can also lead to renal impairment, and should be used with caution in those with renal insufficiency. The risk of bleeding is also increased with diclofenac, and should be assessed preoperatively. Diclofenac, and especially misoprostol, can lead to miscarriage or early labor.

Drug interactions

Diclofenac can lead to displacement of other highly protein-bound drugs, as it is largely protein-bound like most NSAIDS. Drugs such as diuretics may be less effective when being used with diclofenac.

Drug-related adverse events

Common adverse events: nausea, dyspepsia, abdominal pain, headache, constipation, dizziness, rash, urticaria, drowsiness, tinnitus.

Diclofenac, in addition to causing gastric and renal side effects, can have other adverse events. Rare hepatic failure, which is usually reversible, can occur. Occasionally, bone marrow depression will also be seen. Disruption of the normal menstrual cycle can also occur. In 2004, it was shown that selective COX-2 inhibitors may lead to increased cardiac events; however, subsequent studies in 2006 showed no increased adverse events with diclofenac. Susceptible patients with asthma, nasal polyps and mastocytosis may experience severe bronchospasm following exposure to diclofenac.

References

1. Arthrotec Package Insert, Pfizer Inc., 2009

2. Epocrates Essentials. Epocrates, Inc. Drug search: naproxen.

3. Hennekens CH, Borzak S. Cyclooxygenase-2 inhibitors and most traditional nonsteroidal anti-inflammatory drugs cause similar moderately increased risk of cardiovascular disease. *J Cardiovasc Pharmacol Ther* 2008;**13**(1):41–50.

4. Lewis JA, Furst DE. *Nonsteroidal Anti-inflammatory Drugs: Mechanisms and Clinical Uses* 2nd ed., Informa Health Care, 1994, pp. 247–266.

5. Sallmann AR. The history of diclofenac. *Am J Med* 1986;**80**(4B):29–33.

6. Stoelting R, Hillier S. Chapter 19. Drugs used for psychopharmacologic therapy. In *Pharmacology and Physiology in Anesthetic Practice*, 4th ed. pp. 398–406.

54

Diclofenac injectable

Daniel B. Carr and Ryan Lanier

Generic Name: diclofenac sodium for injection

Brand/Proprietary name: Dyloject®

Drug Class: nonsteroidal anti-inflammatory drug

Manufacturer: Javelin Pharmaceuticals, Inc., Cambridge, MA; Javelin was recently acquired by Hospira, Lake Forest, IL

Chemical Structure: see Figure 54.1

Chemical Name: 2-[(2,6-dichlorophenyl)amino] benzeneacetic acid, monosodium (diclofenac sodium)

Molecular Formula: $C_{14}H_{10}Cl_2NNaO_2$

Description

Injectable diclofenac sodium (Dyloject™) was developed to provide a "ready to use" injectable dose in a small volume with prolonged stability at room temperature. Solubilization of diclofenac in this novel formulation is accomplished by the use of hydoxypropyl-β-cyclodextrin ("HPβCD"). HPβCD is a cyclic carbohydrate derivative that is pharmacologically inert and is considered ideal for intravenous (IV) applications due to its high water solubility, excellent solubilizing potential, and favorable safety profile. The new formulation of injectable diclofenac is available as a 37.5 mg/mL solution that can be administered as a rapid IV bolus to provide rapid pain relief. Unlike the earlier formulation of diclofenac for injection (marketed as Voltarol® in the UK), the new formulation does not employ organic solvents to solubilize diclofenac, does not contain sulfites, and has proven less irritating to veins when given IV. The new formulation of injectable diclofenac is provided in the form of a solution that is ready to use without buffering, mixing, or dilution. In contrast, the older formulation requires such preparation prior to IV administration and, even then, its potential for venous irritation requires it to be infused slowly over at least 30 minutes. The new formulation may also be administered IM, in which case its uptake into the circulation is more rapid than after IM injection of the old formulation.

Because the older formulation of diclofenac for parenteral injection was approved in the UK decades ago and marketed there continuously since, with ample experience as to its safety and efficacy, the regulatory pathway for approval of the new formulation in that country as an "essentially similar" product was relatively straightforward. The new formulation was approved and has been marketed in the UK since late 2007 for parenteral use, 75 mg every 12 hours as needed for the treatment of acute moderate to severe pain. This dose, dosing interval, and indication are the same as for the earlier formulation. Other European submissions are planned and our new formulation of injectable diclofenac is currently under clinical development in the USA. Because no injectable diclofenac has previously been approved in the USA, the US clinical development program has been more comprehensive than that in the UK, including clinical trials that have assessed various doses and dose intervals in several pain models and in subjects ranging from healthy normal subjects to post-surgical patients, and patients with renal or hepatic insufficiency.

Mode of activity

Diclofenac is an NSAID with anti-inflammatory, analgesic, and antipyretic activity. It is an amino-phenyl-acetic acid derivative that inhibits prostaglandin biosynthesis to produce analgesic, antipyretic, and anti-inflammatory activity secondary to its nonselective inhibition of the cyclooxygenase (COX) isoenzymes, COX-1 and COX-2. It lies approximately in the middle of the COX-1/COX-2 inhibitory spectrum. Uniquely among NSAIDs, diclofenac opens KCNQ2/3 potassium channels and may inhibit sensory neuronal depolarization. Please refer to the oral diclofenac chapter for additional information.

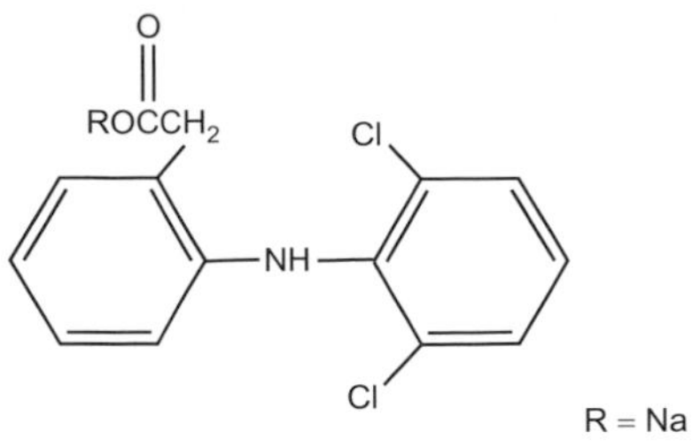

Figure 54.1.

Because the newer formulation of injectable diclofenac can be administered as a rapid bolus IV injection, in comparison to the older formulation which must be infused slowly over 30 minutes, measurable plasma levels of diclofenac are observed almost immediately following IV injection of the newer formulation and peak plasma levels are achieved in approximately 3 minutes. The active substance is 99.7% protein-bound, mainly to albumin (99.4%). "Parenteral administration of diclofenac avoids the first-pass metabolism observed with orally administered diclofenac, whereby only about 60% of the orally administered drug reaches the systemic circulation in unchanged form" [1].

Indications

Pending US regulatory approval of the newer formulation of injectable diclofenac, any discussion of its indications at present refers to the UK, where the approved indications for the newer formulation are broad. For decades, prior injectable formulations of diclofenac sodium have been found effective and safe for the relief of acute pain following a large variety of procedures and conditions, including laparoscopy, laparotomy, thoracotomy, thoracoscopic lung biopsy, joint replacement surgery, cancer, biliary colic, renal colic, migraine, acute sciatic pain, third molar extraction, cesarean section, laparoscopic cholecystectomy, tonsillectomy, upper abdominal surgery, knee-joint arthroscopy, and maxillofacial surgery. Accordingly, IM injection of the newer formulation of injectable diclofenac is indicated for post-operative pain and other types of acute pain including renal colic, exacerbations of osteo- and rheumatoid arthritis, acute back pain, acute gout, acute trauma, and fractures. IV administration of the newer formulation of injectable diclofenac is indicated for the treatment or prevention of acute post-operative pain. Injectable formulations of diclofenac sodium have long been used pre- and intra-operatively as prophylaxis for pain following

major orthopedic surgery, major abdominal surgery, gynecological surgery, dental surgery, day-case laparoscopy, and for children undergoing herniotomy or orchidopexy.

The approved indication of injectable diclofenac for preemptive use contrasts with the more restrictive indication for injectable ketorolac, a relatively COX-1-selective inhibitor that is not approved for the prevention of post-operative pain but only for its treatment. Given the propensity of COX-1-selective NSAIDs such as ketorolac or aspirin to interfere with platelet function, the more restricted indication for ketorolac is understandable. Further, in the USA an unacceptably high incidence of gastrointestinal bleeding during ongoing use of ketorolac has led to a black-box warning that restricts the total duration of treatment with this agent to 5 days regardless of the formulation. No such restriction on the duration of use of diclofenac exists or (to our knowledge) has been proposed in the USA, where diclofenac is marketed in immediate- and controlled-release oral forms as well topical and intraocular formulations.

Contraindications

The contraindications and precautions for injectable diclofenac are the same as described elsewhere in this volume for NSAIDs in general, and such "NSAID class labeling" appears on the UK package insert. More specifically, in the UK all injectable forms of diclofenac are contraindicated in patients with known hypersensitivity to that agent as well as to diclofenac-containing products. Injectable diclofenac should not be given to patients who have experienced asthma, angioedema, urticaria, rhinitis, or other allergic-type reactions after taking aspirin or other NSAIDs. Severe, rarely fatal, anaphylactic-like reactions to diclofenac have been reported in such patients. Parenteral diclofenac should not be used concomitantly with other diclofenac-containing products since they also circulate in plasma as the diclofenac anion.

Potential advantages

The advantages of the newer formulation of injectable diclofenac over the prior formulation available in the UK (as well as in many other countries throughout the world) include both safety and efficacy. In the pivotal UK registration trial (a three-arm, double-blinded RCT in 155 patients with pain after third molar extraction) the incidence of thrombophlebitis was half that in patients who received the newer diclofenac formulation as a rapid IV bolus compared with those who received the older formulation as a 30-minute IV infusion (5.7% vs. 12%, respectively) [2]. Similar results were seen on formal thrombophlebitis assessment at 8 hours post-dosing. Aggregating the total experience with thrombophlebitis in the 531 subjects who received either of the two diclofenac formulations in a total of seven pharmacokinetic and analgesic studies conducted up through that pivotal study, this difference was highly significant ($P < 0.01$) [3].

In that same pivotal registration trial the onset of analgesia following administration of the newer formulation of injectable diclofenac was significantly more rapid compared to the older formulation (see Table 54.1). This finding was consistent across several measures of analgesia including pain intensity, pain relief, and the proportion of patients reporting a 30% or greater reduction of pain intensity. The 30% threshold is generally felt to indicate meaningful pain relief.

The surprisingly rapid onset of analgesia after administration of the newer formulation of injectable diclofenac led us to begin assessing pain and pain relief in our subsequent US dose-ranging studies as early as 5 minutes post-injection, compared with 15 minutes for the first assessment time in the pivotal UK trial. For the US program ketorolac 30 mg IV was included as an active comparator in our first dose-ranging post-molar extraction trial. The doses of the newer formulation of injectable diclofenac tested ranged from 3.75 through 75 mg. The proportion of patients who reported >30% reduction in pain intensity at 5 minutes post-dose was lower (11.8%) in the ketorolac group than in any of the injectable diclofenac dose groups (15.7–31.2%), a significant difference ($P < 0.05$).

Two subsequent large US Phase 3 trials involving multiple doses of injectable diclofenac administered over multiple days in patients following abdominal, pelvic, orthopedic, or other general surgery, have confirmed the safety and efficacy of this product candidate. Detailed results of these studies are being prepared for publication. Notably, these two trials and a large safety observational trial enrolled patients who received routine anticoagulation post-operatively, as well as those with known pre-operative renal or hepatic insufficiency without untoward safety consequences.

To understand better the potential for improved safety of injectable diclofenac compared with ketorolac in terms of their effects upon platelet aggregation, we conducted a preclinical trial in healthy subjects administered IV diclofenac, oral immediate-release diclofenac, IV ketorolac, or oral aspirin [4]. Subjects were exposed to these agents in random sequences of single doses separated by a 2-day washout interval, except that due to its long-lasting effects aspirin was always the final agent tested. Consistent with the prior published literature, injectable or oral diclofenac had minimal (albeit detectable) effects upon platelet aggregation as measured in a standard instrument (PFA-100) that estimates aggregation time in platelets exposed to epinephrine and collagen. In contrast, highly significant interference with platelet function occurred after single doses of ketorolac or aspirin.

Most recently, an investigator-initiated UK case series described the use of the newer formulation of

Table 54.1. Clinical efficacy of a newer formulation of injectable diclofenac (Dyloject) versus an older formulation (Voltarol) in a randomized double-blinded, placebo-controlled pivotal UK registration trial [2]

Primary variable		Secondary variables		
Treatment	Total pain relief over 4-h period post-dose (TOTPAR4)	Pain relief 15 min post-dose (VAS, mm)	>30% reduction in pain intensity in first hour, n (%)	Pain relief over 12-h period post-dose (VAS, mm)
Dyloject® ($n = 53$)	300.6 ± 73.61^a	$40.4^{a,c}$	$49 (92.5)^a$	44.7^b
Voltarol® ($n = 50$)	266.2 ± 91.63^a	19.5^a	$46 (92.0)^a$	46.5^b
Placebo ($n = 52$)	52.5 ± 88.77	5.7	$11 (21.2)$	12.8

TOTPAR4 values presented as mean ± SD; [a]$P < 0.001$ vs. placebo; [b]$P < 0.0001$ vs. placebo; [c]$P < 0.0001$ vs. Voltarol®.

injectable diclofenac in 200 children from 8 months to 16 years undergoing a wide range of surgical procedures including tonsillectomy and appendectomy [5]. A single dose of 0.5 mg/kg IV was given either prior to induction of anesthesia or during surgery, again with an unremarkable safety profile. The authors of that case series cited speed of onset and ability to titrate dose with the newer formulation of injectable diclofenac (compared with fixed, limited dose selections available in diclofenac suppositories) as a factor influencing them to apply it in this setting.

In conclusion, the use of non-opioids as the foundation of a multimodal strategy for acute pain management is now the worldwide standard. NSAIDs such as diclofenac that are of sufficiently high intrinsic efficacy produce an opioid-sparing effect whose magnitude is sufficient to decrease opioid-related side effects, and also enhance the quality of analgesia. The well-understood safety profile (including minimal effects upon platelet aggregation) of a new formulation of injectable diclofenac, together with its speed of onset and paucity of injection site irritation make it an attractive candidate for ongoing development and future availability in the USA.

References

1. McCormack PL, Scott LJ. Diclofenac sodium (Dyloject®) in post-operative pain. *Drugs* 2008;**68**: 123–130.

2. Leeson RM, Harrison S, Ernst CC, Hamilton DA, Mermelstein FH, Gawarecki DG, Moshman M, Carr DB. Dyloject™, a novel injectable diclofenac formulation, offers greater safety and efficacy than Voltarol® for post-operative dental pain. *Reg Anesth Pain Med* 2007;**32**:303–310.

3. Colucci RD, Wright C, Mermelstein F, Gawarecki DG, Carr DB. Dyloject®, a novel injectable diclofenac solubilised with cyclodextrin: reduced incidence of thrombophlebitis compared to injectable diclofenac solubilised with polyethylene glycol and benzyl alcohol. *Acute Pain* 2009;**11**:15–21.

4. Bauer KA, Gerson W, Ruais K, Wang J, McNicol E, Lanier RK, Kramer W, Carr DB. Platelet function following administration of a novel formulation of intravenous diclofenac sodium versus active comparators: a randomized, single dose, crossover study in healthy male volunteers. *J Clin Anesthesia* (in press).

5. Gandhi M, Prosser D. Our experience of Dyloject™ (intravenous diclofenac) in children. *Pediatric Anesthesia* 2009;**19**:908–928.

Section 4 Chapter

NSAIDs

55 Ketorolac

Christopher Wray

Analgesic Agent: ketorolac (injectable)

Trade Name: ketorolac tromethamine (Toradol™, Roche Pharmaceuticals, Nutley NJ)

Chemical Structure: see Figure 55.1

Description

Ketorolac tromethamine is a nonsteroidal anti-inflammatory drug (NSAID) with potent analgesic activity and weaker anti-inflammatory and antipyretic effects. Structurally, ketorolac is a weakly acidic, highly water-soluble pyrrolo-pyrrole, chemically similar to tolmentin and indomethacin. Ketorolac was developed in humans due to its potent analgesic effects demonstrated in animal testing. Ketorolac's analgesic potency was found to be 350 times that of aspirin in animal studies, and was also noted to have a long duration of action, up to 6 hours. The dosages of ketorolac that produced analgesia in animals were well below those

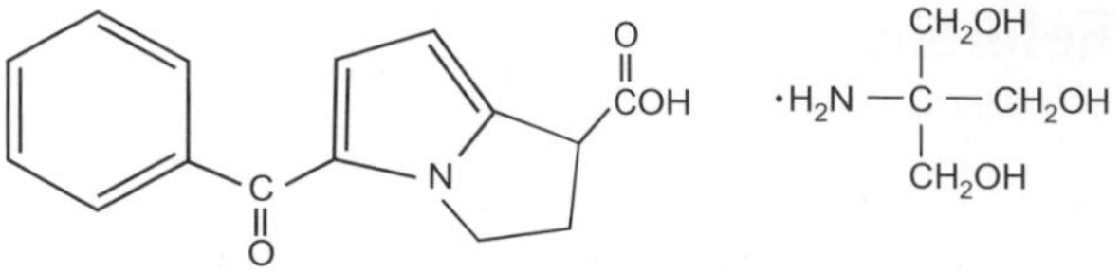

Figure 55.1.

that caused gastrointestinal toxicity. Due to its high potency, high water-solubility, and its potential for causing minimal muscle damage with IM administration compared with other NSAIDs, ketorolac was developed for human analgesia. In 1989, ketorolac became the first NSAID approved for parenteral administration in the U.S.

Mode of activity

Ketorolac is classified as a peripherally acting analgesic. It produces its analgesic effects by its nonspecific inhibition of the enzyme cyclooxygenase-1 (COX-1). It is generally believed that NSAIDs reduce pain by decreasing the enzyme's conversion of arachidonic acid into prostaglandin E2, the inflammatory prostaglandin that directly activates and up-regulates peripheral nociceptors. No other analgesic mechanisms of action have been discovered for ketorolac. Its anti-inflammatory and antipyretic effects are less potent than its analgesic effect. Comparative studies with other NSAIDs suggest that the analgesic activity of ketorolac may be separate from its anti-inflammatory and antipyretic activity. The analgesic potency of ketorolac 30 mg IM is equivalent to approximately 9–12 mg of morphine or 100 mg of meperidine.

Metabolic activity

Oral and parenteral ketorolac demonstrate similar pharmacokinetics. Parenteral ketorolac has a rapid onset (<1 min IV, <10 min IM) due to its rapid absorption and negligible plasma metabolism. Onset of clinical effects occurs within 15 to 20 minutes. Plasma halflife is approximately 6 hours, intermediate in duration compared with other NSAIDs. Ketorolac undergoes mainly renal metabolism. Over half of an entire ketorolac dose is excreted unchanged in the urine with smaller proportions of minimally active polar metabolites. Elimination is minimally affected by age or hepatic function. Renal insufficiency may decrease the clearance of ketorolac. IM ketorolac demonstrates linear pharmacokinetics. Clearance does not change with chronic dosing. Ketorolac does not cross the blood–brain barrier, and there appears to be little central nervous system activity of the drug.

Indications

Ketorolac is indicated for the short-term management of moderately severe acute pain. The primary setting for ketorolac is in post-operative patients that require opioid level analgesia. Duration of therapy should not exceed 5 days of use because of the potential for adverse reactions associated with prolonged therapy (>5 days). Single doses of ketorolac have been shown to be safe and effective in pediatric patients between the ages of 2 and 16 years: however, there are limited data to support the use of multiple doses in pediatric patients.

Contraindications

Absolute: patients with documented allergic reaction to ketorolac or other NSAIDs; patients with complete or partial syndromes of nasal polyps, angioedema, and bronchospastic reactions to NSAIDs.

Relative: patients with advanced renal impairment. Patients with active peptic ulcer disease, recent gastrointestinal bleeding, or gastric perforation. Patients with platelet disorders, coagulation abnormalities, or patients receiving anti-platelet or anti-coagulant medications. Surgical patients at high risk for post-operative bleeding. Labor and delivery patients, due to potential adverse effects of prostaglandin-inhibiting drugs on fetal circulation and inhibition of uterine contractions. Nursing mothers, due to potential adverse effects of prostaglandin-inhibiting drugs on neonates. Patients with or at risk for cerebrovascular bleeding, hemorrhagic diathesis, or incomplete hemostasis. Pre-operative or intra-operative patients having major surgery with a risk of major bleeding

Common doses

Single-dose treatment: IM dosing:

Patients < 65 years of age: 60 mg (0.5–1.0 mg/kg). Patients ≥ 65 years of age, with renal impairment, and/or less than 50 kg: 30 mg.

Single-dose treatment: IV dosing:

Patients < 65 years of age: 30 mg. Patients ≥ 65 years of age, with renal impairment, and/or less than 50 kg: 15 mg.

Multiple-dose treatment (IV or IM):

Patients < 65 years of age: 30 mg every 6 hours. Maximum daily dose should not exceed 120 mg (1.5–2.5 mg/kg per day). Patients ≥ 65 years of age, with renal impairment, and patients less than 50 kg: 15 mg every 6 hours. Maximum daily dose should not exceed 60 mg

Potential advantages

Ketorolac (both IM and IV routes) has been studied in a variety of post-operative patients. Studies assessing single and multiple doses have demonstrated its efficacy in orthopedic, gynecological, abdominal, and dental surgery. One of the major advantages of injectable ketorolac is its use in multimodal analgesia, providing for an opioid-sparing effect. Studies using ketorolac for post-operative pain have noted decreased incidences of side effects when compared with opioids (nausea, vomiting, sedation, respiratory depression, urinary retention, ileus). Low doses of an opioid analgesic at levels below those associated with typical opioid side effects in combination with ketorolac have been shown to provide maximal post-operative pain control in procedures with more severe abdominal pain (abdominal hysterectomy, cholecystectomy).

Cost: inexpensive generic versions are available.
Availability: widely available in most hospitals.

Potential disadvantages

Toxicity: NSAID-induced gastric complications include the potential for hemorrhage and ulcerations. Gastropathy risk is increased in the elderly, patients with a history of peptic ulcer, and concomitant use of anticoagulants or corticosteroids. Ketorolac may cause gastric complications even with short-term therapy, but these are rare when compared to long-term use. Current recommendations limiting ketorolac therapy to 5 days duration are designed to decrease gastric toxicity. Other disadvantages of ketorolac administration include renal impairment and platelet inhibition. The risk of renal impairment is increased with significant reductions in blood volume and in patients with underlying renal dysfunction. NSAID inhibition of platelet aggregation can prolong bleeding time. The risk of peri-operative bleeding may be increased in patients with underlying coagulation abnormalities, in patients receiving anticoagulants, and in surgical settings requiring strict hemostasis. Platelet dysfunction caused by ketorolac is reversible as the drug is eliminated from the body. Platelet function usually returns to baseline levels within 24 hours of administration.

Drug interactions: like other NSAIDs, plasma protein binding of ketorolac is extensive, leading to potential drug interactions due to displacement of other highly protein-bound drugs. Concurrent use of probenicid with ketorolac will decrease its elimination. Concurrent use of furosemide with ketorolac will decrease the diuretic's effect. Concurrent administration of other NSAIDs may increase plasma levels of ketorolac.

Drug-related adverse events

In addition to the gastric, renal, and antiplatelet side effects of ketorolac, other adverse effects of ketorolac have been reported. Ketorolac, like other COX-1 inhibitors, can produce bronchoconstriction in asthmatic patients and in patients with complete or partial syndromes of nasal polyps, angioedema, and allergic reactions to NSAIDs.

References

1. Lewis JA, Furst DE. *Nonsteroidal Anti-inflammatory Drugs: Mechanisms and Clinical Uses*, 2nd ed. Informa Health Care, 1994, pp. 247–266.

2. Della Rocca G, Chiarandini P, Pietropaoli P. Analgesia in PACU: nonsteroidal anti-inflammatory drugs. *Current Drug Targets* 2005;**6**:781–787.

Celecoxib

Joseph Marino

Generic Name: celecoxib

Trade Name: Celebrex

Manufacturer: Pfizer Pharmaceuticals, 235 East 42nd Street, New York, NY 10017

Chemical Structure: see Figure 56.1

Description

Celebrex (celecoxib) is a selective cyclooxygenase (COX)-2 inhibitor nonsteroidal anti-inflammatory drug chemically designated as 4-[5-(4-methylphenyl)-3-(trifluoromethyl)-1-*H*-pyrazol-1-yl)benzenesulfon-amide. It is a diaryl-substituted pyrazole with an empirical formula of $C_{17}H_{14}F_3N_3O_2S$ and a molecular weight of 381.38. The potent anti-inflammatory effects of an original diarylheterocyclic compound, phenyl-butazone, directed scientists to pharmacologically manipulate this chemical scaffold. As a result, celecoxib was the first of the coxibs to be introduced in 1999 by Searle/Pharmacia (now part of Pfizer Inc., USA) [1].

Mechanism of action

Cyclooxygenase (COX) is an enzyme that catalyzes the rate-limiting step in the arachidonic acid cascade involving the conversion of arachidonic acid to prostaglandin H2 (PGH2), the common biosynthetic precursor to prostaglandins and thromboxane. Cyclooxygenase exists in two isoforms: COX-1 and COX-2. COX -1 and COX-2 are monotropic enzymes bound to cellular membranes of the endoplasmic reticulum and nuclear envelope [2].

Non-selective NSAIDs inhibit both COX isoforms. Celecoxib is an NSAID that exhibits antipyretic, analgesic, and anti-inflammatory activities. The mechanism of action of celecoxib is due to inhibition of prostaglandin synthesis via inhibition of COX-2. At therapeutic concentrations in humans, celecoxib does not inhibit the COX-1 isoenzyme. In general terms, COX-1 is the enzyme responsible for basal, constitutive prostaglandin synthesis, whereas COX-2 is important in various inflammatory settings. Celecoxib produces its analgesic effects by blocking the production of prostaglandins, critical to the processing of pain in the periphery and by augmenting the processing of pain information at the spinal cord level.

There is a structural basis for COX-2 selectivity. Although the active sites within both cyclooxygenase isoforms are similar, a single amino acid difference in position 523 accounts for the COX-2 selectivity of celecoxib. The substitution of the smaller valine molecule in COX-2 as opposed to the larger isoleucine molecule in COX-1 provides access to a side-pocket that is the binding site for the phenylsulfonamide moiety of celecoxib (Figure 56.2) [3].

Pharmacokinetics

Absorption

Celecoxib is insoluble in oils and is absorbed throughout the gastrointestinal tract, with most occurring in the jejunum and duodenum. It is well absorbed with peak plasma concentrations being reached within 3 hours after oral administration. With chronic dosing, celecoxib displays linear pharmacokinetics and reaches steady-state conditions on or before day 5 [1].

Distribution

Celecoxib is extensively distributed in tissues and is 97% protein-bound. It is bound primarily to albumin and to a lesser extent alpha-1-acid glycoprotein. The approximate volume of distribution at steady state is 400 liters, suggesting extensive distribution into the tissues. This extensive volume of distribution may be related to the lipophilic nature of celecoxib as well as to its high PKa (11.1). The effective plasma $t_{1/2}$ is approximately 11 hours under fasting conditions [1].

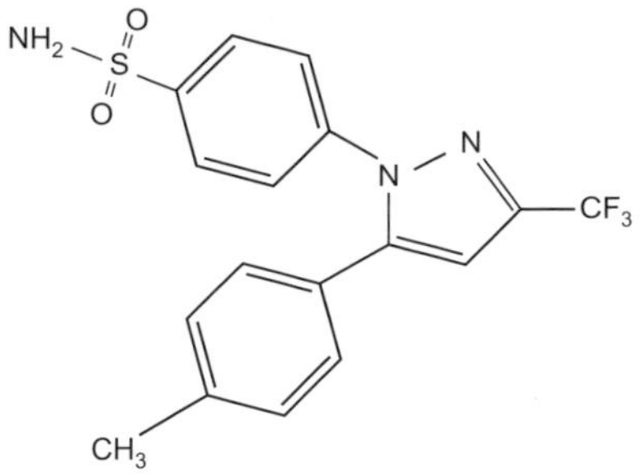

Figure 56.1.

Metabolism

The metabolism of celecoxib involves three steps: (1) oxidative hydroxylation of the methyl group to form a primary alcohol; (2) oxidation to a carboxylic acid (the major metabolite); and (3) conjugation to glucoronic acid, forming the 1-o-glucoronide.

Celecoxib undergoes extensive hepatic metabolism and in vitro studies indicate that it is predominantly mediated via cytochrome P450 (CYP) 2C9. Concomitant administration of celecoxib with drugs known to inhibit CYP2C9 (e.g. fluconazole, lovastatin, fluvastatin) resulted in a two-fold increase in celecoxib plasma concentrations; this is due to the inhibition of celecoxib metabolism via CYP2C9. CYP2C9 genotypes which are known or suspected poor metabolizers should be administered celecoxib with caution as they may have abnormally high levels due to reduced clearance [1].

Excretion

Celecoxib is eliminated predominantly by hepatic metabolism with little unchanged drug recovered in the urine and feces. Fifty-seven percent of the dose was excreted in the feces and 27% was excreted in the urine. As a result, the daily recommended dose of celecoxib should be reduced by 50% in patients with moderate hepatic impairment (Child-Pugh Class B) [1].

Circadian effects

Differences in celecoxib oral bioavailability between morning and evening administration exist. Twelve-hour post-dosing levels were higher in the evening than the morning. These results indicate that in order to maximize control of early morning symptoms, patients on a once-daily dosing schedule should take celecoxib in the evening rather than morning [1].

Indications

Acute surgical pain

Simultaneously utilizing several analgesic approaches rather than one has the potential to provide superior pain control while minimizing side effects. The evidence strongly supports this concept of multimodal analgesia. The American Society of Anesthesiology task force on post-operative pain management, which included members from a spectrum of practice environments, concluded in its practice guidelines that: "all patients should receive an around-the-clock regimen of NSAIDs, coxibs or acetaminophen". Using a comprehensive, preemptive, multimodal, analgesic protocol including celecoxib demonstrated improved peri-operative outcomes including a shortened length of hospital stay, accelerated physiotherapy and a significant reduction in opioid-related side effects [4].

Post-orthopedic surgery, post-general surgery, and post-oral surgery pain studies demonstrated that celecoxib provided significantly greater analgesic efficacy than placebo in terms of onset, magnitude, and/or duration of analgesia. There were lower incidences of dizziness, nausea, vomiting, and somnolence in patients treated with celecoxib than in patients treated with opioid comparator drugs [1].

The recommended dose of celebrex for the management of acute pain in adults is 400 mg initially, followed by an additional 200 mg dose if needed on the first day. On subsequent days, the recommended dose is 200 mg twice a day as needed. At one major medical institution, the following multimodal analgesic regimen is used consisting of:

- continuous perineural/neuraxial blockade where appropriate
- low-dose opioids
- acetaminophen (1 g every 6 hours for 48 hours)
- celecoxib (400 mg) pre-operatively followed post-operatively by 200 mg daily, unless contraindicated by cardiovascular, gastrointestinal, hepatic, or renal comorbidities or allergies to sulfa-containing medications.

If patients manifest inflammatory as well as neuropathic symptoms consider the following multimodal regimen:

- celecoxib 200mg twice daily
- pregabalin (Lyrica) (150 mg twice daily)
- transdermal clonidine (0.1 mg TTS [Transdermal Therapeutic System] skin patch applied weekly).

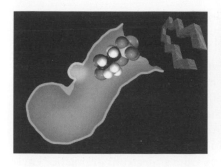 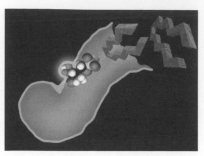

Figure 56.2. Celecoxib bound to COX-2; the phenylsulfamoyl group occupies the side pocket blocking arachidonic acid binding and hence PG synthesis. Adapted from Ref. 3.

Medical pain and common doses

Osteoarthritis: 200 mg once daily or 100 mg twice daily

Rheumatoid arthritis: 100–200 mg twice daily

Juvenile rheumatoid arthritis: 50 mg twice daily in patients 10–25 kg, 100 mg twice daily in patients more than 25 kg

Ankylosing spondylitis: 200 mg once daily single dose or 100 mg twice daily. If no effect is observed after 6 weeks, a trial of 400 mg (single or divided doses) may be of benefit

Primary dysmenorrhea: 400 mg initially, followed by 200 mg dose if needed on first day. On subsequent days, 200 mg twice daily as needed.

Familial adenomatous polyposis (FAP): 400 mg twice daily with food, as an adjunct to usual care. (FAP is a hereditary polyposis syndrome with a progression to colorectal cancer. Increased COX-2 protein was found in the polyp specimens from patients with FAP; in a dose-dependent manner, early treatment with celecoxib significantly reduces the number of colorectal polyps in patients with FAP) [1].

Acute/chronic low back pain

Celecoxib is not approved by the FDA for the treatment of acute/chronic low back pain. Evidence-based data demonstrated greater analgesic efficacy with celecoxib compared to non-opioid comparators for acute and chronic low back pain:

- chronic low back pain: 200 mg daily
- acute low back pain: 200 mg twice daily [1].

Cancer pain

Non-opioid analgesics (NSAIDs, COX-2 inhibitors, APAP), including celecoxib, are part of the World Health Organization's (WHO) analgesic ladder for the treatment of mild to moderate cancer pain. There are no celecoxib dosing guidelines for the treatment of somatic pain associated with cancer.

Contraindications

Absolute: known hypersensitivity to celecoxib or sulfonamides; history of asthma, urticaria, or other allergic-type reactions after taking aspirin or other NSAIDs; for the treatment of peri-operative pain in the setting of coronary artery bypass grafting (CABG) surgery [1].

Routes of administration

Celebrex capsules contain either 50 mg, 100 mg, 200 mg, or 400 mg of celecoxib for oral administration together with inactive ingredients including: croscarmellose sodium, edible inks, gelatin, lactose monohydrate, magnesium stearate, povidone, and sodium lauryl sulfate [1].

Potential advantages

One of the benefits of celecoxib is its convenience and ease of use based on once to twice daily dosing [1].

Peri-operative use of celecoxib in a structured multimodal anesthetic regimen provides both analgesic and opioid-sparing effects for the post-surgical patient resulting in improved patient outcomes [1].

It has been demonstrated clinically that COX-2-selective inhibitors resulted in a lower incidence of gastrointestinal (GI) complications as compared to standard NSAIDs. COX-1 predominates in the gastric mucosa and yields salutary prostaglandins. By sparing COX-1 inhibition GI mucosal integrity is maintained. In a pooled analysis of celecoxib-treated patients with osteoarthritis, rheumatoid arthritis, and ankylosing spondylitis, celecoxib offered the prospect of improved GI tolerability and, in patients not taking aspirin for cardioprophylaxis, a GI safety advantage [1].

Results indicate that even at supratherapeutic doses, celecoxib will not interfere with normal mechanisms of platelet aggregation and hemostasis. Patients treated with celecoxib experienced fewer decreases in hemoglobin/hematocrit than patients treated with comparator NSAIDs [1].

Celecoxib does not demonstrate any adverse effects on bone healing in clinical trials [1].

Celecoxib is not approved by the FDA for the treatment of cancers. However, celecoxib as monotherapy or as part of combination therapy has been demonstrated to suppress tumor growth in a variety of neoplasms and has benefited patients with prostate cancer. Potential mechanisms of anticancer activity of celecoxib include inhibition of endogenous carcinogen formation, modulation of inflammation, increased cellular sensitivity to apoptosis, and inhibition of angiogenesis[1].

There is no known potential for addiction associated with the use of celecoxib.

Prothrombotic potential may be more of a drug-specific effect rather than a COX-2 class effect. Celecoxib is currently the only remaining selective COX-2 inhibitor on the market. Analysis of data from a variety of clinical trials demonstrated an unacceptably high incidence of cardiovascular events with rofecoxib and valdecoxib. As a result, rofecoxib and valdecoxib were voluntarily withdrawn from clinical practice by 2005.While all the coxibs are lipophillic and have a similar volume of distribution, rofecoxib exhibits higher specificity for COX-2 compared to celecoxib (up to 300 times more affinity in contrast to celecoxib, which had up to 30 times more affinity for COX-2 over COX-1). Rofecoxib has a slower almost irreversible dissociation from the active site, and a longer half-life compared to celecoxib. A coxib with a more rapid dissociation from the COX active site might permit recovery of endothelial PGI2 formation and reduce unopposed platelet COX-1-dependent thromboxane formation. There is a greater body of evidence supporting the relative cardiovascular safety of celecoxib when used at the doses prescribed than for any other selective or nonselective cox-2 inhibitor [1,2].

Potential disadvantages

Celecoxib has several drug interactions.

Co-administration with drugs known to inhibit cytochrome P450 (CYP) 2C9 (fluconazole, "statin" drugs) should be done with caution [1].

Co-administration of celecoxib with lithium results in elevated lithium concentrations (mean steady-state levels increased by approximately 17%). Close monitoring of lithium levels is advised when celecoxib is either introduced or withdrawn from patients concomitantly using lithium [1].

Celecoxib co-administration may result in increases in international normalized ratio (INR) in patients who were on warfarin and had stable INRs before the addition of celecoxib [1].

Celecoxib can be used with low-dose aspirin. However, concomitant administration with aspirin may increase the rate of GI ulceration or other complications, compared to the use of celecoxib alone [1].

Drug-related adverse events

Common adverse events: most common adverse reactions in arthritis trials include abdominal pain, diarrhea, dyspepsia, flatulence, peripheral edema, accidental injury, dizziness, pharyngitis, rhinitis, sinusitis, upper respiratory tract infection, and rash [1].

Serious adverse events

The development of COX-2 inhibition as an anti-inflammatory agent without gastric toxicity is based on the premise that COX-1 predominates in the gastric mucosa, producing cytoprotective prostaglandins, while COX-2 is induced in inflammation, leading to hyperalgesia. Selective COX-2 inhibitors decrease vascular prostacyclin (PGI2) production and may alter the balance in vascular homeostasis between prothrombotic (TBXA2) and antithrombotic (PGI2) prostanoids. Celecoxib therapy may be associated with an increased risk of cardiovascular events, but only when used at doses substantially higher than that recommended [1]. The package insert on Celebrex states that Celebrex may cause an increase of serious thrombotic events, myocardial infarction, and stroke, which can be fatal. Patients with known cardiovascular disease/risk factors may be at a greater risk. All NSAIDs may have a similar risk. This risk may increase with duration of use. An analysis of data from two combined colorectal prevention trials (APC: adenoma prevention with celecoxib; and Pre-SAP: prevention of colorectal sporadic adenomatous polyps) showed a nearly two-fold higher risk for the composite of nonfatal heart attack, nonfatal stroke, and death from cardiovascular causes combined, with celecoxib compared to placebo [1].

Serious gastrointestinal (GI) adverse events, which can be fatal. The risk is greater in patients with a prior history of ulcer disease or GI bleeding and in patients at high risk for GI events, especially the elderly [1].

Elevated liver enzymes and, rarely, severe hepatic reactions [1].

New onset or worsening of hypertension [1].

Fluid retention and edema [1].

Renal papillary necrosis and other renal injury with long-term use. Most of the unwanted renal side effects of the class of NSAIDs are related to the inhibiton of prostanoid synthesis. The COX-2 enzyme has been implicated as a mediator of renal blood flow, renin release and sodium excretion. As a result, COX-2 inhibitors may lead to an alteration of renal homeostasis resulting in decreases in glomerular filtration rate, renal blood flow, sodium and water retention, and hyperkalemia [1].

Anaphylactoid reactions: not to be used in patients with the aspirin triad (asthma, aspirin sensitivity, and nasal polyps) [1].

Serious skin adverse events such as exfoliative dermatitis, Stevens–Johnson syndrome, and toxic epidermal necrolysis, which can be fatal and can occur without warning even without known prior sulfa allergy [1,2].

Overdosage

No overdosage of celecoxib was reported during clinical trials. Doses up to 2400 mg/day for up to 10 days in 12 patients did not result in serious toxicity. Symptoms following acute NSAID overdoses are usually limited to lethargy, drowsiness, nausea, vomiting, and epigastric pain which are generally reversible with supportive care. Gastrointestinal bleeding can occur.

Hypertension, acute renal failure, respiratory depression, and coma may occur, but are rare.

Patients should be managed by symptomatic and supportive care following NSAID overdose. There are no specific antidotes. Based on its high degree of plasma protein binding, forced diuresis, alkalinization of urine, dialysis, or hemoperfusion is unlikely to be useful in overdose. Emesis and/or activated charcoal and/or osmotic cathartis may be indicated in patients seen within 4 hours following overdose [5].

References

1. Celecorex® and (celecoxib) package insert.

2. Pairet M, van Ryn J. Cox-2 inhibitors. In *Milestones in Drug Therapy*. Basel: Birkhauser, 2004.

3. Jahr JS, Donkor KN, Sinatra RS, Nonsteroidal anti-inflammatory drugs, Cox-2 inhibitors and acetaminophen for postoperative pain management. In Sinatra R, de Leon-Casasola O, Ginsberg B, Viscusi E, eds. *Acute Pain Management*. New York: Cambridge University Press, 2009, p. 347.

4. Practice guidelines for acute pain management in the perioperative setting. An updated report by the American Society of Anesthesiology Task Force on Acute Pain Management. *Anesthesiology* 2004;**100**:1573–1581.

5. *Physicians desk reference*, 63rd ed. Montvale, NJ: Thomson Reuters, 2009.

NSAIDs

Etoricoxib

Bryan S. Williams and Asokumar Buvanendran

Generic Name: etoricoxib; etoricoxibum; etorikoksib; etorikoksibi; etorikoxib

Chemical Name: 5-chloro-6′-methyl-3-[*p*-(methy-lsulfonyl)phenyl]-2,3′-bipyridine

Proprietary Names: Algix (Gentili, Ital.), Arcoxia (MSD, Arg., Austria, Brazil, Iudon., Irl., Israel, Mex., Philip., Singapore, Swed., UK, Venez.).

Manufacturer: Merck, Whitehouse Station, NJ

Drug Class: selective (cyclooxygenase-2 inhibition) nonsteroidal anti-inflammatory

Chemical Structure: see Figure 57.1

Description

Etoricoxib is a second-generation, highly selective cyclooxygenase 2 (COX-2) inhibitor with anti-inflammatory and analgesic properties [1]. It shows dose-dependent inhibition of COX-2 across the therapeutic dose range, without inhibition of COX-1, does not inhibit gastric prostaglandin synthesis and has no effect on platelet function [2]. Etoricoxib shows 106-fold selectivity for COX-2 over COX-1 [3], compared with 7.6-fold selectivity observed with celecoxib [2,3]. Etoricoxib was first introduced clinically as a medication in 2002 by Merck & Co and is now available in at least 62 countries throughout the world, but still await approval in the USA.

Mode of activity

Traditional nonselective NSAIDs inhibit both COX-1 and COX-2 enzymes. The COX-2 inhibition is associated with anti-inflammatory and analgesic effects, but the COX-1 inhibition is associated with unwanted effects such as gastrointestinal (GI) bleeding. The selective COX-2 inhibitors were developed with the aim of reducing the GI adverse effects associated with COX-1 inhibition.

Major sites of action: inhibition of prostaglandin production.

Minor sites of action: inhibits activation of the transcription factors cyclic adenosine monophosphate response element-binding protein and nuclear factor kappa-B.

Metabolic pathways/drug clearance and elimination: etoricoxib is well absorbed from the gastrointestinal tract after oral doses. Peak plasma concentrations are reached in about 1 hour in fasted adults; food delays absorption by about 2 hours, although it has no effect on the extent of absorption. Plasma protein binding is about 92%. At steady state the half-life of etoricoxib is about 22 hours. Etoricoxib is extensively metabolized with less than 2% of a dose recovered in the urine as the parent drug. The major route of metabolism is via cytochrome P450 isoenzymes including CYP3A4. Excretion is mainly via the urine (70%) with only 20% of a dose appearing in the feces.

Indications (non-approved in the USA)

Etoricoxib is a selective cyclooxygenase (COX-2) inhibitor, approved in Europe for the symptomatic treatment of osteoarthritis, rheumatoid arthritis, ankylosing spondylitis and acute gouty arthritis. Etoricoxib does not have Food and Drug Administration approval.

Medical pain: in osteoarthritis, etoricoxib is given orally in a usual dose of 30 mg once daily, increased to 60 mg once daily if necessary. The recommended dose in rheumatoid arthritis and in ankylosing spondylitis is 90 mg once daily; higher doses of 120 mg once daily are used in gouty arthritis although such doses should only be used for the acute symptomatic period and for a maximum of 8 days [4].

Surgical acute pain: single dose oral etoricoxib (120 mg) has shown usefulness in analgesia after surgery [5].

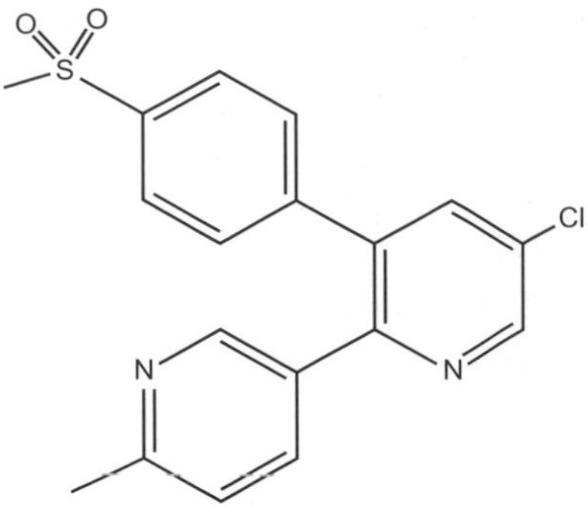

Figure 57.1.

Contraindications

Key contraindications include congestive heart failure (New York Heart Association class II–IV), inadequately controlled hypertension with persistent BP elevation >140/90 mmHg, established ischemic heart disease, peripheral arterial disease and/or cerebrovascular disease, active peptic ulceration or GI bleeding, creatinine clearance <30 mL/min, or severe hepatic dysfunction [4].

Common doses

Etoricoxib is approved in Europe for the treatment of patients with osteoarthritis (recommended dosage 30–60 mg once daily), rheumatoid arthritis (90 mg once daily), acute gouty arthritis (120 mg once daily for a maximum of 8 days) and ankylosing spondylitis (90 mg once daily); although an inhibition of COX-2 by 80% may be reached after the administration of 40 mg, suggesting that the dosage of the drug could be reduced without affecting efficacy [6].

Potential advantages

Nonselective NSAIDs are commonly associated with GI adverse effects and, while NSAIDs that are selective for COX-2 generally have improved GI tolerability, they can be associated with an increased risk of cardiovascular events. COX-2 inhibitors are associated with a reduced risk of GI events compared with nonselective NSAIDs, although the most frequent adverse events with etoricoxib were generally GI in nature. However, etoricoxib was associated with a reduced risk of upper GI events compared with nonselective NSAIDs [1].

Potential disadvantages

The increased risk of cardiovascular events associated with COX-2 inhibitors led to the voluntary withdrawal of rofecoxib and valdecoxib, in 2004 and 2005, respectively. While COX-2 inhibitors as a class are associated with an increased risk of CV adverse events compared with placebo, different agents may be associated with different degrees of risk, especially in those with preexisting risk factors. To date, there have been few large, long-term controlled trials specifically evaluating the relative CV risk with different drugs within the overall NSAID class [2]. The MEDAL (Multinational Etoricoxib and Diclofenac Arthritis Long-term) program was one such evaluation. In this multinational study, composed of three randomized, controlled, double-blind studies involving 34 701 patients, investigators found that etoricoxib was not inferior to diclofenac in terms of the overall rate of thrombotic CV events. After an average duration of 18 months, 320 patients in the etoricoxib group and 323 patients in the diclofenac group experienced thrombotic cardiovascular events, yielding event rates of 1.24 and 1.30 per 100 patient years and a hazard ratio of 0.95 (95% CI 0.81, 1.11) [1]. Additionally NSAIDs should be utilized with caution in patients with renal impairment. Etoricoxib is contraindicated in patients with an estimated renal creatinine clearance <30 mL/min [2].

Drug-related adverse events

Etoricoxib was generally well tolerated in clinical trials in patients with osteoarthritis, rheumatoid arthritis, ankylosing spondylitis, and acute gouty arthritis. The most commonly reported drug-related adverse events were generally GI (e.g. dyspepsia, upper abdominal pain, diarrhea, nausea) or CV (e.g. hypertension and peripheral edema).

References

1. Takemoto JK, Reynolds JK, Remsberg CM, et al. Clinical pharmacokinetic and pharmacodynamic profile of etoricoxib. *Clin Pharmacokinet* 2008;**47**(11):703–720.

2. Croom KF, Siddiqui MA. Etoricoxib: a review of its use in the symptomatic treatment of osteoarthritis, rheumatoid arthritis, ankylosing spondylitis and acute gouty arthritis. *Drugs* 2009;**69**(11):1513–1532.

3. Riendeau D, Percival MD, Brideau C, et al. Etoricoxib (MK-0663): preclinical profile and comparison with other agents that selectively inhibit cyclooxygenase-2. *J Pharmacol Exp Ther* 2001;**296**(2):558–566.

4. Micromedex® Healthcare Series, DrugDex® Evaluations, Thompson Healthcare. Etoricoxib; 2009.

5. Clarke R, Derry S, Moore RA, et al. Single dose oral etoricoxib for acute postoperative pain in adults. *Cochrane Database Syst Rev* 2009;**2**:CD004309.

6. Patrignani P, Tacconelli S, Capone ML. Risk management profile of etoricoxib: an example of personalized medicine. *Ther Clin Risk Manag* 2008;**4**(5):983–997.

Section 4
Chapter

NSAIDs

Parecoxib

Jeff Gudin and Despina Psillides

Generic Name: parecoxib

Trade/Proprietary Name: Dynastat™ (available in EU)

Manufacturer: Pfizer Inc.

Drug class: COX-2 selective inhibitor

Chemical Structure: see Figure 58.1

Chemical Formula: $C_{19}H_{18}N_2O_4S$; molecular wt 370

Introduction

Parecoxib is unique in that it is the first COX-2-specific inhibitor that can be parenterally administered. This feature of parecoxib allows for its role in pre-operative and post-operative analgesia when patients are often unable to take oral pain medications. Parecoxib has a long history in the literature, which will be reviewed below. However, it must be stated that parecoxib is not FDA-approved in the USA, but is available in other countries for short-term peri-operative analgesia.

Parecoxib, N-{[4-(5-methyl-3-phenylisoxazol-4-yl) phenyl]sulfonyl}propanamide, is an inactive prodrug of valdecoxib. After injection, either intramuscular or intravenous, parecoxib rapidly undergoes hepatic metabolism, predominantly via cytochromes P450 3A4 and P450 2C9, to valdecoxib. The peak plasma concentration of valdecoxib occurs 30 minutes after IV and 60 minutes after IM injection of parecoxib [1]. Parecoxib is 100% bioavailable, and is renally excreted in the urine, with 70% as inactive metabolites. The half-life of parecoxib is approximately 22 minutes as opposed to 8 hours for valdecoxib.

Parecoxib and the other COX-2 inhibitors may provide anti-inflammatory effects while still maintaining gastrointestinal integrity and normal platelet functioning. The cyclooxygenases, both COX-1 and COX-2, lead to the production of prostaglandins. The difference between the two forms is that they are expressed at different times and in different cellular locations. Cyclooxygenase-1 (COX-1) is expressed at times of normal physiological functioning and has its main role in the production of prostaglandins in gastric mucosa, kidneys, and platelets [2]. Cyclooxygenase-2 (COX-2), on the other hand, has restricted expression during normal functioning but is induced in response to physiological stress and mediates inflammation and pain.

COX-1 plays a major role in the production of thromboxane A2 (TxA2), which is a prostaglandin that stimulates platelet aggregation. Generally it is believed that inhibition of COX-1 can block the production of TxA2, thus preventing platelet aggregation and prolonging bleeding time. This becomes important when

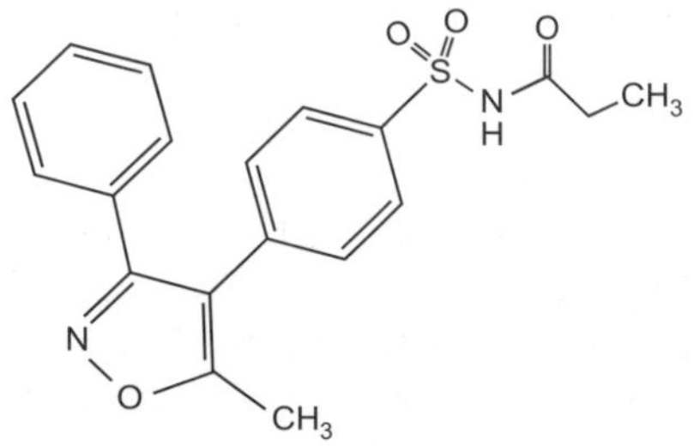

Figure 58.1.

considering the use of nonselective COX inhibitors in the peri-operative setting because they may increase the risk of bleeding. Parecoxib has been studied for its platelet-sparing effects. Noveck et al. [3] studied the effects of parecoxib versus ketorolac or placebo on platelet function and bleeding time in two double-blind active and placebo-controlled trials. In one study involving elderly patients qualified as ages 65–95, there were three groups that received either intravenous parecoxib 40 mg twice daily, intravenous ketorolac 15 mg four times daily intravenously, or placebo for 5 days. Another study evaluated the non-elderly (ages 18–55); the study groups received either 40 mg of parecoxib intravenously twice daily, intravenous ketorolac 30 mg four times daily, or placebo. The two studies evaluated a total of 105 patients, 60 elderly and 45 non-elderly. Both studies showed that parecoxib had no effect on platelet function, while ketorolac significantly reduced platelet aggregation. Also, as compared to parecoxib, ketorolac caused a significant prolongation in bleeding time at 2 and 4 hours after infusion.

Another implication of altered platelet function is the increased risk of gastrointestinal bleeding. As mentioned above, COX-1 plays a protective role in the gastric mucosa and thus inhibition of this enzyme may lead to increased incidence of gastrointestinal ulceration. Parecoxib was evaluated for its role in the gastrointestinal system because of the implication of a peri-operative analgesic that could be administered intravenously, while not increasing the risk of bleeding or gastrointestinal ulceration. There are two studies by Harris et al. [4] that evaluated parecoxib in the settting of upper gastrointestinal complications. In the first study, a randomized, double-blind, double-dummy, placebo-controlled, parallel group study, parecoxib was studied in comparison to ketorolac, naproxen, and placebo. The participants underwent a baseline endoscopy and then qualified subjects were randomized to either intravenous parecoxib 10 mg twice daily, oral naproxen 500 mg twice daily, placebo for 7 days, or

placebo for 2 days with intravenous ketorolac 15 mg four times daily given afterwards for 5 days. The participants had follow-up endoscopies after 7 days. The data collected showed that there were no ulcerations observed in the parecoxib group on follow-up endoscopy, but there were ulcerations observed in all the other active groups. The data were so concerning that the study was terminated early and thus there were no significant data on the safety profile of parecoxib. In 2004, Harris et al. [5] repeated a similar study. The study was again double-blinded and placebo-controlled. The study participants had endoscopic documentation of normal upper intestinal mucosa and were randomized to intravenous parecoxib 40 mg twice daily, placebo for 2 days followed by intravenous ketorolac 30 mg four times daily for 5 days, or placebo for 7 days. In this study, ketorolac showed a statistically significant rate of gastrointestinal complications as compared to placebo and parecoxib ($P < 0.001$). The effects of longer administration of parecoxib were also evaluated in a double-blind placebo-controlled trial. Stoltz et al. [6] evaluated the use of intravenous parecoxib 40 mg administered for 7 days versus intravenous ketorolac 15 mg four times daily for 5 days, or placebo for 7 days. This study demonstrated a statistically significant difference in the incidence of stomach and duodenal ulcers with parecoxib and placebo versus ketorolac. Based on the above studies, the gastrointestinal safety profile of parecoxib appears to be better than that of ketorolac.

The efficacy of parecoxib for analgesia has also been evaluated in clinical trials. The goal was usually to compare parecoxib to other analgesics, such as NSAIDs or opioids. Oral surgery was the model in multiple studies. The outcomes measured included pain relief, pain intensity difference (PID) score, time to onset of analgesia, and time to rescue medication. The overall results were that parecoxib is comparable to ketorolac in providing effective analgesia in the post-operative setting [7]. In one study, the participants were randomized to intramuscular parecoxib 20 mg or 40 mg, intravenous parecoxib 20 mg or 40 mg, intramuscular ketorolac 60 mg, or placebo. There were no statistically significant differences in pain relief or PID scores of patients randomized to parecoxib versus ketorolac. One significant difference was that parecoxib 40 mg had a longer duration of action. Another study [8] compared intravenous parecoxib 20 mg, 40 mg, 80 mg, and placebo given as a one-time dose prior to oral surgery. The time to rescue medication was used as the primary outcome. The 40 mg and 80 mg dosages or parecoxib had a longer duration of action than the 20 mg dose, but there was no significant difference in resue analgesic use between the 40 mg and 80 mg groups.

From early work on the drug, it appears the benefits of parecoxib were promising and had great potential to be used as adjunctive pain management in many situations [9–11]. Studies were conducted with oral surgery, orthopedics, and gynecological models that suggested the COX-2 inhibitor parecoxib offered opioid-sparing attributes. Minimizing opioids in the post-operative period offered obvious benefits, including reduced adverse effects such as nausea and vomiting. However, amidst these promising studies there also emerged data that demonstrated that parecoxib in certain clinical arenas increased the risk of cardiovascular events. The first study by Ott et al. [12] at first demonstrated that parecoxib could be used as an effective analgesic after CABG. An unanticipated side effect of the use of parecoxib in this setting was an increased risk of sternal wound infections, incidence of post-operative myocardial infarction, and severe cerebrovascular events. As the study was not designed primarily to look at adverse events associated with the use of parecoxib, Nussmeier et al. performed another study the results of which were published in the *New England Journal of Medicine NEJM* [13]. The study was a randomized, double-blind study that compared three different 10-day regimens of either intravenous parecoxib use followed by oral valdecoxib, intravenous placebo followed by oral valdecoxib, or all oral placebo. The participants were then examined for a number of predefined adverse events such as cardiovascular events, renal, gastrointestinal, and wound-healing complications. Of all the participants, the two groups that included either parecoxib or valdecoxib treatment did have a higher incidence of adverse events as compared to placebo ($P = 0.02$). The incidence of combined events such as myocardial infarction, stroke, pulmonary embolism, and cardiac arrest was also higher in the treatment groups versus placebo ($P = 0.03$). In 2005, the FDA released a letter of non-approval for parecoxib. Although no official reason was ever documented as to the non-approval, it is likely that the data from the above-mentioned studies were taken into consideration.

The theory behind the increased incidence of cardiovascular thromboembolic events with the use of parecoxib or other COX-2 inhibitors is very interesting. It is thought that the use of these agents causes an "imbalance of pro and anti-platelet aggregation influences though the selective inhibition of COX-2 production of prostacyclin while sparing COX-1 production of thromboxanes" [14]. This theory is fascinating and seems to offer a plausible explanation for the increased risk observed, and also would prove a class effect of COX-2 inhibitors and not just of parecoxib or valdecoxib. However, other authors [14,15] have postulated that this theory is inadequate because in the post-CAGB studies all the patients had already been started on low-dose aspirin, which would effectively negate the postulated COX-1 effect. These authors believe that the bypass procedure itself is what causes increased sheer stress [16], which in turn results in the alteration of the tertiary structure of von Willebrand factor, exposing the site of glycoprotein Ib receptors in platelets and causing aggregation. Much research is still needed in this area to fully understand the mechanism behind adverse cardiovascular events associated with parecoxib and any possible way to decrease this risk.

New studies are now emerging which are evaluating the use of parecoxib in non-cardiac surgery and whether there is increased risk in this patient population [17]. Interestingly, the authors of the original *NEJM* article which evaluated post-CABG patients performed this study. This study was similar in design to the *NEJM* study. The trial was a randomized double-blind study which evaluated the use of parenteral parecoxib for 3 days and oral valdecoxib for 7 days versus 10 days of placebo. The goal was to measure the frequency of predefined adverse events such as cardiovascular thromboembolism, renal, gastrointestinal, and wound-healing complications. No significant difference in adverse events was noted in either group ($P = 0.58$). One of the criticisms of the study is that it was not powered to show significant differences in cardiovascular thromboembolic events because of the low incidence of these events in noncardiac surgery patients.

More study and research is needed to evaluate parecoxib fully and the possible risks and benefits of its use. The benefits of opioid-sparing effects and decreased bleeding risk must be weighed against the cardiovascular risk in certain patient populations. The data available are still not definitive in the absolute risk profile of parecoxib. The possibilities for use in non-cardiac patients, as well as the use of other agents in cardiac patients to temper the physiological mechanisms of

COX-inhibitors and shear stress, still need to be evaluated. Currently, parecoxib is not approved for use in the USA and is not approved for use after cardiac surgery in Europe.

References

1. Cheer SM, Goa KL. Parecoxib (parecoxib sodium). *Drugs* 2001; **61**(8):1133–1141.

2. Kasper DL, Braunwald E, et al., eds. *Harrison's Principles of Internal Medicine*, 16th ed. New York: McGraw-Hill, 2005.

3. Noveck RJ, Laurent A, Kuss M, Talwalker S, Hubbard, RC. Parecoxib sodium does not impair platelet function in healthy elderly and non-elderly individuals: two randomized, controlled tirals. *Clin Drug Investig* 2001;**21**:465–476.

4. Harris SI, Kuss M, Hubbard, RC, Goldstein, JL. Upper gastrointestinal safety evaluation of parecoxib sodium, a new parenteral cyclooxygenase-2-specific inhibitor, compared with ketorolac, naproxen, and placebo. *Clin Ther* 2001;**23**:1422–1428.

5. Harris SI, Stoltz RR, LeComte D, Hubbard RC. Parecoxib sodium demonstrates gastrointestinal safety comparable to placebo in healthy subjects. *J Clin Gastroenterol* 2004;**38**(7):575–580.

6. Stoltz RR, Harris SI, Kuss ME, LeComte D, Talwalker S, Dhadda, S, Hubbard RC. Upper gastrointestinal mucosal effects of parecoxib sodium in healthy elderly subjects. *Am J Gastroenterol* 2002;**97**:65–71.

7. Daniels SE, Grossman EH, Kuss ME, Talwalker S, Hubbard RC. A double-blind, randomized comparison of intramuscularly and intravenously administered parecoxib sodium versus ketorolac and placebo in a post-oral surgery pain model. *Clin Ther* 2001;**23**(7):1018–1031.

8. DesJardins PJ, Grossman EH, Kuss ME, Talwalker S, Dhadda S, Baum D, Hubbard RC. The injectable cyclooxygenase-2-specific inhibitor parecoxib sodium has analgesic efficacy when administered preoperatively. *Anesth Analg* 2001;**93**(3):721–727.

9. Ng A, Smith G, Davidson AC. Analgesic effects of parecoxib following total abdominal hysterectomy. *Br J Anaesth* 2003;**90**:746–749.

10. Malan TP Jr, Marsh G, Hakki SI, Grossman E, Traylor L, Hubbard RC. Parecoxib sodium, a parenteral cyclooxygenase 2 selective inhibitor, improves morphine analgesia and is opioid-sparing following total hip arthroplasty. *Anesthesiology* 2003;**98**: 950–956.

11. Joshi GP, Viscusi ER, Gan TJ, et al. Effective treatment of laparoscopic cholecystectomy pain with intravenous followed by oral COX-2 specific inhibitor. *Anesth Analg* 2004;**98**:336–342.

12. Ott E, Nussmeier NA, Duke PC, et al. Efficacy and safety of the cyclooxygenase 2 inhibitors parecoxib and valdecoxib in patients undergoing coronary artery bypass surgery. *J Thorac Cardiovasc Surg* 2003;**125**:1481–1492.

13. Nussmeier NA, Whelton AA, Brown MT, et al. Complications of the COX-2 inhibitors parecoxib and valdecoxib after cardiac surgery. *NEJM* 2005;**352**:1081–1091.

14. Krotz F, Schiele TM, Klauss V, John H. Selective COX-2 inhibitors and risk of myocardial infarction. *J Vasc Res* 2005;**42**:312–324.

15. Schug S, Joshi G, Camu F, Pan S, Cheung R. Cardiovascular safety of the cyclooxygenase-2 selective inhibitors parecoxib and valdecoxib in the postoperative setting: an analysis of integrated data. *Anesth Analg* 2009;**108**:299–307.

16. Borgdorff P, Tangelder GJ, Paulus WJ. COX-2 inhibitors enhance shear stress-induded platelet aggregation. *J AM Coll Cardiol* 2006;**48**:817–823.

17. Nussmeier NA, Whelton AA, Brown MT, Joshi GP, Langford RM, Singla NK, Boye ME, Verburg KM. Safety and efficacy of the cyclooxygenase-2 inhibitors parecoxib and valdecoxib after noncardiac surgery. *Anesthesiology* 2006;**104**(3):518–526.

59

Meloxicam

Gabriel Jacobs

Generic Name: meloxicam

Trade/Proprietary name: Mobic™

Drug Class: NSAID

Manufacturer: Boehringer Ingelheim Parmaceuticals, Inc., P.O. Box 368, 900 Ridgebury Road, Ridgefield, CT 06877–0368

Chemical Name: 4-hydroxy-2-methyl-N-(5-methyl-2-thiazolyl)-2H-1,2-benzothiazine-3-carboxamide-1,1-dioxide

Chemical Structure: see Figure 59.1

Empirical Formula: $C_{14}H_{13}N_3O_4S_2$ [1]; molecular wt 351

Introduction

Meloxicam is classified as a partially selective COX-2 inhibitor, a subclass of nonsteroidal anti-inflammatory drugs (NSAIDs). It is believed to provide similar anti-inflammatory and analgesic effects similar to nonselective NSAIDs but with a lower gastrointestinal bleeding risk and less effect on platelet aggregation. Meloxicam is an oxicam-type anti-inflammatory drug, chemically related to an earlier released compound, piroxicam. The primary advantage of oxicams is their prolonged elimination half-life (18–20 h) which allows once per day dosing [1]. Meloxicam is approved and primarily prescribed to control pain and inflammation associated with rheumatoid and degenerative joint diseases. Non-approved uses may include control of acute pain related to traumatic injury or following surgery, and chronic low back pain.

Mode of action

The anti-inflammatory nature of NSAIDs is widely attributed to their action of inhibiting the synthesis of prostaglandins. Prostaglandin endoperoxide synthase (PGHS) is a key enzyme involved in inflammation. PGHS has been shown to exist in two isoforms, cyclooxygenase 1 and 2 (COX-1 and COX-2). Most conventional NSAIDs inhibit the cyclooxygenase activity of both COX-1 and COX-2. Meloxicam inhibits the enzyme COX-2, in turn lowering levels of prostaglandins, which are key inflammatory and algesic mediators. The precise degree of meloxicam's ability to inhibit COX-2 selectively over COX-1 is still under investigation but it appears to be less selective than true COX-2 inhibitors such as celecoxib and parecoxib [2].

The Meloxicam Large-scale International Study Safety Assessment (MELISSA) trial evaluated the tolerability of meloxicam, and potential COX-2 selectivity of meloxicam compared to diclofenac [3]. This large-scale (9323 patients), double-blind, prospective trial was conducted over 28 days in patients with symptomatic osteoarthritis. Patients received standard doses of either meloxicam 7.5 mg or diclofenac 100 mg slow release. Significantly fewer adverse events were reported by patients receiving meloxicam. This was attributable to fewer GI adverse events (13%) compared to diclofenac (19%, $P < 0.001$). Of the most common GI adverse events, there was significantly less dyspepsia ($P < 0.001$), nausea and vomiting ($P < 0.05$), abdominal pain ($P < 0.01$), and diarrhea ($P < 0.001$) with meloxicam compared to diclofenac. No endoscopically verified ulcer complication was detected in the meloxicam group compared to four with diclofenac. Patients treated with meloxicam required a total of 5 days hospitalization for drug-related complications versus 121 with diclofenac. On the other hand, patients in the diclofenac group consistently reported lower pain intensity scores. Although differences in analgesic efficacy were small (4.5–9.0% difference), significantly more patients discontinued meloxicam because of lack of efficacy (80 out of 4635 vs. 49 out of 4688; $P < 0.01$).

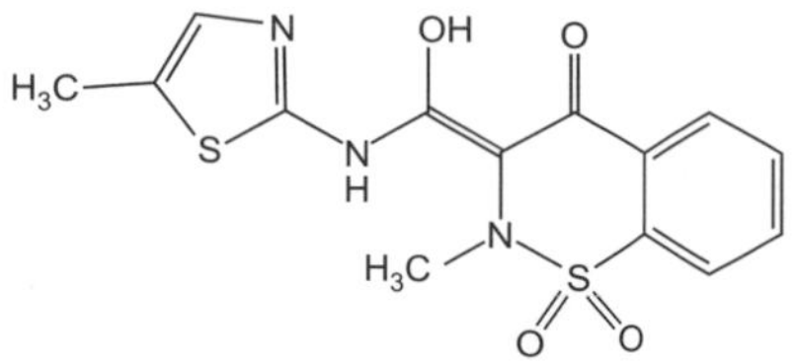

Figure 59.1.

Metabolism

Meloxicam is metabolized in the liver via P450 enzymes and converted into four inactive metabolites [1,3]. The mean $t_{1/2}$ of meloxicam is 15 to 20 hours. Most of meloxicam is excreted in the form of metabolites; very little of the drug is excreted in its unchanged form. Near equal parts of meloxicam's metabolites are excreted in both the urine and feces. Significant billary and enteral secretion has been demonstrated [1].

Indications

Adult indications: osteoarthritis, rheumatoid arthritis, acute musculoskeletal pain, post-operative pain.

Pediatric indications: juvenile idiopathic arthritis.

Potential indication under investigation

Meloxicam is currently under investigation for being used in the treatment of diabetic polyneuropathy. Translational studies from Hokuriku University in Japan demonstrate some positive results. Meloxicam was studied in the treatment of induced diabetic neuropathy in mice. In the study, diabetic mice treated with meloxicam showed improvement in established allodynia when compared with ibuprofen and placebo [4]. These results may lead to further investigation in more animal and human trials. However, with renal impairment and cardiovascular derangements a major concern with many diabetic patients the use of meloxicam in the treatment of diabetic neuropathy could make future human investigation challenging.

Contraindications

Meloxicam should be avoided in patients with known NSAID allergies, pregnancy, and peri-operative period for patients undergoing CABG surgery. Also, meloxicam should be used cautiously in patients with the following: cardiovascular disease, HTN, CHF, history of PUD or GI bleeding, concomitant corticosteroid use, concomitant anticoagulation, tobacco or alcohol use, elderly patients, patients with kidney or liver impairment, and asthmatics. Prolonged use of meloxicam should also be avoided if possible [1,3,5].

Common doses

Meloxicam is available only in oral formularies which include both pill and liquid suspension. Tablet: 7.5 mg and 15 mg. Liquid suspension: 7.5 mg/5mL.

Adult dosing: for osteoarthritis and rheumatoid arthritis dosage is 7.5–15 mg PO qd. Practitioners should prescribe the lower dose of 7.5 mg PO qd and advance to 15 mg PO qd if lower dose proves ineffective in treating symptoms [1,5].

Pediatric dosing (ages 2–17) for juvenile idiopathic arthritis dosing is weight-based at 0.125 mg/kg PO qd with a maximum pediatric dose of 7.5 mg per day [1,5] (Table 59.1).

Potential advantages

Meloxicam has advantages in the treatment inflammatory processes compared to conventional NSAIDs in that it is classified as a selective COX-2 inhibitor. The anti-inflammatory effect of most NSAIDs is attributed to the inhibition of COX-2 enzyme, while many of the deleterious effects such as gastrointestinal bleeding and ulceration have been attributed to the inhibition of COX-1. Though the precise selectivity of meloxicam for COX-2 is still not clear, in vitro studies have shown a 3 to 300 times preferential inhibition of COX-2 over COX-1 [2,6,7]. Long-term data are still lacking with regard to meloxicam's improved side-effect profile, thus the same considerations should be made by a practitioner as with prescribing other NSAIDs. Once-a-day dosing could also help improve patient compliance with meloxicam.

Table 59.1. Juvenile rheumatoid arthritis dosing using the oral suspension should be individualized based on the weight of the child

Dose weight	(1.5 mg/mL)	Delivered dose
12 kg (26 lb)	1.0 mL	1.5 mg
24 kg (54 lb)	2.0 mL	3.0 mg
36 kg (80 lb)	3.0 mL	4.5 mg
48 kg (106 lb)	4.0 mL	6.0 mg
≥60 kg (132 lb)	5.0 mL	7.5 mg

Potential disadvantages

Meloxicam is only available in oral formulations. An IV formulation is not available for human use but has been employed for pain management in veterinary medicine. Despite studies demonstrating improved tolerability, meloxicam, like other NSAIDs, is associated with the potential for serious gastrointestinal and wound site bleeding. Treatment with meloxicam may worsen renal function or precipitate acute renal failure.

Drug interactions

Meloxicam has been shown to have interactions with the following common medications: ACE inhibitors, aspirin, cholestyramine, cimetidine, digoxin, furosemide, lithium, methotrexate, warfarin [1].

Drug-related adverse events

Serious events – meloxicam has been implicated in the following serious adverse events: GI bleeding, MI, stroke, GI ulceration and perforation, anaphylactoid reactions, HTN, CHF, bronchospasm, nephrotoxicity, renal papillary necrosis, hepatotoxicity, exfoliative dermatitis, blood dyscrasias, anemia, toxic epidermal necrosis, Stevens-Johnson syndrome, thromboembolism [1,5].

Common events – meloxicam has been implicated in the following common adverse events: rash, urticaria, dyspepsia, nausea, abdominal pain, elevated liver transaminases, dizziness, somnolence, fluid retention, edema, tinnitus [1,5].

Conclusions

Meloxicam appears to have the advantage of reduced gastrointestinal morbidity; however, it is unclear whether it offers advantages over more selective COX-2 inhibitors such as celecoxib and etoricoxib. Although it offers the convenience of once-a-day dosing, its efficacy in reducing pain intensity appears to be inferior to diclofenac for management of degenerative joint disease. Despite lack of FDA approval, meloxicam has been advocated for acute pain management. Large-scale well-controlled trials will be required to asses its safety and effectiveness in this setting.

References

1. Mobic (meloxicam) Prescribing Information June 2008. U.S. Department of Health and Human Services. http://www.accessdata.fda.gov/drugsatfda_docs/label/2008/020938s018, 02153s006lbl.pdf. June 2008.

2. Van Hecken A, Schwartz JI, Depre M, et al. Comparative inhibitory activity of rofecoxib, meloxicam, diclofenac, ibuprofen, and naproxen on COX-2 versus COX-1 in healthy volunteers. *J Clin Pharmacol* 2000;**40**:1109–1120.

3. Hawkey C, Kahan A, Steinbru, et al. Gastrointestinal tolerability of meloxicam compared to diclofenac in osteoarthritis patients. *Rheumatology* 1998;37:937–945.

4. Kimura Satoko, Kontani Hioshi. Demonstration of antiallodynic effects of the cyclooxygenase-2 inhibitor meloxicam on established diabetic neuropathic pain in mice. *Journal of Pharmacological Sciences. The Japanese Pharmacological Society* 2009.

5. Epocrates Online. https://epocrates.com/u/10a2227/Mobic.

6. Panara M, Giulia R, Sciulli M. Dose-dependent inhibition of platelet cyclooxygenase-1 and monocyte cyclooxygenase-2 by meloxicam in healthy subjects. *J Pharmacol Exp Ther* 1999;290(1).

7. Lipscomb GR, Wallis N. Gastrointestinal tolerability of meloxicam and iroxicam: a double-blind placebo-controlled study. *Br J Clin Pharmacol* 1998;**46**: 133–137.

60

Buffered aspirin and oral salicylate

Jeanna Blitz

Generic Name: aspirin

Trade/Proprietary Name: Bayer Aspirin™, Bufferin™, Ecotrin™, Empirin™, Anacin™

Drug Class: anti-inflammatory drug

Manufacturers: Bayer Health Care, 100 Bayer Road, Pittsburgh, PA 15205; Bristol Myers-Squibb, 5 Research Pkwy, Wallingford, CT 06492–1996

Chemical Name: acetylsalicylic acid

Chemical Structure: see Figure 60.1

Description

Aspirin is a nonsteroidal anti-inflammatory drug (NSAID) that has analgesic and antipyretic properties. It can be used alone to treat minor to moderate acute and chronic pain as well as pain associated with cancer. It is also available as preparations combined with caffeine or with an opioid analgesic to treat moderate to severe acute and chronic pain. Aspirin can be buffered (with calcium carbonate, magnesium oxide, and magnesium carbonate), or enteric coated to decrease the risk of gastric side effects such as dyspepsia, gastritis, bleeding, and ulceration.

Mechanism of action

Aspirin works to decrease pain by inhibiting inflammation at the cellular level. Prostaglandins sensitize pain receptors in afferent nerve endings to histamine and bradykinin, which begin the sensation of pain. Like other NSAIDs, aspirin inhibits cyclooxygenase (COX): the enzyme responsible for converting arachidonic acid to prostaglandin. Aspirin nonspecifically inhibits both COX 1 and 2 by acetylating them. Aspirin is a more potent inhibitor of both prostaglandin synthesis and platelet aggregation than other salicylic acid derivatives. The differences

in activity between aspirin and salicylic acid are thought to be due to the acetyl group on the aspirin molecule.

Pharmacokinetics

Absorption

In general, immediate-release aspirin is well and completely absorbed from the gastrointestinal (GI) tract. Following absorption, aspirin is hydrolyzed to salicylic acid with peak plasma levels of salicylic acid occurring within 1–2 hours of dosing. The rate of absorption from the GI tract is dependent upon the dosage form, the presence or absence of food, gastric pH (the presence or absence of GI antacids or buffering agents), and other physiological factors. Enteric coated aspirin is absorbed in the small intestine, and its absorption is erratic. In clinical studies, enteric coated aspirin was associated with less gastritis and GI bleeding than buffered aspirin or standard aspirin.

Distribution

Salicylic acid is widely distributed to all tissues and fluids in the body including the central nervous system (CNS), breast milk, and fetal tissues. The highest concentrations are found in the plasma, liver, renal cortex, heart, and lungs.

Metabolism

Aspirin is rapidly hydrolyzed in the plasma to salicylic acid such that plasma levels of aspirin are essentially undetectable 1–2 hours after dosing. Salicylic acid is primarily conjugated in the liver to form salicyluric acid. Salicylic acid has a plasma half-life of approximately 6 hours. The clearance of aspirin is limited by the ability of the liver to conjugate salicyclic acid. After conjugation by the liver, the metabolites undergo renal excretion.

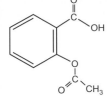

Figure 60.1. Molecular structure image obtained from The Chemical Heritage Foundation website.

Indications

Acute surgical pain

Aspirin is not often used for acute surgical pain due to its inhibition of platelet aggregation; however, it may be prescribed after minor surgery either alone, or in combination with an opioid analgesic such as oxycodone (trade name Percodan™). A common dose would be 1–2 tabs PO Q4h as needed. The combination of butalbital (a mild barbiturate), caffeine, and aspirin (trade name Fiorinol™) is approved for use in nonvascular headache and has been used to treat postdural puncture headache.

Medical pain and chronic non-malignancy pain

Aspirin may be used alone to treat mild to moderate somatic pain, or in combination with an opioid analgesic such as oxycodone or hydrocodone to treat more severe pain. The common dose of 650 mg of aspirin PO or PR has been demonstrated to be as efficacious as 10 mg of morphine administered IM. The maximum dose is 6 g/day in divided doses. It is often prescribed for the treatment of arthritis and other rheumatological pain. The dose of aspirin for the treatment of rheumatological pain is 3–4 g/day in divided doses. With regard to the treatment of migraines, 650 mg of aspirin can also be combined with 65 mg caffeine (trade name Anacin™), but with little increase in efficacy over aspirin alone.

Cancer pain

Aspirin and other NSAIDs are part of the World Health Organization (WHO) analgesic ladder. Doses of 325–650 mg PO or PR q4 hours are recommended for the treatment of mild to moderate somatic pain associated with cancer (Table 60.1).

Contraindications

Absolute

Aspirin is contraindicated in patients with a known allergy to nonsteroidal anti-inflammatory drugs (NSAIDs).

Aspirin also places patients at risk for gastrointestinal bleeding, ulceration and perforation. Patients with a history of significant GI bleeding or peptic ulcer disease should not be prescribed aspirin. Patients who are already taking another type of NSAID should not take aspirin, as this increases the risk for upper GI bleeding even more.

Patients with severe renal or hepatic failure should not be prescribed aspirin.

In addition, it should not be used in children or teenagers with viral infections (with or without fever) because of the risk of Reye's syndrome.

Aspirin is a Pregnancy Category D medication and should not be used in pregnant women.

Relative

Aspirin should be used with caution in patients with asthma or nasal polyps as it may cause urticaria, angioedema, and bronchospasm.

Table 60.1. Aspirin dosing table: acute and chronic pain, cancer pain, and headache

Drug	Dose	Route	Frequency	Maximum daily dose
Aspirin	325–650 mg	PO or PR	q4h	4–6 g
Aspirin + oxycodone (Percodan)	325 mg/4.5 mg	PO	1–2 tabs q4h	4–6 g
Aspirin + hydrocodone	500 mg/5 mg	PO	1–2 tabs q4h	4–6 g
Aspirin + caffeine (Anacin)	650 mg/65 mg	PO	1–2 tabs q4h	4–6 g
Aspirin + caffeine + butalbital (Fiorinol™)	330 mg/40 mg/50 mg	PO	1–2 tabs q4–6h	4 g
Aspirin + caffeine + butalbital + codeine (Fiorinol-C™)	330 mg/40 mg/50 mg /15 mg	PO	1–2 tabs q4–6s	4 g

Patients with preexisting coagulation abnormalities such as liver disease, vitamin K deficiency or hemophilia should avoid aspirin because of its ability to inhibit platelet aggregation.

Patients who are on a sodium-restricted diet should avoid taking buffered aspirin preparations that contain a high concentration of sodium.

Aspirin may increase levels of lithium and enhance toxicity of valproic acid.

The efficacy of oral hypoglycemic medications is also enhanced by moderate to high doses of aspirin.

Renal clearance of methotrexate is inhibited by aspirin; the increased serum levels of methotrexate can lead to bone marrow toxicity.

Fluid retention from an inhibition of renal prostaglandins may exacerbate heart failure. See Table 60.2 for a summary of contraindications.

Drug abuse and dependence

There is no known potential for addiction associated with the use of aspirin.

Common doses and routes of administration

Aspirin may be administered via either the oral (PO) or rectal (PR) route. The common dose is 325–650 mg q4 hours. The maximum dose is approximately 6 g/day. This is due to the fact that aspirin exhibits a ceiling effect, where higher doses do not provide any greater pain relief and are associated with a higher risk of toxicity and side effects.

Potential advantages

- Inexpensive (cost as monotherapy): enteric coated $13.99 for 325-mg tabs 1000/ bottle, buffered aspirin $10.99 for 500-mg tabs 130/ bottle
- Easy to use and administer
- Opioid-sparing as multimodal analgesia
- There is no known potential for addiction associated with the use of aspirin.

Potential disadvantages

- Salicylate toxicity can occur at very high doses (150–500 mg/kg). See below for description of signs, symptoms and treatment of salicylate toxicity.
- Drug interactions occur with many commonly prescribed medications such as oral hypoglycemic agents, valproic acid, methotrexate, lithium, and ACE inhibitors.
- The ceiling effect of aspirin limits the amount of pain relief that can be expected from this agent alone.
- Although enteric coated aspirin is associated with a reduction in gastric side effects, its absorption is less reliable, making consistent dosing difficult.

Drug-related adverse events

Many adverse reactions due to aspirin ingestion are dose-related. Table 60.3 is a list of adverse reactions that have been reported in the literature.

Salicylate toxicity may result from acute ingestion (overdose) or chronic intoxication. Symptoms start to occur at plasma concentrations of 200 μg/mL and increase in severity as plasma levels reach 300–400 μg/mL. Severity of aspirin intoxication is determined by measuring the blood salicylate level. The earliest sign of overdose is usually tinnitus. Respiratory alkalosis is another early sign: the patient's respiratory center is directly stimulated, causing hyperventilation. However, in more severe cases of toxicity, metabolic acidosis ensues, resulting in a raised gap metabolic acidosis: the salicylate overdose inhibits the citric acid cycle and uncouples oxidative phosphorylation, leading to hypercarbia, and an increase in ketones and lactic acid production. The kidneys

Table 60.2. Contraindications to aspirin

Absolute
Known allergy to NSAIDS
Significant GI bleed or peptic ulcer disease
Renal failure
Hepatic failure
Children or teenagers with viral illness (risk of Reye's syndrome)
Pregnant women
Relative
Asthma or nasal polyps (risk of angioedema, bronchospasm)
Preexisiting hypercoaguable state
Sodium-restricted diet
Patients taking lithium or valproic acid
Patients taking oral hypoglycemics
Patients taking methotrexate
Heart failure

Table 60.3. Potential adverse events

Significant adverse events

   Salicylate toxicity

   Reye's syndrome

   GI bleeding, perforation, ulceration and gastritis

Less common adverse events

   General: fever, hypothermia, thirst

   Cardiovascular: dysrhythmias, hypotension, tachycardia

   Fluid and electrolyte: dehydration, hyperkalemia, metabolic acidosis, respiratory alkalosis

   Gastrointestinal: transient elevation of LFTs, hepatitis, pancreatitis

   Hematological: prolongation of prothrombin time, coagulopathy, thrombocytopenia

   Musculoskeletal: rhabdomyolysis

   Metabolism: hyperglycemia, hypoglycemia (in children)

   Reproductive: prolonged labor, low birth weight infants, antepartum and postpartum bleeding

   Urogenital: interstitial nephritis, papillary necrosis, proteinuria, renal insufficiency/failure

secrete potassium, sodium, and bicarbonate, resulting in an alkaline urine. The severe acid–base and electrolyte disturbances may be complicated by hyperthermia and dehydration. The treatment of salicylate toxicity consists of supporting vital functions, increasing salicylate elimination, and correcting the acid–base disturbance: acid–base status should be closely followed with serial blood gas and serum pH measurements. Gastric emptying and/or lavage is recommended as soon as possible after ingestion, even if the patient has vomited spontaneously. After lavage and/or emesis, administration of activated charcoal is beneficial, if less than 3 hours have passed since ingestion. Fluid and electrolyte balance should also be maintained: urinary alkalinization can be performed by administering an IV bolus of sodium barcarbonate 1–2 mEq/kg and then maintaining a constant infusion of D5W with 100–150 mEq/L of sodium bicarbonate and potassium chloride 20–40 mEq/L at 1.5–2.5 mL/kg per h. Serum electrolytes need to be closely monitored along with urine pH. The goal is to maintain alkalinization of the urine at a pH 7.5–8. Serum glucose levels must also be closely monitored: although the patient may at first be hyperglycemic, this may soon lead to hypoglycemia, which will worsen any CNS symptoms of agitation and delirium.

In severe cases, hyperthermia and hypovolemia are the major immediate threats to life.

Dialysis can be performed to reduce the total body drug content. In patients with renal insufficiency or in cases of life-threatening intoxication, it is usually required.

Reye's syndrome is a rare but potentially fatal disease of encephalopathy and hepatitis after ingestion of aspirin. This syndrome most commonly occurs in children (age 4–12) who have recently suffered from influenza, chicken pox, or an upper respiratory infection associated with a fever that was treated with aspirin. The disease usually starts with vomiting that gives way to agitation, lethargy, and coma or seizures. Abnormal LFTs may also occur. Because there is no specific treatment for Reye's syndrome, supportive treatment is recommended.

References:

1. Rainsford KD, ed., Ch 4: Pharmacokinetics and metabolism of the salicylates; Ch 10: Salicylates in the treatment of acute pain. In *Aspirin and Related Drugs*. Boca Raton: CRC Press, 2004, pp. 97–137, 587–607.

2. Barkin RL. Acetaminophen, aspirin, or ibuprofen in combination products, 2001analgesic products. *Am J Ther* 2001;**8**:433–442.

3. Hamilton RJ, ed. *Tarascon Pocket Pharmacopoeia* 2009 Deluxe Edition. Sudbury, MA: Jones and Bartlett, pp. 5–7.

NSAIDs

Acetaminophen oral and rectal

Komal D. Patel

Generic Name: acetaminophen

Proprietary Names: Tylenol[R], Acephen™

Manufacturers: McNeil-ppc, Inc., Fort Washington, PA (Tylenol); Grand W Labs, South Plainfield, NJ (Acephen™)

Drug Class: analgesic and antipyretic, miscellaneous

Chemical Name: *N*-acetyl-para-aminophenol

Chemical Structure: see Figure 61.1

Formula: $C_8H_9NO_2$

Mode of activity

Major and minor sites of action

Acetaminophen produces analgesia by inhibiting prostaglandin synthesis in the central nervous system and peripherally. It produces antipyresis by inhibition of the hypothalamic heat-regulating center, resulting in peripheral vasodilatation and increased dissipation of heat.

Metabolic pathways

Acetaminophen is metabolized primarily in the liver by glucuronidation and sulfation to non-toxic metabolites. Less than 15% is metabolized by the cytochrome P450 enzyme system to a highly reactive intermediate *N*-acetyl-*p*-benzoquinoneimine (NAPQI), which is conjugated with glutathione and inactivated. At toxic doses glutathione conjugation becomes insufficient to meet the metabolic demand, causing an increase in NAPQI concentration, which may cause hepatic cell necrosis.

Clearance and elimination

Peak plasma levels occur between 10 and 60 minutes after oral dose. Elimination half-life is 1–3 hours in adults and 2–5 hours in neonates. Excreted primarily in urine (2–5% unchanged, 55% as glucuronide metabolites, 30% as sulfate metabolites) [1]. The bioavailability of rectal acetaminophen is variable. It is approximately 80% of that of an oral dose and the rate of absorption is slower, with maximum plasma concentrations achieved about 2–3 hours after administration.

Indications (approved/non-approved)

Surgical pain

Oral and rectal acetaminophen is used as a non-opioid analgesic to treat mild to moderate post-operative pain of nonvisceral origin, particularly after ambulatory surgery. Higher doses of rectal acetaminophen (40–60 mg/kg) have been shown to have a morphine-sparing effect in day-case surgery in children [2]. In combination with nonsteroidal anti-inflammatory drugs (NSAIDs) or opioids, acetaminophen is also used in management of moderate to severe post-operative pain and cancer pain [3]. Commonly used analgesic combinations with opioids are Tylenol 1, 2, 3, and 4 (with codeine 10 mg, 15 mg, 30 mg, and 60 mg respectively), Percocet (with oxycodone), Vicodin (with hydrocodone), and Darvocet (with propoxyphene napsylate). These combinations are available only by prescription.

Medical pain

Acetaminophen is commonly used for relief of fever and headaches and is a major ingredient in numerous cold and flu remedies. It is also used in multi-ingredient preparations for migraine headache, tension headache, and vascular headaches.

Chronic non-malignancy pain

Acetaminophen in doses <4 g/day is recommended as a first-line medication for many chronic pains such as back pain and arthritis by the American Pain Society. It is less effective in arthritis pain than NSAIDs.

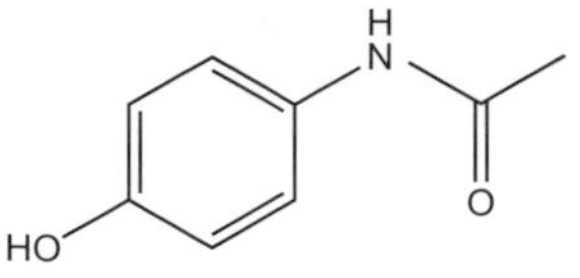

Figure 61.1.

Cancer pain

The World Health Organization's (WHO) three-step analgesic ladder for cancer pain control recommends using acetaminophen alone for mild pain (step 1) and in combination with opioids for moderate pain (step 2).

Contraindications

Absolute: hypersensitivity to acetaminophen or any component of the formulation.

Relative: in patients who consume more than three alcoholic drinks per day, acetaminophen may increase the risk of liver damage. In patients with G6PD deficiency, acetaminophen may induce hemolysis.

Common doses

Adult (oral or rectal): 325–650 mg every 4–6 hours or 1000 mg 3–4 times per day. Maximum dose 4 g/day.

Children < 12 years old (oral or rectal): 10–15 mg/kg/dose every 4–6 hours as needed. Maximum 5 doses in a day.

Renal impairment: Clcr 10–15 mL/minute – administer every 6 hours. Clcr < 10 mL/minute – administer every 8 hours.

Potential advantages

Ease of use, availability: acetaminophen is a readily available over-the-counter medicine. It is available in many different formats (tablet, caplet, liquid suspension, suppository) for self-medication.

Tolerability, reduction of adverse events: in recommended doses, acetaminophen does not irritate the lining of the stomach, affect blood coagulation as much as NSAIDs or affect the function of the kidneys. It is safe in pregnancy and does not affect the closure of the fetal ductus arteriosus as NSAIDs can. Unlike aspirin, acetaminophen is safe in children as it is not associated with a risk of Reye's syndrome in children with viral illnesses. Unlike opioids, acetaminophen does not cause euphoria, alter mood, or pose a risk of addiction, dependence, tolerance, and withdrawal.

Cost: relatively inexpensive generic versions are available over-the-counter as well as in hospitals.

Potential disadvantages

Toxicity: accidental or intentional acetaminophen overdose (7.5–10 g in adults; >150 mg/kg in children) can cause hepatotoxicity, which is the most common cause of acute liver failure in the USA. Toxicity from acetaminophen is not from the drug itself but from one of its metabolites, NAPQI. Normally this metabolite undergoes conjugation with glutathione, but at toxic doses conjugation depletes glutathione. This in combination with direct cellular injury by NAPQI leads to hepatic cell necrosis. It is usually asymptomatic initially. Symptoms related to hepatotoxicity may develop over 1–5 days: anorexia, nausea, vomiting, right upper quadrant pain, diaphoresis, jaundice, hypoglycemia, coagulation defects, encephalopathy, and renal failure. Treatment of acetaminophen overdose includes administration of oral activated charcoal – to decrease absorption of acetaminophen and N-acetylcysteine – as an antidote which acts as a precursor for glutathione. If damage to the liver becomes severe, a liver transplant is often required.

Drug interactions: anticonvulsants (phenytoin, barbiturates, carbamazepine) increase the risk of hepatotoxicity by increasing conversion of acetaminophen to toxic metabolites. Isoniazide also increases risk of acetaminophen hepatotoxicity. Acetaminophen may enhance the anticoagulant effect of warfarin with daily doses > 1.3 g for > 1 week. Phenothiazines may increase risk of severe hypothermia with acetaminophen. Cholestyramine resin may decrease the absorption of acetaminophen.

Drug-related adverse events

Serious adverse events: hypersensitivity – rare. Hepatotoxicity as described above. In patients with G6PD deficiency, acetaminophen can cause hemolysis.

Less common adverse events: other rare adverse reactions with acetaminophen include rash, anemia, neutropenia, pancytopenia; increase in bilirubin, alkaline phosphatase, ammonia, chloride, uric acid, glucose; decrease in sodium, bicarbonate and calcium. Frequency of these adverse reactions not defined.

References

1. McEvoy GK, ed. Acetaminophen. In *AHFS Drug Information 2003*. Bethesda, MD: American Society of Health-System Pharmacists, 2003, pp. 2077–2085.

257

2. Korpela R, Korenoja P, Meretoja OA. Morphine-sparing effect of acetaminophen in pediatric day-case surgery. *Anesthesiology* 1999;91(2).

3. Romsing J, Moiniche S, Dahl JB. Rectal and parenteral paracetamol, and paracetamol in combination with NSAIDs, for postoperative analgesia. *Br J Anaesth* 2002;88:215–226.

Section 4
Chapter

62

NSAIDs

Acetaminophen injectable

Vivian K. Lee and Jonathan S. Jahr

Generic Name: intravenous acetaminophen or paracetamol

Chemical Name: *N*-acetyl-para-aminophenol

Proprietary Name: Perfalgan, Ofirmev™

Manufacturer: Bristol-Myers Squibb Pharmaceuticals (Europe), Cadence Pharmaceuticals, San Diego, CA (USA and Canada)

Distributor: currently submitted for FDA approval, not yet distributed in the USA

Class: antipyretic, analgesic, anesthetic adjunct

Chemical Structure: see Figure 62.1

Description

Intravenous acetaminophen is a synthetic, non-opiate, centrally acting analgesic and antipyretic derived from *p*-aminophenol. It is recommended as a first-line analgesic in mild to moderate acute pain states and is effective in combination with other analgesics for more severe pain. Another available parenteral form is the prodrug propacetamol, which is rapidly hydrolyzed by esterases in the blood to acetaminophen. A dose of 2 g propacetamol is hydrolyzed to 1 g of acetaminophen. Studies have shown these doses to be bioequivalent. However, propacetamol is less favorable because it is associated with pain at the injection site or along the vein where it is infused. Additionally, propacetamol is supplied in powder form and requires reconstitution, whereas IV acetaminophen is supplied in a ready-to-use form.

Mode of activity

Major site of action: the mechanism of action of acetaminophen is not clearly understood. It is a centrally acting inhibitor of cyclooxygenases with weak peripheral effects.

Receptor interactions: the antipyretic and analgesic effects of acetaminophen have been attributed to inhibition of prostaglandin synthesis by blocking the cyclooxygenase-2 pathway in vascular endothelial cells and neurons. Acetaminophen acts as a reducing co-substrate for the peroxidase-active site of the prostaglandin H2 synthase. It has a variable capacity to inhibit prostaglandin production in different tissues and cells, which explains its weak antiplatelet and anti-inflammatory effects at recommended doses. It may also act as an NMDA receptor antagonist and inhibit production of nitric oxide, a molecule important in nociception. Acetaminophen activity has also been associated with the 5-HT3 receptor.

Onset of analgesia: occurs within 5–10 minutes. Peak analgesic effect is obtained in 1 hour and its duration is approximately 4–6 hours.

Onset of antipyretic effects: occurs within 30 minutes. Duration is at least 6 hours.

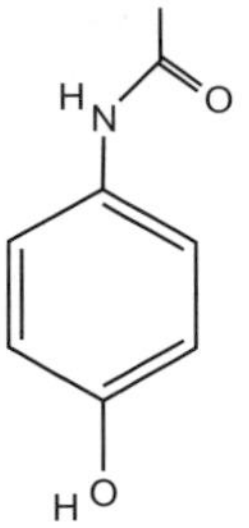

Figure 62.1.

Distribution: readily crosses the blood–brain barrier as well as the placenta (but does not adversely affect the fetus at therapeutic doses). Does not extensively bind to plasma proteins.

Metabolism: acetaminophen is 90–95% metabolized in the liver by conjugation with sulfate and glucuronide to inactive compounds. At higher doses, the drug is metabolized in the liver by the cytochrome P450 enzyme CYP2E1.

Elimination: metabolites are predominantly eliminated in the urine as glucuronide and sulfide conjugates. Less than 5% of the drug is excreted unchanged in the urine, and less than 1% is eliminated in bile.

Half-life: 2.7 hours.

Indications

Intravenous acetaminophen is currently undergoing FDA approval for the short-term treatment of mild to moderate pain and fever in adult and pediatric patients. It has already been in use in numerous countries worldwide since 2002.

In the peri-operative setting, the parenteral form of acetaminophen is preferred because most patients are unable to tolerate oral medications and/or may have unpredictable gastrointestinal function following surgery. Intravenous administration can achieve effective levels in a shorter time with predictable drug levels compared to oral and rectal forms. Additionally, it has demonstrated superior analgesia at least in the first hour after it is administered and a longer duration of action. In clinical trials, it has demonstrated an adverse reaction profile similar to that of placebo, and is therefore an appropriate analgesic option for patients undergoing ambulatory surgery. IV acetaminophen can also be used as an adjunct to other analgesics. In theory, it can reduce the amount of opiates required for post-operative pain, potentially leading to reduced narcotic-related adverse effects, earlier ambulation, and shorter hospital stays.

Contraindications

Absolute: intravenous acetaminophen is absolutely contraindicated in patients in fulminant hepatic failure.

Relative: severe chronic alcohol abusers may be at increased risk of liver toxicity from acetaminophen exceeding the recommended doses. Any disorder leading to glutathione depletion, such as malnourishment or viral illness with dehydration, may decrease the tolerance for acetaminophen. Acetaminophen should be used with caution in patients with severe hepatic impairment, although hepatoxicity has not been shown to occur at the recommended doses. In patients with severe renal impairment, the minimum interval re-dosing of the drug should be increased to 6 hours.

Common doses

General: IV acetaminophen is available as a 1 g infusion that does not require reconstitution. It should be administered over 15 minutes and can be given through a peripheral IV. It is comparable to other IV analgesics for the treatment of moderate post-operative pain (see Table 62.1).

Adults: for adults weighing > 50 kg, the recommended dose is 1 g every 4–6 hours, with a maximum of 4 g per day. For adults weighing < 50 kg, the dose is 15 mg/kg every 4–6 hours, with a maximum of 3 g per day.

Elderly: the pharmacokinetics of IV acetaminophen are unchanged in the elderly. No adjustment in dosage is necessary for older patients.

Pediatric: for children weighing >33 kg, the dose is 15 mg/kg every 4–6 hours, with a maximum of 3 g per day. For children weighing 10–33 kg, the dose is 15 mg/kg every 4–6 hours, with a maximum of 2 g per day. For full-term newborn infants, infants, toddlers and children weighing < 10 kg, the dose is 7.5 mg/kg, with a maximum of 30 mg per kg per day.

Table 62.1. Efficacy of IV acetaminophen 1 g versus other IV analgesics in post-operative pain

Dose	Comparable efficacy
IV acetaminophen 1 g	Ketorolac 30 mg
	Diclofenac 100 mg
	Metamizol 2.5 g
	Morphine 10 mg

Efficacy may depend on type of surgery performed.

Potential advantages

Intravenous acetaminophen has advantages over its prodrug form proparacetamol. Unlike proparacetamol, IV acetaminophen is rarely associated with pain at the infusion site because it has a pH and osmolarity more similar to that of plasma. The lower rate of local intolerance improves patient compliance. Moreover, proparacetamol is supplied as a powder and must be dissolved in saline or glucose immediately before infusion, and is therefore costly, time-consuming, and more prone to dosing or administration error by the healthcare provider. There have also been reports of contact dermatitis in healthcare providers handling the powder, which can be avoided with ready-to-use IV acetaminophen.

Effective blood concentrations of IV acetaminophen can be achieved intra-operatively prior to emergence from anesthesia. This has been the potential for faster discharge for ambulatory surgery. Additionally, intravenous administration is more efficient, faster, and longer-acting than oral administration of acetaminophen. The pharmacodynamic effect appears to correlate well with CSF levels. Achieving an earlier and higher concentration appears to be responsible for the superior early efficacy of IV acetaminophen compared to other routes of administration. Pharmacokinetic modeling suggests that avoidance of first-pass hepatic metabolism by the intravenous route reduces the potential for hepatoxicity.

When used as monotherapy, IV acetaminophen does not cause excessive sedation, biliary spasm, respiratory depression, nausea, vomiting, ileus, or pruritus associated with opioids, nor the harmful cardiovascular, renal, gastrointestinal, and hematological effects associated with NSAIDs and COX-2 inhibitors.

Studies also indicated that differences in the variables studied did not have significant impact on IV APAP's efficacy. A reduction in narcotic requirements has been shown in adult patients undergoing dental, orthopedic, or gynecological surgery (see Table 62.2). For example, in a combined study of three randomized, placebo-controlled trials, acetaminophen 1000 mg given intravenously following major orthopedic surgery significantly reduced both narcotic requirements (by 33 to 63%) and the need for opioid rescue. It is likely that the efficacy as an anesthetic adjunct is also dependent on the type of surgery.

When used in conjunction with opiate analgesics, the narcotic-sparing effect of IV acetaminophen is

Table 62.2. Randomized, controlled trials with IV acetaminophen for post-operative pain

Surgery	Patients	Treatment	Anesthesia	Treatment timing and duration	Scale	Outcome	Ref
Orthopedic	Hospitalized adults 22–87 years	2 g prop vs. 1 g para vs. placebo	General	Given post-op every 6 hours for 24 hours	VAS, VRS	Prop and para both significantly reduced morphine consumption over 24-h period	4
Tonsillectomy	Ambulatory adults 16–40 years	1 g para vs. placebo	General	Given post-op every 6 hours for 24 hours	VAS	Para significantly reduced meperidine consumption over 24-h period	5
Cardiac surgery	Adults 45–79 years	1 g para vs. placebo	General	15 min before end of surgery and every 6 hours for 72 hours	VAS	Para significantly reduced pain at rest and at 12 hours, nonsignficant reduction in morphine consumption	6
Total abdominal hysterectomy	Hospitalized women	1 g para vs. placebo	General	Given once either 30 min before surgery or prior to skin closure	VAS	Preemptive para significantly reduced post-op morphine consumption, no hemodynamic effects	7

prop, proparacetamol; para, paracetamol; VAS, visual analog scale; VRS, visual rating scale.

controversial. Studies seem to indicate that although IV acetaminophen as an adjunct significantly improved patient satisfaction regarding post-operative analgesia, it did not necessarily reduce opioid-related side effects.

Beyond post-operative analgesia, randomized controlled trials have demonstrated that IV acetaminophen 1000 mg administration resulted in a statistically significant reduction in fevers in the post-operative setting compared to placebo. A reduction in fevers represents an indirect measure of IV APAP's efficacy. Additionally, it may also suggest that in the proper clinical setting, IV APAP's use as post-operative pain treatment may lead to a reduction of unnecessary fever workups in the immediate post-operative period.

In aggregate these trials indicate IV acetaminophen (known outside the USA as paracetamol) is an effective analgesic in a variety of surgical procedures. IV acetaminophen was well tolerated and has multiple direct and indirect benefits when used for post-operative pain management.

Potential disadvantages

Adverse events

Adverse reactions related to the use of the intravenous formulation of acetaminophen are extremely rare – less than 1 in 10 000. It has demonstrated a safety profile similar to that of placebo. Adverse events include hypotension, malaise, hypersensitivity reaction, elevated hepatic transaminases, thrombocytopenia, and pain at the infusion site.

Serious adverse events

Hepatotoxicity does not occur at recommended doses of acetaminophen. Administration of 2 g, or twice the recommended dose, of intravenous paracetamol in healthy subjects has been shown to stay far below the threshold of hepatotoxicity. When ingested at high doses, acetaminophen is metabolized to N-acetyl-p-benzoquinone-imine (NAPQI). NAPQI is rapidly conjugated with glutathione to a nontoxic compound. The depletion of glutathione results in the accumulation of NAPQI that is responsible for liver injury. Acetaminophen has a narrow therapeutic window and even minor overdoses may cause severe hepatic injury. Liver necrosis occurs at 7.5–10 g of acetaminophen.

Drug-related adverse events

Drug interactions

The cytochrome P450 enzyme CYP2E1 is responsible for metabolizing acetaminophen to NAPQI. Drugs that induce CYP2E1 may enhance toxicity. Potential drug interactions include alcohol, long-term anticonvulsant use, probenecid, and salicylamide. Caution should be taken and a reduced dose of acetaminophen should be considered when patients are on any of these drugs. Administration of acetaminophen to patients on coumadin may also be associated with elevated international normalized ratio (INR) values. Additional monitoring of INR values for these patients is recommended for up to 1 day after stopping acetaminophen.

Treatment of adverse events

Acetaminophen exceeding the recommended daily doses can be treated with the administration of N-acetylcysteine, and should be given regardless of time of ingestion. N-acetylcysteine is a precursor of glutathione and increases the availability of glutathione for NAPQI metabolism. It is most effective if given within 8–10 hours of acetaminophen ingestion. Progression to fulminant liver failure requires continuously monitoring in an intensive care unit and evaluation for liver transplantation.

References

1. Duggan ST, et al. Intravenous paracetamol (acetaminophen). *Drugs* 2009;**69**(1):101–113.
2. Remy C, et al. State of the art of paracetamol in acute pain therapy. *Curr Opin Anaesthesiol* 2006;**19**:562–565.
3. Jahr JS, et al. Chapter 21: Nonselective nonsteroidal anti-inflammatory drugs, COX-2 inhibitors, and acetaminophen in acute perioperative pain. In Sinatra RS, de Leon-Casasola OA, Ginsberg B, Viscusi ER, eds. *Acute Pain Management*. New York: Cambridge University Press, 2009, pp. 332–365.
4. Sinatra RS, Jahr JS, Reynolds LW, et al. The analgesic efficacy and safety of single and repeated administration of intravenous paracetamol (acetaminophen) 1 g for the treatment of post-operative pain following orthopedic surgery. *Anesthesiology* 2005;**102**:822–831.
5. Atef A, Aly Fawaz A. Intravenous paracetamol is highly effective in pain treatment after tonsillectomy in adults. *Eur Arch Otorhinolaryngol* 2007;**265**(3):351–355.

6. Cattabriga I, et al. Intravenous paracetamol as adjunctive treatment for post-operative pain after cardiac surgery: a double blind randomized controlled trial. *Eur J Cardio-thorac Surg* 2007;**32**(3):527–531.

7. Arici S, et al. Preemptive analgesic effects of intravenous paracetamol in total abdominal hysterectomy. *Agri* 2009;**21**(2):54–61.

8. Göröcs TS, et al. Efficacy and tolerability of ready-to-use intravenous paracetamol solution as monotherapy or as an adjunct analgesic therapy for postoperative pain in patients undergoing elective ambulatory surgery: open, prospective study. *Int J Clin Pract* 2009;**1**:112–120.

9. Jahr JS, Reynolds LW, Royal MA, Pan CP, Breitmeyer JB. A posthoc analysis of a randomized, double-blind, placebo-controlled study of IV acetaminophen for the treatment of postoperative pain after major orthopedic surgery. *Reg Anesth Pain Med* 2009; PS1:10.

10. Royal MA, Gosselin NH, Pan C, Moukassi S, Breitmeyer JB. Route of administration may significantly impact hepatic acetaminophen exposure. *Reg Anesth Pain Med* 2009;PS1:17.

11. Royal MA, Fong L, Pan C, Breitmeyer JB. IV acetaminophen administered to treat postoperative pain significantly decreases the incidence of patient reporting of postoperative fever. *Reg Anesth Pain Med* 2009;PS1:16.

12. Smith HD, Pan C, Breitmeyer JB, Royal MA. Acetaminophen produces clinically meaningful pain response and opioid sparing effect after major orthopedic surgery: Pooled data from three randomized, placebo controlled trials. *Reg Anesth Pain Med* 2009;PS1:21.

13. Breitmeyer JB, Smith HD, Sweeney K, Royal MA. CSF penetration of acetaminophen is an important determinant of efficacy. *Reg Anesth Pain Med* 2009;PS1:4.

14. Macario A, Royal MA. A systematic literature review of randomized clinical trials of intravenous acetaminophen (paracetamol) for acute postoperative pain. *Reg Anesth Pain Med* 2009;PS2:6.

Section 4
Chapter

63

NSAIDs

Fiorinal and Fioricet

Alexander Timchenko

Trade Names: Fiorinal™, Fioricet™

Generic Names: acetaminophen, butalbital, plus caffeine compound; aspirin, butalbital, plus caffeine compound

Manufacturer: Watson Pharmaceuticals, Inc., 311 Bonnie Circle, Corona, CA 92880

Drug Class: anti-headache medication, Rx

Drug Structures: aspirin (Figure 63.1), 2-acetyloxy-benzoic acid, $C_9H_8O_4$; molecular wt 180.16; acetaminophen (Figure 63.2), 4'-hydroxyacetanilide, $C_8H_9NO_2$; molecular wt 151.17; caffeine (Figure 63.3), 1,3,7-trimethylxanthine, $C_8H_{10}N_4O_2$; molecular wt 194.19; butalbital (Figure 63.4), 5-allyl-5-isobutylbarbituric acid, $C_{11}H_{16}N_2O_3$, molecular wt 224.26

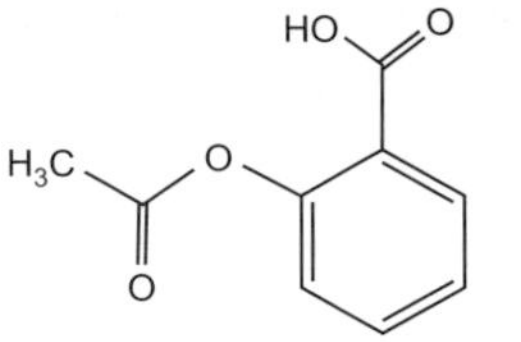

Figure 63.1.

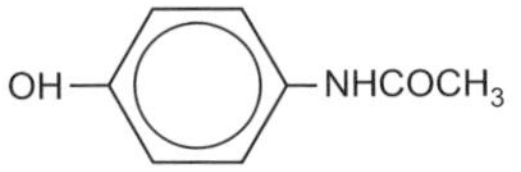

Figure 63.2.

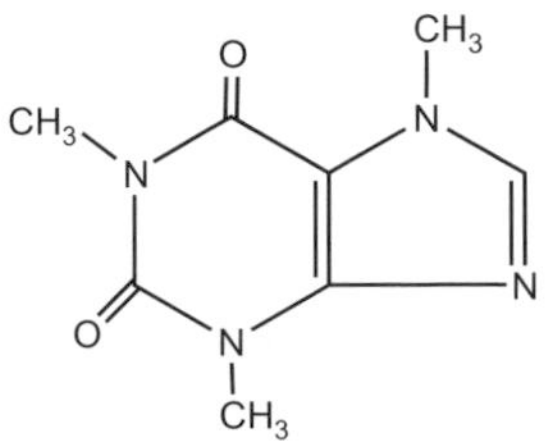

Figure 63.3.

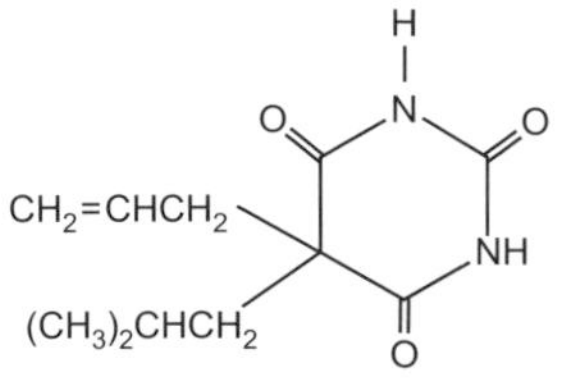

Figure 63.4.

Introduction

Chronic headache represents one of the major medical and socio-economic issues patients face. Approximately 4% of the US population suffers from frequent headaches. Of these, 37% or 1.5% of the population experience daily headaches [1,2].

The pathophysiology of tension-type headache is incompletely understood. Experimental studies suggest that it may be caused by increased excitability of the CNS generated by repetitive and sustained pericranial myofacial input [3]. Peripheral nociceptive factors may play a role in the episodic form of tension headache, whereas central sensitization predominates in the chronic form. Epidemiological studies report an increased familial risk in tension-type headaches [4].

Currently, there is no specific abortive treatment for a tension-type headache (TTH). Self-medication constitutes the most common treatment. Among headache sufferers, 91% of TTH and 90% of migraine patients use non-opioid, over-the-counter analgesics, which are often taken without any other form of treatment and without consulting a physician. A community-based telephone survey demonstrated that 98% of TTH sufferers depend on OTC medications [5–7].

Fiorinal and Fioricet are known as combination analgesics that were introduced to the market as medications for abortive treatment of headache. Fiorinal was formulated in 1950s and contained phenacetin as well as aspirin, caffeine, and butalbital. Later, the phenacetin was withdrawn from the market in the 1960s and compound Fiorinal thereafter consisted of aspirin 325 mg, caffeine 40 mg and butalbital 50 mg. At the time of reformulation, Fioricet was introduced to the market, substituting acetaminophen 325 mg for aspirin [8].

Fioricet is a combination analgesic medication, prescribed as one to two tablets every 4 hours as needed. Each tablet contains:

- acetaminophen USP – 325 mg; non-opiate, non-salicylate analgesic and antipyretic
- butalbital USP – 50 mg; (5-allyl-5-isobutylbarbituric acid) – short-to-immediate acting barbiturate, provides anxiolysis and muscle relaxation
- caffeine USP – 40 mg; (1, 3, 7 – trimethylxanthine) – central nervous system stimulant

Fiorinal is a combination analgesic medication, prescribed as one to two capsules every 4 hours as needed, total daily dose should not exceed 6 capsules. Each tablet contains:

- aspirin USP – 325 mg; analgesic, antipyretic and anti-inflammatory
- butalbital USP – 50 mg; (5-allyl-5-isobutylbarbituric acid) – short- to immediate-acting barbiturate, provides anxiolysis and muscle relaxation
- caffeine USP – 40 mg; (1,3,7-trimethylxanthine) – central nervous system stimulant

Indications

Fioricet and Fiorinal are indicated for the relief of the complex of symptoms known as tension headache. Fioricet is also widely employed for relief of postdural puncture headache (PDPHA), although it is not approved by the FDA for this indication. The mechanism of the drug effect is not completely understood.

Contraindications

Fioricet or Fiorinal are contraindicated in case of known hypersensitivity to any of their components.

263

Fioricet should be prescribed with caution in patients with known liver or kidney insufficiency. Liver and renal function laboratory tests should be performed to ensure safety when using the medication.

Pharmacokinetics and pharmacodynamics

Since Fiorinal and Fioricet are combined medications the brief overview of each component should be given.

Acetaminophen (Fioricet) is rapidly absorbed from the gastrointestinal tract and is distributed throughout most body tissues. The plasma half-life is from 1.25 to 3 hours, but may be increased in liver insufficiency or in the case of medication overdose. Elimination occurs by conjugation in the liver and excretion of conjugates in urine. Acetaminophen 1000 mg provided improvement similar to that of acetylsalicylic acid 650 mg in 269 TTH patients in a controlled study [9]. In well-controlled trials both aspirin (500 and 1000 mg) and acetaminophen (1000 mg but not 500 mg) were superior to placebo in the treatment of TTH [10].

Aspirin (Fiorinal) – systemic availability after oral intake is highly dependent on the dosage form, the presence of food, the gastric pH, antacids, the gastric emptying time, and particle size. During the absorption process and following the absorption, aspirin is mainly hydrolyzed to salicylic acid and distributed to all body tissues and fluids, including fetal tissues, breast milk, and the central nervous system. In plasma, about 50–80% of the salicylic acid and its metabolites are bound to proteins. The elimination of therapeutic doses is through the kidneys in the form of salicylic acid or biotransformation products. Aspirin causes irreversible inhibition of cyclooxygenase. In addition to inhibition of pro-inflammatory mediators, acetylsalicylic acid induces endogenous anti-inflammatory factors. Compared to placebo, aspirin was more effective in reducing headache from severe to mild or in achieving pain relief 1 h after administration. A range of aspirin dosages between 650 mg and 1000 mg proved to be considerably more successful for pain reduction than placebo [9,11].

Caffeine is rapidly absorbed and distributed in all body tissues and fluids, including CNS, fetal tissues, and breast milk. Elimination is by biotransformation in liver and renal excretion of metabolites. Some authors believe that caffeine alone might have analgesic properties for specific types of pain in humans and in human experimental pain models. Caffeine when used in combination with simple analgesics was reported to shift the dose-response curve to the left and enhance analgesic properties of simple analgesics by about 40% [12]. Six randomized, double-blind, two-period crossover studies showed the caffeine-containing analgesics were significantly superior both to placebo and to 1000 mg acetaminophen [13]. Other studies showed that caffeine provided no adjuvant analgesic effect when added to aspirin in patients with post-operative pain [14].

Butalbital is readily absorbed and distributed in most tissues in the body. This component can appear in breast milk and readily cross the placental barrier. Butalbital is excreted in urine as unchanged drug and as metabolites. The effect of butalbital alone has not been studied since butalbital is not available except in combination products. Barbiturates have anti-anxiety and muscle-relaxant properties. Barbiturates do not have analgesic action per se. Another potentially beneficial effect of butalbital is to antagonize the unwanted central stimulant effect of caffeine [8].

Clinical studies of Fiorinal and Fioricet

Information obtained from the Food and Drug Administration's web resource indicates that Fioricet lacks evidence supporting the efficacy and safety of its use. Fiorinal's effectiveness in treatment of tension headache was demonstrated in double-blind, placebo-controlled multicenter studies. Fiorinal was shown to be more effective clinically as compared to its components prescribed separately.

The literature describing randomized double-blind studies of effectiveness of Fiorinal and Fioricet is very limited. In one study Fiorinal PA, aspirin 200 mg and acetaminophen 200 mg (replacing the phenacetin in the old formulation) with caffeine 40 mg and butalbital 50 mg were compared to placebo. Among patients, 84% responded to treatment, compared to placebo response of 27% ($P < 0.05$) [15,16]. In another study, Fioricet (acetaminophen 325 mg, caffeine 40 mg, and butalbital 50mg) was statistically more effective when compared to placebo [17].

Side effects and precautions

The most frequently reported adverse reactions with use of Fiorinal and Fioricet were drowsiness, light-headedness, dizziness, sedation, shortness of breath, nausea, abdominal pain, and intoxicated feeling.

When these drugs were the only ones implicated, there were nine reports presented to the Food and Drug Administration on Fiorinal and 16 attributed to Fioricet. Serious adverse events associated with Fiorinal were one case of acute overdose and two cases of hepatic and renal failure related to prolonged (more than 10 years) use. Serious adverse effects associated with Fioricet use were one case each of pancreatitis and multisystem illness, three deaths due to overdose, three cases of coma (presumably secondary to overdose), and two cases of other encephalopathy due to overdose. Drug dependence was reported twice. In short, serious adverse events were almost always associated with acute overdose (e.g. ingestion of 30 pills) or prolonged (e.g. 10 years) overuse [8].

Caution should be taken when using Fiorinal (aspirin-containing) in patients with hemorrhagic diathesis (e.g. hemophilia, hypoprothrombinemia, von Willebrand's disease, thrombocytopenia, thrombasthenia, and other platelet disorders; severe vitamin K deficiency and severe liver disease) or on anticoagulation therapy. Fiorinal is contraindicated in patients with peptic ulcer or other gastrointestinal lesions. In Fioricet (acetaminophen-containing) use the most serious adverse effect from overdosing is hepatic necrosis; other effects include renal tubular necrosis and hypoglycemic coma.

Caffeine is a CNS stimulant, which may account for such adverse effects as cardiac stimulation, palpitations, irritability, insomnia, delirium, tremor, and hyperglycemia. Toxic dose for adults is 1 g (25 tablets).

Fioricet and Fiorinal can be habit-forming and addicting due to the presence of butalbital as a component [7]. Therefore, extended use is not recommended. As tolerance develops, the amount of medication needed to maintain the same level of response increases. Withdrawal seizures were reported in a 2-day-old infant whose mother had taken butalbital-containing medication during the last 2 months or pregnancy. Butalbital was found in the infant's plasma. Butalbital may impair mental or physical abilities required for the performance of potentially hazardous tasks such as driving a car or operating machinery. Butalbital as a short-acting barbiturate may enhance the CNS depressant effect of narcotic analgesics, alcohol, tranquilizers, and sedative-hypnotics. Toxicity from barbiturate poisoning may include drowsiness, confusion, and coma. The toxic dose of butalbital for adults is 1 g (20 tablets). At present, the main argument for removing butalbital-containing compounds from the market is not the obvious abuse and overuse that may occur with any drug. Rather, it is the insidious overuse that does not cause systemic symptoms, but may cause the evolution of episodic primary headaches to chronic headache [18].

Other serious side effects associated with use of combination analgesics is medication-overuse headache. Medication-overuse headache is an inherent risk of abortive treatment of headache in general and TTH is no exception. Medication-overuse headache implies a consumption of simple analgesics for 15 days/month or more, and opioid or combination analgesics for 10 days/month or more, and therefore represents a challenge in chronic TTH patients suffering from daily headache. Therefore, frequent intake of simple analgesics or NSAIDs should be avoided and patients should be thoroughly informed about this [19, 20].

Summary

Fioricet and Fiorinal are old polypharmaceutical preparations used for abortive treatment of chronic headache and PDPHA unresponsive to "over the counter" analgesics containing aspirin, acetaminophen, or NSAIDs. What was the reason for use of combination analgesics instead of making a separate prescription for each of three components? The advantages of combination analgesics are cost, convenience, and compliance. Clearly, a single pill containing the three components is less expensive than purchasing each component separately [8]. These factors may outweigh the benefits of the cumbersome tailoring of the doses of three drugs to the patient's needs. Although Fioricet may provide greater gastrointestinal safety than Fiorinol, the lack of an anti-inflammatory component may limit its effectiveness in controlling the dural irritative aspects of PDPHA. When clinically indicated, it may be prudent to combine Fioricet and an NSAID (ibuprofen, celecoxib, naproxen) for additive relief of inflammatory pain.

Combination analgesics represent important alternatives for those patients who cannot or should not take vasoconstricting medications or opioids. The acetaminophen compound of Fioricet is also a major alternative to those patients who cannot use NSAIDs. Nevertheless, Fioricet and Fiorinal contain the short-acting barbiturate butalbital and may be habit-forming and addictive. Serious adverse effects may be associated with acute overdose or prolonged overuse.

References

1. Ostergaard S, Russel MB. Comparison of first degree relatives and spouses of people with chronic tension headache. *Br Med J* 1997:**314**:1092–1093.

2. Sher AI, et al. Prevalence of frequent headache in a population sample. *Headache* 1998:**38**:497–506.

3. Lenaerts M. Pharmacotherapy of tension-type headache (TTH). *Expert Opin Pharmacother* 2009:**10**(8):1261–1271.

4. Russel MB, et al. Inheritance of chronic tension-type headache investigated by complex segregation analysis. *Hum Genet* 1998:**102**:138–140.

5. Edmeads J, et al. Impact of migraine and tension-type headache on life-style, consulting behavior, and medication use: a Canadian population survey. *Can J Neurol Sci* 1993;**20**:131–137.

6. Pfaffenrath V, Scherzer S. Analgesics and NSAID in the treatment of the acute migraine attack. *Cephalgia* 1995;**15**(Suppl 5):14–20.

7. Ashina M. Pathophysiology of tension-type headache: potential drug targets. *CNS and Neurol Disord Drug Targets* 2007:**6**:238–239.

8. Solomon S. Butalbital-containing agents: should they be banned? No. *Curr Pain Headache Rep* 2002;**6**:147–150.

9. Farinelli I, Martelletti P. Aspirin and tension-type headache. *J Headache Pain* 2007:**8**:49–55.

10. Lipton RB, et al. Aspirin is efficacious for the treatment of acute migraine. *Headache* 2005;**45**:283–292.

11. Steiner TJ, et al. Aspirin in episodic tension-type headache: placebo-controlled dose-ranging comparison with paracetamol. *Cephalgia* 2003;**23**:59–66.

12. Migliardi JR, et al. Caffeine as an analgesic adjuvant in tension headache. *Clin Pharmacol Ther* 1994;**56**(5):576–586.

13. Laska EM, et al. Caffeine as an analgesic adjuvant. *JAMA* 1984;**251**:1711–1718.

14. Bigal ME, et al. Advances in the pharmacologic treatment of tension-type headache. *Curr Pain Headache Rep* 2008;**12**:442–446.

15. Friedman AP, DiSerio FJ. Symptomatic treatment of chronically recurring tension headache: a placebo-controlled multicenter investigation of Fioricet and acetaminophen with codeine. *Clin Ther* 1987:**10**:69–81.

16. Thorpe P. Controlled and uncontrolled studies on "Fiorinal PA" for symptomatic relief in tension headache. *Med J Aust* 1970:**2**:180–181.

17. Diener HC, et al. The fixed combination of acetylsalicylic acid, paracetamol and caffeine is more effective than single substances and dual combination for the treatment of headache: a multicentre, randomized, double-blind, single-dose, placebo-controlled parallel group study. *Cephalgia* 2005;**25**:776–787.

18. Bigal ME, et al. Acute migraine medication and evolution from episodic to chronic migraine: a longitudinal population-based study. *Headache* 2008;**48**:1157–1168.

19. Lenaerts ME, Couch JR. Medication overuse headache. *Minerva Medica* 2007;**98**:221–231.

20. Mathew NT, et al. Transformation of episodic migraine into daily headache: analysis of factors. *Headache* 1982;**22**: 66–68.

Overview of local anesthetics

Lars E. Helgeson and Raymond S. Sinatra

Introduction

Local anesthetics (LA) represent a class of analgesic compounds that block trans-membrane sodium channels and reduce conduction safely in peripheral, spinal, and cortical axons [1–3]. Local anesthetics were first employed in South American cultures, where coco leaf poultices were found to provide effective topical analgesia when applied to wounds [1]. The active ingredient in coco leaf was later isolated by Albert Niemann in 1860 and named cocaine. Niemann noted that when tasted, small amounts of purified cocaine produced localized numbing of his tongue. In 1884 Carl Koller began using cocaine topically for ophthalmological surgery [1,2]. Since that time, a number of local anesthetics have been developed, utilized and abandoned. Ester-based LAs, including procaine, were first to be commercially developed and utilized in clinical practice. Amide LAs were developed later in the 1950s, the first being lidocaine.

Chemical structure

Local anesthetics all contain a lipophilic aromatic ring, a hydrophilic tertiary amine and an ester or amide linkage. The general chemical structures of amide and ester anesthetics are illustrated in Figure 64.1.

Local anesthetics are broadly classified either as "amide" or "ester" based on the nature of the linkage between the lipophilic aromatic ring and the hydrophilic amine. A simple way to distinguish an amide from an ester is the presence of an "i" in the name of the generic drug (excluding the -caine). For example, lidocaine is an amide, whereas tetracaine is an ester.

There are multiple agents which, when administered appropriately, have safe and effective anesthetic and analgesic effects. Local anesthetics are pharmacologically distinguished by differences in the aromatic ring and/or tertiary amine. Chemical groups attached to the aromatic ring influence speed of onset, while groups attached to the tertiary amine influence lipid/aqueous solubility and anesthetic potency.

Mode of action

In contrast to most drugs used in anesthesia and pain medicine, local anesthetics are only effective when deposited on or in the vicinity of the nerve fibers to be blocked. Local anesthetics act by reversibly interfering with both the initiation and propagation of neuronal action potentials (nerve impulses). They do this by decreasing or eliminating Na^+ influx in the voltage-gated sodium channels at the nodes of Ranvier [2–4]. The result is an inability to raise axonal membrane potential to threshold and conduction blockade. Some local anesthetics (benzocaine, and biotoxins such as tetrodotoxin) physically block the Na^+ channel. Most others diffuse through the axonal plasma membrane and bind to an internal receptor site located on the internal portion of the ion channel [2–5] (Figure 64.2) Local anesthetic binding results in configurational alterations in the ion channel that limit or prevent futher Na^+ conductance. Some local anesthetics (bupivacaine, ropivacaine) can also block the sodium channel directly by a process termed "frequency-dependent blockade". These spindle-shaped amides can fit directly through the ion channel during axonal depolarization. Once they pass the channel they can directly bind to the receptor site and prevent further Na^+ conductance. This process of selective neural blockade is highly efficient and effectively turns off those fibers that are firing most frequently. The ability to selectively block nerve fibers in proportion to their firing frequency underscores the clinical phenomenon termed differential blockade, whereby specific noxious fibers may be blocked to a greater extent than other sensory or motor fibers [2–5]. For example, low concentrations of bupivicaine and levo-bupivicaine block conduction in C fibers with greater selectivity than procaine and tetracaine, which are less effective

The Essence of Analgesia and Analgesics, ed. Raymond S. Sinatra, Jonathan S. Jahr and J. Michael Watkins-Pitchford. Published by Cambridge University Press. © Cambridge University Press 2011.

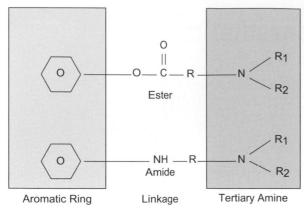

Figure 64.1. Chemical components of ester- and amide-based local anesthetics.

at low concentrations and block all fiber types equally at high concentration. Differential block offers advantages in multiple settings, including the following:

(1) labor analgesia, where selective blockade of noxious fibers and sparing of sensory motor fibers may offer advantages;

(2) upper extremity block, where surgical pain is differentially blocked and perfusion is improved, while motor function is maintained;

(3) treatment of complex regional pain syndrome (CRPS), where autonomic fibers are preferentially blocked over motor fibers.

Other neuroanatomical factors responsible for differential block are discussed in the sections that follow.

Physiochemical correlates of local anesthetic activity

A number of LA physiochemical properties have been classically advocated to explain the pharmacokinetics of this drug class. In recent years a number of investigators have challenged these ideas [2,4,5] as being overly simplistic or incomplete explanations. Nevertheless, some degree of correlation between pKa, lipid solubility, and protein binding and onset/duration of LA effect have been described [3,4]. The pKa of a particular local anesthetic dictates its functionality and onset of activity. If the pKa is approximately physiological pH [7,4] the portion of drug in its uncharged

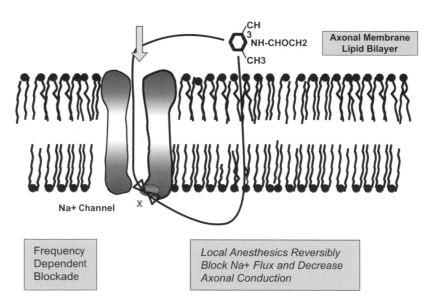

Figure 64.2. Local anesthetics can block sodium conductance and reduce conduction safety by two mechanisms. Most local anesthetics bind to a receptor located on the inner portion of the sodium channel and initiate a conformational change that closes the ion channel. Local anesthetics reach this site by diffusing across the axonal membrane. Highly charged local anesthetics have difficulty crossing this barrier although the charged moiety is able to bind the receptor more efficiently. Local anesthetics having a pKa close to physiological pH have 50% of drug ionized and 50% un-ionized. This optimal ratio allows enough uncharged molecules to pass through the membrane yet provides enough charged molecules to bind at the sodium channel receptor site. Some local anesthetics such as bupivacaine and ropivacaine are spindle-shaped and can penetrate the ion channel directly, but only when it opens during an action potential. These agents can rapidly reach and more efficiently bind to the receptor as they do not have to diffuse through the axonal membrane. This mechanism which allows actively firing nerve fibers to become selectively blocked in the presence of relatively low concentrations of LA is termed frequency-dependent neural blockade.

form is nearly equivalent to the charged form. The drug is therefore less ionized and can more rapidly pass through the internodes or axonal membranes to reach its internal site of action [3,4]. This explains why the onset time of lidocaine (pKa = 7.6) is more rapid than bupivacaine (pKa = 8.5). Lidocaine's time to onset can be further reduced by the addition of bicarbonate. The low pKa of chloroprocaine also implies a slow onset; however, the higher concentration (3%) of drug solution can overcome this drawback, resulting in rapid onset of effect [2,4]. Localized infection decreases the tissue pH, which increases the number of charged molecules and often results in decreased neural penetration. This may explain why LAs are less effective in infected and ischemic tissue.

Local anesthetic potency correlates with increasing lipid solubility, which is influenced by the polar groups attached to the tertiary amine. Like other anesthetics and analgesics, the more lipid-soluble the LA, the more potent it is. In other words, less drug is needed to achieve the desired anesthetic blockade. Highly lipid soluble LAs include tetracaine and bupivacaine [2–4].

Duration of activity has been related to the degree of protein binding of the local anesthetic, the concentration of the local anesthetic, and the addition of epinephrine to LAs that are intrinsic vasodilators (lidocaine, tetracaine). Drugs with high protein binding attach to intra-membrane proteins in axons, Schwann cells, and endoneurium and epineurium, to the extent that a reservoir of LA molecules remains sequestered at the site of deposition and is less likely to be removed by blood circulation in the vasa nervorum. This reservoir is able to maintain prolonged neural blockade by replacing LA that dissociates from the receptor site [3].

Neuro-anatomical correlates of noxious blockade

Certain aspects of neural anatomy and ultrastructure favor LA blockade of noxious impulses [2–5]. To reduce conduction safely in sensory and motor fibers, at least three myelin inter-nodes must be blocked. This "rule of three" favors blockade of thin unmyelinated fibers and also A-delta fibers which have small internodal distances. Larger A-alpha and A-beta fibers are more resistant to blockade because of their size and large distance between nodes of Ranvier (Figure 64.3). Unmyelinated C fibers are easiest to block since LAs can impede Na^+ conductance and action potential propagation at any single site along the course of the nerve fiber.

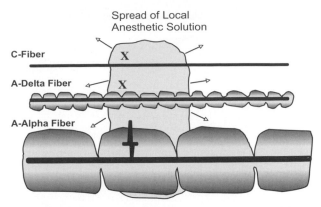

Figure 64.3. The "rule of three" suggests that a minimum of three internodes must be blocked by local anesthetic to reduce salutatory conduction safely to the point that an action potential will no longer be propagated along the nerve fibers. Because of the large internodal distance of thick myelinated A-alpha and A-beta fibers, a relatively large amount of surface must be bathed in local anesthetic solution in order to ensure conduction blockade. Smaller A-delta fibers have relatively small internodal distances, and three or more nodes can be more easily blocked (X). Unmyelinated C fibers do not employ salutatory conduction and are particularly vulnerable to local anesthetic blockade. Propagation of action potentials can be prevented by local anesthetic blockade at any point along the course of the nerve fiber.

Additional factors which have significant impact on LA activity include the thickness of the peripheral or spinal nerve and its epineural and perineural coverings, as well as its microscopic anatomy. Increasing the concentration of a drug will speed its onset and intensity of blockade but may also increase its systemic toxicity. An exception is chloroprocaine, which has a very rapid onset due to its delivery concentration of up to 3%, and its ability to penetrate thick fibrous connective tissues making up the perineurium and epineurium. Epidural administration of 2,4-chloroprocaine is effective in eliminating a commonly observed L5–S1 root anesthetic window, as it can rapidly penetrate into this very thick mixed nerve and establish anesthetic conditions.

The microscopic anatomy of peripheral mixed nerves also has an influence on the fiber types that are blocked. It takes time for LA to diffuse through the nerve and a concentration gradient develops, whereby higher levels of drug occur at the peripheral site of deposition, and progressively lower levels accumulate in the central core. In general, unmyelinated fibers and A-delta fibers are segregated to the outermost regions of the nerve (mantle) and are first to be blocked and last to recover. Motor and larger sensory fibers are located primarily in the core and tend to be more slowly and less effectively blocked, and are first to recover [2–4] (Figure 64.4). This finding as well as the above-described

269

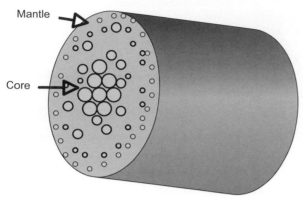

Mixed Sensory Motor Nerve

Mantle

Core

- ○ C-Fibers (unmyelinated)
- ● A-Delta Noxious Fibers
- ◎ A-Beta Sensory Fibers
- ◯ A-Alpha Motor Fibers

Figure 64.4. Anatomical correlates of local anesthetic blockade. In mixed sensory nerves, noxious C fibers and A-delta fibers are generally localized to the outer regions of the nerve (Mantle), while greater numbers of larger motor and sensory fibers are localized in the center of the nerve (Core). Because of a concentration gradient from the site of local anesthetic deposition to the center of the nerve, the mantle fibers are first to be blocked and last to recover. As local anesthetic diffuses further into the nerve, core fibers are blocked; however, they are first to recover. This orientation of fibers favors selective conduction blockade in noxious fibers and analgesic effects that outlast the duration of sensory/motor anesthesia.

"rule of three" help to explain the rapidity and increased intensity of blockade, and prolonged duration of LA effect on smaller-caliber noxious fibers, compared to sensory and motor fibers [2,4,5]. The usual sequence for differential blockade of various fiber types with low to increasing concentrations of local anesthetic is autonomic > noxious > cold > warm > light touch > deep touch > proprioception > motor fibers. In summary, LA blockade of proprioceptive and motor function occurs more slowly and often incompletely due to the greater degree of myelination, large intranodal distances, and core location of these fiber types.

Metabolism

Inactivation of LA clinical effect occurs by diffusion away from the neuronal Na^+ channels and by uptake into the vas nervorum and into the systemic circulation. It is here that metabolic inactivation of the linkage between the aromatic ring and tertiary amine can occur. The mechanism and site are very different for the amide and ester local anesthetics.

Ester linkages are metabolized primarily by pseudocholinesterase, plasma cholinesterase and red

blood cell esterase (minor). Hydrolysis occurs at the ester linkage, resulting in an alcohol and para-aminobenzoic acid (PABA) (or its derivatives). The formation of PABA is a major drawback of ester-linked LAs as it is responsible for mild to severe allergic reactions.

Amide linkages are metabolized in the liver by one of three pathways: aromatic hydroxylation, N-dealkylation, and amide hydrolysis.

Conditions which delay diffusion from the nerve fiber into the vasculature will prolong the duration of action of these drugs. The most common method to prolong LA duration is by the addition of a vasoconstrictor (epinephrine, clonidine) [6–8]. The microvasculature constricts resulting in a decreased blood flow and slowed drug uptake by the blood. Decreased uptake can also occur with hypothermia, hypotension and hypovolemia [3–5].

Site of injection is an important determinant in uptake and is dependent on tissue vascularity. The more vascular tissues have a faster drug uptake than less vascular tissue. Sites of injection with faster to slower uptake are noted as follows: intercostal > caudal > epidural > brachial plexus > femoral/sciatic > intrathecal.

Indications

Local anesthetics are used to locally anesthetize a wide range of specific body parts or areas to allow painless surgery. Local anesthetics are most commonly used for dental procedures and repair of lacerations. They can also be used to provide neural blockade for larger, more painful procedures. Sites of LA application include localized injection, peripheral nerve blocks as well as central nerve blockade. The only safe agents which can be utilized for intravenous regional anesthesia (Bier block) are lidocaine and prilocaine. Other typical indications are outlined in Table 64.1.

Contraindications

An allergic reaction to specific agents is an obvious contraindication. Allergy to para-aminobenzoic acid (PABA) is a contraindication to use of ester local anesthetics due to the fact that PABA is a metabolic product of ester metabolism. Methylparaben is a common preservative chemically similar to PABA and likewise can cause an allergic reaction. Metabisulfite is a commonly used preservative that may also cause allergic reactions but more notably is neurotoxic when used intrathecally. Local anesthetics containing any preservative should not be used intrathecally. Ester local

Table 64.1. Local anesthetic applications

		Drugs
Topical	Ophthalmic	Tetracaine
	Nasal	Cetacaine
	Skin – intact and abrasions	EMLA
	Oral	Cetacaine
	Laryngeal	Cetacaine
	Uretheral	Lidocaine
Infiltration	Field block	Lidocaine
		Ropivacaine
		Bupivacaine
		Levobupivacaine
	Specific nerve block (brachial plexus, ankle, intrabulbar, dental, etc.)	Lidocaine
		Bupivacaine
		Ropivacaine
		Levobupivacaine
	Intravenous regional	Lidocaine
Neuraxial	Intrathecal	Bupivacaine
		Tetracaine
	Epidural	Lidocaine
		Bupivacaine
		Ropivacaine
		Levobupivacaine
Other	Trigger point	Bupivacaine
	Chronic regional pain syndrome	Lidocaine

Table 64.2. Temporal sequence of lidocaine toxicity

Numb tongue
Lightheadedness
Visual/auditory (ringing sound)
Muscle twitching
Unconsciousness
Seizures
Coma
Respiratory arrest
Cardiovascular depression

The addition of morphine and fentanyl to intrathecal and epidurally administered local anesthetics decreases local anesthetic dose requirements while reducing surgical and post-operative pain intensity. One exception is chloroprocaine, which may antagonize epidural opioid analgesic effects.

Dosages

Correct dosing of LAs is primarily dependent on the particular agent, total amount of drug administered (mg/kg), and nerve or area to be injected. Descriptions of specific nerve blocks and appropriate LA dosages are described elsewhere. The onset duration and toxic doses of specific LAs are presented in Table 64.3.

Advantages

These agents reliably un-bind from their sites of action leaving no lasting effects. They are well tolerated and considered to be very safe when administered properly.

They are generally predictable regarding their individual onset times and durations of action. Varying the concentration and volume coupled with the addition of vasoconstrictors allows the duration and degree of blockade to be customized to whatever specific surgical or patient requirements present.

In the immediate post-operative period, patients can experience little to no pain, allowing for significant narcotic sparing, thereby minimizing narcotic-associated adverse effects.

Conduction blockade prior to incision can lessen the imprinting in the spinal cord of the nociceptive pathways thereby lessening the level of pain experienced over the next several days. The exact nature of this "wind-up" is being investigated.

anesthetics should be avoided in patients with atypical plasma cholinesterase due to slowed metabolism that can lead to enhanced local anesthetic toxicity. Total dosage must be monitored, with attention to avoiding the toxic dose and continous monitoring of symptoms. The clinical symptomatology of lidocaine toxicity is presented in Table 64.2.

Local anesthetic + opioid – additive analgesic

There is an additive anesthetic effect when combining local anesthetics with opioid analgesics. There are well-documented spinal opioid receptors in the dorsal horn, and up-regulation of opioid receptors has been described in chronically inflamed peripheral nerves.

Table 64.3. Onset of action (infiltration)

		Onset (minutes)	Duration (hours)	Prolongation with epinephrine	Toxic dose with single administration
Ester	Procaine	3–5	½–1	++	10–12 mg/kg
	Chloroprocaine	10	½–1	++	10–12 mg/kg
	Tetracaine	<15	2–3+	++	2 mg total
	Benzocaine (topical)	<2	½+	++	200 mg total
Amide	Lidocaine	<2	½–1	++	4–5 mg/kg (7 with epinephrine)
	Bupivacaine	5	2–4	+/−	1.7 mg/kg (2 with epinephrine)
	Mepivacaine	<5	¾–1½	++	4–5 mg/kg (7 with epinephrine)
	Prilocaine	<2	1		8–10 mg/kg
	Ropivacaine		1½–3	+/-	3 mg/kg

Pre-incision conduction blockade may also decrease the incidence of developing a surgical site chronic pain syndrome.

These agents are available at low cost and can present significant cost savings, especially when considering the pharmacological costs of general anesthesia, shorter PACU times and less management time needed to address pain post-operatively. Additionally, some patients are able to be discharged sooner with fewer (immobility) complications such as deep venous thrombosis, ileus, and pulmonary atalectisis.

LAs may be combined neuraxially with opioids to gain additive analgesic benefits.

Esters are less cardiotoxic and neurotoxic than amides due to their rapid metabolism by plasma cholinesterase.

Amides offer several clinical advantages over esters, particularly fewer allergic reactions and easier titratability.

Disadvantages

These agents must be delivered directly to the desired nerve bundle. The delivery is often a problem due to technical issues accessing these anatomical sites, particularly cervical, brachial plexus, lumbar plexus, sciatic, and popliteal blocks. This is commonly the reason for inadequate neural blockade. There may be other issues precluding needle or catheter placement, such as patient cooperation, infection, or coagulation concerns.

All of these agents have some degree of neurotoxicity, which is dose and exposure duration dependent; particularly the amide agents.

Systemic dosage toxicity is related to several factors (Table 64.4). In addition to dosage and rapid vascular uptake, toxicity may also be metabolism-dependent. Rapidly metabolized agents such as chloroprocaine are less toxic. Agents (especially in a large dose) placed in highly vascular tissues are more rapidly absorbed by the blood which can quickly reach toxic levels, compared to less vascular tissues [8].

Adverse events

Situations which affect the level or efficacy of pseudo-cholinesterase can significantly alter the duration of action and toxicity of ester local anesthetics. This is more likely in premature infants, individuals with atypical pseudocholinesterase production or advanced liver disease.

Allergic reactions are very rare, but occur more commonly with the ester local anesthetics. Ester local anesthetics should be avoided in known PABA-allergic patients. Other allergic reactions may be due to the preservative methylparaben, which is chemically similar to PABA.

Table 64.4. Factors affecting systemic toxicity of local anesthetics

Site of injection	High perfusion tissues results in faster blood uptake
Dosage	Larger dosage results in faster uptake
Vasoconstrictors	Decreases blood flow with decreased uptake
Metabolism	Minimal, except in liver failure (amides)

Toxicity is a concern with either unintentional IV administration or rapid vascular uptake from tissue [8]. Central nervous system symptoms are the most common type of toxic reaction to local anesthetics. Initial symptoms are excitatory (dizziness, visual, and auditory) followed by CNS depression such as unconsciousness, seizures, and coma. Some agents are reasonably benign such as lidocaine, prilocaine or chloroproacaine, but others such as bupivicaine or tetracaine can result in seizures or fatal ventricular arrhythmias. Depending on the agent, dosage and injection location, treatment of toxicity may not be necessary. For example, symptoms may rapidly resolve without required treatment, such as lidocaine-associated dizziness or numb lips. Other agents may only require supportive care such as oxygen. Required supportive care may be airway and ventilatory support, seizure treatment, blood pressure support, and arrhythmia control. In cases of systemic toxicity due to bupivicaine, IV administration of a fat emulsion is effective [9]. Refer to Table 64.5.

Prilocaine can result in methemoglobinemia, when the total dose exceeds 600 mg.

Lidocaine and mepivicaine when given intrathecally have been associated with transient neurological syndrome, causing intrathecal nerve injury resulting in prolonged pain radiating to one or both legs. Although usually of short duration, it can last up to several months.

Chloroprocaine when administered intrathecally may result in prolonged sensory or motor deficits. This is most probably due to the bisulfate preservative and/or its very low pH.

Cauda equine syndrome is associated with intrathecal micro-catheters delivering a high concentration of lidocaine (and perhaps the preservatives). It consists of prolonged neural injury with motor weakness, significant pain and other sensory changes. These catheters are no longer in use.

Clinical presentation of systemic toxicity is variable, depending on the specific agent. Several agents are so rapidly metabolized that toxicity symptoms are very rarely seen, as with procaine and chloroprocaine. Different drugs present toxic symptoms in different sequence. For example, lidocaine first presents with dizziness or a numb tongue whereas bupivicaine is generally associated with dose-dependent depression of myocardial contractility and conduction and may result in fatal ventricular dysrhythmias.

Table 64.5. Treatment of bupivacaine cardiac toxicity

- Fat emulsion 20% (Intralipid™)
- Bolus 1.5 mL/kg over 1 minute – may repeat 1×
- Infusion 0.25 mL/kg per min until stable

Maximum total 8 mL/kg

References

1. Calatayud J, Gonzalez A. History of the development and evolution of local anesthesia since the coca leaf. *Anesthesiology* 2003;**98**:1503–1508.

2. Butterworth J. Local anesthetics in regional anesthesia and acute pain management. In Sinatra RS, de Leon-Casasola OA, Ginsberg B, Viscusi ER, eds. *Acute Pain Management.* London: Cambridge University Press, 2008.

3. Arthur GR. Pharmacokinetics. In Strichartz GR, ed., *Local Anesthetics. Handbook of Experimental Pharmacology*, vol. 81. Berlin: Springer, 1987, pp. 165–186.

4. Strichartz GR, Sanchez V, Arthur GR, et al. Fundamental properties of local anesthetics. II. Measured octanol:buffer partition coefficients and pKa values of clinically used drugs. *Anesth Analg* 1990;**71**:158–170.

5. Butterworth J, Ririe DG, Thompson RB, et al. Differential onset of median nerve block: randomized, double-blind comparison of mepivacaine and bupivacaine in healthy volunteers. *Br J Anaesth* 1998;**81**:515–521.

6. Chambers WA, Littlewood DG. Anesthesia with hyperbaric bupivacaine: effect of added vasoconstrictors. *Anesth Analg* 1982;**61**:49.

7. Ilfeld BM, Morey TE, Thannikary LJ, et al. Clonidine added to a continuous interscalene ropivacaine perineural infusion to improve postoperative analgesia: a randomized, double-blind, controlled study. *Anesth Analg* 2005;**100**:1172–1178.

8. Mather LE, Copeland SE, Ladd LA. Acute toxicity of local anesthetics: underlying pharmacokinetic and pharmacodynamic concepts. *Reg Anesth Pain Med* 2005;**30**:553–566.

9. Rosenblatt MA, Abel M, Fischer GW, et al. Successful use of a 20% lipid emulsion to resuscitate a patient after a presumed bupivacaine-related cardiac arrest. *Anesthesiology* 2006;**105**:217–218.

Generic Name: bupivacaine

Trade/Proprietary Names: Marcain, Marcaine, Sensorcaine and Vivacaine

Manufacturer: AstraZeneca, London, UK, and Södertälje, Sweden

Drug Class: local anesthetic (amino amide)

Chemical Structure: see Figure 65.1

Chemical Name: 1-butyl-N-(2,6-dimethylphenyl)piperidine-2-carboxam: $C_{18}H_{28}N_2O$

Mode of activity

Major and minor sites of action: nerve cells, sodium channels, pain nerve fibers.

Receptor interactions: bupivacaine binds to the intracellular portions of sodium channels and blocks sodium influx into nerve cells which therefore prevents nerve cell depolarization. Since pain-transmitting nerve fibers tend to be thinner (small diameter) and either unmyelinated or only lightly myelinated (myelin is non-polar and lipophilic), the local anesthetic agent can diffuse more readily into them than into thicker and more heavily myelinated nerve fibers such as touch and proprioception.

Metabolic pathways/drug clearance and elimination: bupivacaine is bound to plasma proteins in varying degree. It undergoes hepatic metabolism (via conjugation with glucuronic acid) and renal excretion (4–10% unchanged).

Indications (approved/non-approved)

Surgical acute pain: bupivacaine is indicated as a local anesthetic and used for infiltration, peripheral nerve block, nerve plexus blockade, epidural, and intrathecal (spinal) anesthesia and analgesia. It can be used as a single-shot injection or administered through a catheter for prolonged anesthesia and/or analgesia.

For example: bupivacaine often is administered by epidural injection before total hip arthroplasty. It also is commonly injected into surgical wound sites to reduce pain for up to 20 hours after the surgery. Bupivacaine is often co-administered with adrenaline to prolong the duration of its action. It may be combined with opioids for epidural and subarachnoid analgesia. Bupivacaine may also be combined with glucose (dextrose), resulting in a hyperbaric (increases density of the local anesthetic solution above that of cerebrospinal fluid) solution; sterile water resulting in a hypobaric (decreases density of the local anesthetic solution above that of cerebrospinal fluid, "floats") solution; and mixed with cerebrospinal fluid prior to injection to create an isobaric (commercially available solutions are commonly formulated with sodium chloride) solution for spinal anesthesia. An understanding of the baricity of the combined local anesthetic solution will permit an ability to direct the solution in the subarachnoid space toward the appropriate spinal nerves innervating the surgical site. For obstetrical procedures, only the 0.25% and 0.5% concentrations are indicated for obstetrical anesthesia.

Medical pain: oral surgery procedures as well as diagnostic and therapeutic procedures where a local anesthetic is necessary.

Chronic non-malignancy pain: as an anesthetic and analgesic option when patients present with medical pain or for acute surgical pain needs.

Cancer pain: useful for somatic, visceral, or neuropathic pain.

Contraindication

Absolute: bupivacaine is contraindicated for IV regional anesthesia (IVRA, Bier block) because of the potential risk of tourniquet failure and systemic absorption of a toxic volume of the drug. Bupivacaine is contraindicated in obstetrical paracervical block anesthesia as its use in this technique has resulted in

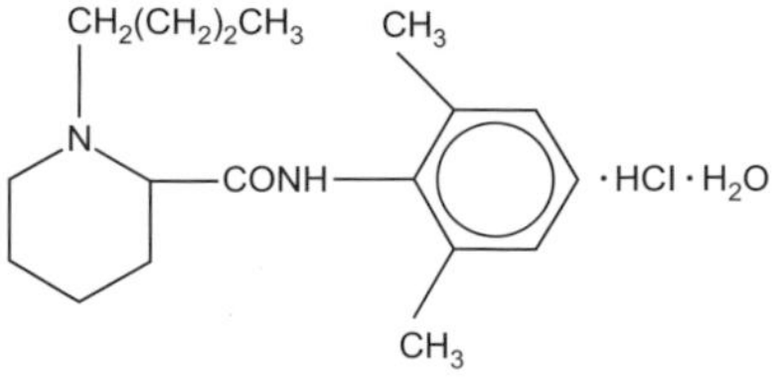

Figure 65.1.

fetal bradycardia and death. Bupivacaine is contraindicated in patients with a known hypersensitivity to it or to any agent of the amide type or to other components of bupivacaine solutions.

Relative: the dose of bupivacaine varies with the anesthetic procedure, the area to be anesthetized, the vascularity of the tissues, the number of neuronal segments to be blocked, the depth of anesthesia and degree of muscle relaxation required, the duration of anesthesia desired, individual tolerance, and the physical condition of the patient. Dosages of bupivacaine should be reduced for young, elderly and/or debilitated patients and patients with cardiac and/or liver disease. The rapid injection of a large volume of local anesthetic solution should be avoided.

Common doses

Parenteral and topical routes of administration: maximum single dose for an average 70 kg adult is 175 mg. Local infiltration 0.25–0.75%, peripheral nerve block 0.25% and 0.5%, retrobulbar block 0.75% (15–30 mg), and sympathetic block 0.25% (50–125 mg).

Neuraxial: dose is determined by vertebral level of initial block placement and desired dermatome level of anesthesia/analgesia. Sympathetic block 0.25%, spinal 0.25–0.75% (6–15 mg), lumbar and thoracic epidural (25–150 mg) 0.25%, 0.5%, and 0.75% (non-obstetrical), caudal 0.25% and 0.5% (35–150 mg), epidural test dose (3 mL 0.25%). Use only the single-dose ampoule and single-dose vials for spinal, caudal, or epidural anesthesia as the multiple-dose vials contain a preservative and, therefore, should not be used for these procedures.

Potential advantages

Ease of use, tolerability, opioid sparing. Bupivacaine provides clinically useful differential block particularly when dilute infusions are employed. It is associated with frequency-dependent blockade whereby noxious nerve fibers that conduct action potentials most frequently are first to be blocked, while larger-caliber less active sensory motor fibers are relatively spared. The rapid injection of a large volume of bupi-

vacaine should be avoided and fractional (incremental) doses should be used.

Reduction in adverse events: the smallest dose and concentration required to produce the desired result should be administered.

Drug interactions: intravenous administration of a benzodiazepine will provide sedation and hypnosis for patient comfort during anesthetic procedures and also serve to raise the seizure threshold, thus minimizing the adverse CNS affect of bupivacaine.

As monotherapy: bupivacaine blocks the generation and the conduction of nerve impulses by increasing the threshold for electrical excitation in the nerve, slowing the propagation of the nerve impulse, and reducing the rate of elevation of the action potential.

As used for multimodal analgesia: bupivacaine regional anesthesia/analgesia plays a vital role as the center of a multimodal pain management protocol.

Potential disadvantages

Toxicity: compared to other local anesthetics, bupivacaine is markedly cardiotoxic.

Drug interactions: bupivacaine solutions containing epinephrine or norepinephrine administered to patients receiving monoamine oxidase inhibitors or tricyclic antidepressants may produce severe, prolonged hypertension. Concurrent administration of vasopressor drugs added to bupivacaine/vasoconstrictor solutions and of ergot-type oxytocic drugs may cause severe, persistent hypertension or cerebrovascular accidents.

Phenothiazines and butyrophenones may reduce or reverse the pressor effect of epinephrine added to bupivacaine.

Adverse events: bupivacaine can be neurotoxic and/or cardiotoxic, although adverse drug reactions are rare when it is administered correctly. Most adverse drug events relate to the administration technique used or direct pharmacological effects of bupivacaine, which may result in a toxic systemic exposure. Although rare, allergic reactions can occur with bupivacaine. Systemic exposure to excessive quantities of bupivacaine mainly results in central nervous system (CNS) and/or cardiovascular effects. The CNS effects usually occur at lower blood plasma concentrations and the additional cardiovascular effects present at higher concentrations (it has been reported that cardiovascular collapse may also occur with low concentrations). CNS effects may include CNS excitation (nervousness, tingling around the mouth, tinnitus, tremor, dizziness, blurred vision, seizures) followed by depression (drowsiness, loss of consciousness, respiratory depression and apnea). Cardiovascular effects include hypotension, bradycardia, arrhythmias, and/or cardiac arrest (some of which may be due to hypoxemia secondary to respiratory depression). It has been reported that bupivacaine was determined to be the cause of death when the intended epidural anesthetic drug (bupivacaine) dose was accidentally administered intravenously.

Drug-related adverse events

Common/serious adverse events: CNS effects such as nervousness, tingling around the mouth, tinnitus, tremor, dizziness, blurred vision, seizures, drowsiness, loss of consciousness, respiratory depression, and apnea. Cardiovascular effects such as hypotension, bradycardia, and cardiac arrhythmias are also possible.

Less common adverse events: injection site reaction, allergic reactions, cardiovascular collapse and asystole.

Treatment of adverse events: benzodiazepines (IV), addition of vasoconstrictors that cause blood vessel contraction that may reduce vascular absorption, and IV fluid hydration prior to neuraxial blockade should all be considered.

Lipid rescue as a treatment of bupivacaine overdose: there is evidence with animal studies [1] that Intralipid, a commonly available intravenous lipid emulsion, is effective in treating the severe cardiotoxicity that may result secondary to local anesthetic overdose. In addition, there are human case reports of successful use of Intralipid for rescue from cardiotoxic and cardiovascular collapse from systemic bupivacaine overdose [2] as well as a widespread campaign to publicize Intralipid as an available drug for emergencies in all anesthetizing locations where bupivacaine is used.

References

1. Weinberg G, Ripper R, Feinstein DL, Hoffman W. Lipid emulsion infusion rescues dogs from bupivacaine-induced cardiac toxicity. *Reg Anesth Pain Med* 2003;**28**:198–202.

2. Rosenblatt MA, Abel M, Fischer GW, et al. Successful use of a 20% lipid emulsion to resuscitate a patient after a presumed bupivacaine-related cardiac arrest. *Anesthesiology* 2006;**105**:217–218.

Section 5 Chapter

66

Local Anesthetics

Ropivacaine

Neesa Patel

Generic Name: ropivacaine HCl

Brand Names: Naropin, Naropin Polyamp, Naropin SDV

Ropivacaine Strength Descriptions: 0.2%; 0.5%; 0.75%; 1%

Chemical Name: (*S*)-1-propyl-2′,6′-dimethyl-anilino-formoxy1piperidine, monohydrochloride, monohydrate

Chemical Structure: see Figure 66.1

Description

Ropivacaine is part of the amino amide class of long-acting local anesthetics. It is a pure *S*-(−)-enantiomer, and is an optically pure solution. Ropivacaine is very similar to bupivacaine in its pKa and molecular weight, but is much less lipophilic. Ropivacaine is primarily used both as a local anesthetic for surgical anesthesia and for acute pain management. The onset, duration, and depth of sensory blockade is similar to that of bupivacaine; however, the motor blockade is much less for ropivacaine.

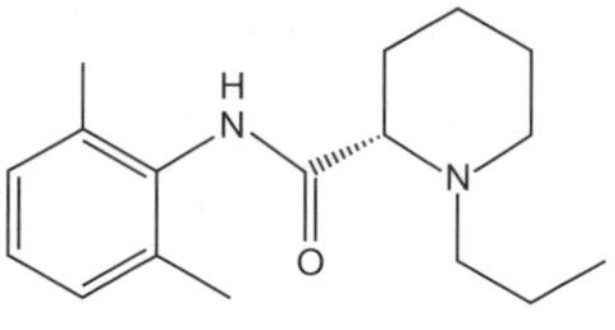

Figure 66.1. Molecular structure image obtained from en/wikipedia.org.

Mechanism of action

Like all local anesthetics, ropivacaine binds directly to the intracellular voltage-dependent sodium channels. It blocks primarily open and inactive sodium channels. Thus, this blocks the generation and conduction of nerve impulses. Lipid solubility appears to be the primary determinant of intrinsic anesthetic potency and toxicity. The more lipid-soluble, the greater is the potency of the local anesthetic. Hence, ropivacaine is less potent and less toxic than bupivacaine. In addition, the progression of blockade is affected by the diameter, myelination, and conduction velocity of the nerve fibers.

Pharmacokinetics

Absorption

Ropivacaine follows linear pharmacokinetics and the maximum plasma concentration is proportional to the dose. In general, the systemic concentration is dependent on multiple factors, including the route of administration, vascularity of the administered site, total dose and concentration given, and the patient's medical condition. Ropivacaine is primarily used for epidural and peripheral nerve blockade. From the epidural space, ropivacaine shows complete and biphasic absorption, half-life of the two phases being 14 ± 7 minutes and $4.2 \pm .9$ h.

Distribution

Ropivacaine is 94% bound to alpha-1 glycoprotein and is mainly protein-bound. After intravascular infusion, steady-state volume of distribution is 41 liters. In addition, ropivacaine readily crosses the placenta and unbound concentration equilibrium is quickly reached. The degree of plasma protein binding in the fetus is less than in the mother. This results in lower total plasma concentrations in the fetus than in the mother. The ratios of umbilical vein to maternal vein total and free concentrations are 0.31 and 0.74, respectively.

Metabolism

Like all amide local anesthetics, ropivacaine is metabolized extensively in the liver via aromatic hydroxylation mediated by cytochrome P4501A. The metabolite is 3-hydroxy ropivacaine.

Elimination

Ropivacaine metabolites are excreted by the kidney. If given intravenously, only 1% is excreted unchanged in the urine.

Indications

Ropivacaine is indicated for both surgical anesthesia, and acute pain management.

Epidural administration for surgical anesthesia: 25 clinical studies with 900 patients were done to evaluate the use of epidurally administered ropivacaine for surgical anesthesia. Median onset time to T10 sensory level was 10 minutes and the median duration at the T10 level was 4 hours. Higher doses produced more profound blockade and duration of effect.

Epidural for labor and delivery: many studies have shown that in comparison to bupivacaine, ropivacaine produced equally adequate pain relief. In addition, detailed evaluation of the delivered newborns demonstrated no difference in clinical outcome.

Epidural for cesarean section: in general, ropivacaine provides adequate muscle relaxation for surgical anesthesia. Many studies have evaluated ropivacaine at a concentration of 0.5% in doses up to 150 mg, with median onset time to T6 level of 11 to 26 minutes.

Epidural for post-operative pain control: most studies have tested ropivacaine 0.2% for post-operative epidural infusion. Infusion rates of 6–14 mL per hour of 0.2% ropivacaine provide adequate analgesia with only slight and non-progressive motor block in cases of moderate to severe pain. Most studies have dosed ropivacaine for up to 72 hours.

Peripheral nerve blockade: for surgical anesthesia, 0.5% to 0.75% concentrations are routinely used, with an onset time depending on technique. The median duration of anesthesia ranged from 11.4 and 14.4 hours.

Two clinical trials were done to verify the safety of ropivacaine in the intrathecal space, both with doses of 3 mL. Both studies showed that 3 mL doses did produce an adequate spinal anesthesia blockade with no

Table 66.1. Dosing recommendations

	Conc. (mg/mL)	(%)	Volume (mL)	Dose (mg)	Onset (min)	Duration (hours)
Surgical anesthesia						
Lumbar epidural	5.0	(0.5%)	15–30	75–150	15–30	2–4
Administration	7.5	(0.75%)	15–25	113–188	10–20	3–5
Surgery	10.0	(1%)	15–20	150–200	10–20	4–6
Lumbar epidural	5.0	(0.5%)	20–30	100–150	15–25	2–4
Administration	7.5	(0.75%)	15–20	113–150	10–20	3–5
Cesarean section						
Thoracic epidural	5.0	(0.5%)	5–15	25–75	10–20	n/a
Administration	7.5	(0.75%)	5–15	38–113	10–20	n/a
Surgery						
Major nerve block	5.0	(0.5%)	35–50	175–250	15–30	5–6
(eg. Brachial plexus block)	7.5	(0.75%)	10–40	75–300	10–25	6–10
Field block	5.0	(0.5%)	1–40	5–200	1–15	2–6
Labor pain management						
Lumbar epidural administration						
Initial dose	2.0	(0.2%)	10–20	20–40	10–15	.5–1.5
Continuous infusion	2.0	(0.2%)	6–14	12–28	n/a	n/a
Incremental	2.0	(0.2%)	10–15	20–30	n/a	n/a
Injections (top-up)			mL/h	mg/h		
Post-operative pain management						
Lumbar epidural administration						
Continuous	2.0	(0.2%)	6–14	12–28	n/a	n/a
Infusion			Ml/h	Mg/h		
Thoracic epidural	2.0	(0.2%)	6–14	12–28	n/a	n/a
Administration			mL/h	mg/h		
Continuous infusion						
Infiltration	2.0	(0.2%)	1–100	2–200	1–5	2–6
eg. Minor nerve block	5.0	(0.5%)	1–40	5–200	1–5	2–6

serious adverse event. The drug has not been studied for use in paracervical block and retrobulbar blockade.

Contraindications and warnings

Systemic toxicity may occur due to inadvertent intravascular administration or excessively high doses. Signs of toxicity are either central nervous system (CNS) or cardiovascular in origin.

Use of ropivacaine with other local anesthetics should be monitored closely as the toxic effects are additive.

CNS toxicity: initial signs are usually excitatory in nature, as there is a preferential block of inhibitory central pathways. These include shivering, muscle twitching, and tremors. Patients may report dizziness, ear disorder and deafness, tinnitus, speech disorders, circumoral paresthesia, and taste perversion.

After a certain plasma concentration is reached, toxicity manifests as CNS depression, with respiratory depression, hypoventilation, and convulsions.

Cardiovascular toxicity: CV toxicity can also be excitatory in nature at first due to activation of the sympathetic nervous system, followed by arrhythmias and profound myocardial depression. Ropivacaine shows a dose-dependent prolongation of cardiac conduction, with an increase in the PR interval and QRS duration. These effects are explained by the persisting block of sodium channels into diastole, predisposing to re-entrant arrhythmias. In addition, the conductivity of potassium channels is affected, increasing the QTc interval and enhancing the block of the inactivated state of the sodium channel.

Given bupivacaine's high lipid solubility, it is more toxic and has greater CV affects than ropivacaine.

Dosing and timing

Ropivacaine, like all other local anesthetics, should never be rapidly infused, but given in incremental dosing with adequate monitoring of hemodynamic and mental status, and functional intravenous access. Dosage varies depending on: anesthetic procedure and area to be anesthetized, vacularity of surrounding tissues, number of neuronal segments to be blocked, degree of muscle relaxation required, individual tolerance, and physical condition of the patient (Table 66.1).

Clinical recommendations

As compared with bupivacaine, ropivacaine has the clinical advantage of a stronger differentiation between sensory and motor blocks. This is particularly useful when doing peripheral nerve blockade for post-operative pain control when early mobilization is important for recovery. Ropivacaine is 40–50% less potent than bupivacaine because of its lower lipid solubility. However, the duration of blockade is very similar to bupivicaine, making it ideal as a long-acting local anesthetic with a better toxicity profile. This is especially meaningful for long-term infusions.

References

1. Leone, Stefania et al. Pharmacology, toxicology, and clinical use of new long acting local anesthetics, ropivacaine and levobupivacaine. *Acta Biomed* 2008;**79**:92–105.

2. Avery P, Redon D, Schaenzer G, Rusy B. The influence of serum potassium on cerebral and cardiac toxicity of bupivacaine and lidocaine. *Anesthesiology* 1984;**61**:134–138.

3. Naropin (ropivacaine HCL) injection package insert and ; APP Pharmaceuticals, Llc.

Section 5 Chapter 67

Local Anesthetics

Lidocaine for neural blockade

Mary Hanna Bekhit

Lidocaine's chemical name is 2-(diethylamino)-N-(2,6-dimethylphenyl)ethanamide (IUPAC). Its other chemical names include: N-diethylaminoacetyl-2,6,xylidine hydrochloride, 2-(diethylamino)-N-(2,6-dimethylphenyl)acetamide, 2-diethylamino-2′,6′-acetoxylidide, and omega-diethylamino-2′,6′-dimethylacetanilide.Lidocaine is also known as lignocaine (former British Approved Name).

Its proprietary names include Akten, Xylocaine, Xylotox, Leostesin, EMLA, Rucaina, Isicaine, Lidoderm, Cuivasal, Duncaine, Sylestesin, Anestacon, Gravocain, Lidothesin, Xylocitin, and Xylestesin.

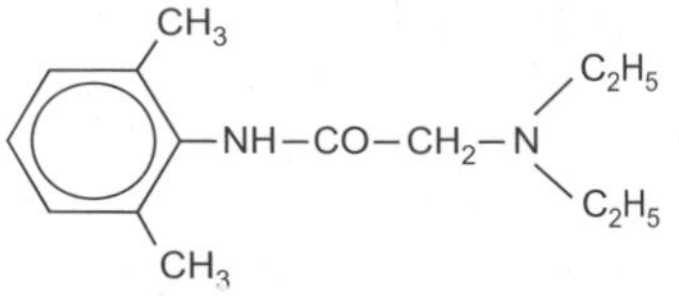

Figure 67.1.

Lidocaine in its generic form is manufactured by many different pharmaceutical companies worldwide.

Chemical structure/properties (Figure 67.1): lidocaine's aromatic group, a benzene ring, confers its lipophilic properties, and its tertiary amine group possesses hydrophilic properties. The two groups are linked by an amide bond. Lidocaine has a molecular weight of 234 g/mol, melting point of 68°C, and a pKa of 7.9. It is usually prepared as lidocaine hydrochloride, a white, odorless, crystalline powder.

Historical development

Lidocaine is the most widely used and first synthesized amide local anesthetic. Nils Lofgren, a Swedish chemist who later became a professor of organic chemistry at the University of Stockholm, synthesized the chemical in 1943 and named it xylocaine. His coworker Bengt Lundqvist first tested the chemical on himself via injection prior to marketing the drug in 1948 [1–3].

Mode of activity/pharmacodynamics

Lidocaine, like other local anesthetics, binds axonal membrane voltage-gated fast Na^+ channels and thus prevents Na^+ transport across the channels, thus inhibiting cell membrane depolarization. It is by this same mechanism that lidocaine exerts its effect as a class Ib antiarrhythmic to inhibit cardiac smooth muscle excitability and as an anti-epileptic drug to inhibit cortical excitability. Its lipophilic aromatic group allows the molecule to penetrate the nerve membrane, while its hydrophilic charged amine group is the portion of the molecule that actually binds the Na^+ channel [1–3].

Pharmacokinetics

Lidocaine undergoes primarily (>90%) hepatic metabolism via CYP3A4 and CYP1A2 enzymes to the pharmacologically active metabolite monoethylglycinexylidide, the majority of which is hepatically converted to the inactive metabolite glycinexylidide. Both metabolites are renally excreted, so adverse side effects from metabolite accumulation may present in patients with renal failure, despite normal serum lidocaine levels. Its elimination half-life ranges from 1 to 1.5 hours in healthy patients, but can exceed 2 hours in patients with congestive heart failure or 5 hours in patients with hepatic dysfunction [1,4].

Lidocaine is 65–70% protein-bound in serum. Albumin accounts for about 30% of the protein binding, while alpha-1-acid glycoprotein (AGP) accounts for the other 70%. Since AGP synthesis may increase as an acute-phase reactant during physiological stresses such as trauma, myocardial infarction, or infection, the protein-bound fraction of lidocaine can significantly increase in these situations to 85–90%. Thus, the drug's clearance can be dramatically reduced, with potentially higher serum concentrations in patients receiving infusions for longer than 24 hours [1,4].

Metabolism

In the same way that a number of disease processes can impair lidocaine's hepatic metabolism by the cytochrome P450 enzymes, surprisingly so can hormone replacement therapy. Gawronska-Sklarz and colleagues in 2006 studied in a randomized controlled trial 18 women who received hormone replacement therapy for 6 months [5]. They followed their pharmacokinetic response 360 minutes after an intravenous injection of lidocaine 1 mg/kg before initiation of hormone therapy, at 3 months and at 6 months. They found that the patients showed accelerated drug elimination after 3 months of oral (not transdermal) hormone replacement therapy, which resolved at the 6-month mark. Further studies with larger patient populations are needed to further elucidate this interaction between hormone replacement therapy and lidocaine's hepatic metabolism.

Onset of action

Lidocaine has a rapid onset of action of 5–7 minutes, but can even approach 3 minutes depending on added adjuvants such as sodium bicarbonate, the volume and concentration of drug injected, and the site of peripheral nerve blockade. Alkalinization of the drug to a pH closer to its pKa to increase the nonionized fraction, higher concentration such as 2%, larger volume, and the nerve sheath lying within a confined space (such as the supraclavicular brachial plexus which passes between the clavicle and first rib) all help to speed the local anesthetic saturation of Na^+ channels and thus onset of action [2,3].

Mixtures of lidocaine with long-acting local anesthetics such as bupivacaine or ropivacaine for peripheral nerve blockade have long been common in clinical practice. Lidocaine's rapid onset of action has been noted clinically to decrease the time to attainment of surgical anesthesia, thus improving efficiency when a peripheral nerve block functions as the sole anesthetic. Cuvillon and colleagues in 2009 sought to demonstrate a clear benefit to adding lidocaine to peripheral nerve blocks, in terms of improving onset of block without significant adverse effects [6].

In a randomized controlled trial involving 82 patients undergoing lower extremity surgery, they demonstrated faster onset of sensorimotor blockade as well as shorter duration of action in patients receiving a mixture of lidocaine with a long-acting local anesthetic for femoral and sciatic nerve blocks, compared with patients receiving a long-acting local anesthetic alone. The patients who received a mixture of local anesthetics did demonstrate higher lidocaine plasma concentrations. These patients also had higher morphine PCA cumulative doses during the 48 hours post-operatively, compared to the patients who received long-acting local anesthetics only. The mixed results in Cuvillon et al.'s study suggest addition of lidocaine to local anesthetic mixtures for peripheral nerve blockade clearly improves time to onset of the block, but with significant serum lidocaine concentrations, decreased duration of sensory blockade, and increased post-operative requirement for other analgesics [6].

Duration of action

Its duration of action is 60–120 minutes, depending on the vascularity of the site blocked as well as added adjuvants such as epinephrine. The drug is 70% protein-bound, with 30% in the free unbound form. It is this 30% that is rapidly cleared by the systemic circulation for hepatic metabolism. The vasoconstrictive properties of epinephrine help to decrease this systemic uptake of the drug and thus to prolong its duration of action. Other adjuvants such as the alpha-2 receptor agonists clonidine and dexmedetomidine have been studied recently and found to prolong the duration of action of lidocaine. Their mechanism of action (specific receptor vs. pharmacokinetic/pharmacodynamic interaction with local anesthetics) and site (central vs. peripheral) of action have not been fully elucidated [6–8].

Bernard and Macaire in 1997 demonstrated improved onset, quality, and duration of sensory blockade from addition of clonidine to lidocaine for axillary brachial plexus blockade [7]. In a randomized controlled trial, they assigned 56 patients undergoing carpal tunnel surgery to receive an axillary block with either lidocaine 400 mg or lidocaine 400 mg with varying doses of clonidine (30, 90, or 300 µg). They found that the addition of clonidine dose-dependently reduced the time to onset of sensory block, prolonged the duration of post-operative analgesia, and extended the field of anesthesia. They found that the patients receiving lidocaine with clonidine 300 µg had more hypotension (MAP < 55 mmHg) and arterial oxyhemoglobin desaturation < 90% than the other three groups, in some cases preventing discharge from the recovery room.

Pratap and colleagues in 2007 studied the effects of clonidine when added to lidocaine during subcutaneous infiltration of the forearm in a randomized controlled trial on 20 healthy volunteers [8]. They used lidocaine 0.5% on one forearm and lidocaine 0.5% with clonidine 10 µg on each patient's contralateral forearm. They found that clonidine significantly prolonged the duration of sensory blockade to pinprick (median time at least 6 hours) when compared to the lidocaine alone (median time 3.5 hours).

Dexamethasone has also been postulated to prolong the duration of action of lidocaine, with mechanism unknown. Movafegh and colleagues in 2006 enrolled 60 patients undergoing hand and forearm surgery under axillary brachial plexus blockade in a randomized controlled trial assessing the efficacy of dexamethasone in prolonging lidocaine's duration of action [9]. Patients received either lidocaine 1.5% (34 mL lidocaine with 2 mL saline) or lidocaine 1.5% with dexamethasone 8mg (34 mL lidocaine with 2 mL dexamethasone). They found that patients receiving dexamethasone as an adjuvant had significantly longer duration of sensory (242 minutes) and motor (310 minutes) blockade compared to the patients receiving lidocaine only (98 and 130 minutes, respectively). They also demonstrated no difference in onset of action between the two groups.

Differential blockade

Lidocaine's differential blockade has been examined with peripheral and neuraxial administration [10–11]. Peripheral nerve fibers seem to respond differently to lidocaine than dorsal nerve roots. Epidural lidocaine seems to block small unmyelinated C fibers (supplying temperature sensation) more effectively than larger myelinated A fibers (A-beta supplying touch, and A-delta supplying pinprick sensation). Wildsmith and colleagues [10] postulated that perhaps the myelinated axons of A fibers in the epidural space may not have a large number of consecutive nodes of Ranvier exposed and bound by lidocaine (at least three nodes needed [11]) to effectively block electrical transmission, while the small unmyelinated C fibers have more exposed axon for effective blockade.

However, these results contradict long-accepted in vitro studies on mammalian peripheral nerve fiber axon diameter. These studies suggest that larger myelinated A fibers which conduct with higher velocity may be more susceptible to peripheral nerve blockade with local anesthetics than smaller unmyelinated C fibers which conduct more slowly [12,13]. Jaffe and Rowe in 1996 [14] actually found no difference in sensitivity to lidocaine based on axon diameter. Many mechanisms in addition to axon diameter have been proposed for lidocaine's differential neural blockade, such as differences in Na⁺ channel block (state-dependent vs. frequency-dependent) between different nerve fiber types. Further research is needed to elucidate the underlying mechanism as well as the discrepancy between the differential blockade witnessed in epidural and peripheral nerve blocks.

Indications

Lidocaine is commonly administered for peripheral neural blockade when rapid onset of surgical anesthesia is desired. It is also routinely administered intrathecally for outpatient gynecological and urological procedures. It is frequently administered in labor epidurals to provide rapid surgical conditions in emergency cesarean section deliveries, and is the most commonly used local anesthetic for topicalization of the airway prior to awake fiberoptic intubation. The transdermal lidocaine patch has also been approved by the FDA for treatment of post-herpetic neuralgia, and has gained popularity with several other off-label conditions such as chronic low back pain and osteoarthritic knee pain [15]. Lidocaine is classified under Pregnancy Category B.

Contraindications

Patients with hypersensitivity reactions to amide local anesthetics should not receive lidocaine. Lidocaine should be used with caution in patients with severe hepatic dysfunction or congestive heart failure, both of which may impair hepatic metabolism and lead to toxic serum levels of the drug.

Common doses/uses

For intravenous regional anesthesia, lidocaine is administered in 0.5% solution. For peripheral neural blockade, the 2% solution with or without epinephrine is most commonly administered to provide fastest onset of action as well as maximal surgical motor blockade. More dilute concentrations such as 1–1.5% may also be administered, but provide less motor blockade than the 2% solution.

Potential advantages

Lidocaine's rapid onset of action makes it an ideal choice for peripheral neural blockade that will function as the sole surgical anesthetic. Its relatively safe cardiotoxicity profile also increases its attractiveness when compared to other local anesthetics such as bupivacaine or ropivacaine. It is also widely available commercially in generic form for low cost. A 20-mL vial of lidocaine 2% with epinephrine 1:200k costs between $4 and $6 [1,2].

Potential disadvantages

Lidocaine's short duration of action makes it a poor candidate as the local anesthetic for peripheral nerve blockade for surgical anesthesia when the surgery will last longer than 2 hours, or for post-operative analgesia when maximal duration of effect is desired after highly painful surgery. Its potential for neurotoxicity presenting with seizures also limits the total dose that may be used in combined nerve blocks. Lidocaine should be used with caution in patients with significant hepatic impairment or renal disease, due to potential toxic metabolite accumulation.

Adverse events

Most of the adverse events related to lidocaine are associated with serum toxicity, with various symptoms presenting at different serum levels. Symptoms such as lightheadedness, perioral numbness, tinnitus, nausea, or metallic taste in the mouth may occur when plasma lidocaine concentrations are 1–5 µg/mL. Dysarthria, local muscle twitches, hallucinations, or nystagmus may present at plasma concentrations from 5 to 8 µg/mL. Seizures may occur at 8–12 µg/mL, followed by respiratory depression or coma at levels higher than 20 µg/mL. Hypotension, bradycardia, cardiac arrest, and arrhythmias may also occur at serum levels greater than 20 µg/mL. Intralipid remains the only available treatment for adverse events related to serum toxicity.

References

1. Bauer LA. *Applied Clinical Pharmacokinetics*, 2nd ed. New York: McGraw Hill Professional Publishing, 2008, pp. 356–397.

2. www.Xylocaine@3dchem.com./.

3. Wang JS, Backman JT, Taavitsainen P, Neuvonen PJ, Kivistö KT. Involvement of CYP1A2 and CYP3A4 in lidocaine N-deethylation and 3-hydroxylation in humans. *Drug Metab Dispos* 2000;**28**(8):959–695.

4. Hersh EV. In Fonseca RJ, ed. *Oral and Maxillofacial Surgery: Local Anesthetics*. Elsevier Health Sciences, 2000, pp. 58–78.

5. Gawronska-Szklarz B, Zarzycki M, Musial HD, Pudlo A, Loniewski I, Drozdzik M. Lidocaine pharmacokinetics in postmenopausal women on hormone therapy. *Menopause* 2006;**13**(5):793–798.

6. Cuvillon P, Nouvellon E, Ripart J, Boyer JC, Dehour L, Mahamat A, L'hermite J, Boisson C, Vialles N, Lefrant JY, de La Coussaye JE. A comparison of the pharmacodynamics and pharmacokinetics of bupivacaine, ropivacaine (with epinephrine) and their equal volume mixtures with lidocaine used for femoral and sciatic nerve blocks: a double-blind randomized study. *Anesth Analg* 2009;**108**(2):641–649.

7. Bernard JM, Macaire P. Dose-range effects of clonidine added to lidocaine for brachial plexus block. *Anesthesiology* 1997;**2**:277–284.

8. Pratap JN, Shankar RK, Goroszeniuk T. Co-injection of clonidine prolongs the anesthetic effect of lidocaine skin infiltration by a peripheral action. *Anesth Analg* 2007;**104**:982–983.

9. Movafegh A, Razazian M, Hajimaohamadi F, Meysamie A. Dexamethasone added to lidocaine prolongs axillary brachial plexus blockade. *Anesth Analg* 2006;**102**(1):263–267.

10. Wildsmith JAW, Brown DT, Paul D, Johnson S. Structure-activity relationships in differential nerve block at high and low frequency stimulation. *Br J Anaesth* 1989;**63**:444–452.

11. Tasaki, I. *Nervous Transmission*. Springfield: CC Thomas, 1953.

12. Gissen AJ, Covino BG, Gregus J. Differential sensitivities of mammalian nerve fibers to local anesthetic agents. *Anesthesiology* 1980; **53**:467–474.

13. Mama KR, Steffey EP. In Adams HR, ed. *Veterinary Pharmacology and Therapeutics: Local Anesthetics*, 8th ed, Blackwell, 2001, pp. 343–359.

14. Jaffe RA, Rowe MA. Differential nerve block: direct measurements on individual myelinated and unmyelinated dorsal root axons. *Anesthesiology* 1996;**84**:1455–1464.

15. Sakai T, Tomiyasu S, Yamada H, Ono T, Sumikawa K. Quantitative and selective evaluation of differential sensory nerve block after transdermal lidocaine. *Anesth Analg* 2004;**98**:248–251.

**Section 5
Chapter**

Local Anesthetics

Topical local anesthetics

Steven J. Weisman

Generic Names: topical lidocaine/prilocaine, topical lidocaine/tetracaine, tetracaine gel, 4% liposomal lidocaine, 1,1,1,3,3-pentafluoropropane and 1,1,1,2-tetrafluoroethane

Trade/Proprietary Names: EMLA™ (Eutectic Mixture of Local Anesthetics), Synera™, Ametop Gel™, LMX-4™, PainEase (vapocoolant spray)

Manufacturers: (EMLA) Ferndale Laboratories, Ferndale, MI; (Synera) ZARS Pharma, Salt Lake City, UT; (LMX-4) APP Pharmaceuticals, LLC, Schaumburg, IL; (Ametop) Smith and Nephew, St-Laurent, Quebec; (Vapocoolant) Gebauer, Cleveland, OH

Chemical Structure: lidocaine (lignocaine), see Figure 68.1; prilocaine, see Figure 68.2

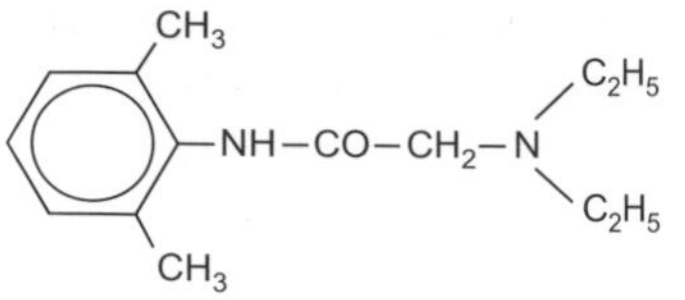

Figure 68.1.

$C_{14}H_{22}N_2O$ M.W. 234.3

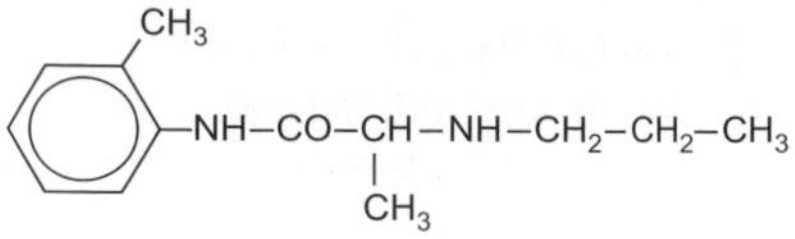

Figure 68.2.

$C_{13}H_{20}N_2O$ M.W. 220.3

EMLA

Description

EMLA is a eutectic mixture of 2.5% lidocaine and 2.5% prilocaine, which, when mixed, form a liquid that is formulated into a water-oil emulsion. EMLA is available as a cream, a gel and an anesthetic disc. Only the cream and gel are available in the USA. The cream is approved for use on intact skin for local anesthesia or genital mucosa for superficial minor surgery and as pretreatment for infiltration anesthesia. The gel is approved for adults who require localized anesthesia in periodontal pockets during scaling and/or root planning [1].

Mode of action/pharmacology

The cream is applied to the skin and is usually contained under a transparent dressing for 45–60 minutes. Local anesthesia persists for 60 to 120 minutes after removal of the occlusive dressing [1,2]. The amount of EMLA that should be applied to the skin is age- and weight-based as follows: age 0–3 months or < 5 kg should receive 1 g over 10 cm² skin for up to 1 hour; age 3–12 months and > 5 kg should receive 2 g over 20 cm² skin for up to 4 hours; age 1–6 years and > 10 kg should receive 10 g over 100 cm² skin for up to 4 hours; and age 7–12 years and > 20 kg should receive 20 g over 200 cm² skin for up 4 hours (see Table 68.1).

How to use

EMLA has been used in practice for many years. It has been studied and used for venipuncture, intravenous cannulation, needle immunizations, subcutaneous port access, subcutaneous reservoir access, circumcision, chest tube removal, lumbar puncture, bone marrow aspiration, and laser treatment of port-wine stains. Significant treatment effect has been demonstrated in individual as well as meta-analysis study of EMLA. Initially, a 30 min application time was recommended. However, 60 minutes will ensure significantly more anesthesia and even longer duration (90 min) and produce improved pain relief [1,3].

Inherent in these observations lies the major drawback of EMLA cream. In busy clinical practice, anticipatory application of the cream is challenging. Most often, when decisions to perform minor needle-based procedures are made, they are in an acute clinical setting. Therefore, time will often preclude application. In addition, the cream is available in 5 g (2–4 applications) and 30 g tubes with a significant cost associated with use. As noted below, there are some additional constraints associated with use.

Nonetheless, application before anticipated procedures, such as bone marrow aspiration, lumbar puncture or planned venipuncture/IVcannulation can be

Table 68.1. EMLA cream maximum recommended dose, application area, and application time by age and weight for infants and children based on application to intact skin

Age and body weight requirements	Maximum total dose of EMLA cream	Maximum application area	Maximum application time
0 up to 3 months or < 5 kg	1 g	10 cm²	1 hour
3 up to 12 months and > 5 kg	2 g	20 cm²	4 hours
1 to 6 years and > 10 kg	10 g	100 cm²	4 hours
7 to 12 years and > 20 kg	20 g	200 cm²	4 hours

Please note: if a patient greater than 3 months old does not meet the minimum weight requirement, the maximum total dose of EMLA cream should be restricted to that which corresponds to the patient's weight.
For more individualized calculation of how much lidocaine and prilocaine may be absorbed, physicians can use the following estimates of lidocaine and prilocaine absorption for children and adults: the estimated mean (±SD) absorption of lidocaine is 0.045 (±0.016) mg/cm² per h; the estimated mean (±SD) absorption of prilocaine is 0.077 (±0.036) mg/cm² per h.

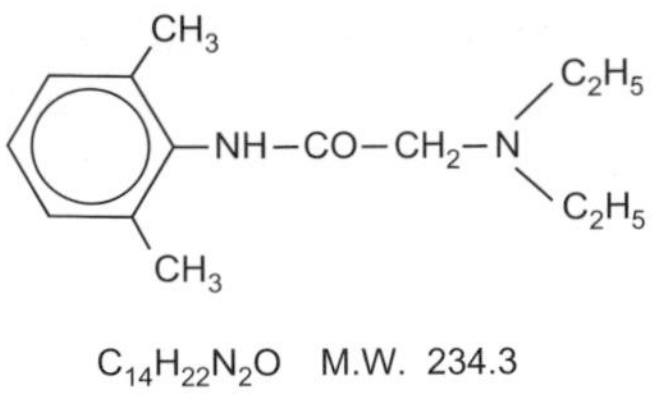

Figure 68.3.

$C_{14}H_{22}N_2O$ M.W. 234.3

readily incorporated into the healthcare workflow. In the peri-operative environment, the cream can be applied while the patient is undergoing check-in and pre-operative preparation. Patients can also apply the cream at home, if it is dispensed before a planned intervention.

Potential advantages

This product has been safely employed across the age continuum, from birth to the elder years, with excellent efficacy. It is totally non-invasive and easy to apply.

Potential disadvantages

Application to open wounds will result in significantly higher plasma levels of the local anesthetics. Since this is a product that is most commonly employed in children, extreme care must be taken to avoid accidental oral ingestion. Prilocaine has been associated, in susceptible individuals, with methemoglobinemia. This may be more common in the very young and the product should probably be avoided in infants less than 37 weeks gestation. Concomitant use of phenytoin or acetaminophen may predispose to methemoglobinemia in those susceptible.

Another well-known limitation of EMLA is that it causes vasoconstriction with observable skin blanching. This can lead to more difficult visualization of superficial veins.

Contraindications

Known history of methemoglobinemia or in patients with a known history of sensitivity to amide local anesthetics.

LMX4 (Liposomal Lidocaine 4%)

Chemical structure: see Figure 68.3

Description

This is an over-the-counter product of 4% lidocaine formulated in biocompatible, non-immunogenic vesicles. The liposomes are multilamellar vesicles of phospholipids and cholesterol that enclose an aqueous compartment. This technology leads to protection of the active agent (lidocaine) from degradation and to enhanced absorption with better penetration through the statum corneum.

Mode of action/pharmacology

This product is also applied to the skin with an occlusive clear dressing. It is effective without the covering, but as the cream warms, it will drip off the desired location. After a 30 min application, analgesia is comparable to that achieved with a 60 min application of EMLA. The local anesthetic effect lasts for 60 min after a typical 30 min application. LMX-4 application should be limited to 100 cm² in children weighing ≤ 10 kg or between 10 kg and 20 kg for each use. There are limited data in children under 2 years of age, but adverse reaction in small infants has generally not been reported.

How to use

Use of LMX4 is identical to that for EMLA. LMX is recommended for treating pain, itching, soreness, and discomfort of the skin or mucous membranes due to certain conditions such as eczema, scratches, minor burns, insect bites, and hemorrhoids. Thus the guidelines allow for application even to open skin.

Potential advantages

This, surprisingly, is an over-the-counter pharmaceutical. There is more rapid onset with LMX4 than EMLA. Clinically efficacy appears to be comparable to EMLA, as well as buffered lidocaine injections for IV cannulation. Methemoglobinemia is not a problem with lidocaine alone. Blanching, vasoconstriction, and loss of visibility of veins is not commonly seen with LMX4.

Potential disadvantages

Care to avoid oral ingestion by small children is needed.

Contraindications

Allergy or sensitivity to lidocaine.

Synera (lidocaine/tetracaine topical patch)

Chemical structure: lidocaine, see Figure 68.4; tetracaine, see Figure 68.5

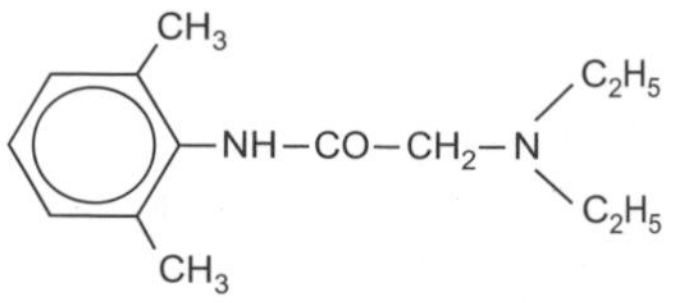

Figure 68.4.

$C_{14}H_{22}N_2O$ M.W. 234.3

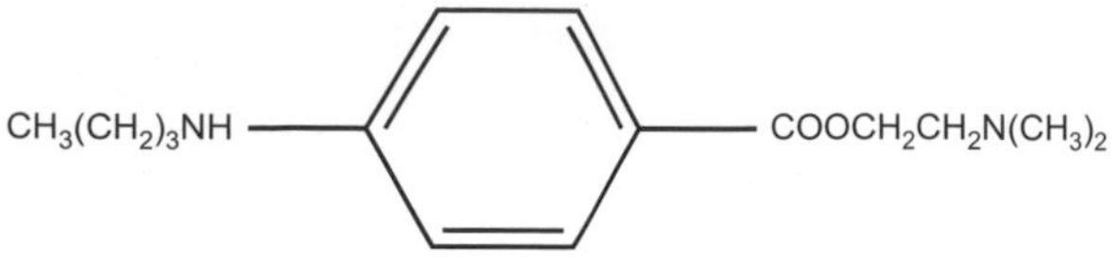

Figure 68.5.

Description

Since absorption of local anesthetics through the skin is enhanced by heat, a topical patch with an intrinsic heating system was developed [4]. This incorporates a controlled heat-assisted delivery system that is physically separated from a eutectic mixture of 70 mg of lidocaine and 70 mg of tetracaine. The surface area of the entire Synera patch is approximately 50 cm², 10 cm² of which is active.

Mode of action/pharmacology

The patch adheres to the skin and when it is exposed to air, the contained heating element is activated and through oxidation releases heat. Local skin temperature remains between 39 and 41°C during the heating phase of application. Systemic absorption is minimal and even with sequential or simultaneous applications of up to four patches, lidocaine plasma levels were low (9–12 ng/mL in adults) and tetracaine levels were essentially non-detectable. The product insert indicates that application of one Synera patch for up to 30 minutes in children 4 months to 12 years of age produced maximum peak plasma concentrations of lidocaine and tetracaine of 63 ng/mL and 65 ng/mL, respectively. Application of two Synera patches for up to 30 minutes to children 4 months to 12 years of age produced peak lidocaine levels of up to 331 ng/mL and tetracaine levels of less than 5 ng/mL.

How to use

Application is recommended for 20–30 min to the area that will be punctured. It too can be used for the

same procedures as EMLA. Application to open skin is not recommended. The product is approved for use by the FDA in children over 3 years of age. In fact, application to a small child can be challenging due to the size of the patch.

Potential advantages

Like LMX4, onset of clinically important anesthesia is much more rapid than EMLA. The local anesthetics used are not as likely to induce methemoglobinemia. The use of heat enhances vasodilatation and may facilitate venous identification.

Potential disadvantages

The patch must stick to the skin and bring the local anesthetics into contact with the skin. In a small limb in a child, the patch can often not fit very well. Once the application time has elapsed, the patch must then be peeled off. Although it might seem minor, some children become quite upset with removal of the patch, much like when a Band-aid is removed. In my opinion, the major deterrent to use of this otherwise efficacious system remains the cost ($12–20/application).

Contraindications

Synera™ is contraindicated in patients with a known history of sensitivity to lidocaine, tetracaine, or local anesthetics of the amide or ester type. Synera is also contraindicated in patients with para-aminobenzoic acid (PABA) hypersensitivity.

Amethocaine (tetracaine) gel (Ametop)

Chemical structure: tetracaine, see Figure 68.6

Description

This is a 4% (w/w) gel formulation of tetracaine approved for use in Canada, Europe, New Zealand, Australia and many other parts of the world to be used for dermal analgesia.

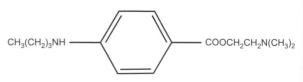

Figure 68.6.

Mode of action/pharmacology

Approximately 1 gram of the gel will cover 30 cm² when used under an occlusive dressing. The gel actually contains solid tetracaine particles which melt when applied to the skin and then form an oil emulsion that penetrates the stratum corneum. A 30 (venipuncture) to 45 (IV cannulation) minute application is recommended. Anesthesia will last 4–6 hours, as tetracaine has a considerably longer elimination half-life. It appears to have clinical comparability in providing anesthesia/analgesia when compared to EMLA.

How to use

Approximately 1 gram (packaged in 1.5 g tubes) is applied to the skin and covered with a clear occlusive dressing. As with EMLA and LMX4, a variety of cutaneous invasive procedures can be accomplished after the requisite waiting time. It should only be applied to intact skin. It also should not be applied to mucous membranes or the conjunctivae.

Potential advantages

Tetracaine gel appears to have an excellent safety profile. Its extended duration of action could lend some advantage when the time of the procedure is not easily determined. Tetracaine is also vasodilating and even associated with some transient erythema at the application site. This then avoids the vasoconstricting effects of EMLA. The product may be used in infants as young as 1 month of age.

Potential disadvantages

As with all the other aforementioned topical products, care to prevent ingestion by children is required. Erythema and skin rash may occur at application site

Contraindications

Use in premature babies or full-term infants less than 1 month of age, in whom the metabolic pathway for tetracaine may not be fully developed, is not recommended. In addition, it should be avoided if patients have known hypersensitivity to any of the local anesthetics of the ester type.

Vapocoolant spray (PainEase)

Chemical structure: $CF_3CH_2CHF_2$ (1,1,1,3,3-pentafluoropropane); CH_2FCF_3 (1,1,1,2-tetrafluoroethane)

Description

PainEase is a mixture of two fluorocarbons dispensed in spray cans. PainEase is a vapocoolant (skin refrigerant) spray for topical application to skin, intact mucous membranes (oral cavity, nasal passageways and the lips) and minor open wounds [5]. PainEase controls pain associated with injections (venipuncture, IV starts, cosmetic procedures), minor surgical procedures (such as lancing boils, incisions, drainage of small abscesses and sutures) and the temporary relief of minor sports injuries (sprains, bruising, cuts and abrasions). PainEase can also be used for myofascial release procedures employed in physical therapy or physiatry to manage myofascial pain.

Mode of action/pharmacology

The product is non-flammable. The spray is directed to the area that will be manipulated and the vapocoolant properties offer cutaneous analgesia. The analgesic effect is quite transitory, so the operator must be prepared to proceed with the procedure expeditiously.

How to use

Vapocoolant sprays have been shown to be beneficial for immunization pain, venipuncture, as well as intravenous cannulation.

Potential advantages

There is immediate onset of action. The cost per application and personnel time is minimal.

Potential disadvantages

The main disadvantage is the brief duration of action. This requires precise orchestration of the brief procedure. The cold spray can be startling and even upsetting to younger children.

Contraindications

PainEase is contraindicated in individuals with a history of hypersensitivity to 1,1,1,3,3-pentafluoropropane and 1,1,1,2-tetrafluoroethane

References

1. Koh JL, Harrison D, Myers R, Dembinski R, Turner H, McGraw T. A randomized, double-blind comparison study of EMLA and ELA-Max for topical anesthesia in children undergoing intravenous insertion. *Paediatr Anaesth* 2004;**14**:977–982.

2. Taddio A, Stevens B Craig K, Rastogi, P, Ben-David S, Shennan A, Mulligan P, Koren G. Efficacy and safety of lidocaine-prilocaine cream for pain during circumcision. *N Engl J Med* 1997;**336**:1197–1201.

3. Zempsky WT. Pharmacologic approaches for reducing venous access pain in children. *Pediatrics* 2008;**122**:S140–153.

4. Sethna NF, Verghese ST, Hannallah RS, Solodiuk JC, Zurakowski D, Berde CB. A randomized controlled trial to evaluate S-Caine patch for reducing pain associated with vascular access. *Anesthesiology* 2005;**102**:403–408.

5. Cohen Reis E, Holubkov R. Vapocoolant spray is equally effective as EMLA cream in reducing immunization pain in school-aged children. *Pediatrics* 1997;**100**: e5 at www.pediatrics.org/cgi/content/full/100/6/e5.

**Section 5
Chapter**

69

Local Anesthetics

Lidocaine transdermal

Maggy G. Riad

Generic Name: lidocaine transdermal patch

Trade Name: Lidoderm Patch 5%

Manufacturer: Endo Pharmaceuticals, Chadds Ford, PA

Chemical Structure: see Figure 69.1

Description

Lidoderm is a 10 cm × 14 cm patch containing 50 mg of lidocaine per gram of adhesive material. Each patch contains a total of 700 mg of lidocaine, the only active ingredient.

Mode of activity and pharmacology

Lidocaine or lignocaine is an amide-type local anesthetic and anti-arrhythmic agent that was first synthesized and marketed in the 1940s. Lidocaine acts by blocking the fast voltage-gated Na channels in neurons by decreasing the frequency of their opening. As a consequence, depolarization and transmission of action potential in neurons is blocked, thereby decreasing both the peripheral nociceptor sensitization as well as the central nervous system hyperexcitability. In small doses lidocaine inhibits nerve discharges at aberrant or ectopic foci generated as a result of nerve injury, without interfering with normal neuronal conduction.

Bioavailability after topical administration of lidocaine via the Lidoderm patch is only 3%, which is about only 10% of its bioavailability after oral ingestion. With 70% of lidocaine being bound to plasma proteins, the blood lidocaine concentration after application of Lidoderm patch remains very low (average concentration 128 ng/mL). These low blood lidocaine levels are sufficient to produce topical analgesia without causing a complete sensory block, thus preserving skin sensation to light touch and pinprick. This effect represents a key difference between the Lidoderm patch and other topical lidocaine formulations (Table 69.1).

Lidocaine is primarily metabolized by the cytochrome P450 hepatic enzyme system into active but less potent metabolites, mainly monoethyl-glycinexylidide (MEGX). Lidocaine has a half-life of 1.5–2.5 hours and is excreted mainly via the renal system.

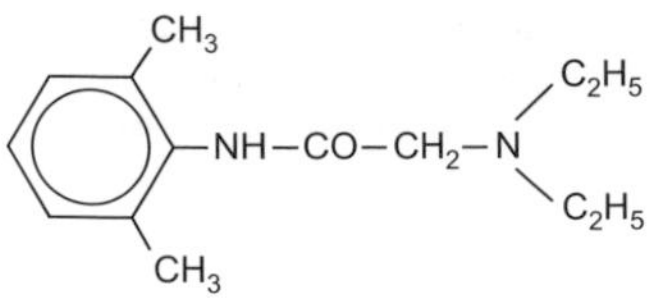

Figure 69.1.

How to use this drug in pain management

Lidoderm patch was approved by the FDA in 1999 for the treatment of post-herpetic neuralgia (PHN) based on its efficacy, tolerability, and safety. PHN is the most frequent complication of shingles (herpes zoster), the most common neurological ailment in the USA, affecting as many as 850 000 people annually. PHN is the result of sensory nerve damage by the varicella zoster virus causing development of abnormal sodium channels and the generation of ectopic or aberrant nerve discharges. Clinically it manifests as sharp, shooting or dull aching pain, usually associated with allodynia along the dermatomal distribution of affected nerve fibers.

Evidence-based treatment guidelines recommend Lidoderm patch and Pregabalin as first lines of treatment for neuropathic pain associated with PHN.

Other unapproved uses: other conditions associated with neuropathic pain. Randomized controlled multi-center European studies evaluated Lidoderm for the treatment of neuropathic pain associated with diabetic polyneuropathy. Results show Lidoderm to be as efficacious as systemic analgesics, with substantially fewer systemic side effects.

A recent randomized double-blind controlled study examined Lidoderm patch efficacy for relief of post-surgical pain after unilateral knee arthroplasty and found it to be beneficial in relieving post-operative pain and consequently improving early joint mobility. This application of Lidoderm patch is of particular benefit to elderly patients who cannot tolerate side effects of systemically administered analgesics.

There is evidence of the usefulness of low doses of lidocaine, such as obtained by using the Lidoderm patch, in the termination and early relief of migraine headache that is preceded by an aura. This application is based on lidocaine's effectiveness in the suppression of clinical and electrographic manifestations of seizures at low blood concentrations (below 5 µg/mL).

Lidoderm is also reported to work well for relief of mild to moderate pain resulting from localized conditions such as carpal tunnel syndrome, chronic bursitis, muscle sprains and arthritic joint pain.

Potential advantages

Drug is delivered directly to the site of pain, minimal systemic absorption and risk of toxicity, decreased incidence of drug–drug interactions, no need to titrate dosage, ease of use.

Potential disadvantages

It is seldom effective in conditions associated with moderate to severe pain when used alone. Studies show no significant difference between Lidoderm and placebo when used as a sole analgesic in cases of PHN or other causes of neuropathic pain.

Contraindications

Known sensitivity to amide-type local anesthetics.

Table 69.1. Other lidocaine preparations: indications and dosage

Lidocaine form	Dosage	Common clinical application (including off-label uses)
Local infiltration	5 mg/kg (7 mg/kg if used with epi)	Preemptive analgesia, post-op pain management
Peripheral nerve block	200–450 mg	Surgical anesthesia, post-op pain management
Neuroaxial block	200–500 mg	Surgical anesthesia, post-op pain management
Intravenous infusion	1–4 mg/kg per h	Diagnostic tool, treatment of fibromyalgia, post-op pain, chronic pain syndromes, neuropathic pain
Subcutaneous infusion	80–150 mg/h	Neuropathic pain, localized post-op pain, palliative care
Topical patch	700–2100 mg for 12 h	PHN, neuropathic pain, localized pain
Topical gel/ointment	2%, 4%, 5%	Localized minor pains, topicalization prior to procedures
Oral	200–300 mg TID	Treatment of fibromyalgia, neuropathic pain

Table 69.2. Pharmacokinetics of Lidoderm patch

Lidoderm dose	Site	Duration	Dose absorbed	Blood concentration
2100 mg	Back	12 hours	32–96 mg	0.07–0.19 µg/mL

Caution: use only if necessary during pregnancy (Pregnancy Category B) and lactation. The clinical effects on humans during pregnancy and nursing have not been studied. Lidocaine crosses the placenta and is known to be secreted in milk at a milk/plasma ratio of 0.4/1. Lidoderm use in the pediatric population has not been studied and is not recommended.

Dosing

Each Lidoderm patch may be used only once for up to 12 hours/day. Lidoderm patches should be applied to the most painful area, only if the skin is intact. No more than three patches are to be applied at a time. Average blood concentration achieved with this dosing is between 0.13 and 0.25 µg/mL of lidocaine, depending on the site of application (Table 69.2). Lidocaine toxicity coincides with a lidocaine blood level at or above 5 µg/mL.

Drug-related adverse events

Lidoderm may cause transient skin irritation, blistering or burning at the application site. Wearing transdermal drug patches with backings that contain even a small amount of aluminum or other metals in the MRI suite may result in severe skin burns at the application site. Even though the Lidoderm patch backing consists of a non-woven polyester felt, devoid of visible metals, it is currently the FDA's recommendation to temporarily remove all transdermal patches while undergoing MRI examinations or procedures. The FDA is currently conducting a formal investigation to examine the safety and compatibility of all transdermal patches with the MRI environment.

Patients with known allergic reactions to methylparaben or propylparaben may develop allergic reactions to the lidoderm patch. Severe hypersensitivity-types of reactions to lidoderm are rare.

Complications related to increased blood lidocaine concentrations

Lidocaine overdose from transdermal absorption only is rare but possible. Conditions that result in increased lidocaine absorption and hence increase its blood concentrations include:

- Application of a lidoderm patch for longer than 12 hours/day
- Application of more than three patches at a time
- Patients with low body mass index
- Application to areas where the skin barrier is violated
- Concomitant administration of other medications containing lidocaine
- Concomitant administration of other local anesthetics
- Concomitant administration of drugs that decrease hepatic blood flow
- Decreased metabolism due to severe liver impairment
- Concomitant administration with cytochrome P450 hepatic enzyme inhibitors, e.g. macrolide antibiotics, antifungal agents, verapamil, cimetidine, ciprofloxacin, enoxacin, fluvoxamine, amiodarone
- Patients with decompensated congestive heart failure
- Decreased elimination due to renal failure
- Accidental ingestion of discarded patches by children or pets

Systemic effects of lidocaine overdose include:

- CNS: tremors, dizziness, restlessness, agitation, dysarthria, confusion, hallucinations, tinnitus, nystagmus, blurred vision, seizures
- Respiratory: increased airway tone, airway narrowing, bronchospasm, respiratory arrest
- Cardiovascular: hypotension, sinus bradycardia, asystole, cardiovascular collapse
- Gastrointestinal: nausea, vomiting

Treatment of overdose: life support and symptomatic treatment for acute lidocaine toxicity. Most of the cases present with mild symptoms that respond to temporary discontinuation of treatment and decreasing the dosage. Dialysis was found to play no role in the treatment of lidocaine overdose.

Caution should be exercised with the disposal of used lidoderm patches, since about 95% of its lidocaine content could still be found in each used patch. It is therefore imperative to discard used patches after folding them so that the medication side of the patch is covered in order to avoid accidental ingestion by small children or pets.

References

1. Transdermal drug patches with metallic backings www.fda.gov/safety/medwatch/safetyinformation/safety.

2. Lidoderm: Endo Pharmaceuticals Inc. 2008.

3. Efficacy and safety of 5% lidocaine medicated plaster in comparison with pregabalin in patients with postherpetic neuralgia and diabetic polyneuropathy. *Clin Drug Investig* 2009;**29**:231–241.

Neuropathic pain caused by injury and sensitization of the peripheral or central nervous system does not generally respond to traditional pain therapies such as opioids and nonsteroidal-anti-inflammatory drugs. Neuronal sensitization and ectopic noxious transmission resemble to some degree the abnormal, easily triggered neural circuits associated with seizure disorders. Drugs acting to reduce such ectopic activity, anticonvulsants, or anti-epileptic drugs (AED), date from 1910–1970, and include "first-generation" agents such as benzodiazepines, barbiturates, phenytoin (Dilantin), ethosuximide (Zarontin), carbamazepine (Tegretol, Carbatrol), and valproic acid (Depakon, Depakene). Second-generation agents are represented by felbamate (Felbatol), gabapentin (Neurontin), lamotrigine (Lamictal), levateracetam (Keppra), oxcarbazepine (Trileptal), pregabalin (Lyrica), tiagabine (Gabitril), topiramate (Topamax), vigabatrin (Sabril), and zonisamide (Zonegran). The adoption of anti-convulsant drugs into mainstream neuropathic pain therapy has been a long process, as many were developed for very different applications. In general, first-generation agents had great patient intolerability, higher toxicity, and variable effectiveness. Second-generation drugs, often termed "gabapentinoids", offer greater tolerability and selectivity [1,2]. The mechanism of action of first- and second-generation drugs is often multiple, with the major sites of action summarized in Table 70.1.

Some anticonvulsants appear to exhibit anti-inflammatory effects. The wound-healing effects of phenytoin and its associated gingival hypertorophy may reflect its action on fibroblast activity. It appears in animal studies that gabapentin and lamotrigine have peripheral analgesic effects, suggesting an effect on peripheral neurotransmission.

Applications of first-generation AEDs

Carbamazepine: trigeminal neuralgia, migraine prophylaxis, post-herpetic neuralgia, diabetic neuropathy

Valproic acid: migraine prophylaxis, chronic pain

Phenytoin: diabetic neuropathy, cancer pain

Clonazepam: trigeminal neuralgia, myofascial pain, migraine prophylaxis

Currently the most commonly prescribed anticonvulsants for pain control are gabapentin and pregabalin [1,2]. Gabapentin is an aminobutyric acid analog that received Food and Drug Administration approval in 1993 for adjunctive treatment of partial seizures in adults. Soon after its release a number of case reports and uncontrolled trials were published attesting to its safety and effectiveness in controlling intractable neuropathic pain in patients presenting with reflex sympathetic dystrophy, post-herpetic neuralgia, migraine, and trigeminal neuralgia. In a letter to the editor Mellick was one of the first to report remarkable effectiveness of gabapentin in relieving pain associated with reflex sympathetic dystrophy [3]. These authors reported that the drug was very well tolerated but that dose adjustments (300–2400 mg/day) and upwards titration were required to compensate for significant variabilites in patient response. Subsequently, a number of well-controlled gabapentin trials were performed which validated earlier anecdotal observations, and secured FDA approval for its use in the management of neuropathic pain.

Despite extensive studies, gabapentin's mechanism of action is unknown. While it was initially believed to function as a GABA analog, it does not appear to act on GABA receptors. However, muscular relaxation associated with gabapentin has been related to indirect presynaptic activation of GABA pathways. It is now recognized that gabapentin and pregabalin have high binding affinity for the 2 subunit of presynaptic voltage-gated calcium channels [4]. Their analgesic effects may be related to inhibition of calcium influx and release of excitatory neurotransmitters in spinal and supraspinal pain pathways. They also appear to reduce the excitability of irritated and injured peripheral noxious fibers.

The Essence of Analgesia and Analgesics, ed. Raymond S. Sinatra, Jonathan S. Jahr and J. Michael Watkins-Pitchford. Published by Cambridge University Press. © Cambridge University Press 2011.

Table 70.1. AED modes of action

Sodium channel blockade	Carbamazepine, felbamate, lamotrigine, oxcarbazepine, phenytoin, topiramate, zonisamide
Calcium channel blockade	Carbamazepine, ethosuximide, felbamate, gabapentin, lamotrigine, levitiracetam, oxcarbazine, pregabilin, topiramate, valproic acid, zonisamide
Glutamate release reduction and action on NMDA / AMPA receptors	Carbamazepine, felbamate, gabapentin, lamotrigine, oxcarazine, phenytoin, pregabalin, topiramate, valproic acid
Peripheral anti-inflammatory and fibroblast activity	Phenytoin, gabapentin, lamotrigine

Both gabapentin and pregabalin are commonly employed in neuropathic pain and are approved for post-herpetic neuralgia and diabetic neuropathy. The commonest side effects with therapeutic doses are dizziness and sedation, which are often tolerable if doses are started low. Renal elimination requires that dosage be reduced significantly in patients with renal impairment. Gabapentin has complex pharmacokinetics, requiring dosage three times daily, gradually increasing up to 3600 mg/day until pain relief is achieved or intolerability limits further increase of dosage. Finding optimal dosage can take 3 months or more.

In contrast to gabapentin, the more recently approved gabapentinoid, pregabalin, was conceived, developed, and marketed as an analgesic as well as an anticonvulsant [5]. Pregabalin has neurochemical and therapeutic similarities to gabapentin, but is more selective, has greater tolerability, and is simpler to dose. Commonly, 75–150 mg/day is given in two divided doses, increasing to 300 mg/day after a week or two as tolerated. Higher does have been used, up to 600 mg/day, generally without much benefit but increased side effects [5].

Gabapentin and pregabalin and, to a lesser extent, lamotrigine have displaced almost all first-generation anticonvulsants for the management of neuropathic pain, perhaps the only exception being carbamazepine, which is still prescribed for poorly controlled trigeminal neuralgia-related pain. They are approved for diabetic neuropathy and post-herpetic neuralgia, and while there are no controlled trials to attest safety and efficacy, they are frequently prescribed to control neuropathic symptoms associated with reflex sympathetic dystrophy, sciatica, polyneuropathy, and phantom limb. Other off-label uses include management of migraine, nystagmus, and restless leg syndrome. Pregabalin effectively reduces spinal cord sensitization and centrally mediated neuropathic pain, and has recently been approved for management of fibromyalgia [6].

In addition to their use in chronic pain both gabapentin and pregabalin have been advocated for use as post-operative analgesic adjuvants [7,8]. Pre- and post-operative dose of gabapentin (900 mg) and pregabalin (150 mg) significantly reduced opioid consumption in several post-surgical models. While they do not improve pain intensity scores, they do appear to reduce wound site hyperalgesia. There is also evidence to suggest that peri-operative dosing may reduce central sensitization and the development of persistent pain.

Adverse effects

Early side effects such as drowsiness are often tolerated as time passes. Later side effects are often more serious and an indication for cessation of the AED. The frequency of side effects of AEDs is classified and listed in the product inserts according to Food and Drug Administration (FDA) guidelines. Adverse reactions are classified as frequent (>1/100), infrequent (<1/100), or rare (<1/1000). Most of the frequent adverse events are dose-related, CNS-mediated side effects. Non-neurological side effects are hirsutism and gingival hyperplasia with phenytoin, leukopenia and hyponatremia with carbamazepine, and weight gain and hair loss with valproate. Some of the most severe and life-threatening adverse events do not affect the CNS (e.g. Stevens–Johnson syndrome [SJS], aplastic anemia, and hepatic failure). These are rare and early recognition is essential.

While there are ample studies to confirm the efficacy of gabapentin and pregabalin, there is a dearth of comparisons with established antidepressant drugs such as amitriptyline and other tricyclics. Other concerns include the possible ability of gabapentin to cause neuropathy, so reassurance would be welcome that the benefits outweigh the risks in differing clinical circumstances, particularly in the long term.

293

Conclusion

The mechanisms by which these different agents work in the pain setting, often far from their original purpose, remain unclear though progress is rapid. The efficacy is undoubted, while the frequency of side effects and adverse reactions continue to diminish. Their marketing has legally tested the limits of "off-label" prescription, and still their acceptance increases. Gabapentin and now pregabalin offer new and exciting therapeutic options for mostly adjuvant treatment of neuropathic pain and may have a future role in acute pain management.

References

1. http://en.wikipedia.org/wiki/Gabapentin. Accessed January 16, 2010.

2. Goa KL, Sorkin EM. Gabapentin: a review of its pharmacological properties and clinical potential in epilepsy. *Drugs* 1993;**46**(3):409–427.

3. Mellick GA, Mellick LB. Gabapentin in the management of reflex sympathetic dystrophy. *(Letter) J Pain Symptom Manage* 1995;**10**:265–266 .

4. Lou ZD, Calcutt NA, Higuera ES, et al. Injury type-specific calcium channel alpha2delta-1 subunit up-regulation in rat neuropathic pain models correlates with antiallodynic effects of gabapentin. *J Pharmcol Exp Ther* 2002;**303**:1199–1205.

5. http://en.wikipedia.org/wiki/Pregabalin. Accessed January 16, 2010.

6. Crofford LJ, Rowbotham MC, Mease PJ, et al. Pregabalin for the treatment of fibromyalgia syndrome: results of a randomized, double-blind, placebo-controlled trial. *Arthritis Rheum* 2005;**52**(4):1264–1273.

7. Gilron I, Orr E, Tu DS, O'Neill JP, Zamora JE, Bell AC. A placebo-controlled randomized clinical trial of perioperative administration of gabapentin, rofecoxib and their combination for spontaneous and movement-evoked pain after abdominal hysterectomy. *Pain* 2005;**113**:191–200.

8. Dahl JB, Mathiesen O, Moiniche S. A review of gabapentin and pregabalin in the treatment of post-operative pain. *Acta anaesthesiologica Scandinavica* 2004;**48**:1130–1139.

9. Kroenke K, Krebs EE, Bair MJ. Pharmacotherapy of chronic pain: a synthesis of recommendations from systematic reviews. *Gen Hosp Psychiatry* 2009; **31**:206–219.

10. O'Connor AB, Dworkin RH. Treatment of neuropathic pain: an overview of recent guidelines. *Am J Med* 2009;**122**(10A) S22–32.

Section 6 Chapter 71

Anticonvulsant-Type Analgesics

Gabapentin

Boris Gelman and Eric S. Hsu

Generic Name: gabapentin

Trade Name: Neurontin

Manufacturer: Pfizer Inc.

Class: anticonvulsant analgesic

Chemical Structure: see Figure 71.1

Description

Gabapentin is an analgesic commonly used in the treatment of neuropathic pain. It is described as 1-(aminomethyl)cyclohexaneacetic acid with a molecular formula $C_9H_{17}NO_2$. It has a molecular weight of 171.24 and a pKa1 of 3.7 and pKa2 of 10.7. It is freely soluble in water and both basic and acidic aqueous

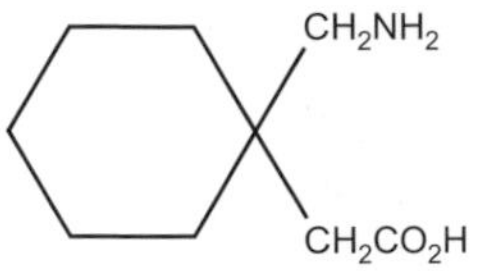

Figure 71.1.

solutions. Gabapentin is currently only available in the oral form as capsules (100 mg, 300 mg, and 400 mg), tablets (600 mg and 800 mg), or oral solution (250 mg/5 mL).

Mode of activity

Pharmacodynamics

The mechanism by which gabapentin exerts its analgesic action is unknown. It has been shown in animal models to prevent allodynia (pain-related behavior in response to a normally innocuous stimulus) and hyperalgesia (exaggerated response to painful stimuli). Particularly, gabapentin has been shown to attenuate pain-related responses in several animal models of neuropathic pain (diabetes, spinal nerve ligation, spinal cord injury, acute herpes zoster infection) and also decreases pain-related responses after peripheral inflammation. However, gabapentin did not alter immediate pain-related behaviors in animal models.

Gabapentin is structurally related to the neurotransmitter GABA (gamma-aminobutyric acid) but it does not modify GABAA or GABAB radioligand binding. Gabapentin is not converted metabolically into GABA or a GABA agonist, and it is not an inhibitor of GABA uptake or degradation. Gabapentin was shown to activate the descending noradrenergic system after pre-operative oral administration at the time of surgery. Therefore, a central mechanism of oral gabapentin in modulation of post-operative pain was proposed and this could be magnified by treatments that boost the effect of norepinephrine release.

It was proposed that gabapentin may modulate the central voltage-gated calcium channels similarly to pregabalin as a potential mechanism of clinical efficacy in neuropathic pain. Pregabalin binds with high affinity to the alpha$_2$-delta site (an auxiliary subunit of voltage-gated calcium channels) in CNS tissues of animal models. Although the exact mechanism of action of pregabalin is unknown, results with genetically modified mice and with compounds structurally related to pregabalin (such as gabapentin) suggest that binding to the alpha$_2$-delta subunit

may be involved in antinociceptive and antiseizure effects of pregabalin in animal models. Pregabalin reduces the calcium-dependent release neurotransmitters (glutamate, substance P) via possible modulation of calcium channel function.

Pharmacokinetics

The bioavailability of gabapentin is approximately 60%, 47%, 34%, 33%, and 27% following 900, 1200, 2400, 3600, and 4800 mg/day given in three divided doses, respectively. The bioavailability is not dose-proportional (as the dose is increased, bioavailability decreases). In contrast, pregabalin offers a more linear pharmacokinetic profile over gabapentin and a consistent >90% bioavailability. Pregabalin may result in a shorter course of titration and quicker response in clinical application.

Less than 3% of gabapentin is protein-bound, therefore it has insignificant drug interactions. The elimination half-life of gabapentin is 5–7 hours and follows linear kinetics even with multiple doses. Because of its short half-life, gabapentin may be administered either twice or three times daily. Gabapentin is not appreciably metabolized in the body and is excreted in urine unchanged. The elimination rate constant, plasma and renal clearance of gabapentin are all directly proportional to the creatinine clearance.

Drug interactions

There was a slight degree of inhibition (14–30%) of P450 CYP2A6 observed only at the highest concentration (approximately 15 times the C_{max} at 3600 mg/day). No inhibition of any of the other isoforms (CYP1A2, CYP2C9, CYP2C19, CYP2D6, CYP2E1, and CYP3A4) tested was observed. Gabapentin is not appreciably metabolized in liver nor does it inhibit any cytochrome P450 enzymes in standard clinical dosing. Gabapentin does not interfere with the metabolism of commonly co-administered anti-epileptic drugs.

Indications

There are only two US FDA-approved indications for gabapentin:
1. Post-herpetic neuralgia (PHN)
2. Partial seizures

However, gabapentin has been commonly prescribed for off-label uses such as neuropathic pain and chronic pain syndromes. Here are some examples.

Post-operative pain

The administration of gabapentin to patients undergoing craniotomy for supratentorial tumor resection was effective for acute post-operative pain. It also decreased other analgesic consumption after surgery.

Gabapentin appears safe and well tolerated when used for persistent post-operative and post-traumatic pain in thoracic surgery patients despite minor side effects. Gabapentin may relieve refractory chest wall pain especially in those patients with more severe pain.

Reduce chronic post-operative neuropathic pain

Although pre-operative gabapentin did not modify immediate pain relief in thyroidectomy patients receiving superficial cervical plexus block, it did prevent the delayed neuropathic pain at 6 month follow-up.

Phantom pain

Gabapentin monotherapy was better than placebo in post-amputation phantom limb pain after 6 weeks. There were no significant differences in mood, sleep interference, or activities of daily living.

Complex regional pain syndrome (CRPS)

Gabapentin was shown to significantly reduce the sensory deficit in the affected limb in CRPS despite only modest relief of pain. Therefore, a subpopulation of CRPS patients may benefit from gabapentin as part of timely and comprehensive intervention.

Cancer pain

Neuropathic cancer pain can be relieved by gabapentin as part of the multimodal treatment following WHO's three-step analgesia guidelines since the majority of cancer pain involves various etiologies of pathophysiology.

Contraindications

Absolute contraindication: hypersensitivity to gabapentin.

Relative contraindication:

1. Renal insufficiency: gabapentin is excreted via the kidneys thus dose should be adjusted based on creatinine clearance.
2. Suicidal behavior and ideation: all anti-epileptic drugs (AEDs) including gabapentin may increase the risk of suicidal thoughts or behavior in patients taking these drugs for any indication. Patients should be monitored for the emergence or worsening of depression, suicidal thoughts or behavior, and/or any unusual changes in their mood or behavior.

Common doses

Post-herpetic neuralgia (PHN): gabapentin therapy may be initiated as a single 300-mg dose on day 1, 600 mg/day on day 2 (divided BID), and 900 mg/day on day 3 (divided TID). The dose can subsequently be titrated up as needed for pain relief up to a target daily dose of 1800 mg (divided TID). In clinical studies, efficacy was also demonstrated over a range of doses

Table 71.1. Gabapentin dosage based on renal function

Renal function (mL/min)	Total daily dose range (mg/day)	Dose regimen (mg)				
≥60	900–3600	300 TID	400 TID	600 TID	800 TID	1200 TID
>30–59	400–1400	200 BID	300 BID	400 BID	500 BID	700 BID
>15–29	200–700	200 QD	300 QD	400 QD	500 QD	700 QD
15[a]	100–300	100 QD	125 QD	150 QD	200 QD	300 QD
Post-hemodialysis supplemental dose (mg)[b]						
Hemodialysis		125[b]	150[b]	200[b]	250[b]	300[b]

[a]For patients with creatinine clearance < 15 mL/min, reduce daily dose in proportion to creatinine clearance (e.g. patients with a creatinine clearance of 7.5 mL/min should receive one-half the daily dose that patients with a creatinine clearance of 15 mL/min receive).

[b]Patients on hemodialysis should receive maintenance doses based on estimates of creatinine clearance as indicated in the upper portion of the table and a supplemental post-hemodialysis dose administered after each 4 hours of hemodialysis as indicated in the lower portion of the table.

from 1800 mg/day to 3600 mg/day with comparable effects across the dose range. Additional benefit related to doses higher than 1800 mg/day of gabapentin was not demonstrated. Gabapentin needs to be tapered over 7 days when discontinuing.

Dosage in renal impairment: creatinine clearance is difficult to measure in outpatients. In patients with stable renal function, creatinine clearance (CCr) can be reasonably well estimated using the equation of Cockcroft and Gault: for females CCr = (0.85) × (140−age) × (weight)/[(72) × (SCr)] for males CCr = (140−age) × (weight)/[(72) × (SCr)] where age is in years, weight is in kilograms and SCr is serum creatinine in mg/dL.

Dosage adjustment in patients ≥12 years of age with compromised renal function or undergoing hemodialysis is recommended as shown in Table 71.1.

Potential advantages

1. Gabapentin presents with minimal drug interaction so it appears versatile in combination with other neuropathic pain medications in clinical use.
2. Gabapentin is affordable with generic form and available in outpatient and hospital settings.

Potential disadvantages

Abrupt discontinuation and withdrawal of gabapentin may precipitate seizure (status epilepticus). The most frequently reported events following abrupt discontinuation were anxiety, insomnia, nausea, pain, and sweating.

Precaution and instruction for patients: patients should be instructed to take gabapentin only as prescribed since gabapentin may cause dizziness, somnolence, and other CNS depression. Patients should be advised neither to drive a car nor to operate other complex machinery until they have gained sufficient experience on gabapentin to gauge whether or not it affects their mental and/or motor performance adversely.

Drug-related adverse events

The most commonly observed adverse events associated with the use of gabapentin versus placebo in adults with PHN were dizziness, somnolence, and peripheral edema. In the two controlled studies in PHN, 16% of the 336 patients who received gabapentin and 9% of the 227 patients who received placebo discontinued treatment because of an adverse event.

Postmarketing and other experience: these data are insufficient to support an estimate of their incidence or to establish causation. The listing is alphabetized: angioedema, blood glucose fluctuation, breast hypertrophy, erythema multiforme, elevated liver function tests, fever, hyponatremia, jaundice, movement disorder, and Stevens–Johnson syndrome.

Overdose and treatment: acute oral overdoses of gabapentin up to 49 grams have been reported. In these cases, double vision, slurred speech, drowsiness, lethargy, and diarrhea were observed. All patients recovered with supportive care. Gabapentin can be removed by hemodialysis. Although hemodialysis was not performed in the few overdose cases reported, it may be indicated by the patient's clinical state or in patients with significant renal impairment.

References

1. *Gabapentin.* Micromedex Healthcare Series. Thompson Healthcare, 2009.
2. Gabapentin prescribing information. New York: Pfizer. Revised April 2009.
3. Hayashida K, et al Gabapentin activates spinal noradrenergic activity in rats and humans and reduces hypersensitivity after surgery. *Anesthesiology* 2007;**106**(3):557–562.
4. Sills GJ. The mechanisms of action of gabapentin and pregabalin. *Curr Opin Pharmacol* 2006;**6**(1):108–113.
5. Rice AS, Maton S. Postherpetic Neuralgia Study Group. Gabapentin in postherpetic neuralgia: a randomized, double blind, placebo controlled study. *Pain* 2001;**94**(2):215–224.
6. Rowbotham M, Harden N, Stacey B, et al. Gabapentin for the treatment of postherpetic neuralgia: a randomized controlled trial. *JAMA* 1998;**280**(21):1837–1842.

72

Pregabalin

Neil Sinha

Generic Name: pregabalin

Trade Name: Lyrica™

Drug Class: anticonvulsant analgesic

Manufacturer: Pfizer Pharmaceuticals, 235 East 42nd Street, New York, NY

Chemical Structure: see Figure 72.1

Chemical Name: (S)-3-(aminomethyl)-5-methyl-hexanoic acid

Chemical Formula: $C_8H_{17}NO_2$; molecular wt 159.2

Introduction

Pregabalin (Lyrica) is an anti-epileptic drug used for the treatment of neuropathic pain, fibromyalgia, post-herpetic neuralgia, and as an adjunct therapy for partial seizures. The systemic (IUPAC) description of pregabalin is (S)-3-(aminomethyl)-5-methylhexanoic acid and its molecular formula is $C_8H_{17}NO_2$. It has a molecular weight of 159.23. Pfizer, Inc. introduced this drug (under the trade name Lyrica) and it was approved in the European Union in 2004 and by the FDA (initially for the treatment of epilepsy, diabetic neuropathic pain, and post-herpetic neuralgia) in December 2004 [1,2].

Mechanism of action

Voltage-gated calcium channels (VGCC) are cell membrane glycoproteins that regulate action potential of neurons. VGCC consist of four subunits (designated α_1, α_2-δ, α_2-β, and α_2-γ) present in equal ratios with six transmembrane helices each. Calcium entry into neurons through the VGCC results in the release of neurotransmitters into the synaptic cleft. Certain physiological states such as epilepsy or neuropathy may have "hyper-excited" VGCCs resulting in the continuous influx of calcium ions and the sustained release of excitatory neurotransmitters as glutamate, norepinephrine, and substance P [2,3].

Pregabalin, like gabapentin, binds to the α_2-δ subunit of the presynaptic voltage-gated calcium channels in the dorsal horn of the spinal cord and the brain, causing conformational changes that prevent the influx of calcium and the subsequent release of excitatory neurotransmitters. In particular, pregabalin has higher affinity to "hyper-excited" neurons, selectively targeting the pathological neurons. Although pregabalin is structurally a GABA analog, it has no affinity to the $GABA_A$ or $GABA_B$ receptors. In addition, it has no affinity to the cardiac or vascular calcium receptors.

Pharmacokinetics

After oral intake, pregabalin is transported across the gastrointestinal tract by the L-amino acid transport system and displays linear pharmacokinetics across and even above clinical dosing regimens. Maximal absorption (>90% bioavailability) after oral administration in fasting subjects occurs in 1 to 1.5 hours. With chronic dosing, pregabalin reaches a steady state in 24–48 hours [2,3]. Pregabalin is not appreciably bound to plasma proteins and has a volume of distribution of 0.56 L/kg after oral administration. In animal models, pregabalin has been shown to cross the blood–brain barrier by the L-amino acid transport system. The half-life of pregabalin under fasting conditions and in patients with normal renal function is 6 hours.

Pregabalin undergoes negligible metabolism in humans. Approximately 90% of radiolabeled pregabalin is detected in urine after single-dose administration. The major metabolite, N-methylated pregabalin, was found in urine at 0.9% of original administered does.

In humans, pregabalin is primarily excreted from systemic circulation by the renal system as an unchanged drug. Renal clearance of pregabalin, in young healthy

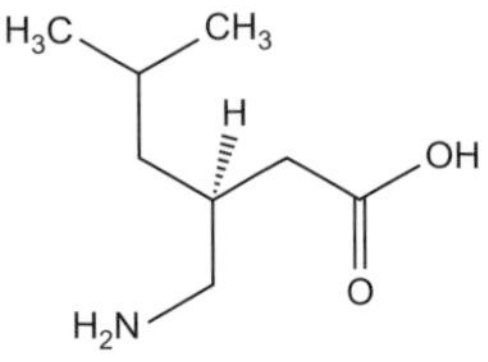

Figure 72.1.

volunteers with normal functions, is estimated to be 67.0 to 80.9 mL/min. Because pregabalin is only negligibly metabolized and does not bind to plasma proteins, its elimination is nearly proportional to creatinine clearance [3].

Routes of administration

Pregabalin is currently available as an oral administered drug. It is supplied in 25 mg, 50 mg, 75 mg, 100 mg, 150 mg, 200 mg, 225 mg, and 300 mg tablets. The capsule shell is composed of gelatin and titanium dioxide [2,3].

Contraindications

The only contraindication to pregabalin is known hypersensitivity to pregabalin or any of its components.

Indications

The FDA has approved the use of pregabalin for the following classes of pain.

1. Neuropathic pain associated with diabetic peripheral neuropathy

Diabetes mellitus is a worldwide disease that, according to estimates by the World Health Organization, affects at least 171 million people; by 2030, this number is expected to double. Diabetic peripheral neuropathy (DPN) is a frequent complication, occurring in approximately 20–24% of patients with diabetes and in 50% of those with diabetes for greater than 25 years. The symptoms of DPN range from mild tingling to deep, severe lacinating and burning pain. DPN may have a profoundly devastating effect on the quality of life and the psychological well being of those affected. Multiple multi-center, double-blind, randomized controlled trials have demonstrated that pregabalin use in patients with diabetes results in an early and sustained decrease in pain scores and a beneficial effect on sleep [3,4].

Pregabalin dosing for DPN should begin at 50 mg three times a day and may be increased to a maximum of 100 mg three times a day over the period of a week in patients with normal renal function. Higher doses (greater than 300 mg/day) have not shown any additional benefits [5].

2. Post-herpetic neuralgia

Post-herpetic neuralgia (PHN) is persistent pain that continues 3 months after the resolution of the herpes zoster eruption. In the USA, approximately 1 million individuals develop herpes zoster; of those, 20% develop PHN. The symptoms are variable in nature – ranging from mild discomfort to a very severe burning or stabbing sensation that is typically confined to a single dermatome of skin. Multiple multi-center, double-blind, randomized controlled trials have demonstrated that pregabalin use in PHN results in an early and sustained decrease in pain scores.

Pregabalin dosing for PHN should begin at 50 mg three times a day (or 75 mg times twice a day) in patients with normal renal function [3]. Dosing may be increased to 300 mg per day within 1 week. If sufficient pain relief is not achieved by 2–4 weeks, the pregabalin dose may be increased to 600 mg per day (administered in twice a day or thrice a day schedule). However, doses above 300 mg a day should only be reserved for those with ongoing pain despite pregabalin therapy of 300 mg per day [3].

3. Fibromyalgia

Fibromyalgia is a rheumatological condition that is characterized by widespread pain in all four quadrants of the body lasting for more than 3 months; in addition, in fibromyalgia, patients experience tenderness in at least 11 of 18 designated trigger points. Approximately 2% of Americans suffer from fibromyalgia, with a strong female preponderance (9:1 by ACR criteria). Pregabalin, in a randomized controlled trial, has shown a 50% reduction in pain (NNT is 6). The Cochrane Database analysis concludes that "A minority of patients will have substantial benefit with pregabalin, and more will have moderate benefit. Many will have no or trivial benefit, or will discontinue because of adverse events".

Pregabalin dosing for fibromyalgia should begin at 75 mg twice a day and may be increased to 150 mg twice a day within a week in patients with normal renal function. In those patients who do not exhibit sufficient benefits, the pregabalin dose may be increased to 225 mg twice a day [3]. Doses higher than

450 mg a day have not been shown to confer any additional benefits.

Although these are the only FDA-approved uses, pregabalin is often used for "off-label" adjunctive analgesia for moderate to severe acute pain (including surgery and dental procedures), and also for non-DPN/PHN neuropathic pain.

Potential advantages

1. Pregabalin displays linear pharmacokinetics across its therapeutic range and has high bioavailability resulting in predictable dose-dependent responses.
2. It has a short titration period as the dose may be increased after 1 week.
3. It is well tolerated; less than 10% of patients will discontinue the use of pregabalin as a consequence of adverse side effects.
4. Pregabalin is largely excreted unchanged in the urine and does not bind to plasma proteins, resulting in minimal drug–drug interactions.
5. Pregabalin may be taken with or without food.
6. It is a schedule V controlled substance.

Disadvantages

1. Pergabalin requires dose modification in patients with renal dysfunction
2. Pregabalin is a relatively expensive medication; (but in some areas of the country, pregabalin remains cheaper than Neurontin™ and generic gabapentin).
3. Pregabalin has not demonstrated *superiority* to alternative treatments.
4. There are limited studies demonstrating the long-term safety of pregabalin.
5. Pregabalin should be gradually tapered for a period of at least 1 week; abrupt discontinuation may result in insomnia, headache, nausea, and diarrhea
6. Pregabalin crosses the placenta and is present in breast milk. It has been designated a Pregnancy Category C drug by the FDA.

Drug-related adverse effects

The most frequent adverse effects of pregabalin are dizziness and drowsiness; other common effects include visual disturbances, ataxia, dysarthria, tremor, lethargy, memory impairment, euphoria, constipa-tion, dry mouth, peripheral edema, a decrease or loss in libido, and weight gain.

Special precautions should be taken for:

- Angioedema, which may occur with initial or chronic treatment with pregabalin and may occur at higher rates with patients on ACE inhibitors and those with a history of angioedema. Pregabalin should be immediately stopped and supportive care instituted.
- Hypersenstivity, which typically presents as rash, hives, dyspnea, and wheezing. Pregabalin should be immediately stopped and supportive care instituted.
- Suicidal ideation, which may occur within a week of initiation or at any stage of treatment. Pregabalin, like all AEDs, may increase the risk of depression and suicidal thoughts and behaviors and special care should be given to patients with preexisting depression and/or suicidal ideation before starting pregabalin.
- Peripheral edema, which occurred in 6% of patients administered pregabalin in controlled trials (compared to 2% in the placebo arm). The peripheral edema is not a consequence of congestive heart failure, or renal or hepatic insufficiency. The thiazolidinedione class of oral hypoglycemics may increase the risk of fluid retention. In addition, because of limited data, pregabalin should be administered cautiously in patients with NYHA class III or IV cardiac status.
- Dizziness, which may occur in up to 31% of pregabalin treated patients. Hence, caution with driving should be taken.
- Weight gain of over 7% of baseline weight occurred in 9% of patients in controlled trials.

Overdose

The highest reported accidental overdose of pregabalin has been 8 grams of pregabalin, which resulted in no long-term consequences. In the case of overdose, emesis or gastric lavage can be used to eliminate unabsorbed drug (if down within 1–1.5 hours). In addition, the patient should be carefully monitored and supportive care is indicated. Hemodialysis may be attempt in patients with severe renal compromise, which significantly eliminates pregabalin from systemic circulation (50% in 4 hours with standard hemodialysis).

References

1. Bellioti T, Capiris T, Wustruw D, et al. Structure–activity relationships of pregabalin and analogues that target the α2-δ protein. *J Med Chem* 2005;**48**(7):2294–2307.

2. Kavoussi R. Pregabalin: from molecule to medicine. *Eur Neuropsychopharmacol* 2006;**16**(S2):S128–S133.

3. Lyrica (pregabalin). Prescribing information. New York: Pfizer, 2006. http://www.pfizer.com/products/rx/rx_product_lyrica.jsp. Accessed August 25, 2009.

4. Lesser H, Sharma U, LaMoreaux L, Poole RM. Pregabalin relieves symptoms of painful diabetic neuropathy: a randomized controlled trial. *Neurology* 2004;**63**:2104–2110.

5. Thomas J, Walker R. Pregabalin (Lyrica) for the management of pain associated with diabetic neuropathy. *Steps New Drug Rev* 2006;**74**(12): 2093–2094.

Section 6 Chapter

73

Anticonvulsant-Type Analgesics

Carbamazepine

Keren Ziv

Trade Names: Atretol® (Athena, USA Neurosciences), Carbatrol® (Shire Richwood, USA), Equetro® (Shire Richwood, USA), Tegretol Chewable® Tablets, Tegretol® Suspension, Tegretol®-XR (Novartis, USA)

Clinical Class: anticonvulsant

Chemical Class: iminostilbene

Chemical Name: 5H-Dibenz[b,f]azepine-5-carboxamide

Chemical Structure: see Figure 73.1

Description

Carbamazepine is an anticonvulsant that is structurally related to tricyclic antidepressants such as amitriptyline and imipramine. Carbamazepine is effective in the treatment of psychomotor and grand mal seizures and pain from trigeminal neuralgia and, in combination with other drugs, for psychiatric disorders such as mania and extreme aggression. Carbamazepine is also occasionally used to control pain in persons with cancer. Carbamazepine was first mar-keted as an anti-seizure medication and as a first-line treatment for trigeminal neuralgia. Because it was later noted to be effective in patients with certain psychiatric disorders, psychiatrists began combining it with other drugs such as lithium and major tranquilizers in severe cases of bipolar disease and aggressive behavior that could not be managed with single-drug therapy.

Mode of activity

Although not fully understood, animal studies have shown that carbamazepine blocks voltage-sensitive sodium channels resulting in stabilization of hyperexcited neural membranes, inhibition of repetitive neuronal firing and inhibition of the spread of discharges. Pain relief is believed to be due to reduction in ectopic nerve discharges and stabilization of neural membranes. Seizure control is due to reduction of post-tetanic potentiation of synaptic transmission in the spinal cord.

Absorption: oral, extended-release tablets: time to peak concentration, 3 h to 12 h; oral, regular-release tablets: time to peak concentration, 4 h to 5 h; oral, suspension, time to peak concentration, 1.5 h. Bioavailability:

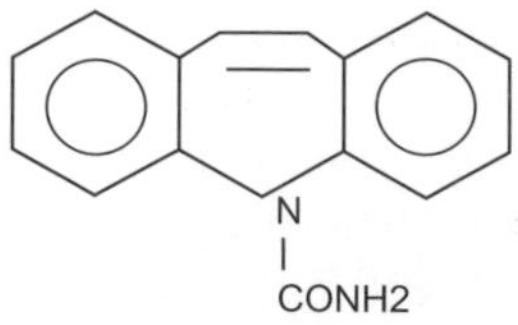

Figure 73.1.

oral, 70–80% and is increased by the presence of food in the stomach.

Distribution: Vd: 0.8 to 2 L/kg. Protein binding: 76%.

Metabolism: hepatic (98%); via cytochrome P450 isoenzyme CYP3A4. During prolonged treatment, carbamazepine induces its own metabolism. Active metabolites: carbamazepine-10,11-epoxide (CBZ-E).

Excretion: 72% renal and 28% fecal. Half-life of a single dose is 25–65 hours initially, then 12 to 17 hours after repeated doses (3 to 5 weeks) due to autoinduction. Dialyzable: yes via hemodialysis.

Indications

FDA-labeled indications: epilepsy: partial, generalized and mixed episodes; trigeminal neuralgia; glossopharyngeal neuralgia; bipolar 1 disorder, acute manic and mixed episodes.

Epilepsy

Carbamazepine is indicated for use as an anticonvulsant drug. Evidence supports the use of carbamazepine in the control of partial seizures with complex symptomatology (psychomotor, temporal lobe), generalized tonic-clonic seizures (grand mal), and mixed seizure patterns which include the above. Absence seizures (petit mal) do not appear to be controlled by carbamazepine.

Trigeminal neuralgia

Carbamazepine is indicated in the treatment of the pain associated with trigeminal neuralgia. Most of the studies that have examined its use in this disorder were conducted in the 1960s and 1970s. On review, in a 5-day placebo-controlled trial, using dose titration to a maximum of 1 g/day, 19/27 participants had a complete or very good response on 5 days' treatment of trigeminal neuralgia. A higher dosage of up to 2.4 g/day was used in a 2 week trial in which 15/20 patients achieved a good or excellent response. Although most of these studies were conducted with a small number of patients in short-term trials, the quality of the studies is rated as level 1 (good quality, patient-oriented

evidence). Beneficial results have also been reported in glossopharyngeal neuralgia.

Glossopharyngeal neuralgia

Carbamazepine has also been shown to be effective in the treatment of glossopharyngeal neuralgia. Like trigeminal neuralgia, original studies were performed in the 1960s and recent studies have confirmed the use of carbamazepine as initial treatment for glossopharyngeal neuralgia.

Diabetic neuropathy

Small placebo-controlled studies have demonstrated improvement in parasthesias and pain in patients with diabetic neuropathy treated with carbamazepine. In a 30-day comparison of carbamazepine and nortriptyline for the treatment of painful diabetic neuropathy, no difference in pain reduction was observed.

Other forms of neuropathic pain

Small studies have shown moderate benefit in the treatment of post-herpetic neuralgia and post-stroke pain. Treatment of other neurogenic pain syndromes with carbamazepine is considered a non-FDA-labeled indication.

Black-box warning

Serious dermatological reactions and HLA-B*1502 allele

Serious, sometimes fatal dermatological reactions have been reported, including Stevens–Johnson syndrome and toxic epidermal necrolysis. The risk is 10 times greater in some Asian countries due to a strong association with the HLA-B*1502 allele, which is found almost exclusively in Asian patients. Genetically at-risk patients should be screened prior to receiving carbamazepine, and carbamazepine should not be given to patients who test positive for the allele.

Aplastic anemia/agranulocytosis

Aplastic anemia and agranulocytosis have been reported. Complete hematological testing should be obtained pretreatment. If a patient during the course of treatment exhibits low or decreased white blood cell or platelet counts, the patient should be monitored closely. Discontinuation of carbamazepine should be considered if any evidence of significant bone marrow depression develops.

Contraindications

Carbamazepine should not be used in patients with a history of previous bone marrow depression, or known hypersensitivity to carbamazepine or tricyclic compounds. It is contraindicated with concomitant use of an MAOI or within 14 days of discontinuing an MAOI. Co-administration of carbamazepine and nefazodone may result in insufficient plasma concentrations of nefazodone and decreased drug effectiveness. Co-administration of carbamazepine with nefazodone is contraindicated.

Cautions

As listed above in Warning and Contraindications as well as:

- Caution if hepatic porphyria history; acute attacks reported
- Caution if hypersensitivity to other anticonvulsants; risk of cross-sensitivity
- Caution if absence, atonic, or myoclonic seizures; may increase generalized convulsion frequency
- Caution if increased intraocular pressure; may cause exacerbation due to cholinergic antagonism
- Caution if hepatic or renal impairment
- Caution if cardiac disease, or cardiac conduction disturbances; increased risk of atrioventricular heart block
- Caution in SLE
- Caution in elderly; may cause confusion or agitation
- Caution in mental illness history; risk of latent psychosis activation or increased risk of suicidality
- Caution in pregnancy (FDA Pregnancy Category D)

Common doses

Monitoring of blood levels has increased the efficacy and safety of anticonvulsants. Complete pretreatment blood counts, including platelets and possibly reticulocytes and serum iron, should be obtained as a baseline. If a patient during treatment exhibits low or decreased white blood cell or platelet counts, the patient should be monitored closely. Discontinuation of the drug should be considered if any evidence of significant bone marrow depression develops (see Warning). Baseline and periodic evaluations of liver function, especially in patients with a history of hepatic disease, must be performed during treatment with this drug since liver damage may occur. Car-

bamazepine should be discontinued if indicated by newly occurring or worsening clinical or laboratory evidence of hepatic dysfunction.

Dosage should be adjusted to the needs of the individual patient. A low initial daily dosage with a gradual increase is advised. As soon as adequate control is achieved, the dosage may be reduced very gradually to the minimum effective level. Tablets should be taken with meals. Sudden discontinuation of this drug is not advised. Patients should not take carbamazepine suspension with other liquid medications or diluents, as precipitation may occur. Patients should not eat grapefruit or grapefruit juice while taking this medication.

Conversion of patients from oral carbamazepine tablets to carbamazepine suspension: patients should be converted by administering the same number of mg per day in smaller, more frequent doses (i.e., BID tablets to TID suspension). No adjustment for renal dosing.

Adult dosing
Seizure disorder

Immediate-release form: 800–1200 mg/day PO divided BID-QID; start: 200 mg PO BID, increase 200 mg/day per week; max: 1600 mg/day; rare patients may require up to 2400 mg/day.

Extended-release form: 400–600 mg ER PO bid; start: 200 mg ER PO BID, increase 200 mg/day per week; max: 1600 mg/day ER; do not cut/crush/chew ER form.

Trigeminal neuralgia

Immediate-release form: 200–400 mg PO BID; start: 100 mg PO BID, increase 200 mg/day divided BID; max: 1200 mg/day.

Extended-release form: 200–400 mg ER PO BID; start: 100 mg ER PO BID, increase 200 mg/day; max: 1200 mg/day ER; do not cut/crush/chew ER form.

Glossopharyngeal neuralgia

Regular-release tablets: initial, 100 mg PO every 12 hours, may increase by 200 mg/day (divided into two doses) as needed for pain control (max dose 1200 mg/day).

Extended-release tablets: initial 100 mg PO every 12 hours, may increase by 200 mg/day (divided into two doses) as needed for pain control (max dose 1200 mg/day).

Maintenance: 400–800 mg/day PO (range 200–1200 mg/day); at least once every 3 months throughout the treatment period, attempts should be made to reduce the dose.

Cost guide

Generic: $6–15, branded, $14–35. Extended release $36–196, per month treatment.

Potential advantages

In addition to the treatment of partial and secondarily generalized tonic-clonic seizures, carbamazepine has a long history of use in the treatment of trigeminal neuralgia. It has been studied in the treatment of patients with trigeminal neuralgia since the 1960s and is considered the drug of choice for this condition. A 100 mg tablet may produce significant and complete relief within 2 hours, and for this reason it is a suitable agent for initial trial of treatment. So predictable and powerful is the relief that if the patient does not respond at least partially to carbamazepine, the diagnosis of trigeminal neuralgia may need to be reconsidered. Satisfactory pain relief may be achieved in 70% or more of patients. Carbamazepine is one of the oldest medications in its class and therefore inexpensive. Although rare life-threatening adverse reactions are possible (see warnings), most side effects are mild and carbamazepine is usually well tolerated. Baclofen may be added to carbamazepine as adjunct therapy. In addition there is no evidence of abuse potential associated with carbamazepine, nor is there evidence of psychological or physical dependence in humans.

Potential disadvantages

In addition to the warning/contraindications as discussed above, consider the following disadvantages of carbamazepine: increased risk of contraceptive failure in women with concomitant use; risk of congenital malformations especially spina bifida; increasing dosage may be necessary with prolonged treatment.

Acute toxicity: lowest known lethal dose: adults, 3.2 g.

Signs and symptoms: the first signs and symptoms appear after 1–3 hours. Neuromuscular disturbances are the most prominent. Cardiovascular disorders are generally milder, and severe cardiac complications occur only when very high doses (>60 g) have been ingested. Other signs and symptoms include: respiratory depression, tachycardia, hypotension or hypertension, shock, conduction disorders, coma, convulsions, ataxia, nausea, vomiting, anuria, or oliguria,

Treatment: the prognosis in cases of overdose is dependent upon prompt elimination of the drug, by inducing vomiting, gastric lavage, activated charcoal. There is no specific antidote. Dialysis is indicated only in severe poisoning associated with renal failure.

Drug interactions

Carbamazepine levels are increased by CYP3A4 inhibitors (cimetidine, macrolides, diltiazem, fluoxetine, ketoconazole, verapamil, valproate); levels are decreased by CYP3A4 inducers (cisplatin, doxorubicin, felbamate, phenobarbital, phenytoin, primidone, rifampin, theophylline). Carbamazepine may increase levels of clomipramine, phenytoin, and primidone and lithium toxicity; may decrease levels of phenytoin, warfarin, oral contraceptives, doxycycline, theophylline, haloperidol, alprazolam, clozapine, ethosuximide, and valproate; may interfere with other anticonvulsants.

Adverse reactions

If adverse reactions are of such severity that the drug must be discontinued, the physician must be aware that abrupt discontinuation of any anticonvulsant drug in a responsive epileptic patient may lead to seizures or even status epilepticus.

The most severe adverse reactions have been observed in the hematopoietic system, the skin, (see Warning), liver, and the cardiovascular system.

The most frequently observed adverse reactions, especially during initial therapy, are dizziness, drowsiness, unsteadiness, nausea, and vomiting. Therapy should be initiated at the low dosage recommended to minimize such reactions.

The following additional adverse reactions have been reported:

Hemopoietic system: aplastic anemia, agranulocytosis, pancytopenia, bone marrow depression, thrombocytopenia, leukopenia, leukocytosis, acute intermittent porphyria.

Skin: pruritic and erythematous rashes, urticaria, toxic epidermal necrolysis, Stevens-Johnson syndrome (see Warnings), photosensitivity reactions, erythema multiforme, aggravation of disseminated lupus erythematosus.

Cardiovascular system: congestive heart failure, edema, aggravation of hypertension, hypotension, syncope, aggravation of coronary artery disease, arrhythmias and AV block.

Liver: abnormalities in liver function tests, cholestatic and hepatocellular jaundice, hepatitis, very rare cases of hepatic failure.

Respiratory system: pulmonary hypersensitivity characterized by fever, dyspnea, pneumonitis, or pneumonia.

Genitourinary system: urinary frequency, acute urinary retention, oliguria with elevated blood pressure, azotemia, renal failure.

Nervous system: dizziness, drowsiness, ataxia, confusion, headache, fatigue, blurred vision, visual hallucinations, transient diplopia, oculomotor disturbances, nystagmus, abnormal involuntary movements, peripheral neuritis and paresthesias, depression with agitation, and tinnitus.

Gastrointestinal system: nausea, vomiting, gastric distress and abdominal pain, diarrhea, constipation, anorexia, and dryness of the mouth, pancreatitis.

Eyes: scattered punctate cortical lens opacities, conjunctivitis.

Musculoskeletal system: aching joints and muscles, and leg cramps.

Metabolism: fever and chills, syndrome of inappropriate antidiuretic hormone (ADH) secretion, water intoxication with decreased serum sodium (hyponatremia) and confusion.

Other: multi-organ hypersensitivity reactions occurring days to weeks or months after initiating treatment have been reported in rare cases. Signs or symptoms may include fever, skin rashes, vasculitis, lymphadenopathy, disorders mimicking lymphoma, arthralgia, leukopenia, hepatosplenomegaly, and abnormal liver function tests. These signs and symptoms may occur in various combinations and not necessarily concurrently. Signs and symptoms may initially be mild.

References

1. Micromedex Healthcare Series: http://www.thomsonhc.com/hcs/librarian/ND_T/HCS/ND_PR/Main/CS/A 9C255/DUPLICATIONSHIELDSYNC/08B79F/ND_PG/PRIH/ND_B/HCS/SBK/1/ND_P/Main/PFActionId/hcs.common.RetrieveDocumentCommon/DocId/106598/ContentSetId/100/SearchTerm/carbamazepine/SearchOption/BeginWith.

2. Wiffen PJ, McQuay HJ, Moore RA. Carbamazepine for acute and chronic pain in adults. *Cochrane Database Syst Rev* 2005;**3**:CD005451. DOI: 10.1002/14651858. CD005451.

3. Eisenberg E, River Y, Shifrin A, et al. Antiepileptic drugs in the treatment of neuropathic pain. *Drugs* 2007;**67**(9):1265–1289.

Lamotrigine

Laurie Yonemoto

Generic Name: lamotrigine

Brand/Proprietary Names: Lamictal™, Lamictin, Lamogine

Drug Class: anticonvulsant analgesic

Manufacturer: GlaxoSmithKline, 980 Great West Road, Brentford, Middlesex, TW8 9GS, UK

Chemical Structure: see Figure 74.1

Chemical Name: 3,5-diamino-6-(2,3-dichloro-phenyl)-as-triazine

Chemical Formula: $C_9H_7Cl_2N$

Inroduction

Lamotrigine is an anticonvulsant drug developed by GlaxoSmithKline in 1994 as an adjunctive treatment of seizures, both generalized and partial seizures as well as seizures associated with Lennox–Gastaut syndrome. Lamotrigine was later approved in 2003 as an alternative to lithium maintenance therapy to prevent and treat depressive symptoms in bipolar I disorder without triggering mania, hypomania, or rapid cycling. Lamotrigine may also possess antinociceptive and antineuropathic properties. Several recent clinical evaluations have found that lamotrigine is effective in controlling neuropathic pain associated with diabetic neuropathy, phantom limb pain, trigeminal neuralgia, HIV polyneuropathy and complex regional pain syndrome [1–3].

Mode of activity

Although the exact mechanism of action is not known, in vitro pharmacological studies suggest that lamotrigine, like other anticonvulsant-class analgesics, acts by inhibiting voltage-sensitive sodium channels thus blocking the release of excitatory and noxious neurotransmitters such as glutamate and aspartate. In animal studies lamotrigine was found to inhibit selective NMDA subunits (NR2B) without important sensory or motor impairment [2,3].

Eisinberg and colleagues [4] evaluated clinical investigations of lamotrigine for the treatment of various forms of neuropathic pain. They identified five open trials and six out of seven controlled trials that identified measurable analgesic efficacy. Many of these trials were hypothesis-driven clinical evaluations performed in patients with either intractable pain or in those not responding to standard anti-neuropathic therapy. Some were small randomized studies that were not well controlled, or individual case reports.

Duvulder and De Laat [5] evaluated 20 patients with chronic, neuropathic pain not responding to interventional therapy who were treated with lamotrigine, as monotherapy or in combination with oral morphine. The latter occurred in patients who lost pain relief from morphine after time. Ten patients did not respond to the drug; four were temporary responders and six patients obtained sustained pain relief. These authors noted that five patients regained opioid responsiveness and that lamotrigine plus morphine combination produced excellent pain relief for more than 5 months. The most compelling case was a patient with spinal cord tumor, who was using 3600 mg oral morphine, yet complained of inadequate relief. After receiving lamotrogine (200 mg/day) morphine consumption was reduced significantly and and pain relief was improved. Based on these observations, the authors recommended follow-up control trials to evaluate the possible synergy between lamotrigine and opioids.

Radicular pain syndromes caused by disk herniation are often difficult to treat.

In a patient with severe radicular pain and central cord syndrome, the addition of lamotrigine 100–200 mg/day over a period of 6 weeks reduced pain intensity scores from 100mm down to 20mm and greatly improved quality of life [6].

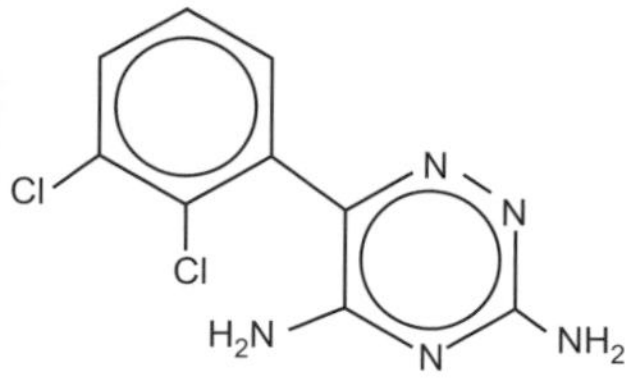

Figure 74.1.

The safety and efficacy of lamotrigine was evaluated in 68 patients with chronic neuropathic pain who had failed at least two or more other anti-neuropathic medications [7]. Patients were started on lamotrigine at a dose of 50 mg/day for 2 weeks, increased to 100 mg/day for 2 weeks and titrated upward by 50 mg/day at weekly intervals. The target dose was 200 mg/day. Thirty-eight percent of patients responded to lamotrigine and reported reductions in pain intensity. It was most effective in patients with diabetic neuropathy, followed by post-herpetic neuralgia, trigeminal neuralgia, peripheral neuropathy and central pain. Most patients with radiculopathy were non-responders as were patients with atypical head pain and failed back syndrome. The average dose of lamotrigine in responders was 300 mg/day while the average dose in non-responders was 160 mg/day. Four patients discontinued due to side effects.

One negative trial was published by Silver and co-workers [8]. They performed a double-blind, placebo-controlled study which was undertaken to evaluate the efficacy and tolerability of lamotrigine added to gabapentin, a tricyclic antidepressant, or a non-opioid analgesic in patients with inadequately controlled neuropathic pain. Patients were randomized to receive doses of lamotrigine 200, 300, or 400 mg daily ($n = 111$) or placebo ($n = 109$) for up to 14 weeks, in addition to their prestudy analgesic regimen. No statistically significant difference in the mean change in pain-intensity score from baseline to week 14 (primary endpoint) was detected between lamotrigine and placebo ($P = 0.67$). Lamotrigine was generally well tolerated but did not demonstrate efficacy as an adjunctive treatment of neuropathic pain.

Metabolic clearance/elimination

Lamictal is well absorbed when given orally with negligible first-pass metabolism. Lamictal has a bioavailability of 98% which is not affected by food with peak plasma concentrations occurring 1.4–4.8 hours following drug administration. In vitro studies show that lamotrigine is approximately 55% bound to plasma proteins, suggesting that clinically significant interactions with other drugs through competition for protein binding sites is very unlikely [2,3,9].

Lamotrigine is metabolized by glucuronic acid conjugation resulting in the production of an inactive metabolite 2-N-glucoronide. The majority of lamotrigine's clearance is via renal excretion as glucuronide conjugates with a minor amount excreted in feces. Lamotrigine has an elimination half-life of 25–33 hours. This elimination half-life is increased in patients with renal failure and hepatic impairment [9].

Contraindications

Absolute contraindications to lamotrigine include any hypersensitivity reaction to Lamictal or any component for the formulation. Relative contraindications or concerns to administration of lamotrigine include hypersensitivity to antiepileptic drugs, in patients with renal or hepatic impairment, and in patients on valproic acid, as this has been shown to increase the incidence of rash. Lamotrigine inhibits dihydrofolate reductase. In studies on pregnant rats, administration of Lamictal resulted in decreased concentrations of fetal and maternal folate levels, which are frequently associated with teratogenesis and fetal abnormalities such as cleft lip or palate. Due to the potential increased risk of teratogenesis, lamotrigine is not advised for use during the first trimester of pregnancy [2,9].

Table 74.1. Lamictal doses

Disorder	Recommended dosage
Partial and generalized seizures	Initial dose: 25 mg/day for first 1–2 weeks, increasing dose by 50 mg/day for weeks 3–4. Titrate dose to effect. Maintenance dose: 225–375 mg/day divided into two doses
Bipolar disorder	Initial dose: 25 mg/day for first 1–2 weeks, increasing dose by 50 mg/day for weeks 3–4. Increase dose to 100 mg/day for week 5. Maintenance dose: 200 mg/day
Neuropathic pain	Initial dose: 50 mg/day for first week with weekly increases of 50 mg/day titrate to effect. In many patients analgesia is observed with doses up to 300–400 mg/day.

Table 74.2. Adverse effects

System	Adverse reaction
Cardiovascular	Chest pain (5%), peripheral edema (2–5%), atrial fibrillation (<1%), tachycardia (<1%)
CNS	Somnolence (9%), fatigue (8%), anxiety (5%), ataxia (2–5%), suicidal ideation (2–5%), agitation (1–5%), emotional lability (1–5%)
Dermatological	Rash (non-serious 7%), dermatitis (2–5%), dry skin (2–5%), acne (<1%), alopecia (<1%), Stevens–Johnson syndrome (<1%)
Endocrine	Dysmenorrhea (5%), increased libido (2–5%), menorrhagia (<1%)
Gastrointestinal	Nausea (7–14%), vomiting (5–9%), dyspepsia (7%), xerostomia (2–6%), constipation (5%), weight loss (5%), weight gain (1–5%), anorexia (2–5%), flatulence (1–5%)
Genitourinary	Urinary frequency (1–5%), urinary incontinence (<1%), hematuria (<1%)
Neuromuscular and skeletal	Back pain (8%), weakness (2–5%), myalgia (1–5%), paresthesia (1%), rhabdomyolisis (<1%)
Ocular	Nystagmus (2–5%), photophobia (<1%), conjunctivitis (<1%), dry eyes (<1%)
Hematological	Disseminated intravascular coagulation, hemolytic anemia, leukopenia, neutropenia, pancytopenia, red cell aplasia, thrombocytopenia (<1%)

Table 74.3. Cost

	Brand	Generic
25 mg	$4.67/tab	$3.86
100 mg	$5.33	$4.00
150 mg	$5.83	$4.95
200 mg	$6.50	$5.39

Common doses/uses

Lamotrigine (Lamictal™) is available as an oral regimen in 25 mg, 100 mg, 150 mg and 200 mg tablets. Only whole tablets are recommended for use and doses should be rounded down to the nearest whole tablet. It is recommended that Lamictal therapy be initiated at low doses and slowly escalated over the first 4 weeks of therapy to minimize adverse side effects such as skin rash (see Table 74.1).

Potential advantages

Lamotrigine is relatively easy to use, is well tolerated and has a safe pharmacological profile. The high bioavailability with oral administration adds to lamotrigine's easy administration and, unlike other anti-epileptic drugs, it has no significant metabolic or neurological effects and does not require laboratory testing of plasma concentrations. Lamotrigine can be used as a monotherapy in the treatment of chronic neuropathic pain syndromes such as diabetic neuropathy and trigeminal neuralgia by inhibiting neuronal transmission of pain signal and sparing the use of opioids in these types of pain syndromes.

Adverse events

See Table 74.2.

Cost

See Table 74.3.

References

1. Barash PG, Cullen BF, Stoelting RK, Cahalan MK, Stock MC. *Clinical Anesthesia*, 6th ed. Philadelphia: Lipincott Williams & Wilkins, 2009.

2. Maizels M, McCarberg B. Antidepressants and antiepileptic drugs for chronic non-cancer pain. *Am Fam Physician* 2005;**71**:483–490.

3. Sadok B, Sadok V. *Concise Textbook of Clinical Psychiatry*, 3rd ed. Philadelphia: Lippincott Williams & Wilkins, 2008, pp. 51–514.

4. Eisenberg E, Shifrin A, Krivoy N. Lamotrigine for neuropathic pain. *Expert Rev Neurother* 2005;**5**(6):729–735.

5. Devulder J, Martine De Laat M. Lamotrigine in the treatment of chronic refractory neuropathic pain. *J Pain Symptom Manage* 2000;**19**:398–406.

6. Titlik M, Junuk I, Tonkic A, et al. Lamotrigine therapy for resistant pain in radicular lesions. *Acta Clinica Croat* 2009;**48**:157–160.

7. Gabriela-Gregory M, Semenchuck RM. Lamotrigine is effective in refractory neuropathic pain 2002; Poster presentation, 10th World Congress on Pain.

8. Silver M, Blum D, Grainger J, et al. Double-blind, placebo-controlled trial of lamotrigine in combination with other medications for neuropathic pain. *J Pain Symptom Manage* 2007;**34**:446–454.

9. Stoelting R, Hiller S. *Pharmacology & Physiology in Anesthetic Practice*, 4th ed. Philadelphia: Lippincott Williams & Wilkins, 2006, pp. 569–579.

75

Overview of NMDA receptors and antagonists

R. Todd Rinnier, Michael E. Goldberg and Marc C. Torjman

NMDA receptors and receptor agonists

General description of the receptor

The *N*-methyl-D-aspartate (NMDA) receptor is classified as part of the larger family of glutamate receptors often referred to as a superfamily. The primary role of the glutamate receptor is to process rapid synaptic transmission of an excitatory nature throughout the nervous system. It performs this function utilizing a group of receptors located on the cell membrane. These can be divided into ionotropic and metabotropic receptors. The primary ionotropic receptors in the glutamate superfamily are the alpha-amino-3-hydroxy-5-methyl-4-isoxazole propionic acid (AMPA) receptors, kainate receptors, and *N*-methyl-D-aspartate (NMDA) receptors. The nomenclature for these receptors is derived from the synthetic agonists that result in activation of said receptors [19].

The NMDA receptor, along with the AMPA receptor, have been implicated in the processing and mediation of acute and chronic pain [20]. The NMDA receptor is associated with persistent changes within neurons of patients with pain. The activation of these receptors leads to removal of a magnesium ion "plug" followed by calcium entry into the postsynaptic neuron along with other biochemical events such as c-Fos transcription and G-protein activation. These events allow development of CNS plasticity at a cellular level which is expressed as long-term potentiation. The NMDA receptor is a ligand-gated ion channel recognized for some of its unique characteristics. It exerts its effects on a cation channel that is very permeable to calcium and monovalent ions. In order to activate the receptor, simultaneous binding of glutamate and glycine are required. In its resting state the NMDA receptor is blocked by magnesium [7]. Activation of this receptor may also occur via polyamine stimulation. NMDA receptor modulation can occur through arachidonic acid, while it is inhibited by zinc ions [19].

The receptor will only open when both binding of agonist and simultaneous depolarization occur.

Receptor structure

Structurally, the NMDA receptor has been described to contain four transmembrane (helical domains) channels that utilize both glycine and glutamate for activation. The primary result of this activation is transmembrane influx of calcium ion. Additionally when the NMDA receptor membrane channel is isoelectric, the receptor is blocked by magnesium. The magnesium block will only be released by "simultaneous depolarization and receptor agonist binding" [20]. By exploiting the receptor activation and inactivation through the use of various compounds, the NMDA receptor can be manipulated to facilitate pain relief.

NMDA receptors are further divided into three subunits: NR1, NR2 (subunits: A, B, C, D) and NR3 (subunits: A, B). A combination of the essential channel-forming subunit NR1 and one or more of the NR2 subunits is vital for the expression of a functional NMDA receptor. Studies have demonstrated that the NR2B subunit has specifically been most involved in the process of nociception, and thus a target for drug therapy aimed at reducing pain [20] (Figure 75.1).

Receptor function

These receptors function in the excitatory neurotransmission pathway in the CNS, together with various excitatory amino-acid receptors. The activity of glutamate excitatory neurotransmission is a complex process that involves co-transmission and summation. The effectiveness of the active transporter mechanisms responsible for clearing glutamate from the synaptic cleft heavily influences the activity of these receptors. At a cellular level, the permeability of calcium in the CNS is controlled by excitatory neurotransmission. This explains why excitatory neurotransmission exerts its

The Essence of Analgesia and Analgesics, ed. Raymond S. Sinatra, Jonathan S. Jahr and J. Michael Watkins-Pitchford. Published by Cambridge University Press. © Cambridge University Press 2011.

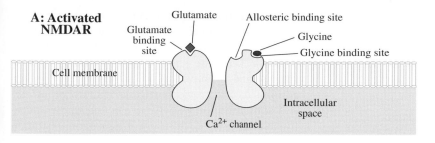

A: Activated NMDAR

Glutamate
Glutamate binding site
Allosteric binding site
Glycine
Glycine binding site
Cell membrane
Intracellular space
Ca^{2+} channel

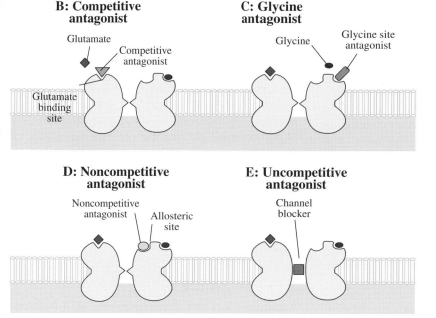

B: Competitive antagonist

Glutamate
Competitive antagonist
Glutamate binding site

C: Glycine antagonist

Glycine
Glycine site antagonist

D: Noncompetitive antagonist

Noncompetitive antagonist
Allosteric site

E: Uncompetitive antagonist

Channel blocker

Figure 75.1. Activated NMDA receptor and assorted NMDA receptor blockers. (With permission from Kim AH, Kerchner GA, Choi DW. (2002). Blocking excitotoxicity. In *CNS Neuroproteciton.* Marcoux FW Choi DW, eds. Springer, New York. Pages 3–36.)

effects immediately, but over the long term induces synaptic plasticity. Synaptic plasticity is the process by which neural circuits modify their strength or efficacy of synaptic transmission at preexisting synapses [8]. Several mechanisms exist that make this possible, including changes in the quantity of neurotransmitters in the synapse, and the effectiveness of the cell's ability to respond to these neurotransmitters. Synaptic plasticity is a fundamental neurobiological process involved in learning and memory development. The basic mechanism behind these processes bears a striking resemblance to those involved in the processing of pain transmission [7]. NMDA receptors also play an integral role in the CNS, such that antagonists to these receptors can have serious neurological consequences, including psychotomimetic effects, memory impairment, motor impairment, and ataxia to name a few [20].

NMDA receptors also appear in the spinal dorsal horn where, with NMDA receptor activation, ion channels are opened, intracellular calcium levels rise leading to increased levels of protein kinase C. There is a concomitant decrease in the sensitivity of the mu opioid receptor [13]. Protein kinase C activation, in vitro, occurs following the activation of mu opioid receptors, resulting in NMDA activation and increased glutamate response. It is these excitatory neurotransmitters, glutamate and aspartate, that work on the NMDA receptors to create and maintain continued chronic pain states [18]. Multiple and intense stimulation causes the NMDA receptor to become activated. This can create a long-term rise in cell excitability due to calcium influx, thereby initiating the second-messenger effect. In the spinal cord dorsal horn, NMDA receptors are heavily expressed at nociceptive synapses. Both chronic pain and opioid tolerance can sensitize the central pain pathways and result in an NMDA receptor-mediated increase in dorsal horn synaptic efficacy [14]. NMDA receptor antagonists reduce central sensitization, which has been shown to prevent the development of persistent pain in animal studies [1]. NMDA receptors are found not only centrally but also in the periphery, encompassing both visceral and somatic structures [20].

Clinical pharmacology

Clinical studies have shown that activation of the NMDA receptor results in increased pain and the development of neuropathic pain, including opioid-resistant pain [6]. NMDA receptors have a substantial role in synaptic plasticity including CNS facilitation of the pain processing pathway [7]. N-Methyl-D-aspartate receptor antagonists are known to modulate central sensory processing, are potent antihyperalgesics, potentiate opioid-induced analgesia, and prevent the development of opioid tolerance [1]. Many compounds including ketamine, amantidine, memantine, dextromethorphan, and magnesium ions have been utilized in both clinical practice and research protocols for pain modulation. Several of these clinical effects will be described in greater detail by other authors. It is through varied receptor activation and inactivation mechanisms that these compounds are able to exert their effect to modulate the pain response.

Ketamine

Ketamine, a phenyl-piperidine derivative, is a noncompetitive NMDA receptor antagonist which exerts its effect through a conformational change resulting in release of the magnesium block and transmembrane influx of calcium [20]. The compound is rapidly distributed in the brain and other highly perfused tissues, with about 10% of the drug bound to plasma. The bioavailability of ketamine is dependent on the route of administration, being as high as 93% for an intramuscular dose, 20–50% for an intranasal dose, and approximately 20% for an oral dose. Recent treatment with anesthetic doses of ketamine for severely ill, generalized chronic regional pain syndrome (CRPS) patients has shown some efficacy and prompted its use in less severely ill patients by low-dose infusion [22]. Goldberg et al. also showed that a 4 hour infusion of sub-anesthetic doses of ketamine over a 10 day period in the outpatient setting resulted in a significant reduction of pain with increased mobility, and a tendency to decreased autonomic dysregulation. Numerous studies involving animals and humans have demonstrated its opioid-sparing effect and potentiation of opioid-induced analgesia, as well as ability to decrease phantom limb pain after lower

limb amputation [1,3]. A recent systematic review concluded that out of the 24 studies that examined ketamine, 58% demonstrated a positive effect in blocking pain. IV ketamine showed positive results in nine studies, and negative results in seven studies when administered to provide analgesia. Epidural or intrathecal administration was effective in four studies, negative in three studies, while subcutaneous administration showed positive results in one study [17]. With respect to pediatric use, a recent study suggested a ketamine-related opioid-sparing effect. Eight out of eleven children or adolescents with advanced cancer who were taking high-dose opioids had positive results with the addition of a low-dose ketamine infusion (0.1–1 mg/kg per h) for 1–75 days. There was a concomitant reduction in opioid consumption, improved pain control, and improved alertness and interactiveness [18]. Moreover, these patients did not experience psychotropic effects, attributable to 0.025 mg/kg lorazepam given every 12 hours to protect against these untoward effects. Ketamine has therefore demonstrated some promise in the area of chronic pain and future studies are needed with focus on route of administration, timing of dose, and more interestingly, the effect of ketamine metabolites.

S-(+)-Ketamine

Ketamine exists as a chiral compound with two optical enantiomers: S-(+) and R-(−) ketamine. The analgesic potency of the dextro- S- (+) form is two- to four-times that of the levo- R-(−) form.[27]. In addition, animal model receptor studies have shown that S-(+)-ketamine displays a four-fold greater affinity on the NMDA receptor phencyclidine binding sites compared to R-(−)-ketamine [28]. The S-(+) enantiomer inhibits serotonin transport half as much as the enantiomer. Compared to racimic ketamine, the S-(+) form has a significantly higher elimination rate. S-(+)-Ketamine has a therapeutic index (LD_{50}/ED_{50}) 2.5 greater than that of racimic or R-(−)-ketamine. Even though the potency is greater allowing for a decreased effective dose, evidence for a lowered side-effect profile is lacking between S-(+) and that of racemic ketamine. However, due to the decreased effective dose and higher elimination rate for S-(+)-ketamine, the recovery time seems to be faster [28]. Recently, S-(+)-ketamine was shown to decrease acute pain in CRPS patients, with long-term effects lasting beyond the infusion period when drug levels were well below the analgesic threshold [27].

Amantidine

Amantidine was first approved in 1966 as an antiviral agent that works by disrupting the function of the transmembrane domain of the viral M2 protein effectively blocking the release of infectious viral nucleic acid into the host cell. It has also been shown in some cases to interrupt virus replication by stopping virus assembly. Amantidine was later found to possess anti-parkinsonian properties through its direct and indirect effects on dopamine neurons, as well as its effects on NMDA receptors. Recent interest for its use in pain management is attributed to its weak noncompetitive NMDA antagonism (K_i = 10 µM) [25] which may be useful in decreasing pain and analgesic requirements by preventing post-operative central sensitization, opioid-induced hyperalgesia, and acute opioid tolerance. Interestingly, it displays anticholinergic-like side effects (dry mouth, urinary retention, and constipation) [25]; however, animal studies have yet to show direct anticholinergic activity [26]. One study showed that given pre- and post-operatively, amantidine was able to decrease opioid consumption in post-operative radical prostatectomy patients [15]. Another study showed that when compared to lidocaine, it failed to decrease sciatic-related pain effectively. There are conflicting data regarding amantidine's use in pain management and it appears that this agent may be better suited as an antiviral and antiparkinsonian therapy.

Dextromethorphan and derivatives

Dextromethorphan, administered intravenously, intramuscularly, or orally has been used for over 40 years [1]. It is a central antitussive agent that exerts its effect by increasing the cough threshold in the medulla oblongata [23]. It is the D-isomer of the codeine analog levorphanol [7]. Dextromethorphan's active metabolite, dextrorphan, is a low-affinity noncompetitive NMDA receptor antagonist. It has a weak affinity for the mu opioid receptor and, according to several investigations, has either very weak or no analgesic properties [6,7]. The drug has extensive first-pass metabolism and the oral bioavailability of the drug is low [7]. In experimental animal studies, dextromethorphan's use exhibited inhibited expression of central sensitization including a facilitated response to sensory inputs, hyperalegsia, and wind-up pain. There are conflicting data concerning dextromethorphan's use in the acute pain (peri-operative) setting as post-operative pain relief studies have not shown much benefit [7]. More importantly, in a recent review of 12 studies that examined dextromethorphan, 67% demonstrated clinically significant analgesia. The positive studies (pain relief) used both oral and IV/IM routes, while the negative studies used only the oral form. The dosage given did not appear to be associated with success of treatment, varying from 0.5 mg/kg to 150 mg [17]. Dextromethorphan's use in chronic pain has demonstrated mixed results. Therefore its role in chronic pain is still uncertain. The dose necessary for effective pain management increases its side-effect profile, raising concerns of its potential for abuse [23]. Aside from antitussive use, and mixed results in chronic pain, dextromethorphan has shown some additional usefulness in the treatment of cancer-related pain, as well as methotrexate-induced neurotoxicity [23].

Magnesium

Magnesium is a naturally occurring mineral and is the fourth most abundant mineral in the body. Magnesium is a vital component of homeostasis and is responsible for maintaining normal nerve and muscle function, supporting immune system functions, regulating blood sugar, supporting healthy bones, promoting normal blood pressure, maintaining a normal heart rhythm, and is a key component in energy metabolism and protein synthesis [21]. Magnesium ions function as noncompetitive NMDA receptor antagonists that modulate NMDA receptor activation by preventing extracellular calcium from gaining entry into the cell. Experimental animal models of tissue injury and central sensitization have shown that magnesium, in combination with morphine, created an increased analgesic effect greater than either drug alone [9]. There is also evidence that when administered intrathecally, in combination with morphine, magnesium sulfate potentiated morphine antinociception, suggesting that it also works on spinal NMDA receptors [10]. Clinical studies have shown conflicting evidence on intravenous magnesium administration to reduce analgesic requirements or post-operative pain. Recently, it was shown that intravenous magnesium given as a bolus, followed by continuous infusion after extubation in cardiac surgery patients, moderately decreased remifentanil dose required for post-operative pain management [24]. A current review of IV magnesium's clinical efficacy concluded that none of the four studies examined demonstrated a preventative analgesic effect greater than standard therapies [17]. One possible explanation of magnesium's lack of efficacy is that it may be removed from the extracellular space too rapidly, or that the ion is specific to the NMDA channel, but not to the receptor site where other NMDA receptor antagonists bind and exert their effect [17]. Another explanation is that the dose may be insufficient, as studies using bolus dosing have not shown magnesium to be as efficacious as those using bolus and continuous infusions. Based on available data, magnesium's potential seems to be as an adjuvant as opposed to monotherapy.

Memantine

Memantine is an oral long-acting voltage-dependent uncompetitive NMDA receptor antagonist with a high therapeutic index approved for the treatment of Alzheimer's disease [14]. In addition, it acts as an uncompetitive antagonist at the $5HT_3$ receptor and as a noncompetitive antagonist at different neuronal nicotinic acetylcholine receptors which may also be responsible for the processing of pain. There is also a weak to negligible affinity for adrenergic, benzodiazepine, dopamine, GABA, glycine, and histamine receptors, in addition to voltage-dependent Ca^{2+}, Na^+ or K^+ channels [25].

Its greatest potency is achieved as compared to other NMDA antagonists when given intrathecally as demonstrated in animal studies [1]. Memantine may have several advantages compared to ketamine, displaying a higher potency, longer elimination half-life (60–80 hours vs. 2.5 hours), and a decreased side-effect profile [1]. Memantine's adverse effects are much milder than ketamine's, including dizziness and restlessness which disappear with discontinuation [14]. Memantine's tolerability may be explained by its low affinity to the receptor-associated ion channel with resultant decreased dwell-time in the channel, in addition to preferential blockade of pathologically over-activated channels [14]. One study has shown memantine (30 mg/day for 4 weeks) to decrease phantom limb pain, citing a four-fold decrease 6 months after amputation [4]. One unique application has been described in a recent case report of a patient with metastatic liposarcoma and opioid-refractory pain that responded to low-dose IV ketamine, and then was successfully transitioned to oral memantine for long-term outpatient pain management [14]. Memantine, although useful for Alzheimer's disease, has demonstrated some clinical usefulness in acute and chronic pain management and warrants further study.

Neramexane

Neramexane is an oral moderate-affinity, strong voltage-dependent, open-channel, uncompetitive NMDA receptor antagonist [29]. This drug prevents pathological activation of the NMDA receptor, but maintains the physiological activity relating to its minimal side-effect profile. Like memantine, neramexane displays rapid blocking/unblocking kinetics leading to its minimal side-effect profile at therapeutic doses. Currently, neramexane is under development for various central CNS disorders as a potential neuroprotectant. Neramexane was recently shown to have a marked analgesic effect in response to intradermal capsaicin injection which represented a surrogate model of neurogenic hyperalgesia [30]. It is currently in various phases of drug trials for Alzheimer's disease, drug and alcohol abuse, depression, tinnitus, and chronic pain.

Methadone

Methadone is a synthetic opioid agonist that may have some potential as it also functions as a weak NMDA antagonist [6]. Several authors will discuss these drugs as well as other drugs in greater detail in following chapters.

References

1. Suzuki Manzo. Role of N-methyl-D-asparate receptor antagonists in post-operative pain management. *Curr Opin Anaesthesiol* 2009;22.

2. Michelet P, Guervilly C, Helaine A, et al. Adding ketamine to morphine for patient-controlled analgesia after thoracic surgery: influence on morphine consumption, respiratory function, and nocturnal desaturation. *Br J Anaesth* 2007;**99**:396–403.

3. Wilson JA, Nimmmo AF, Fleetwood-Walker SM, Colvin LA. A randomized double blind trial of the effect of preemptive epidural ketamine on persistent pain after lower limb amputation. *Pain* 2008;**135**: 108–118.

4. Schley M, Topfer S, Weich K, et al. Continuous brachial plexus blockade in combination with NMDA receptor antagonist memantine prevents phantom limb pain in acute traumatic upper limb amputees. *Eur J Pain* 2007;**11**:299–308.

5. Jantus D, Lason, W. Different mechanisms of NMDA-mediated protection against neurinal apoptosis: a stimulus-dependant effect. *Neurochem Res* 2009; 10.1007/s11064–009–9991-y.

6. Lucas L, Lipman A. Recent advances in pharmacotherapy for cancer pain management. *Cancer Practice* 2002;**10**:suppl. 1.

7. Kock M, Lavand'homme P. The clinical role of NMDA receptor antagonists for the treatment of postoperative pain. *Best Pract Res Clin Anesth* 2007;**21**:85–98.

8. Malenka R. Synaptic plasticity. In *Neuropsychopharmacology: 5th Generation of Progress.* Nashville, TN: American College of Neuropsychopharmacology, 2002.

9. Begon S, Pickering G, Eschalier A, Dubray C. Magnesium increases morphine analgesic effect in different experimental models of pain. *Anesthesiology* 2002;**96**:627–632.

10. Kroin JS, McCarthy R, Von Roenn N, et al. Magnesium sulfate potentiates morphine at the spinal level. *Anesth Analg* 2000;**90**:913–917.

11. Liu HT, Hollmann M, Lui WH, et al. Modulation of the NMDA receptor function by ketamine and magnesium: Part 1. *Anesth Analg* 2001;**92**:1173–1181.

12. Ilkjaer S, Bach LFL, Nielsen PA, et al. Effect of perioperative oral dextromethorphan on immediate and late postoperative pain and hyperalgesia after total abdominal hysterectomy. *Pain* 2000;**86**:19–24.

13. Suzuki M, Kinoshita T, Kikutani T, et al. Determining the plasma concentration of ketamine that enhances epidural bupivacaine-and-morphine-induce analgesia. *Anesth Analg* 2005;**101**:777–84.

14. Grande LA, O'Donnell BR, Fitzgibbon DR, Terman GW. Ultra-low dose ketamine and memantine treatment for pain in an opioid-tolerant oncology patient. *Int Anesth Res Socy* 2008;107(4).

15. Snijdelaar DG, Koren G, Katz J. Effects of perioperative oral amantadine on postoperative pain and morphine consumption in patients after radical prostatectomy: results of a preliminary study. *Anesthesiology* 2004;**100**(1):134–141.

16. Galer BS, Lee D, Ma T, et al. MorphiDex (morphine sulfate/ dextromethorphan hydrobromide combination) in the treatment of chronic pain: three multicenter, randomized, double-blind, controlled clinical trials fail to demonstrate enhanced opioid analgesia or reduction in tolerance. *Pain* 2005;**115**:284–295.

17. McCartney C, Sinha A, Katz J. A qualitative systematic review of the role of N-methyl-D-aspartate receptor antagonists in preventive analgesia. *Anesth Analg* 2004;**98**:1385–1400.

18. Finkel JC, Pestieau SR, Quezado ZM. Ketamine as an adjuvant for treatment of cancer pain in children and adolescents. *J Pain* 2007;**8**(6):515–521.

19. (EBIDatabasesInterPro) http://www.ebi.ac.uk/interpro/IEntry?ac=IPR001508.

20. Petrenko AB, Yamakura T, et al. The role of N-methyl-D-aspartate (NMDA) receptors in pain: a review. *Anesth Analg* 2003;**97**:1103–1116.

21. http://dietary-supplements.info.nih.gov/factsheets/magnesium.asp.

22. Schwartzman RJ, Popescu A. Reflex sympathetic dystrophy. *Curr Rheumatol Rep* 2002;**4**:165–169.

23. Siu A, Drachtman R. Dextromethophan: a review of N-methyl-D-aspartate receptor antagonism in the management of pain. *CNS Drug Rev* 2007;**13**:96–106.

24. Steinlechner B, Dworschak M et al. Magnesium moderately decreases remifentanil dosage required for pain management after cardiac surgery. *Br Jour Anesth* 2006;**4**:444–449.

25. http://www.rxlist.com/namenda-drug.htm.

26. http://www.rxlist.com/symmetrel-drug.htm.

27. Sigtermans M, et al. An observational study on the effect of S(+)-ketamine on chronic pain versus experimental acute pain in Complex Regional Pain Syndrome type 1 patients. *Eur J Pain* 2009; doi:10.1016/j.ejpain.2009.05.012

28. Kohrs R, Durieux M. Ketamine: teaching an old drug new tricks. *Anesth Analg* 1998;**87**:1186–1193.

29. Rammes G. Neramexane: a moderate-affinity NMDA receptor channel blocker: new prospects and indication. *Exp Rev Clin Pharm.* 2009;**2**(3):231–238.

30. Klein T, Margerl W, Hanschmann A, et al. Antihyperalgesia and analgesic properties of the N-methyl-D-aspartate (NMDA) receptor antagonist neramexane in a human surrogate model of neurogenic hyperalgesia. *Eur J Pain* 2008;**12**:17–29.

76

Ketamine

Carsten Nadjat-Haiem

Generic Name: ketamine hydrochloride

Trade Names: Anesject™, Brevinaze™, Keiran™, Keta™, Ketaject™, Ketalar™, Ketalin™, Ketamax™

Drug Class: NMDA receptor antagonist, central-acting analgesic

Manufacturers: Pfizer Pharmaceuticals, 235 East 42nd Street, New York, NY

Chemical Structure: see Figure 76.1

Chemical Name: (RS)-2-(2-chlorophenyl)-2-methylaminocyclohexan-1-one

Chemical Formula: $C_{13}H_{16}ClNO$; molecular wt 238

Introduction

Ketamine is a central-acting anesthetic and analgesic. It was developed by Calvin Stevens at Parke-Davis in 1962 in an effort to synthesize a drug with fewer side effects than phencyclidine and cyclohexamine. Ketamine was originally named C1581, and was patented in 1965 and sold under the trade name Ketalar. Ketamine was officially released for human use in 1970 and was used extensively during the Vietnam War [1].

Ketamine has a molecular weight of 238 and is partially soluble at pH 7.4 (pKa 7.5). All commercial ketamine is composed of a racemic mixture of the R- and S- enantiomers, and is prepared in an acidic solution with a pH between 3.5 and 5.5.

Mode of activity

Ketamine (2-(O-chlorophenyl)-2-methylamino cyclohexanone) is a nonbarbiturate anesthetic/analgesic agent structurally related to phencyclidine and cyclohexamine. The drug is water-soluble, and has a lipid solubility about 10 times that of thiopental. Ketamine is the only single-agent anesthetic capable of producing "dissociative" anesthesia [1,2]. The agent provides potent analgesia even at sub-anesthetic doses. It is believed that analgesic and anesthetic actions are due to different mechanisms. There are many hypotheses proposed to explain the clinical effect of ketamine. These include binding and antagonism at the N-methyl-D-aspartame (NMDA) receptors in the central nervous system, interactions with opiate receptors at both the spinal and central levels, and interactions with muscarinic cholinergic, serotoninergic, and norepinephrine receptors. This is evidenced by the fact that some of the effects of ketamine are reversed by antagonists at the opioid level (naloxone), and the muscarinic cholinergic level (4-aminopyrdine and physostigmine).

Ketamine is a rapidly acting anesthetic and analgesic. It can be given intravenously, intramuscularly, nasally, orally, rectally, epidurally, spinally, and topically. The initial anesthetic response if given intravenously is seen after 30–40 seconds, while a response after intramuscular administration is seen after 3–4 minutes. Nasal administration results in a response after 8–12 minutes. Analgesic effects after intramuscular, oral, and epidural injection are 10–15, within 30, and within 15–30 minutes, respectively.

Bioavailability of ketamine is 90–93% after intramuscular injection, 16% after oral administration, and 77% after epidural injection. Protein binding of ketamine is 47%, and it is initially distributed to highly perfused tissues such as brain, heart, and the lungs. There the concentration can reach up to five times the plasma concentration. Redistribution is similar to thiopental. The distribution half-life after intravenous administration is 7 to17 minutes, and the volume of distribution is 2 to 3 L/kg.

Ketamine is extensively metabolized in the liver via N-demethylation via the cytochrome P450 system to yield norketamine. This metabolite has one-third the activity of the parent compound, and is subsequently hydroxylated and conjugated to become a

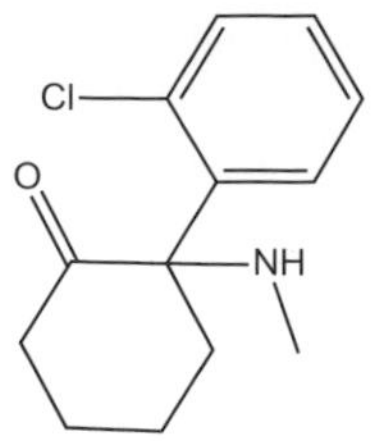

Figure 76.1.

water-soluble compound. Subsequently, the metabolites (hydroxylated and conjugated compounds, 3% unchanged as norketamine) are cleared by the kidney. The clearance rate is 12–17 mL/min per kg, yielding a mean residence time of about 3 hours in adults, which also reflects the approximate elimination half-life.

Indications

Ketamine has many indications and uses, but is only FDA-approved as an adjunct for general anesthesia and procedural sedation. Ketamine is useful for short procedures due to its relatively rapid induction and emergence, and is particularly helpful in the management of patients in whom cardiovascular depression is to be avoided (pericardial tamponade, cardiogenic or hypovolemic shock, non-ischemic cardiomyopathy, and constrictive pericarditis). It can be used for induction of general anesthesia for cesarean sections. The potential ketamine-induced emergence reactions can be minimized with concomitant administration of a benzodiazepine, and cardiovascular effects of potential tachycardia and hypertension can be well managed with the use of beta-blockers and clonidine. The use of glycopyrrolate as an antisialagogue is also advisable. Ketamine is approved for short-term procedural sedation not requiring skeletal muscle relaxation, and has been used extensively in children undergoing cardiac interventional procedures, either as the sole agent, or with the use of propofol, midazolam, opioids, and others.

The non-FDA-approved indications are discussed below. One of the most encountered clinical scenarios is the use of ketamine as an analgesic for sedation (gastroenterological procedures, biopsies, painful emergency room procedures, burn dressing changes, lumbar punctures, etc.), especially in patients with a history of bronchospasm. It is frequently used as an adjunct to local anesthesia alone, or with the use of propofol and midazolam.

Ketamine potentiates opioid-induced analgesia and hence has an opioid-sparing effect [2]. Co-administered with an opioid it can reduce the incidence of opioid side effects such as respiratory depression and psychotropic side effects. One successful combination if used in patient-controlled analgesia (PCA) is ketamine and morphine sulfate in a 1:1 ratio on a milligram basis with a dosing interval of 8 minutes. If patients continue to experience pain despite this regimen it is inadvisable to increase the dose further because excessive sedation and psychotropic side effects due to ketamine may arise. One has to realize that this dosing regimen may need to be altered taking into account patient factors, use of adjunct analgesics, and anesthetic regimen used during surgery. Another way to potentiate opioid analgesia is to provide for a ketamine infusion. The target serum concentration of ketamine is probably anywhere between 50 and 100 ng/mL. This corresponds to a continuous infusion to reach 2 mg/kg per day. One must realize that the contribution of ketamine to analgesia in both the PCA and continuous infusion regimen to analgesia is probably small, but coupled with a multimodal approach (epidural use, peripheral nerve blocks, NSAIDs, tramadol) pain relief can be excellent. This multimodal approach may also reduce the risk of opioid-induced hyperalgesia due to overall reduced opioid requirements.

Ketamine may be ideal to treat post-operative pain after adenotonsillectomy. It avoids the feared risks of bleeding with NSAIDs and respiratory depression with opioids. Ketamine at a dose of 0.5 mg/kg IV reduces post-operative pain and need for other analgesics. Peritonsillar infiltration at the same dose has a similar effect to the intravenous dose. The time of administration either before the start or the conclusion of surgery has no bearing on the analgesic effect. If prolonged pain is anticipated a ketamine infusion of 0.3 6 mg/kg per h can be started after the administration of a loading dose of 0.5 mg/kg.

Ketamine may play a role in the prevention of post-amputation pain and development of phantom limb pain if given epidurally over a period of 48 hours at a dose of 0.03 mg/kg per h. Ketamine can be used as second-line treatment in refractory status asthmaticus in both adults and children should conventional treatment have failed.

Ketamine may be a good alternative to conventional treatment of bronchospasm on mechanical ventilation.

There are some limited data showing the use of ketamine in the treatment of chronic pain. Ketamine in a topical gel is used in the treatment of neuropathic pain. It has some limited use if administered IV in terminal cancer patients, but increases duration of action of epidural morphine in the same group of patients.

Ketamine may be used to decrease the duration of a migraine with aura in patients with familial hemiplegic migraine, and can be used to decrease opioid withdrawal symptoms. It can decrease phantom limb pain if given IV.

Ketamine has been used extensively in the realm of electroconvulsive therapy due to its seizure-prolonging effect.

Other off-label indications are second-line treatment for refractory priapism, pruritus of the skin secondary to erythroderma, and restless leg syndrome.

Contraindications

The only absolute contraindication is use in patients who have a hypersensitivity or allergy to ketamine products.

Relative contraindications:

1. Mild to severe hypertension, a history of congestive heart failure, tachyarrythmias, and myocardial ischemia
2. Acute alcohol intoxication or history of alcohol abuse
3. Sole use of ketamine in airway surgery
4. Use in the presence of intracranial mass lesions, head and globe injuries, hydrocephalus, and increased intracranial pressure
5. Preexisting respiratory depression.

Common doses

Ketamine as an adjunct for induction of general anesthesia in adults is given at a dose of 1–4.5 mg/kg IV as a single dose, or as an infusion of 1–2 mg/kg at a rate of 0.5 mg/kg per min in addition to small doses of diazepam or midazolam [2]. Alternatively, it can be given IM at a dose of 6.5–13 mg/kg. Maintenance can be accomplished either with an infusion of 0.01–0.03 mg/kg per min, or by repeated half or full initial induction doses.

Procedural sedation doses are 1–2 mg/kg IV over 1–2 minutes, followed by 0.25–0.5 mg/kg IV every 5–10 minutes.

The rapid-sequence induction dose is 2 mg/kg.

Ketamine is used extensively in the pediatric population, but does not have FDA approval for children under 16 years of age. Doses for the indications above are similar for older children, but may be much higher in younger children.

Oral and rectal administration is less predictable than the IV and IM routes. A dose for anxiolysis would be 0.5–10 mg/kg depending on age.

Topical ketamine gel for neuropathic pain would be administered at a dose of 0.24–0.37 mg/kg, and a typical dose for epidurally administered drug for cancer pain would be 0.20 mg/kg.

Potential advantages

Ketamine is an excellent anesthetic, analgesic, and sedative in specialized settings. It can be used in patients who cannot tolerate barbiturates, in settings where cardiovascular depression must be avoided, and in patients with refractory bronchospasm. It is useful in one-lung ventilation, asthmatic patients, or when there is need for an intramuscular route of administration. It is very helpful in specific situations such as the need for anesthesia in uncontrollable, mentally retarded patients. It can be simply mixed with syrup if oral premedication is desired.

Ketamine, in contrast to opioid medications, does not cause significant respiratory depression.

Ketamine is available in a generic form as either 10 mg/mL or 100 mg/mL solution. It is inexpensive, and widely available. It can be used either as an adjunct to the use of opioids or alone, and certainly has an opioid-sparing effect by all routes of administration.

Ketamine caries the Pregnancy Risk Classification A, and is compatible with breast feeding according to the WHO. The Thompson Lactation Rating, however, does not rule out risk to infants.

Nephrotoxicity or hepatotoxicity have not been reported.

Potential disadvantages

Although no human studies exist, the use of ketamine beyond the recommended doses carries some risk. The LD_{50} in rats for intraperitoneal ketamine is 100 times the typical intravenous dose and 20 times the typical human intramuscular dose.

Concomitant ketamine and neuromuscular blocking agent administration causes increased neuromuscular blockade. The use of metrizamide or theophylline and ketamine increases seizure risk, and use of St Johns Wart can potentially lead to hypotension and delayed emergence. The combination of tramadol and ketamine has the potential for respiratory and central nervous system depression.

Drug-related adverse events

Ketamine can certainly cause tachycardia, systemic and pulmonary hypertension, and an increased vascular resistance if not attenuated by appropriate drugs. It can cause injection site pain and a transient rash, and hyperglycemia. Anorexia, nausea, and emesis are relatively common after administration of the drug, but their incidence can be significantly reduced by the concomitant use of propofol. Salivary and tracheobronchial secretions can be well managed by premedication with an anticholinergic. Ketamine can cause skeletal muscle hyperactivity, and myoclonus, twitching, vocalization, fasciculations, and rigidity are not uncommon. Emergence reactions such as vivid dreams, hallucinations, delirium, and confusion are common, and can be prevented by premedication with a benzodiazepine or barbiturate, or stopped after their occurrence.

The effect of ketamine on intracranial pressure remains controversial, but the drug should certainly be avoided in patients with refractory intracranial hypertension. Ketamine may cause nystagmus, diplopia, and lacrimation. It may transiently increase intraocular pressure.

It is a potent bronchodilator, but there have been few cases of laryngospasm.

Ketamine is considered to be a drug of potential abuse, and is listed as a Schedule III narcotic.

References

1. Micromedex® Healthcare Series, DrugDex® Evaluations, Thompson Healthcare. Ketamine, 2009. http://www.thomsonhc.com/hcs/librarian/ND_T/HCS/ND_PR/Main/CS/C37C33/DUPLICATIONSHIELDSYNC/88B073/ND_PG/PRIH/ND_B/HCS/SBK/2/ND_P/Main/PFPUI/U41ex6J2SR7kKR/PFActionId/hcs.common.RetrieveDocumentCommon/DocId/0425/ContentSetId/31#all.
2. Suzuki M. Role of NMDA receptor antagonists for postoperative pain management. Pending publication.

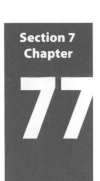

Section 7
Chapter

NMDA Antagonists

Memantine

Bryan S. Williams and Asokumar Buvanendran

Generic Name: memantine hydrochloride

Proprietary Names: Nemenda™, Abixa™ (Lundbeck, Philipp.), Akatinol

Drug Class: *N*-methyl-D-aspartate (NMDA) receptor antagonist

Manufacturers: Forest Pharmaceuticals, St Louis, MO; Grunenthal GmbH 52099 Aachen, Germany

Chemical Structure: see Figure 77.1

Chemical Name: 1-amino-3,5-dimethyladamantane hydrochloride

Chemical Formula: $C_{12}H_{21}N$; molecular wt 179.3

Introduction

Memantine was first synthesized in the 1960s and found to antagonize the NMDA receptor in the 1980s.

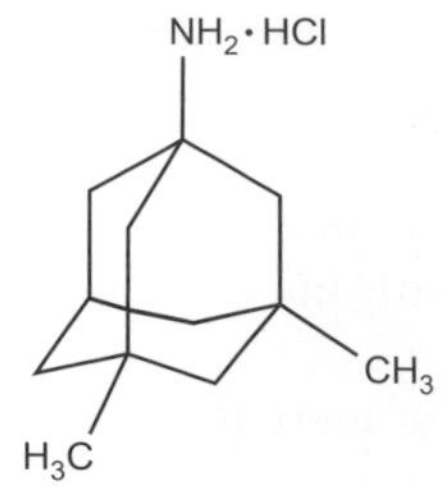

Figure 77.1.

Ketamine is one of the most widely known and medically used NMDA receptor antagonists (NMDAR) and memantine is similar in that it is a noncompetitive NMDA antagonist but is better tolerated in patients because of multiple theorized properties including the ability to bind only (or preferentially) to open channels; the tendency to inhibit faster, or with higher affinity, at higher agonist concentrations; a relatively low affinity of inhibition; being an open channel blocker with a fast off-rate compared with ketamine [1,2].

Mode of activity

Major sites of action: blockade of current flow through the NMDA receptor channel.

Minor sites of action: at high concentrations memantine affects many CNS targets, including serotonin and dopamine uptake, nicotinic acetylcholine receptors (nAChRs), serotonin receptors, sigma-1 receptors, and voltage-activated Na^+ channels [2,3].

Metabolic pathways, drug clearance and elimination

Memantine is completely absorbed from the gastrointestinal (GI) tract with maximal plasma concentration occurring between 3 and 8 hours after oral administration. Food does not influence the bioavailability of memantine [2]. Approximately 80% of the administered dose remains as the parent drug. The mean terminal elimination half-life is 60–100 h.

Indications

Memantine has Food and Drug Administration approval for Alzheimer's disease (moderate to severe), but has been used in painful medical conditions such as neuropathic pain.

Contraindications

Hypersensitivity to memantine hydrochloride.

Relative contraindications

1. Concomitant use of drugs that make the urine alkaline
2. Concomitant use of other NMDA antagonists
3. Genitourinary conditions that raise urine pH; may increase plasma levels of memantine
4. Moderate to severe renal impairment
5. Seizure disorder

Common doses

The recommended initial dose of memantine hydrochloride for the treatment of moderate to severe dementia of Alzheimer's type is 5 mg orally once daily. The dose should be increased in 5 mg increments to 10 mg/day (given as 5 mg twice daily), 15 mg/day (given twice daily in separate doses of 5 mg and 10 mg), and 20 mg/day (given as 10 mg twice daily). The minimum recommended interval between dose increases is 1 week. The recommended maintenance dose is 10 mg twice daily (20 mg/day). There is not an established dose for the treatment of chronic pain states, but case reports and medication trials have started at 5–10 mg BID and increases at 1 week intervals to 30 mg/day have been examined [3–5].

Clinical use in neuropathic pain

Early placebo-controlled trials of memantine for patients with established chronic neuropathic pain demonstrated limited effectiveness. In a randomized, crossover study on 15 patients with chronic pain for 1–28 yr after amputation, the analgesic efficacy of memantine could not be demonstrated at a dose of 20 mg/day versus placebo on any of the measured outcomes: pain scale and allodynia [4]. In contrast, a more recent randomized, double-blind, placebo-controlled trial with memantine 20–30 mg/day initiated immediately after upper limb amputation ($n = 19$) for 4 weeks post-operatively demonstrated a nearly four-fold decrease in the incidence of phantom limb pain at 6 months from 38% to 10% [6]. After cessation of ropivacaine infusion, patients maintained on memantine 30 mg/day had reduced intensity (0–100 mm visual analog scale [VAS] scoring) of phantom limb pain at 4 weeks (VAS of 3 mm in the memantine group vs. 24 in the placebo group) and 6 months (VAS of 7 in the memantine group vs. 17 in the placebo group). This trial exemplifies the benefit of preventive administration of memantidine, and that intervention may be best initiated before surgery.

Potential advantages

Ketamine causes memory deficits; reproduces with impressive accuracy the symptoms of schizophrenia; is widely abused; and induces vacuoles in neurons at moderate concentrations and cell death at higher concentrations. Memantine, on the other hand, is well tolerated; although instances of psychotic side effects have been reported, in placebo-controlled clinical studies the incidence of side effects is remarkably low. Memantine improves memory in Alzheimer dementia patients and in some (but not all) studies in animals [1].

Drug-related adverse events

In a randomized double-blind trial for the treatment of Alzheimer dementia, the most common adverse events were agitation, insomnia, diarrhea, and urinary incontinence and infection. Additionally hypertension and tachycardia have been reported with the use of memantine [5].

References

1. Johnson JW, Kotermanski SE. Mechanism of action of memantine. *Curr Opin Pharmacol* 2006;**6**(1):61–67.

2. Micromedex® Healthcare Series, DrugDex® Evaluations, Thompson Healthcare. Memantine; 2009.

3. Jarvis B, Figgitt DP. Memantine. *Drugs Aging* 2003;**20**(6):465–476; discussion 477–468.

4. Wiech K, Kiefer RT, Topfner S, et al. A placebo-controlled randomized crossover trial of the N-methyl-D-aspartic acid receptor antagonist, memantine, in patients with chronic phantom limb pain. *Anesth Analg* 2004;**98**(2):408–413.

5. Sinis N, Birbaumer N, Gustin S, et al. Memantine treatment of complex regional pain syndrome: a preliminary report of six cases. *Clin J Pain* 2007;**23**(3):237–243.

6. Hackworth RJ, Tokarz KA, Fowler IA, Wallace SC, Stedje-Larsen ET. Profound pain reduction after induction of memantine treatment in two patients with severe phantom limb pain. *Anesth Analg* 2008;**107**:1377–1379.

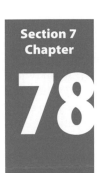

Section 7
Chapter

78

NMDA Antagonists

Dextromethorphan

Muhammad Anwar

Generic Names: dextromethorphan, dextromethorphan hydrobromide

Brand Names/Trade Names: Tussionex™, Polistirex™ Extended Release suspension, Robitussin™ DM

Manufacturer: Covidien Pharmaceuticals (a division of Malinckrodt), 15 Hampshire Street, Mansfield, MA 02048; Wyeth Healthcare, P.O. Box 26609, Richmond, VA 23261–6609

Drug Class: antitussive, *N*-methyl-d-aspartate (NMDA) receptor antagonist

Chemical Structure: see Figure 78.1

Chemical Name: 3-methoxy-17-methyl-9-(alpha),13(alpha),14(alpha)-morphinan hydrobromide monohydrate

Chemical Formula: $C_{18}H_{25}NO \cdot HBr \cdot H_2O$; molecular Wt 271; dextromethorphan is the *d* isomer of levophenol; it occurs as white crystals, is sparingly soluble in water, and freely soluble in alcohol

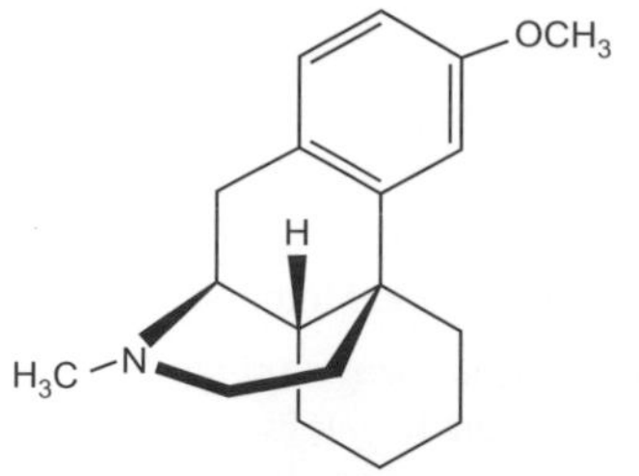

Figure 78.1.

Introduction

Dexromethorphan is a synthetically produced substance that is chemically related to codeine and morphine. It is not classified as an opioid, is non-habituating, and is not associated with respiratory depression. The FDA approved this drug as a cough suppressant in 1954 and it has gradually replaced codeine as the most widely used cough suppressant in the USA. Dextromethorphan is currently an ingredient in more than 140 over-the-counter cough and cold medications.. It is marketed alone or in combination with other drugs such as analgesics (e.g. acetaminophen), antihistamine (e.g. chlorpheniramine), decongestants (e.g. pseudo-ephedrine) and/or expectorants (e.g. guaifenesin). Experimental evidence suggests that dextromethorphan is a low-affinity NMDA receptor antagonist and may provide relief of somatic and neuropathic pain.

Mode of activity

Neuropathic pain often presents a management dilemma for patients and their caregivers, because of its severity, chronicity, and resistance to conventional analgesics. Important pathophysiological mechanisms associated with neuropathic pain include sodium and calcium channel up-regulation, spinal hyperexcitability, facilitation of noxious transmission and aberrant sympathetic nervous system activity. Central sensitization is the result of NMDA receptor activation in the central nervous system and is triggered by barrages of noxious input from the periphery. Hence, one strategy for relieving post-operative pain is to block NMDA receptors before the induction of central sensitization.

Several studies have provided evidence that NMDA antagonists, alone or in combination with opioids, attenuate sensitization induced by noxious stimulation, and result in improved pain relief with few side effects. Nonspecific NMDA receptor antagonists such as ketamine have been shown to reduce the intensity

of post-operative pain and certain neuropathic pain conditions. Like ketamine, dextromethorphan is a low-affinity, nonspecific NMDA receptor antagonist that also has weak affinity for the μ opioid receptor. Controversy exists as to whether dextromethorphan is as effective as ketamine, since some clinical trials demonstrate reductions in pain intensity and opioid requirements while others have failed to demonstrate measurable analgesic effects.

Dextromethorphan is usually taken orally and is well absorbed from the gastrointestinal tract. It is metabolized in the liver by various hepatic enzymes and subsequently undergoes O-demethylation into an active metabolite dextrophan, N-demethylation, and partial conjugation with glucuronic acid and sulfate ions. One well-known metabolic catalyst involved is a specific cytochrome P450 enzyme known as 2D6, or CYP2D6. The therapeutic activity of dextromethorphan is believed to be caused by both the drug and this metabolite. Dextromethorphan and its metabolites are excreted via kidney.

Efficacy in acute and chronic pain

Recent human and animals studies have found that dextromethorphan reduces the intensity of post-surgical pain [1–4]. A meta-analysis of preemptive administration of dextromethorphan for acute post-operative pain management demonstrated proof of efficacy (reduction in opioid requirements) [1]. A study performed by Henderson and coworkers [4] found that dextromethorphan reduces post-operative pain intensity and morphine dose requirements in patients recovering from abdominal hysterectomy. Fifty patients were randomized to receive a preemptive oral dose of dextromethorphan 40 mg, then 40 mg three times per day for the next 2 days, or placebo solution at identical times. Median pain scores at rest were significantly lower at 48 and 72 hrs and mean IV-PCA morphine consumption was reduced in the dextromethorphan group (1.1 vs 1.5 mg/h); $P = 0.54$.

Chia and coworkers [5] evaluated the effectiveness of dextromethorphan in 60 patients recovering from major abdominal surgery. Thirty patients received an IV infusion of dextromethorphan 5 mg/kg before anesthetic induction (Pre group), whereas the remaining 30 patients received the same volume of saline solution, followed by a post-operative IV infusion of dextromethorphan 5 mg/kg (Post group). Patients in the Pre group received the same volume of saline solution post-operatively. All patients were then treated with IV-PCA morphine. The mean visual analog pain score during cough or movement and at rest were similar in the two groups in the first 3 days post-operatively. However, Post group patients consumed more morphine than Pre group patients during the first 2 days ($P < 0.01$). The sedation scores, patient satisfaction, and the incidence of morphine-related side effects were similar between the two groups. The authors concluded that the pre-operative administration of dextromethorphan 5 mg/kg reduces post-operative morphine consumption compared with post-operative administration.

A randomized double-blind study on day-surgery patients examined the effects of pre-incisional oral dextromethorphan and epidural lidocaine for post-operative pain reduction and morphine sparing. Dextromethorphan-treated patients reported significantly ($P < 0.05$) less pain and sedation, and reported greater satisfaction with their pain control [6].

In nonsurgical settings, patients suffering neuropathic and cancer pain treated with dextromethorphan had a reduced need for morphine and experienced less sedation. Dextromethorphan was found to be effective in patients presenting with neuropathic pain; however, dose requirements are high [7,8]. Carlsson and coworkers [7] found that a single dose of dextromethorphan (270 mg) was effective in treating post-traumatic neuropathic pain; however, the effect varied among test subjects and was determined to be useful only in patients who could experience the pain-relieving effect without significant side effects.

Nelson and co-workers [8] also evaluated high doses of dextromethorphan in patients with neuropathic pain. They performed two randomized, double-blind, crossover trials comparing 6 weeks of oral dextromethorphan to placebo in two groups of patients with painful neuropathy (14 patients with one distal symmetrical diabetic neuropathy and 18 with post-herpetic neuralgia). Dextromethorphan dose was titrated in each patient to the highest level reached without disrupting normal activities; mean doses were 381 mg/day in diabetics and 439 mg/day in post-herpetic neuralgia patients. In diabetic neuropathy, dextromethorphan decreased pain by a mean of 24% (95% CI: 6% to 42%, $P = 0.011$), relative to placebo. In post-herpetic neuralgia, dextromethorphan did not reduce pain (10% decrease in pain, $P = 0.72$). Five of 31 patients who took dextromethorphan dropped out due to sedation or ataxia during dose escalation.

Contraindications

Dextromethorphan is contraindicated in patients taking selective serotonin reuptake inhibitors and monoamine oxidase inhibitors.

Alcohol and CNS depressants should not be used with dextromethorphan.

Dextromethorphan should not be taken for persistent or chronic cough or when cough is accompanied with excessive secretions such as in COPD.

Dextromethorphan may be associated with release of histamine and should not be used in atopic children.

Common doses/uses

Adults: oral doses of 20 to 40 mg every 4 hours or 30–60 mg every 6 to 8 hours not to exceed 180 mg daily. Long-acting preparation: 60 mg twice a day. The extended-release oral Polistirex™ suspension delivers dextromethorphan from an ion-exchange complex over a period of 9 to 12 hours. One 60-mg dose of Polistirex™ suspension delivers a plasma concentration similar to two 30-mg doses of immediate-release dextromethorphan given every 6 hours. For preemptive surgical pain control doses between 90 and 120 mg have been used in different clinical trials. Doses employed for control of neuropathic pain are considerably higher (200–300 mg) as tolerated.

Children: dextromethorphan is not generally recommended in children less than 2 years of age unless under medical supervision. Children aged 2 to 6 years 2.5 to 5.0 mg every 4 hours or 7.5 mg every 6 to 8 hours not to exceed 30 mg daily. Children aged 6 to 12 years may be given 5 to 10 mg every 4 hours or 15 mg every 6 to 8 hours, not to exceed 60 mg daily.

Dextromethorphan is available in different forms such as capsule, liquid, liquid gelatin capsule, lozenge, tablets, intramuscular, as well as in powdered forms (available on the internet).

Potential advantages

Although dextromethorphan is not a potent analgesic drug, it may be useful as an adjunct drug as a part of multimodality treatment in chronic neuropathic as well as in acute pain management. There does not appear to be any evidence of physical dependence or habit-forming from this drug when used in therapeutic doses. The advantage of dextromethorphan preparation over those containing codeine was the lack of physical addiction potential and sedative side effects, although, as with most cough suppressants, studies show that its effectiveness is highly debatable.

Potential disadvantages

Adverse events are very uncommon with therapeutic doses (40–160 mg); however, dextromethorphan can cause some side effects such as dizziness, drowsiness, lightheadedness, nervousness, restlessness, nausea and vomiting, and stomach pain.

There is also an illicit use of dextromethorphan. Teenagers and young adults commonly abuse this drug. When dextromethorphan is abused in higher doses, it acts as a dissociative anesthetic, similar to PCP and ketamine. Slang terms for dextromethorphan include DM, DXM, Dex, skittles, Triple C, Tussin, robo, rojo, and velvet.

Poison control experts point to a four-fold increase in abuse cases since 2000, mostly involving school-aged youth and young adults, particularly among those who are part of the dance club or "rave" scenes. Intoxications come from swallowing large doses of cough syrup or cough-suppressant pills. Visual and/or auditory hallucinations, euphoria, disorientation, insomnia, confusion, dizziness, double or blurred vision, slurred speech, impaired physical coordination, abdominal pain, nausea, and vomiting have been reported. In children there are cases of ataxia, stupor, transient fever, lethargy, tachycardia, high blood pressure, headache, numbness of fingers and toe, loss of consciousness, seizures, and nystagmus. The main target organ is the central nervous system. Coma and death have also been reported with high-dose abuse. Dextromethorphan is not an illegal or controlled drug; nevertheless, increasing reports of abuse and intoxification have resulted in monitoring by the DEA, and the drug could be added to the Controlled Substances Act if warranted.

Drug interactions

Concomitant use of monoamine oxidase inhibitors has caused toxicity leading to coma and death. There are serious life-threatening serotonergic syndrome interactions between dextromethorphan and serotonin reuptake inhibitors. Alcohol and other CNS depressant drugs should be avoided when taking dextromethorphan.

Treatment of acute poisoning

Oral ingestion is the most common route of acute poisoning. The most common clinical effects involve the central nervous system. General principles are assessment and support of airway, ventilation, and circulation. Naloxone may antagonize respiratory depression and CNS effects of dextromethorphan. Patients with respiratory depression may require admission to an intensive care unit. Other patients can be observed in the emergency facility for 4 to 6 hours and then discharged. Patients with minor symptoms may be sent home under supervision. Children who have ingested a long-acting preparation should be hospitalized for 24 hours observation.

Gastric decontamination is recommended for a recent ingestion of more than 10 mg/kg. If a long-acting dextromethorphan preparation has been ingested, whole bowel lavage may be considered.

References

1. Helmy SAK, Bali A. The effects of the preemptive use of the NMDA receptor antagonist dextromethorphan on postoperative analgesic requirements. *Anesth Analg* 2001;**92**(3):739–744.

2. Aoki T, Yamagauchi H, Naito H, Shiiki K, Ota Y, Kaneko A. Dextromethorphan premedication reduced postoperative analgesic consumption in patients after oral surgery. *Oral Surg Oral Med Oral Pathol Oral Radiol Endodontology* 2006;**102**(5);591–595.

3. Talakoub R, Molaeinasab F. Premedication with oral dextromethorphan reduces intra-operative morphine requirement. *J Res Med Sci* 2005;**10**(5);281–284.

4. Henderson DJ, Withington BS, Wilson JA, et al. Perioperative dextromethorphan reduces postoperative pain after hysterectomy. *Anesth Analg* 1999;**89**:399.

5. Chia YY, Liu K, Chow LH, et al. The preoperative administration of intravenous dextromethorphan reduces postoperative morphine consumption. *Anesth Analg* 1999;**89**:748–753.

6. Weinbroum AA. Dextromethaphan reduces immediate and late postoperative analgesic requirement and improves patients' subjective scoring after epidural lidocaine and general anesthesia. *Anesth Analg* 2002;**94**(6):1547–1552.

7. Carlsson KC, Hoem NO, Moberg ER. The effect of Dextromethorphan in neuropathic pain. *Acta Anesthesiologica Scand* 2004;**48**:328–336.

8. Nelson, KA, Park KM, Robinovitz, E et al. High-dose oral dextromethorphan versus placebo in painful diabetic neuropathy and postherpetic neuralgia. *Neurology* 1997;**48**:1212–1218.

79

NMDA antagonists: magnesium and amantadine

Clinton Kakazu, John Charney and Yaw Wu

Generic Name: magnesium, Epsom salts

Trade/Generic Name: magnesium sulfate injectable, topical gel

Manufacturer: HOSPIRA, Inc., Chicago, IL

Chemical Structure: see Figure 79.1

Chemical Name: magnesium sulfate

Chemical Formula: $MgSO_4$ molecular wt 120.3

Generic Name: amantadine, see Figure 79.2

Trade/Proprietary Name: Symmetrel®

Manufacturer: Endo Pharmaceuticals, Inc., Chadds Ford, PA

Chemical Structure: see Figure 79.3

Chemical Name: adamantan-1-amine

Chemical Formula: $C_{10}H_{17}N$; molecular wt 159

Introduction

Magnesium and amantidine are nonspecific inhibitors of the NMDA receptors. Both have been advocated as analgesic adjuvants for pain management. Several small-scale studies have demonstrated measurable efficacy as well as safety in selected settings.

Magnesium: mode of activity

Magnesium (Mg^{2+}) has multiple mechanisms of action. At the neurocellular level within the CNS, Mg^{2+} acts as a noncompetitive antagonist of the N-methyl-D-aspartate (NMDA) receptor and its associated ion channels in a voltage-dependent manner. It has been postulated that NMDA receptor activation is one of the mechanisms causing central sensitization, and inhibition of its primary agonist (i.e. glutamate and aspartate) by Mg^{2+} may attenuate peripheral hypersensitive nociception. While intravenous (IV) Mg^{2+} has been demonstrated to attenuate post-operative pain [1,3], its ability to effectively cross the blood–brain barrier remains unclear [2].

A study by Tramer et al. [1] demonstrated no increase in CSF Mg^{2+} concentration with peri-operative IV Mg^{2+} infusion, and conversely, no post-operative analgesic effects. Thus, there are limitations of IV Mg^{2+} for modulation of antinociception via central NMDA blockade due to insufficent Mg^{2+} transference into the CNS at effective concentrations.

Direct Mg^{2+} administration into the CNS intrathecally (IT) has been demonstrated to augment fentanyl spinal analgesia [4].

In addition to NMDA blockade, Mg^{2+} has calcium channel blockade properties resulting in direct effects on smooth muscle causing peripheral vasodilatation, bronchial dilatation, and uterine relaxation.

At the neuromuscular junction Mg^{2+} reduces the amount of acetylcholine release, thus explaining its role in treatment of convulsions and seizures by blocking neuromuscular transmission.

Indications

While not FDA-approved, IV and IT Mg^{2+} has been studied as an analgesic adjuvant and does not have the equianalgesic potency of narcotics. IT Mg^{2+} slightly prolongs the duration of spinal narcotics.

Topical Mg^{2+} in gel (Epsom gel) or solution form has anecdotal evidence for use in minor myalgias and arthalgias in osteoarthritis, osteoperosis, rheumatoid arthritis and fibromyalgia.

Contraindications

IV Mg^{2+} is contraindicated in patients with heart block or myocardial damage.

Doses

IV

The original study claiming analgesic adjuvant activity was at loading doses of 50 mg/kg pre-operatively, with 8 mg/kg per h given intra-operatively [1].

325

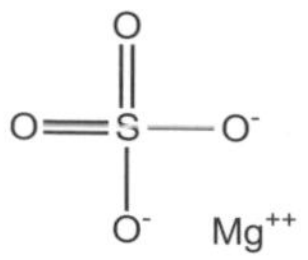

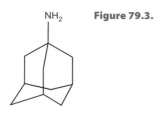

Figure 79.1.

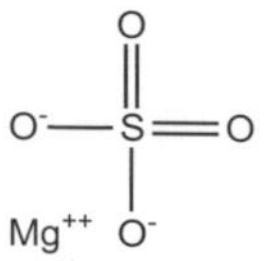

Figure 79.2.

Figure 79.3.

IT

As an adjuvant for spinal narcotics the original study used 50 mg of Mg^{2+} in 3 mL of preservative-free 0.9% sodium chloride [4].

Potential advantages

Intra-operative IV Mg^{2+} is also associated with improved patient comfort and better quality of sleep but without increased adverse effects [1].

IV Mg^{2+} has many other potential advantages which can benefit patients with other co-existing disease states such as: treatment of psychiatric illness (depression, bipolar disease); obstetrics (preeclampsia, tocolytic); cardiac ventricular dysrhythmias (torsade de pointes).

Moreover, in animal models, Mg^{2+} has been shown to improve neurological outcome in brain and spinal cord injury. Studies demonstrating neuroprotective effects in humans are ongoing. The basis for neuroprotection is the ability of Mg^{2+} to block both the NMDA receptor and calcium ion channels, thereby reducing the excitatory amino acid stimulatory effect and calcium ion influx into the cell.

Potential disadvantages

Mg^{2+} is eliminated solely by renal excretion and plasma concentration is directly proportional to glomerular filtration rate. Thus, in patients with renal dysfunction caution is advised. Unintentional high levels of serum magnesium may be obtained.

Increase in serum magnesium concentrations may lead to less desirable effects intra-operatively such as prolongation of muscle relaxants, peripherial vasodilatation, cardiac conductivity disorders, and gastric hypomotility.

Related adverse events

GI: diarrhea

Skeletal muscle: muscle weakness, delayed deep tendon reflex

Cardiac effects: cardiac arrhythmia, congestive heart failure

Respiratory effects: respiratory depression, bronchodilation, pulmonary edema

CNS effects: antiseizure, sedation, stupor, coma

Amantadine: mode of activity

Amandatine is an N-methyl-D-aspartate (NMDA) receptor antagonist. It is an uncompetitive antagonist; it blocks the ion channel of the receptor by accelerating its closure. The drug exhibits substantial protein binding. Hepatic metabolism is negligible. The drug undergoes renal excretion. Its half-life is 10 to 14 hours, which is prolonged in the event of renal failure [5].

Indications

Amantadine is indicated for the treatment of chronic neuropathic pain related to cancer and other pathologies such as diabetes. It has also been used to treat musculoskeletal pain and post-surgical pain [5–7].

Contraindications

Absolute: amantadine is contraindicated for patients with a history of hypersensitivity to the drug.

Relative: amantadine is relatively contraindicated for use in patients with a history of seizures, substance abuse, or psychiatric illness since the drug may exacerbate symptoms related to these disorders.

Doses

Amantadine hydrochloride is available in tablet form (100 mg/tablet) and as an oral suspension (10 mg/mL). The usual dose for the treatment of pain is one tablet per day for 7 to 14 days.

An intravenous solution of amantadine sulfate (PK Merz®), 200 mg in 500 mL of normal saline, is not approved for use in the USA.

Potential advantages

Amantadine is generally well tolerated. The drug can be used either as monotherapy or as an adjunct to other pain medications.

Since its hepatic metabolism is minimal amantadine would not be expected to interact with other drugs. However, it has been shown to increase morphine levels, probably by interfering with 3-glucuronidation in the kidneys. Thus, amantadine may reduce the dosage of morphine required for pain relief when administered with this opioid.

Potential disadvantages

Amantadine may exacerbate central nervous system effects in disorders. Dosages must be adjusted for patients with renal disease or congestive heart failure. Since amantadine interacts with morphine caution is required when these two drugs are administered together.

Related adverse events

Adverse reactions related to the administration of amantadine include:

1. Central nervous system: insomnia, depression, anxiety, ataxia, hallucinations
2. Gastrointestinal: nausea, diarrhea, constipation
3. Cardiovascular: arrhythmias, orthostatic hypotension, cardiac arrest
4. Other: dizziness, neuroleptic malignant syndrome

References

1. Tramer MR, et al. Role of magnesium sulfate in postoperative analgesia. *Anesthesiology* 1996;**84**: 340–347.

2. Seong-Hoon Ko, et al. Magnesium sulfate does not reduce postoperative analgesic requirements. *Anesthesiology* 2001;**95**:640–646.

3. Koinig H, Wallner T, Marhofer P, Andel H, Hörauf K, Mayer N. Magnesium sulfate reduces intra- and postoperative analgesic requirements. *Anesth Analg* 1998;**87**:206–210.

4. Buvanendran A, et al. Intrathecal magnesium prolongs fentanyl analgesia: a prospective, randomized, controlled trial. *Anesth Analg* 2002;**95**:661–666.

5. Blanpied T, Clark R, Johnson J. Amandatine inhibits NMDA receptors by accelerating channel closure during channel block *J Neurosci* 2005;**25**(13): 3312–3322.

6. Pud E, Eisenberg E, Spitzer A, et al. The NMDA antagonist amantadine reduces surgical neuropathic pain in cancer patients: a double blind, randomized, placebo controlled trial. *Pain* 1998;**75**(2–3): 349–354.

7. Snijdelaar D, Koren G, Katz J. Effects of perioperative oral amantadine on postoperative pain and morphine consumption in patients after radical prostatectomy: results of a preliminary study. *Anesthesiology* 2004;**100**(1):134–141.

80

Overview of adrenergic and serotoninergic pain suppression

Frederick Conlin and Shamsuddin Akhtar

Introduction

Norepinephrine and serotonin are ubiquitous endogenous neurotransmitters in the human body. They exert their effect via their receptors and are intricately involved in nociception and antinociception pathways. Both the adrenergic and serotoninergic systems consist of numerous distinct receptor subtypes that are located throughout the periphery, the spinal cord, and supraspinally. Stimulation of the same receptor at different locations in the body can lead to dramatically different effects. While activation and inhibition at each of these sites play an important role in the perception of pain, it is in the descending inhibitory pain pathways where these transmitters appear to have their most significant influence. The understanding of these interactions and anatomic pathways affords the clinician the opportunity to utilize various methods of pharmacological interventions to alleviate pain.

Descending pain pathways

The descending modulation of pain involves many neurotransmitters, neuromodulators and pathways. Descending pathways arise from a number of brainstem structures that include periaqueductal gray matter (PAG), nucleus raphe magnus (NRM), nucleus paragigantocellularis and locus coerulus (LC). The frontal lobes and the amygdala also exert a descending influence via their projections to the PAG and the hypothalamus. The interactions are varied and complex. In animals, stimulation of the PAG has long been recognized to produce analgesia. It has large concentrations of opioid receptors and appears to modulate pain through both opioid and non-opioid (serotoninergic) induced antinociception. Receiving input from the frontal and insular cortex, thalamus, cerebellum, and limbic system, the PAG projects to NRM in the medulla. The NRM then projects to the dorsal horn via serotoninergic fibers in the dorsolateral funiculus.

Similar to the PAG, stimulation of the NRM can produce analgesia, confirming its importance in descending inhibition.

Activation of the serotoninergic, or 5-hydroxytryptamine (5-HT), receptors in the dorsal horn can inhibit nociception. Indeed, intrathecally administered serotonin has been shown to possess some analgesic properties. These beneficial results are most probably achieved by serotonin-induced release of spinal GABA and opioids, and not via direct action of serotonin itself, as the degree of antinociception was diminished when 5-HT agonists were given in the presence of naloxone or a GABA antagonist. The effect of intrathecal serotonin is not exclusively antinociceptive and it may have pro-nociceptive effects in some situations. The potential explanation of this observation is that there are seven different families of serotonin receptors. While the serotonin receptors share many common properties, the unique qualities of each receptor and its location (presynaptic versus postsynaptic), may contribute to the variable response to serotonin.

The locus coeruleus, which contains large concentrations of adrenergic neurons, also contributes to descending inhibition of nociception. Serving as the adrenergic center of the brain it communicates with the dorsal horn of the spinal cord (substantia gelatinosa) through the descending bulbospinal noradrenergic pathway. Stimulation of the bulbospinal pathway leads to the release of norepinephrine, which acts on the alpha-2-adrenergic receptors located on the primary afferents (C and A-delta fibers) and second-order neurons. Activation of the alpha-2-adrenergic receptors inhibits the release of primary afferent neurotransmitters and hyperpolarizes the second-order neurons, resulting in decreased pain transmission and antinociception. These actions serve as the basis for the analgesic properties seen with neuraxial use of alpha-2-adrenergic agonists such as clonidine. It should be pointed out that these effects can be amplified when opioids are present but may also be seen independent of concomitant opioid administration. The locus coeruleus also projects to the cerebral cortex, thalamus, hypothalamus, hippocampus, amygdala, and PAG. Stimulation of cortical α-1 receptors regulates attention and wakefulness, while α-2 agonism there results in sedation. Conversely, noradrenergic fibers traveling from the locus coeruleus and terminating in the PAG may actually promote nociception when stimulated, further highlighting the complexity of the system.

Serotonin

As discussed above, serotonin has many different receptor subtypes to which it may bind. The seemingly contradictory properties of serotonin have made it difficult to develop specific pharmacological agents that carry out the desired effect on the intended receptor subtype. However, selective serotonin reuptake inhibitors and tricyclic antidepressants are two classes of medications that can be used clinically to modulate pain. It is believed that at least some of the analgesic properties displayed by tricyclic antidepressants and serotonin reuptake inhibitors are through potentiation of the serotoninergic pathways described earlier. The antinociceptive properties of tricyclic antidepressants, which have noradrenergic and anticholinergic effects as well, are more profound than the modest analgesia seen with primarily serotonin reuptake inhibition. Further complicating the issue is that, in the periphery, serotonin functions largely as a pronociceptive transmitter. Injury to peripheral tissue causes platelets to release their serotonin stores, which then stimulates nociceptors and initiates pain signals. In addition, serotonin is involved in the inflammatory response to injury, which may further contribute to pain, further demonstrating the dual effects of serotonin.

Norepinephrine

Pain is modulated by norepinephrine via its effect on alpha-adrenergic receptors, specifically the alpha-2-adrenergic receptor. The adrenergic system consists of alpha and beta receptors with multiple subtypes within each class. While there may be a role for modulating the β receptor to produce analgesia this is currently not widely accepted. However, recent years have seen increasing attention being given to the ability of the alpha receptor, and more specifically the alpha-2-adrenergic receptor, to modulate nociception. The alpha-2-adrenergic receptor is found throughout the body and the response to its stimulation differs based on location. Centrally it results in analgesia and sedation as discussed above, while in the periphery it can yield bradycardia, diuresis, and vasoconstriction or vasodilatation. Clinically, the alpha-2 agonists clonidine and dexmedetomidine are available and can be utilized systemically or intrathecally (clonidine) for their analgesic and sedative properties. A second mechanism whereby descending noradrenergic pathways can be employed to enhance spinal and supraspinal analgesia is to inhibit the synaptic reuptake, thereby increasing local concentrations of norepinephrine. Norepinephrine released at synaptic endings of descending fibers binds to alpha-2-adrenergic receptors located on postsynaptic pain transmission cells. Activation of these receptors inhibits neuronal depolarization and pain transmission. The effects of norepinephrine are short-lived since molecules either diffuse away from the synapse or are actively taken up by a norepinephrine reuptake protein. Tricyclic antidepressants described above provide measurable antinociception by blocking this key protein and increasing concentrations of norepinephrine at the pain transmission synapse.

We have described above the mechanisms by which alpha-2-adrenergic stimulation can produce both sedation and spinal and supraspinal analgesia. However, alpha-1-adrenergic stimulation at sites in the medulla and the periphery may be responsible for some opposing actions, which may actually facilitate nociception. After injury to a peripheral nerve, alpha-adrenergic stimulation can increase the frequency of impulses by the surrounding nerves leading to pain, and actually potentiate the development of chronic pain states. Oddly enough, there appears to be both alpha-1- and alpha-2-adrenergic contributions to this phenomenon. The pronociceptive properties of the adrenergic system can also be seen in CRPS, which is mediated by the reaction to an elevated adrenergic tone.

References

1. Terman GW, Bonica JJ. Chapter 4: Spinal mechanisms and their modulation. In Loeser JD, Butler SH, Chapman R, Turk DC, eds. *Bonica's Management of Pain*, 3rd ed. Philadelphia: Lippincott Williams & Wilkins, 2001, pp. 125–138.

2. Lubenow TR, Ivankovich AD, Barkin RL. Chapter 55: Management of acute postoperative pain. In Barash PG, Cullen BF, Stoelting RK, eds. *Clinical Anesthesia*, 5th ed. Philadelphia: Lippincott, Williams & Wilkins, 2006, pp. 1407–1416.

3. Carroll I, Mackey S, Gaeta R. The role of adrenergic receptors and pain: the good, the bad, and the unknown. *Semin Anesth Periop Med Pain* 2007; **26**:17–21.

4. Giordano J, Schultea T. Serotonin 5-HT3 receptor mediation of pain and anti-nociception: implications for clinical therapeutics. *Pain Physician* 2004;**7**: 141–147.

5. Chiari A, et al. Clonidine as the sole analgesic agent during first stage of labor: a dose-response study. *Anesthesiology* 1999;**91**:388–396.

Section 8 Chapter

81

Alpha-Adrenergic Analgesics

Clonidine (transdermal and parenteral)

Anahat Kaur Dhillon

Generic Name: clonidine hydrochloride

Trade Names: Catapres™, Catapres-TTS™

Manufacturer: Boehringer Ingelheim Pharmaceuticals, Inc., Ridgefield, CT 06877

Chemical Structure: see Figure 81.1

Description

Clonidine is an alpha-2-adrenoreceptor agonist as well as an imidazoline. Ahlquist's 1948 classification of adrenoreceptors into alpha and beta receptors was followed by a description of receptors that decrease the release of neurotransmitters that were labeled alpha-2 and thought to be presynaptic. Clonidine was initially synthesized in 1962 as a nasal decongestant. When tested in the first human, intranasal clonidine caused hypotension, significant bradycardia and reportedly the subject was asleep for 24 hours. Since then clonidine has played an important role in the treatment of hypertension and a smaller role for anesthesia and analgesia. It produces sedation, anxiolysis, potent analgesia, hemodynamic stability as well as a reduction in post-operative shivering and nausea and vomiting.

Mode of activity

Major and minor sites of action: alpha-2-adrenoreceptors in the CNS and periphery, as well as non-adrenergic imidazoline binding sites.

Receptor interactions: clonidine interacts at the G protein-coupled alpha receptors with a greater affinity for the alpha-2 receptors. The activation of the alpha-2 receptors results in decreased cAMP, K^+ efflux as well as Ca^{2+} entry into the nerve terminals. Activation of receptors in the sympathetic nerve endings and in the noradrenergic neurons in the CNS inhibits release of norepinephrine and may release acetylcholine. The locus coeruleus is an important modulator of alertness and may be the major site for the hypnotic effects of clonidine. Additionally, the G protein pathway has a similar transduction pathway to the opioids, explaining some of the cross-tolerance and synergy between the two classes of drugs.

Clonidine also binds to the imidazole receptors found in the brain, kidney and pancreas. These receptors

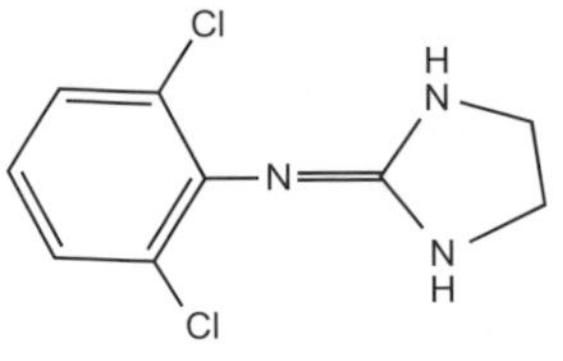

Figure 81.1.

Clonidine

mediate a central hypotensive and anti-arrhythmogenic response.

Metabolic pathways/drug clearance and elimination: clonidine is highly lipophilic and has excellent bioavailability. Peak plasma levels are achieved in 60–90 minutes after oral administration. Transdermal preparations take 24 hours to achieve levels. It is less than 50% metabolized in the liver with the remaining drug excreted unchanged in the kidney. The elimination half-life is 6–20 hours.

Indications (approved/non-approved)

Surgical acute pain: although not FDA-approved, clonidine is a potent analgesic and has been used for postoperative pain control. Pre-operative administration provides anxiolysis and some sparing effect on anesthetics. This effect can translate into decreased postoperative pain and use of opioids.

Medical pain: clonidine is a potent analgesic and may be particularly helpful in the management of patients with opioid tolerance. It can be used as an adjunct or monotherapy.

Chronic non-malignancy pain: oral or transdermal clonidine is less commonly used in the chronic setting for pain control due to the increased level of sedation. However, it may be helpful in managing patients who have been on high-dose narcotics as it has some efficacy in withdrawal syndromes. It can also be used for migraines.

Contraindications

Absolute: patients with documented severe allergic reactions to clonidine.

Relative: use with caution in patients with preexisting bradycardia or sinus node dysfunction, hypotension, cerebrovascular disease, chronic renal impairment.

Common doses

Clonidine has excellent bioavailability, making the oral and parenteral doses almost equivalent.

Oral: tablets are supplied in 0.1 mg, 0.2 mg and 0.3 mg forms. Starting doses of 2 μg/kg with titration up to 5 μg/kg are recommended.

Parenteral: in one study 150 μg of clonidine was equivalent to 5 mg of morphine for pain control. Starting with 2 μg/kg and careful titration is suggested.

Transdermal patches are generally started at the 0.1 mg dose and titrated over several days.

Potential advantages

Monotherapy: the combination of anxiolysis and potent analgesia is very desirable in some patients.

Multimodal therapy: clonidine seems to have a synergistic effect with opioids. This provides for more intense analgesia with the minimization of some of the adverse effects of either class of drugs. There is some cross-tolerance with opioids; however, for patients with high opioid tolerance clonidine is an excellent adjunct.

Cost and availability: relatively inexpensive generic versions are readily available at most hospitals.

Reduction in adverse side effects: one of the major advantages of clonidine is its minimal effect on respiratory drive. Additionally, the bradycardia and decrease in sympathetic outflow can be protective in patients with cardiac disease.

Potential disadvantages

Significant sedation can occur with clonidine. While direct respiratory depression is not common, sedation can result in hypopnea and subsequent hypoxemia. Another limiting factor in its use has been the hemodynamic profile that includes initial hypertension followed by hypotension and bradycardia. Orthostatic hypotension in particular can limit its use in both the acute and chronic settings.

Drug-related adverse events

Common/serious adverse events: central nervous system mediated sedation, dizziness and fatigue are common. Xerostomia is a common side effect that can be prohibitive in some patients. Patients should also be monitored for hypothermia, bradycardia and hypotension.

Less common adverse events: respiratory depression and apnea are not common but have been reported with large doses. Sinus and AV node blocks are also rare but serious side effects seem to occur more frequently with the transdermal administration.

331

Treatment of adverse events: the treatment is generally supportive. Volume resuscitation, norepinephrine, and atropine are effective for management of hypotension and bradycardia. The initial hypertension noted with administration is generally transient and should be treated cautiously with short acting medications.

Naloxone does not seem to be effective in reversing the sedative effects but may be helpful if opioids have been co-administered.

References

1. Khan Z, Ferguson C, Jones R. Alpha-2 and imidazoline receptor agonists: their pharmacology and therapeutic role. *Anaesthesia* 1999;**54**:146–165.

2. Micromedex® Healthcare Series, DrugDex® Evaluations, Thompson Healthcare. Clonidine.

Section 8 Chapter

82

Alpha-Adrenergic Analgesics

Neuraxial clonidine hydrochloride

Richard W. Hong

Generic Names: clonidine-HCl

Brand Name: Duraclon™

Manufacturer: Roxane Laboratories, Inc., Columbus, OH

Drug Class: analgesic agent

Chemical Structure: see Figure 82.1

Chemical Name: *N*-(2,6-dichlorophenyl)-4,5-dihydro-1*H*-imidazol-2-amine

Description

Alpha-adrenergic mechanisms had been unknowingly utilized for analgesia since the first forays into neuraxial analgesia were made by August Bier in the late 1800s. However, more focused explorations into the effects of alpha-2 agonism in the CNS only started to gain serious momentum late last century, as effective adjuncts to more commonly employed regional anesthetics were sought. Gradually, it became known that clonidine appears to be safe for neuraxial use in humans, is most potent when given

spinally, and is more potent epidurally than intravenously or intramuscularly [1]. In larger doses, or in combination with other analgesics, neuraxial clonidine can provide profound analgesia. However, safe doses of neuraxial clonidine employed as a monotherapy have not been found adequate for surgical anesthesia.

Mode of activity

Major and minor sites of action: alpha-2-adrenoreceptors, non-adrenergic imidazoline-preferring binding sites.

Receptor interactions: clonidine acts at postsynaptic alpha-2-adrenoreceptors in the CNS, mimicking the effects of norepinephrine to produce analgesia in animals and humans. Clonidine also stimulates release of the inhibitory neurotransmitters acetylcholine and norepinephrine in the dorsal horn. Stimulation of postsynaptic alpha-2-adrenoceptors in the brainstem and sympathetic preganglionic neurons in the spinal cord decreases sympathetic outflow, causing hypotension and bradycardia depending on the extent of spread. Alpha-2-adrenergic activity in the

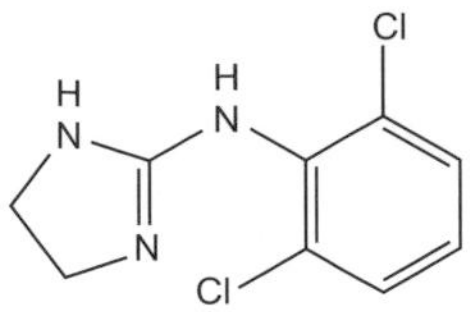

Figure 82.1.

periphery, the result of systemic uptake, may cause vasorelaxation. Non-adrenergic activity in the lateral reticular nucleus may also produce hypotension. Sedation can result from effects in the locus coeruleus of the brainstem. Clonidine's neuraxial effects differ from its effects on peripheral nerves, which are devoid of alpha-2-adrenergic receptors, where clonidine instead appears to have a direct effect on nerve conduction [1].

Metabolic pathways: due to its lipophilicity, epidural clonidine is quickly absorbed into systemic circulation, with peak arterial concentrations after 10 minutes, peak venous concentrations after 30–45 minutes, and peak CSF concentrations after 30–60 minutes. The liver is responsible for metabolism of 50% of clonidine into inactive metabolites. Approximately two-thirds of clonidine, metabolized and unmetabolized, are excreted renally. While the effects of epidural clonidine may last only 3–5 hours, elimination takes longer. The plasma elimination half-life of clonidine is 22 ± 15 hours and can be prolonged in renal failure [1,2].

Indications

Black-box warning: clonidine-HCl is not recommended for routine obstetrical, post-partum or peri-operative pain management due to risk of hemodynamic instability, especially hypotension and bradycardia, from epidural administration. However, in rare obstetrical, post-partum or peri-operative patients, the potential benefits may outweigh the risks.

Cancer pain: neuraxial clonidine can be utilized as an analgesic for patients with intractable cancer pain, particularly neuropathic pain [1,2]. Clonidine is less likely to be effective for diffuse, visceral or poorly localized pain secondary to cancer. Preservative-free clonidine-HCl (Duraclon™) has an orphan drug designation and has only been approved by the FDA for epidural administration in cancer patients with intractable pain.

Surgical acute pain: neuraxial clonidine is not approved for but can be used to relieve intra-operative and post-operative pain, as an adjunct or as monotherapy.

Labor pain: epidural clonidine has been shown to have a dose-sparing effect on local anesthetic requirements of laboring women but there are insufficient data to determine adverse neonatal effects.

Chronic pain: because its activity differs from that of opioids, neuraxial clonidine is potentially useful as an analgesic adjunct to opioids or as monotherapy in patients developing opioid tolerance. In limited studies, there is no histopathological evidence against its use; however, there are insufficient data regarding long-term clonidine administration in chronic pain patients.

Contraindications

Absolute: patients with documented severe allergic reaction or hypersensitivity.

Relative: anticoagulant therapy, bleeding diathesis, infection at the site of injection, and any other relative contraindication to placement of neuraxial analgesia; epidural use above the C4 dermatome (insufficient data regarding safety).

Common doses

Black-box warning: the 500 µg/mL strength product should be diluted in sterile, preservative-free 0.9% sodium chloride to a final concentration of 100 µg/mL prior to use.

Adjunct, cancer pain, epidural infusion, adult: 30 µg/h infusion titrated up to 40 µg/h (experience is limited with infusion rates exceeding 40 µg/h)

Adjunct, cancer pain, epidural infusion, pediatric: 0.5 µg/kg per h, titrated to response

Adjunct, pain, epidural bolus, adult: 75–700 µg

Adjunct, labor pain, patient-controlled epidural analgesia, adult: bupivacaine 0.0625% with fentanyl 2 µg/mL + clonidine 4.5 µg/mL

Adjunct, post-operative pain following total knee arthroplasty, intrathecal bolus, adult: bupivacaine 15 mg + clonidine 75 µg or bupivacaine 15 mg + clonidine 25 µg + morphine 250 µg

Adjunct, post-operative pain following coronary artery bypass graft, intrathecal bolus, adult: clonidine 1 µg/kg + morphine 4 µg/kg

Potential advantages

Monotherapy: neuraxial clonidine has not been associated with sensory or motor blockade when used as a single agent. The sedative and hemodynamic effects are sometimes desirable, depending on the clinical situation.

Adjunct therapy: epidural clonidine as an analgesic adjunct enhances both sensory and motor block caused by local anesthetics (mechanism unclear). It also enhances the effect of other spinal analgesics, including intrathecal opioids. Both quality and duration are enhanced when clonidine is combined with these other neuraxial analgesics

Reduction in adverse events: the dose-sparing effect of clonidine on other neuraxial medications can potentially minimize the overall side effects of the analgesic regimen. Micturition is not delayed by neuraxial clonidine as it is with the most commonly used neuraxial analgesics, namely local anesthetics and opioids.

Potential disadvantages

Adverse events: sedation is frequently a limiting side effect of neuraxial clonidine, particularly in the larger doses necessary for epidural analgesia. Significant, direct respiratory depression is not common, but significant sedation can result in transient decreases in oxygen saturation during sleep, encouraging continuous pulse oximetry when larger (epidural) doses are given. As stated in the black-box warning, hemodynamic effects may preclude its use in laboring patients (to preserve uteroplacental perfusion) and in peri-operaive patients for whom hemodynamic stability is of great concern. (That being said, some centers successfully employ epidural clonidine as an intra-operative/post-operative analgesic monotherapy for thoracoabdominal aortic aneurysm surgery.)

Limited approved indications: despite safety and efficacy demonstrated in a variety of neuraxial applications, most of clonidine's neuraxial potential uses are not FDA-approved, and it remains a Pregnancy Class C drug.

Drug-related adverse events

Common adverse events: clonidine has a centrally mediated sedative effect. Other CNS depressants, such as benzodiazepines and opioids, may enhance the sedative effects of clonidine. Neuraxial clonidine can also affect the sympathetic nervous system, resulting in hypotension and bradycardia. When clonidine is used as a neuraxial adjunct analgesic, its hemodynamic effects may be enhanced by other neuraxial medications, particularly as local anesthetics. All effects are dose-dependent.

Less common adverse events: serious respiratory depression appears to be rare, and the documented arrhythmogenic effects of clonidine (most notably bradyarrhythmias and atrioventricular block) are unlikely to result from appropriate neuraxial dosing.

Treatment of adverse events: for co-administration of clonidine with other agents, one or both doses should be reduced as necessary to avoid adverse events. Treatment of these adverse events is typically supportive, though it should be noted that intrathecal neostigmine appears to counteract clonidine-induced spinal hypotension and that yohimbine has been used to counteract clonidine-induced sedation in postoperative patients. Hemodialysis is not likely to be effective for complications from neuraxial clonidine administration.

References

1. Product information: *Duraclon™, clonidine hydrochloride injection.* Roxane Laboratories, Inc., Columbus, OH, 2000.

2. Eisenach J, De Cock M, Klimscha, W. Alpha 2 adrenergic agonists for regional anesthesia: a clinical review of clonidine (1984–1995). *Anesthesiology* 1996;**85**(3):655–674.

Alpha-Adrenergic Analgesics

Dexmedetomidine

David Burbulys and Kianusch Kiai

Generic Name: dexmedetomidine hydrochloride

Proprietary Name: Precedex®

Manufacturers: Abbott Laboratories, Hospira and InterMed

Class: selective α_2-adrenergic agonist with sedative, hypnotic, anxiolytic, analgesic and sympatholytic effects

Chemical Name: (S)-4-[1-(2,3-dimethylphenyl) ethyl]-1H-imidazole monohydrochloride

Chemical Structure: see Figure 83.1

Mode of activity

Precedex®, dexmedetomidine hydrochloride, is a selective α_2-adrenergic agonist with sedative, hypnotic, anxiolytic, and analgesic properties as well as marked sympatholytic effects with little or no respiratory depression. It is an imidazole derivative and the refined active d-isomer of medetomidine, an agent used in veterinary medicine as an anesthetic.

Its mechanism of action is not well understood, but probably resembles the central effects of clonadine. Compared to clonadine, it binds more selectively to the α_2 over the α_1 receptor and has approximately eight times the affinity. Like clonadine, it produces sedation, reduced salivation and initially raises and then significantly lowers the heart rate and blood pressure. This is probably due to the overall stimulation of both the central and peripheral pre- and postsynaptic α_1 and α_2 receptors. The α_1-mediated hypotension and bradycardia may be pronounced with large doses or rapid infusions. It also has marked intrinsic anesthetic and analgesic properties that clonadine does not possess. This is probably due to the enhanced stimulation of central and spinal postsynaptic α_2 receptors as well as peripheral antinociception via

release of an enkephalin-like substance. It has been shown that the anesthetic effects are blocked by the centrally acting α_2 antagonist atipamexole but not a peripherally acting analog. The analgesic effects have been shown to be blocked by antipamezole but not naloxone.

It is highly protein-bound and has a very large volume of distribution. In animal studies, it has been shown to cross the placenta and is distributed into breast milk. It undergoes almost complete hepatic biotransformation with direct glucuronidation, aliphatic hydroxylation and N-methylation via the CYP2A6 and P450 systems. The metabolites are then excreted in the urine. In patients with hepatic dysfunction mean clearance values are reduced 50 to 75% and doses should be adjusted accordingly. Patients with significant renal insufficiency may experience the accumulation of metabolites and long-term infusions should be avoided.

Indications

Dexmedetomidine was approved in 1999 by the FDA for the sedation of mechanically ventilated adult patients in the critical care setting for 24 hours or less. Subsequently, it has received approval for procedural sedation in non-intubated adult patients.

Despite its recent FDA approval, it has also been studied and used off label in several other circumstances. Peri-operatively, it has been beneficial in the management of critically ill patients and patients at high cardiovascular risk undergoing vascular surgery, in bariatric patients, in patients to facilitate awake fiberoptic intubation or during awake craniotomy, and in pediatric patients. It also has potential to be used as an anesthetic adjunct to decrease dosages of other common anesthetic agents. Its use reduces intraocular pressure, attenuates the tachycardic response to endotracheal intubation, and blunts the adverse anesthetic shivering reaction. It has been used to treat post-operative pain, cyclical vomiting syndrome, and

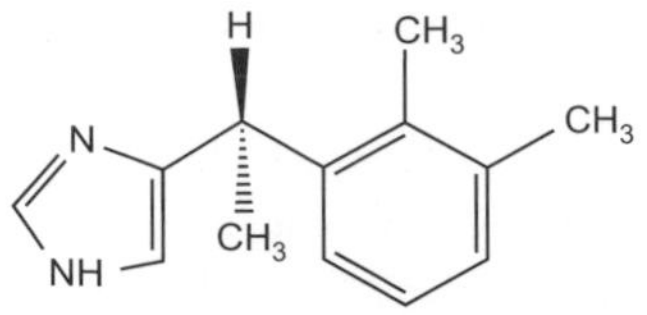

Figure 83.1.

various drug withdrawal states. It may have potential as a neuroprotective agent and as an adjunct to extend peripheral nerve block.

Contraindications

Absolute: Precedex® is contraindicated in patients with known allergy to dexmedetomidine.

Relative: avoid use during pregnancy, breast-feeding or if pregnancy is planned. Use with caution in geriatric patients or in patients with advanced heart block, significant hypertension, severe ventricular dysfunction, diabetes mellitus, hypovolemia, hepatic or renal insufficiency.

Common doses and uses

Dexmedetomidine is commonly administered by the IV route. Intramuscular, transdermal or intranasal routes have also been described. It has a rapid onset of action with sedative effects observed within 5 minutes of IV administration and a terminal half-life of approximately 2 hours.

It is supplied as a preservative-free concentrate of 100 μg/mL in a 2 mL clear glass vial. This should be diluted in 48 mL normal saline prior to its use. It is compatible with most commonly administered IV drugs and infusions, with the exception of amphotericin B and diazepam. It should not be infused through the same IV line as blood or plasma.

Sedation for intubated and mechanically ventilated patients is generally achieved with a loading dose of 1 μg/kg infused over 10 minutes followed by a continuous infusion 0.2 to 0.7 μg/kg per h. Over this range, dexmedetomidine exhibits linear effects and pharmacokinetics when administered for up to 24 hours in individuals with normal hepatic and renal function.

Procedural sedation in non-intubated patients is generally achieved with a loading dose of 1 μg/kg infused over 10 minutes followed by a continuous infusion 0.6 μg/kg per h. Less stimulating procedures may only require 0.5 μg/kg as a loading dose. The continuous infusion may be titrated to the desired clinical effect with doses ranging from 0.2 to 1 μg/kg per h.

As a general anesthesia adjunct, 0.5–0.6 μg/kg may be given as a bolus over 1 minute, in 5–10 mL of normal saline, 10 to 15 minutes prior to induction. Glycopyrrolate is often used to minimize the bradycardic effects. Alternatively, an IM dose of 0.5–1.5 μg/kg may be administered 60 minutes prior to induction. With IM dosing sedation may be prolonged and significant bradycardia has been observed with higher doses (1–1.5 μg/kg).

Awake fiberoptic intubation may be facilitated with a loading dose of 1 μg/kg infused over 10 minutes followed by a continuous infusion 0.7 μg/kg per h until intubation is achieved.

Potential advantages

Dexmedetomidine does not alter respiratory rate or oxygen saturation at the recommended dosages and it is not necessary to discontinue the drug prior to extubation.

Its use attenuates sympathetic activity and leads to a dose-dependent decrease in systolic and diastolic blood pressure and heart rate during its use and in the immediate post-operative period. This is related to both the dose and rate of administration.

There are no clinically important effects on neuromuscular blockade and, despite being highly protein-bound, there is little displacement of other highly protein-bound agents such as digoxin, fentanyl, lidocaine, NSAIDS, phenytoin, theophylline, or warfarin.

It has potential as an anesthetic adjunct to decrease dosages of other common anesthetic agents. It can reduce intraocular pressure, decrease intracranial pressure, be neuroprotective, attenuate the tachycardic response to endotracheal intubation, and blunt the adverse anesthetic shivering reaction.

It has an excellent safety profile.

Potential disadvantages

Transient hypertension has been reported with IV loading doses and IM administration but treatment is generally not required.

Hypotension and bradycardia are more pronounced in geriatric patients or those with hypovolemia, diabetes mellitus, or chronic hypertension. Consider lower initial loading and maintenance infusion doses in these patients. If treatment is required, consider slowing or stopping the dexmedetomidine infusion, increasing IV fluids and/or administering vasopressors or anticholinergic agents to modify vagal tone.

Bradycardia and sinus arrest have been reported in young, healthy adults with high vagal tone and with large or rapid IV administration. Safety and efficacy have not been established in children under 18 years of age. Despite this, numerous trials have shown its use in pediatric patients.

Supraventricular and ventricular tachycardia, atrial fibrillation, extrasystoles, and cardiac arrest have been rarely reported. These generally respond to standard therapies and discontinuation of dexmedetomidine. Dexmedetomidine should be used with caution in patients with advanced heart block or severe ventricular dysfunction.

It has been shown to have additive effects when used with other anesthetic agents, narcotics, benzodiazepines, vasodilators, and negative chronotropic agents. Reduced dosage should be considered when used with these agents.

Potential withdrawal manifestations such as nervousness, agitation, insomnia, tremor, palpitations, headaches, rapid rise in blood pressure, and elevated plasma catecholamine levels are possible with prolonged administration (>24 hours) and abrupt discontinuation of therapy. Despite this warning, dexmedetomidine has been used for longer periods of time with little withdrawal or tolerance noted.

Cortisol response to corticotropin stimulation has been shown to be decreased by 40% in animals following continuous infusion for 1 week but no changes have been observed with single-dose administration.

The effects on cortisol response have not been well studied in humans.

Dexmedetomidine is a Pregnancy Category C agent and its use during pregnancy, labor and delivery, including cesarean section deliveries, is not recommended. It is also excreted into milk in animal studies and caution should be used in nursing women.

Drug-related adverse events

Hypotension (28%), hypertension (16%), bradycardia (7%), tachycardia (3%), atrial fibrillation (4%), hypoxia (4%), nausea (11%), vomiting (4%), xerostomia (4%), fever (5%), and anemia (3%).

References

1. Abbott Laboratories. *Precedex® (dexmedetomidine) injection prescribing information.* North Chicago, IL, 2008.

2. Khan ZP, Ferguson CN, Jones RM. Alpha-2 and imidazoline receptor agonists. *Anaesthesia* 1999;**54**:146–165.

3. Kamibayashi T, Harawawa K, Maze M. Alpha-2 adrenergic agonists. *Canad J Anaesth* 1997;**44**:R13–R18.

4. DynaMed®, EBSCO Publishing. Dexmedetomidine, 2009.

5. Micromedex®Healthcare Series, DrugDex® Evaluations, Martindale – The Complete Drug Reference, and Posindex®, Tompson Healthcare. Dexmedetomidine, 2009.

84 Overview and use of antidepressant analgesics in pain management

Paul M. Peloso

Introduction

It is evident from the literature that pain and depression commonly coexist in the setting of severe post-surgical pain and chronic pain [1,2]. Given that pain represents the number one reason that patients visit general practitioners, with 45% of visits related to pain, and that depression is the most common mental health disorder, with 10–15% of all clinic visits having depression present, and further that both increase with age, their co-occurrence would not be surprising. In fact, pain and depression co-exist in 30–50% of those with either disorder, and their adverse effects are additive in terms of healthcare outcomes and reduced quality of life. However, as clinicians managing chronic pain can attest, pain leads to depression and depression leads to pain. Recent evidence, which will be briefly reviewed, also corroborates the clinical impression that managing either well requires managing the other well concurrently. Further, antidepressants have pain-relieving properties, in addition to their mood-altering properties, as will also be discussed.

The monoamine inhibitors and the tricyclic antidepressants were first discovered in the 1950s and were not originally intended for the treatment of depression. The name "tricyclic" refers to the chemical structure of this class, consisting of two benzene rings joined by a seven-member ring, containing nitrogen, oxygen, and carbon. Since the tricyclic antidepressants (TCA) family includes drugs with tetracyclic structures, some prefer the term "heterocyclics" although "tricyclics and TCA" are deeply embedded within the physician's lexicon. Given their serendipitous discovery, it is not surprising that TCAs interact with a wide variety of brain receptors, including norepinephrine, serotonin, histamine 1, muscarinic, cholinergic and alpha-2-adrenergic receptors, to varying degrees, with slight differences in side effects related to this. Major adverse events include QT prolongation, conduction abnormalities, hypotension, dry mouth, urinary retention, weight gain, sedation, lowered seizure threshold and given their narrow therapeutic margin, a risk of overdose (Table 84.1).

The monoamine oxidase inhibitors (MAOIs) work through augmented activity of dopamine, as monoamine oxidase normally degrades norepinephrine and serotonin. The MAOIs are rarely used clinically due to their adverse effects, notably orthostatic hypotension, peripheral edema, myoclonic jerks, weakness, and insomnia. Hypertensive crisis can result when combined with sympathomimetics, including over-the-counter products such as ephedrine and pseudoephedrine. Further, MAOIs are known to contribute to the serotonin syndrome and use of meperidine must be avoided in such patients. Patients on MAOI need to restrict tyramine-rich foods, as well [1,2].

The selective serotonin reuptake inhibitors (SSRIs) are highly selective agents, with limited off-target activity, and are among the most commonly prescribed antidepressants, due to the superior tolerability. It is worthwhile to point out that no single class of antidepressants appears to have superior efficacy, and newer agents are preferred principally for enhanced tolerability. The most frequent adverse event is nausea, typically occurring on initiation of therapy. Following that, sexual side effects tend to predominate. Inhibition of platelet function can lead to clinically important gastrointestinal bleeding, and interactions with NSAIDs and warfarin do occur. There is also a risk of serotonin syndrome, which consists of mental status changes, autonomic abnormalities (elevated pulse, blood pressure, and temperature) and neuromuscular hyperactivity, with rigidity, clonus, and heightened reflexes.

The Hunter criteria for serotonin syndrome have an 84% sensitivity and 96% specificity for the diagnosis, and require exposure to a drug known to cause the syndrome and at least one of (a) spontaneous clonus,

Table 84.1. Common drug interactions for the antidepressants

Tricyclic antidepressants (TCA)

Examples	Amitryptyline, desipramine, imipramine, doxepine, nortyptiline maprotyline.
Major actions	Serotonin and norepiphrine, reuptake inhibitors with additional effects via anticholinergic and alpha-2 antagonism.
Primary metabolism	Multiple CYP pathways, with the CYP2D6 pathway being the major route.
Potential interactions and clinical result	Acetylcholinesterase inhibitors can have diminished effects.
	May enhance QTc effects with alfuzosin, ciprofloxacin, cisapride, dronedaron, lumefantrine, nilotinib, quinidine, tetrabenazine: thioridazine, ziprasidone.
	Alpha-/beta-agonists may have enhanced vasopressor effects.
	Aspirin, NSAIDs, COX-2 inhibitors: may enhance antiplatelet effects and increase anticoagulation (including with vit K antagonists).
	May decrease TCA metabolism with terbinafine, cimetidine.
	Lithium can enhance neurotoxic effects.
	May enhance CNS effects, including propoxyphene.
	Sulfonylureas can have enhanced hypoglycemic effects.
	Tramadol can further enhance seizure potential.

Selective serotonin reuptake inhibitors (SSRI)

Examples	Citralopram, fluoxetine, paroxetine, sertraline.
Major actions	Inhibit serotonin reputake.
Primary metabolism	Citralopram - CYP2C19 is a major path.
	Fluoxetine - CYP2C9 CYP2D6 and other CYP.
	Paroxetine - CYP2D6.
	Sertraline - CYP2C19 CYP2D6.
Potential interactions and clinical result	ASA, NSAIDs, COX-2 selective inhibitors, pentoxifylline, drotrecogin alfa, pentosan polysulfate sodium, omega-3-acid ethyl ester can have enhanced antiplatelet effects and increased bleeding.
	Beta-blockers may have enhanced bradycardic effects.
	Selective serotonin reuptake inhibitors may decrease metabolism of alpha/beta blockers, benzodiazepines, carbamazepine, cimetidine, clozapine, fesoterodine, haloperidol, methadone, mexiletine, phenytoin, propafenone, respiradone, tamoxifen, galantamine, respiradone, thioridazine.
	May enhance the adverse effect of other CNS depressants, like methotrimeprazine.
	Cyproheptadine can compete with binding sites and limit the therapeutic effects.
	Macrolide antibiotics can decrease the metabolism of SSRI.
	Desmopressin, dextromethorphan may enhance adverse effects.
	Tramadol can enhance lowered seizure thresholds.
	Disulfiram can enhance adverse effects of sertraline, due to alcohol content.

Selective norepinephrine and serotonin reuptake inhibitors (SNRI)

Examples	Duloxetine, venlafaxine
Major actions	Serotonin and norepinephrine reuptake inhibitor.
Primary metabolism	Duloxetine - CYP1A2, CYP2D6.
	Venlafaxine - multiple CYP, mostly CYP2D6 CYP3A4.
Potential interactions and clinical result	Alpha/beta-agonists: may enhance tachycardic, vasopressor effects.

Table 84.1. (cont.)

	Alpha 2 agonists: may have diminished antihypertensive effects.
	Aspirin, NSAIDs, COX-2 inhibitors - can enhance antiplatelet effects and anticoagulant effects (vit K antagonists).
	Dasatinib, voriconazole - may increase serum concentration of venlafaxine.
	Can enhance orthostatic effects of the MAOI.
	May enhance CNS depressant effects of other CNS depressants.
	Metoclopramide can increase risk of serotonin syndrome.
	Propafenone: may increase serum levels of venlafaxine.
Buproprion	
Major Actions	Dopamine, norepinephrine uptake inhibitor.
Primary metabolism	CYP2B6.
Potential interactions and clinical result	Buproprion: can decrease TCA metabolism.
	Can enhance other CNS depressants effects, including with methotrimeprazine.
Mirtazapine	
Major actions	5-hydroxy-tryptophan 2A receptor antagonist.
Primary metabolism	CYP2D6, CYP1A1, CYP2C19
Potential interactions and clinical result	May diminish hypotensive effect of alpha2-agonists.
	Darunavir - may increase serum concentration of CYP2D6 substrates.
	May enhance CNS depressive effects of other CNS depressants, including methotrimeprazine.
Monoamine oxidase inhibitors (MAOI)	
Examples	Phenelzine, trancylcypromine, isocarboxazid, moclobemide, seleginline.
Major actions	Monoamine oxidase blocked (reversibly or irreversibly), with inhibition of dopamine and norepinephrine action.
Primary metabolism	Substrates or inhibitors of various CYP enzymes, metabolism not well studied.
	Tranylcypromine is a relatively potent inhibitor of CYP2C19.
	Moclobemide inhibits CYP2D6, CYP2C19, CYP1A2.
Potential interactions and clinical result	Acetylcholinesterase inhibitors can have reduced effects.
	Succinylcholine: phenelzine may enhance neuromuscular blockade.
	Alpha/beta-agonists have enhanced vasopressor effects.
	May enhance orthostatic effects of altretamine-antihypertensives.
	May enhance hypertensive effects of buspirone, levodopa, methylphenidate, and the rauwolfia alkaloids.
	May enhance neurotoxic and central effects of atomoxetine, buproprion, tapentadol.
	tramadol, may further lowered seizure-threshold.
	Drugs must be weaned off to avoid syndrome.

Table 84.2. Commonly used drugs implicated in the serotonin syndrome

Drug implicated	Purported mechanism
Monoamine oxidase inhibitors	Inhibits serotonin metabolism
Buspirone	Direct serotonin agonist
Triptans (e.g. sumatriptan)	Direct serotonin agonist
Ergot alkaloids	Direct serotonin agonist
Fentanyl	Direct serotonin agonist
Sibutramine	Direct serotonin agonist
Cocaine, ecstasy	Impairs reuptake
Meperidine	Direct serotonin agonist
Selective serotonin reuptake inhibitors	Direct serotonin agonist
Serotonin norepinephrine reuptake inhibitors	Direct serotonin agonist
Tricyclic antidepressants	Direct serotonin agonist
St. John's wort	Direct serotonin agonist
Ondansetron, granisetron	Direct serotonin agonist
Dextromethorphan	Direct serotonin agonist
Trazadone	Direct serotonin agonist

Emergency consultation with a medical toxicologist available at US Poison Control Network 1–800–222–1222, or find a poison control center at the World Health Organization's list of international poison centers at www.who.int/ipcs/poisons/centre/directory/en.

(b) inducible clonus plus agitation or diaphoresis, (c) ocular clonus plus agitation or diaphoresis, (d) tremor and hyperreflexia, (e) hypertonia, or (f) temperature above 38°C plus ocular clonus or inducible clonus. Table 84.2 outlines those drugs that might contribute to the development of serotonin syndrome and which may be used concurrently with antidepressant therapy.

The serotonin and norepinephrine reuptake inhibitors, or SNRIs, have both serotonin and norepinephrine inhibition, and are less selective than the SSRIs. They also have nausea as a common adverse event on initiation, and can have dizziness, drowsiness, sweating, and dry mouth, as well as sexual dysfunction, as occur with the SSRI and have been associated with serotonin syndrome.

Caregivers prescribing antidepressant medications should consider the following key questions:

1. How good is the clinical evidence for antidepressant effects on pain?
2. Are there differences among the antidepressant classes with respect to pain control?
3. What has the recent evidence taught us about the intersection of pain and depression?
4. Does recognizing and treating depression have any impact on the acute post-operative period,

with respect to pain control, morbidity and mortality?

In order to address these questions, focused literature reviews were carried out in Medline through 2009. In keeping with the established hierarchy of clinical evidence, meta-analyses of randomized controlled trials and large randomized controlled trials were afforded the highest level of evidence, and are preferentially represented here. Large, well-controlled cohort designs were considered of lesser, but important, evidence. Cohort studies are far more common designs than randomized trials when the clinical questions are concerned with prognosis. The reader should be aware that there is a large and growing literature on these key questions, and this chapter cannot represent all of it, in its entirety. The interested reader is referred to the references herein and to the primary literature for greater detail.

How good is the clinical evidence for antidepressant effects on pain?

Clinical experience and randomized trial evidence shows that antidepressant medications have pain-relieving properties [1–4]. Is this pain relief related to

341

Table 84.3. Evidence for effectiveness of antidepressants in musculoskeletal and neuropathic pain conditions

	OA	CLBP	FMS	Diabetic PN	PHN	Painful polyneur
TCA	n.t.	MA	MA	MA	MA	MA
SSRI	n.t.	Neg	Neg.	Contra	n.t.	Contra
Venlafaxine	RCT	nt	nt	RCT	Neg.	RCT
Duloxetine	RCT	RCT[a]	MA	RCT	n.t.	RCT
Milnacipran	n.t.	n.t.	RCT	n.t.	n.t.	n.t.

TCA, tricyclic antidepressants; multiple tested include amitriptyline, desipramine, imipramine, nortryptiline, maprotyline; SSRI, selective serotonin reuptake inhibitors (tested are citralopram, paroxetine, fluoxetine); Venlafaxine, Duloxetine, Milnacipran (selective serotonin norepinephrine reuptake inhibitors, SNRIs).

RCT, randomized controlled trial with positive results; MA, metaanalysis of RCTs with positive results; OA, osteoarthritis; CLBP, chronic low back pain; FMS, fibromyalgia syndrome; Diabetic PN = diabetic peripheral neuropathy; PHN, post-herpetic neuralgia; Painful polyneur, painful polyneuropathy; n.t., not tested; Neg., negative results in ≥ 1 RCT; Contra, contradictory evidence.

[a]Short-term effects on pain and sleep, but not sustained longer-term.

mood alteration (i.e. amelioration of depressive symptoms), or to direct pain-relieving properties? This question was unanswerable when the TCAs alone were used for pain, but the advent of the SSRIs and the SNRIs allows an ability to probe this issue further. Since the SSRIs are highly effective antidepressants, yet appear to have limited analgesic effects, modulation of mood is probably not sufficient. The SNRIs, with inhibition of both serotonin and norepinephrine reuptake, and demonstrated efficacy for depression and multiple pain states, suggested that modulation of multiple receptor targets is necessary for pain relief. Some authors suggest that inhibition of norepinephrine reuptake may be required for pain relief, since TCAs and SNRIs both inhibit NE reuptake, while others have suggested that fully adequate doses of SSRIs for pain have not been tested. The quality and consistency of evidence for antidepressants as pain-relieving agents is reviewed, in brief, in Table 84.3.

Several high quality meta-analyses of randomized controlled trials have been published on the value of antidepressants and pain control, in a variety of chronic painful musculoskeletal conditions, including low back pain, fibromyalgia, osteoarthritis, etc. [2–4]. The SNRIs continue to be developed for pain indications. There is clear evidence of benefit for antidepressants in fibromyalgia, for the TCAs and the SNRIs (duloxetine, milnacipran), osteoarthritis (duloxetine, venlafaxine), and low back pain (TCAs, duloxetine).

In the setting of chronic musculoskeletal pain, such as osteoarthritis and low back pain, most guidelines recommend beginning with acetaminophen/paracetamol or nonsteroidal anti-inflammatory agents. If these agents are not sufficient, antidepressants can be added or substituted. Opiates are recommended only after failure of multiple other agents. In fibromyalgia, where NSAIDs have limited utility, the TCA and SNRI antidepressants are preferred therapy, where multiple randomized trials demonstrate the effects of TCAs and SNRIs, including duloxetine, venlafaxine, and milnacipran. If these agents are not effective, there is some evidence of effectiveness of tramadol, whereas opiates are not recommended for fibromyalgia (Table 84.3).

In the setting of neuropathic pain, there are multiple randomized trials demonstrating the effectiveness of TCAs and the SNRIs, venlafaxine and duloxetine [5,6]. Efficacy is demonstrated for TCAs and SNRIs in several neuropathic pain subtypes, including diabetic peripheral neuropathy, post-herpetic neuropathy and painful polyneuropathy, as reviewed in Table 84.3. Milnacipran, an SNRI, has not been tested in the setting of neuropathic pain. As reviewed in Sindrup et al, [5], the tricyclic antidepressants can have important treatment effects, with numbers-needed-to-treat (NNT) in the range of 1.2 to 2.4, where any NNT less than 4 is generally regarded as having important pain effects beyond placebo. SNRIs such as venlafaxine and duloxetine also have effects, with NNT in the range of 5 to 7. The SSRIs citalopram, fluoxetine and paroxetine have also been tested in painful polyneuropathy, and it would appear in small trials that these agents do have some efficacy, although this effect is less predictable and further studies are clearly needed to fully quantify the role of SSRIs in neuropathic pain states. Recent US guidelines support the use of TCAs and SNRIs antidepressants as first-line agents in the treatment of neuropathic pain, prior to the use of opioid agents, for instance [6].

Are there differences among the antidepressant classes for pain control?

As reviewed above, there is strong evidence of efficacy for the TCAs and for the SNRIs in fibromyalgia, osteoarthritis, low back pain, diabetic neuropathy, and chronic neuropathic pain. Deciding whether there might be differences among agents or classes is not straightforward. There are few head-to-head trials, and proper studies examining the dose-response relationship for pain have not been conducted for the TCAs or the SSRIs. In addition, TCA dosing is often limited by tolerability. For instance, it is not clear whether TCAs, as they are currently used, are being under-dosed for pain. In short, deciding on what doses to contrast in head to head trials, among TCAs, SSRIs and SNRIs, is not a trivial undertaking. Some have suggested that the SSRIs are not effective in pain, yet others argue that the proper doses for SSRIs in pain have not been established. Unfortunately, there is limited clinical trial information with the SSRIs. This is disappointing in part, since pain is a common symptom accompanying depression, and it can be part of the diagnostic criteria, yet pain in the depression trials was not well quantified, limiting the opportunity to draw pain efficacy conclusions. The prior discussion notwithstanding, the limited data that are available suggest that SSRIs, like fluoxetine, are not effective analgesics per se, although some trials do demonstrate positive effects with paroxetine.

However, managing depression is integral to managing pain well. Thus if the goal is to manage pain in patients who do not have concomitant depression, then the TCAs or the SNRIs are preferred for their demonstrated pain-relieving qualities. If the goal is to manage depression in someone with concurrent pain, then the SSRIs or the SNRIs are both sensible choices, and preferred over the TCAs for their superior tolerability profiles.

What has the recent evidence taught us about the intersection of pain and depression?

Recent experimental evidence suggests that pain and depression share common biological pathways. The excellent systematic review by Kroenke and colleagues outlines the evidence, in detail, that suggests depression and pain follow the same descending pathways of the CNS [1,2,4]. Focus has been on the descending system of pain modulation. Several areas appear to be key to pain modulation and in particular the periaqueductal gray (PAG). The amygdala, hypothalamus, and frontal neocortex all send fibers there, with further relays into the pons and medulla. These relay systems contain serotonergic neurons in the rostral ventromedial medulla, and norepinephrine neurons in the dorsolateral pontine tegmentum. The rostral ventromedial medulla has two types of cells, "on cells" which facilitate pain transmission, and "off cells" which inhibit it, and serve to modulate peripheral sensory input. Interestingly, opiates tend to excite off cells and inhibit on cells, dampening peripheral nociceptive input. With the attendant reductions in serotonin and norepinephrine that accompany depression, minor peripheral signals can be amplified, and this is consistent with the observation that patients with depression often describe multiple symptoms, including unexplained pain. Of note, serotonin and norepinephrine administered intrathecally can block pain transmission. As reviewed in Perrot et al. [3], some studies have suggested peripheral mechanisms for TCAs in pain reduction for musculoskeletal pain, including inhibition of local nitric oxide and prostaglandin production.

It is well appreciated clinically that current and persistent pain can lead to depression. What is not clear is, "what is the chicken, and what is the egg?" Is there clinical research evidence to suggest that pain leads to depression, supporting the clinical experience? Does depression lead to pain? Are both events predicted by the presence of the other? There is evidence from a variety of sources that acute trauma and its associated pain can lead to future depression. To cite one example, a 2000 *New England Journal of Medicine* publication reported on a population-based cohort of 7463 individuals who had whiplash post motor vehicle collision and who were then followed until symptom resolution [7]. Pain severity, size of body area with pain, and depressive symptomatology were strongly related with both time to recovery and probability of recovery. Those individuals who had whiplash pain but who did not report being depressed prior to the whiplash event were followed for future symptoms of depression, using the Epidemiological Studies Depression Scale [8]. In this follow-up, 42% of whiplash subjects who had not been previously depressed met the definition for depression over the next 6 weeks. The majority (60%) of these 42% experienced resolution within the subsequent year, with a median recovery time of 92 days, whereas 19% experienced recurrent bouts of

343

depression and 19% experienced persistent depression throughout the next one year. Kroenke and coworkers [1,2,4], in their systematic review, show that 2% to 100% of patients attending specialized pain clinics have depression and, when population-based studies and general practitioner clinics are considered, a median of 20% of patients in pain are depressed. Differences in rates depend on the clinical setting, the underlying pain condition, and the instrument used to detect depression. However, in sum, there is strong, consistent evidence from cohort studies that pain leads to depression.

Several, large, general-practice-based randomized controlled trials have been completed, examining the effect of managing with both pain and depression, on depression outcomes. The Stepped Care for Affective Disorders and Musculoskeletal Pain (SCAMP) conducted a randomized trial in general medicine clinics in 250 patients with low back, hip, or knee pain and moderate depression severity [2]. Patients were randomized to a 12 week, three-step program of optimized antidepressant therapy (step 1) then a 12 week pain self-management program (step 2), followed by 6 months of ongoing therapy continuation (step 3). This three-step program was contrasted with usual care. At 12 months, 37.4% of those in the three-step program had a 50% or greater reduction in depression severity, compared to baseline, as contrasted with 16.5% reduction in the usual care patients. Importantly, a clinically significant reduction in pain, defined as $\geq$ 30% reduction from baseline, occurred in 41.5% of patients in the three-step program, as compared to 17.3% in usual care. Combining improvement in both depression and pain, 26.0% in the three-step program improved versus 7.9% in the usual care group. There was a variety of antidepressants used in the study, including the SNRIs, the SSRIs, buproprion, mirtazipine and the TCAs. Therefore the effects on pain improvement cannot be ascribed solely to the choice of antidepressant alone, but are more likely to reflect the benefit of good depression management.

In another study, conducted in the US Veterans Affairs healthcare system, in adults over 60 years with depression, an examination of whether pain severity and interference with normal work activities moderated the effects of depression treatment response was undertaken [9]. In this study, patients were randomized to integrated care (care delivered in the primary care clinic, by a mental health professional) versus enhanced specialty referral care (care delivered in the subspecialty clinic office) and results were examined at 3, 6, and 12 months. The trial showed that both groups had improvement in their depression symptomatology, but that higher levels of pain severity and interference with work activities blunted the improvements in depressive symptoms. The authors concluded that pain interference accounted for the moderating effects of pain severity on changes in depressive symptoms over time.

In a randomized controlled trial, designed to examine whether enhancing the care for depression improves pain and functional outcomes in older adults with concomitant osteoarthritis, a total of 1001 patients were randomized to antidepressant medications with or without an additional six to eight psychotherapy sessions [10]. Both groups had improvement in depressive symptoms from baseline. The group receiving antidepressants and psychotherapy had lower mean (SE) scores for pain intensity (5.62 [0.16] vs. 6.15 [0.16]) measured on a 0–10 numerical rating scale; less interference with daily activities due to arthritis (4.40 [0.18] vs. 4.99 [0.17]) as measured on a 0–10 numerical rating scale, and less interference with daily activities due to pain (2.92 [0.07] vs. 3.17 [0.07]) as measured by two questions from the SF-12, on a 0–4 scale. A variety of antidepressants were allowed, and 66% of the enhanced care group and 52% of the usual care group used antidepressants over the 12 months. The authors concluded that in a diverse population of older adults with osteoarthritis and comorbid depression, benefits of improved depression care extended beyond reduced depressive symptoms and included decreased pain as well as improved functional status and quality of life.

In summary, these recent trials illustrate that enhancing depression care has important impacts on pain control, independently of the antidepressant class. Interference with function, related to pain, appears to be a major determinant of depression response. There is a tight intertwining of response to both pain and depression, based on improving both simultaneously.

Does recognizing and treating depression have any impact on the acute post-operative period, with respect to pain control, morbidity and mortality?

Finally, we will consider evidence that depression has an influence on the outcome of major illnesses, including recovery in the post-operative setting. It has been long understood that depression has an influence on coronary artery bypass grafting. This continues to be an area of active investigation. In a 2008 study, 1319 patients who had 2496 grafts had baseline angiography and were then followed up angiographically, over a median of 4.2 years [11]. Those who were depressed, as assessed by a Centers for Epidemiologic Studies Depression scale (CES-D) score ≥ 16, were statistically more likely to have graft progression (OR 1.50, 95% CI 1.08 to 2.10, $P < 0.02$), after adjusting for age, gender, race, treatment, and years since surgery. Additional statistical adjustment for past medical history, blood pressure, and renal function did not materially alter these results. These authors conclude that depressive symptoms are associated with a higher risk of atherosclerotic progression among patients with saphenous vein grafts.

In a 2009 study, 1238 patients scheduled for CABG were assessed for depression using the Patient Health Questionnaire (PHQ-9) [12]. Of these, 21.6% had elevated depression scores. Predictors for pre-operative depression were dyspnea at rest and exertion, previous myocardial infarction, multiple comorbidities, as well as younger age, female gender, lower educational attainment, and living alone. This study demonstrated that active screening of pre-operative depression is feasible, and can be suspected based on clinical features. Knowledge of depression status could lead to improved post-operative management.

Oncologists believe that psychological variables influence the course of cancer. A 2009 meta-analysis evaluated the literature on depression and mortality in cancer patients [13]. The 25 studies included in this meta-analysis showed that mortality rates were up to 39% higher in depressed patients (RR = 1.39; 95% CI, 1.10–1.89; $P < 0.03$). This analysis also showed that adjusting for known clinical prognostic factors had no influence on the predictive ability of depression on mortality, suggesting that the relationship between depression and cancer mortality could be cause and effect. While few would deny the value of treating pain and depression in the setting of cancer, managing depression could influence the ultimate prognosis.

Data that depression can influence disease outcome are just beginning to appear in the setting of total knee replacement (TKR). In a 2009 cohort study 43 patients undergoing TKR were followed for 12 months post-operatively [14]. Depression was studied as a prospective predictor of post-operative pain. The authors reported that depressive symptoms predicted global pain complaints, and postulated that interventions designed to reduce depressive symptoms have the potential to improve joint replacement outcomes.

In a 2003 cohort study designed to identify factors predicting excessive post-operative pain, 116 patients were followed for 1 year [15]. Importantly, greater pre-operative pain predicted greater post-operative pain, and pre-operative depression and anxiety were associated with elevated pain levels at 1 year. The study also showed that one in eight patients report moderate to severe pain 1 year after surgery, with no evidence of abnormalities on clinical exam or radiographs. The authors recommend that office-based pre-operative screening for depression could improve patient-perceived outcomes.

Although the evidence is not presented in its entirety, it is clear that post-operative depression can influence disease outcome, as illustrated in the setting of CABG, and cancer mortality, as well as post-operative recovery, as shown in the setting of TKR. It is also increasingly apparent that pre-operative depression can predict post-operative pain control, and authors are increasingly advocating depression screening. To this end, a simple, four-item instrument, the Ultra-Brief Screening Scale for Anxiety and Depression, Patient Health Questionnaire, PHQ-4, is presented with its scoring schema [16]. This instrument has two questions focused on anxiety and two on depression, and has shown validity in population-based samples. As argued, given the structured pre-operative assessment process, an assessment of depression would facilitate planning for the post-operative recovery.

References

1. Bair MJ, Robinson RL, Katon W, Kroenke K. Depression and pain comorbidity. A literature review. *Arch Intern Med* 2003;**163**:2433–2445.

2. Kroenke K, Krebs EE, Bair MJ. Pharmacotherapy of chronic pain: a synthesis of recommendations from systematic reviews *Gen Hosp Psychiatry* 2009;**31**: 206–219.

3. Perrot S, Javier RM, Marty M, et al. and the CEDR (Cercle d'Etude de la Douleur en Rhumatologie France), French Rheumatological Society, Pain Study Section. Is there any evidence to support the use of

anti-depressants in painful rheumatological conditions? Systematic review of pharmacological and clinical studies. *Rheumatology* 2008;**47**: 1117–1123.

4. Kroenke K, Bair MJ, Damush TM, Wu J. Optimized antidepressant therapy and pain self-management in primary care patients with depression and musculoskeletal pain: a randomized controlled trial. *JAMA* 2009;**301**(20):2099–2110.

5. Sindrup SH, Otto1 M, Nanna B, et al. Antidepressants in the treatment of neuropathic pain. *Basic Clin Pharmacol Toxicol* 2005;**96**:399–409.

6. O'Connor, AB, Dworkin RH. Treatment of neuropathic pain: an overview of recent guidelines. *Am J Med* 2009;**122**: S22–S32.

7. Cassidy JD, Carroll LJ, Cote P, et al. Effect of eliminating compensation for pain and suffering on the outcome of insurance claims for whiplash injury. *N Engl J Med* 2000;**342**:1179–1186.

8. Carroll LJ, Cassidy JD, Cote P. Frequency, timing, and course of depressive symptomatology after whiplash. *SPINE* 2006;**31**(16): E551–E556.

9. Mavandadi S, Ten Have TR, Katz IR, Nalla U, Durai B, Krahn DD, Llorente MD, Kirchner JA, Olsen EJ, Van Stone WW, Cooley SL, Oslin DW. Effect of depression treatment on depressive symptoms in older adulthood: the moderating role of pain. *J Am Geriatr Soc* 2007;**55**:202–211.

10. Lin EHB, Katon W, Von Korff M, Tang l., Williams Jr JW, Kroenke K, Hunkeler E, Harpole L, Hegel M, Arean P, Hoffing M, Della Penna R, Langston C, Unutzer J, for the IMPACT Investigators. Effect of improving depression care on pain and functional outcomes among older adults with arthritis: a randomized controlled trial. *JAMA* 2003;**290**:2428–2434.

11. Wellenius GA, Mukamal KJ, Kulshreshtha A, et al. Depressive symptoms and the risk of atherosclerotic progression among patients with coronary artery bypass grafts. *Circulation* 2008;**117**:2313–2319.

12. Dunkel A, Kendel F, Lehmkuhl E, et al. Predictors of preoperative depressive risk in patients undergoing coronary artery bypass graft surgery. *Clin Res Cardiol* 2009;**98**:643–650.

13. Jillian R, Satin JR, Linden W, Phillips MJ. Depression as a predictor of disease progression and mortality in cancer patients: a meta-analysis. *Cancer* 2009; 5349–5361.

14. Edwards RR, Haythornthwaite JA, Smith MT. Catastrophizing and depressive symptoms as prospective predictors of outcomes following total knee replacement. *Pain Res Manag* 2009;**14**(4): 307–311.

15. Brander VA, Stulberg SD, Adams AD, et al. Predicting total knee replacement pain: a prospective, observational study. *Clinic Orthop Rel Res* 2003;**416**:27–36.

16. Löwe B, Wahl I, Rose M, et al. A 4-item measure of depression and anxiety: validation and standardization of the Patient Health Questionnaire-4 (PHQ-4) in the general population. *J Affect Disord* 2009. http://dx.doi.org/10.1016/j.jad.2009.06.019.

85

Tricyclic antidepressants

Carly Miller and Alan Miller

Tertiary Amines

Generic Name: amitriptyline-HCl

Trade Name: Elavil™

Manufacturer: Astra Zeneca Pharmaceuticals, Wilmington, DE

Generic Name: doxepin-HCl

Trade Name: Sinequan™

Manufacturer: Pfizer U.S. Pharmaceuticals, New York, NY

Generic Name: imipramine-HCl

Trade Name: Tofranil™

Manufacturer: Novartis Pharmaceuticals, East Hanover, NJ

Secondary Amines

Generic Name: desipramine-HCl

Trade Name: Norpramin™

Manufacturer: Aventis Pharmaceuticals, Inc., Bridgewater, NJ

Generic Name: nortriptyline-HCl

Trade Name: Pamelor™

Manufacturer: Novartis Pharmaceuticals, East Hanover, NJ

Generic Name: protriptyline-HCl

Trade Name: Vivactil™

Manufacturer: Odyssey Pharmaceuticals, East Hanover, NJ

Chemical Structure: tertiary amine (amitriptyline), see Figure 85.1; secondary amine (nortriptyline), see Figure 85.2

Description

Tricyclic antidepressants (TCAs) can be effective monotherapy for pain, or as an adjuvant to other analgesics [1]. They are particularly effective for neuropathic pain and their efficacy for post-herpetic neuralgia may be greater than that of the newer pregabalin [2]. Tricyclics are commonly used to treat headaches, fibromyalgia, neck and low back pain. The mechanism of the antinociceptive activity of the tricyclic antidepressants is largely unknown, and appears to be distinct from their antidepressant properties. It may be related to sodium channel blockade. Analgesic effects are achieved with lower doses and quicker onset than antidepressant effects.

Traditionally the tertiary amine amitriptyline has been favored for pain management over nortriptyline, despite increased side effects and interactions and no proven analgesic benefit of tertiary amines over secondary amines.

Mode of activity

Major sites of action: serotonin and norepinephrine receptors in the CNS.

Minor sites of action: cholinergic (muscarinic), alpha-1- and alpha-2-adrenergic, histaminic-1 and dopaminergic receptors; CNS and cardiac sodium channels.

Receptor interactions: the tricyclic antidepressants inhibit the postsynaptic reuptake of serotonin and norepinephrine, and increase concentrations in the spinal cord. Norepinephrine binds to, and activates, postsynaptic alpha-adrenergic receptors, thereby suppressing pain transmission. Norepinephrine reuptake blocks dopamine activity in the frontal cortex, and by inhibiting this process tricyclics increase dopaminergic activity in this area. Depending on the tricyclic agent, there is postsynaptic blockade of histamine-1, dopaminergic, cholinergic, alpha-1-adrenergic and alpha-2-adrenergic receptors (concentrated in CNS and cardiac tissue due to high lipophilicity). This activity is largely responsible for side effects and drug interactions of these medications.

347

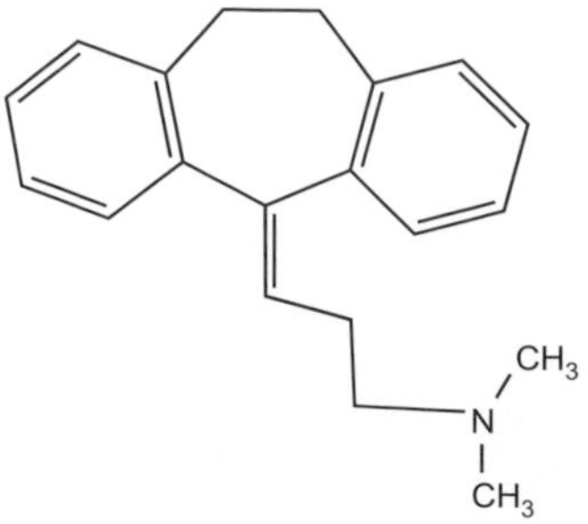

Figure 85.1.

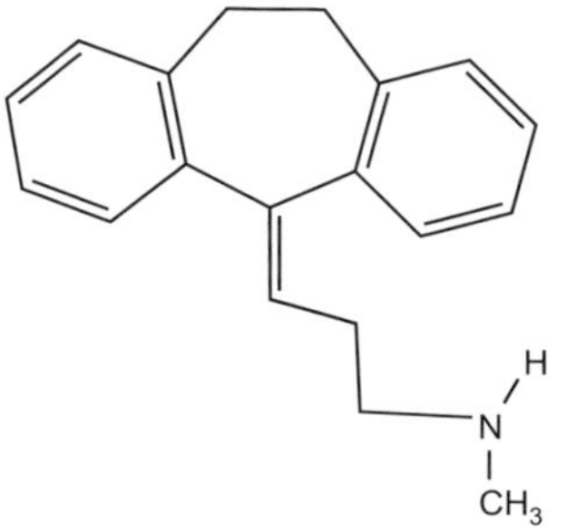

Figure 85.2.

Metabolic pathways/drug clearance and elimination: there is significant first-pass effect, with roughly 50% bioavailability. Most tricyclics are greater than 90% plasma-bound. The mean half-lives of amitriptyline and nortriptyline (an active metabolite of amitriptyline) are about 21 and 32 hours, respectively. Peak levels occur from 2 to 12 hours, although analgesic effects are not achieved for at least 3 to 10 days. Elimination is 98% renal for amitriptyline and 67% renal for nortriptyline. Tricyclic antidepressants are substrates of the cytochrome P450 2D6 system, which is inhibited by several medications, including selective serotonin reuptake inhibitors. Interactions may lead to significant increases in plasma concentration.

Indications (non-approved)

Tricyclic antidepressants are not FDA-approved for any pain indications.

Surgical acute pain: amitriptyline may be beneficial for adjunctive use for pain control as well as nighttime sedation. Patients recovering from amputation, traumatic or surgical nerve injuries (intercostal nerves, branches of the brachial plexus, inguinal and genitofemoral nerve, etc.). Consider starting dose of 12.5–25 mg qhs and increase to 50 mg as tolerated. Monitor for urinary retention/constipation that may coincide with post-operative symptoms. Consider nortriptyline or desipramine to reduce side effects.

Medical and chronic non-malignant pain: amitriptyline and nortriptiline are useful for controlling diabetic neuropathic pain, post-herpetic neuralgia, neck and back radicular pain, as well as pain from conditions including HIV, complex regional pain syndrome (CRPS; RSD), and autoimmune disorders (RA, SLE). Migraine and tension headaches, fibromyalgia, temporomandibular joint disorder, interstitial cystitis, irritable bowel syndrome, premenstrual, pelvic and phantom limb pain may also respond to tricyclics. Consider starting amitriptyline 25–50 mg qhs and increase to 300 mg qhs as side effects (dry mouth, constipation, daytime sedation, urinary retention, etc.) permit. Titrate with weekly dosage increases. As the active metabolite of amitriptyline, consider starting nortriptyline at 25 mg. Consider discontinuing amitriptyline if no pain benefits by 150 mg or nortriptyline if no benefit by 75 mg. Again, fewer side effects occur with nortriptyline (Table 85.1), although amitriptyline is sometimes preferred for its sedative effects. Use caution prescribing TCAs for patients with fibromyalgia and interstitial cystitis where agents such as SSRIs are commonly used.

Cancer pain: tricyclic antidepressants may be a helpful adjuvant in treating visceral and neuropathic pain of malignancy. Consider using them alone or as adjuncts to opioid analgesics for neuropathic symptoms in cancer pain such as burning, tingling, electric shock and sharp sensations. If minimal medical comorbidities are present, consider a rapid titration to maximum effective dose with tolerable side effects (150 mg/day for amitriptyline or nortriptyline).

Contraindications

Absolute: documented allergy to tricyclics, recent myocardial infarction, history of QTc prolongation or cardiac arrhythmia, and unstable heart failure. Do not use in conjunction with substances known to significantly prolong QTc such as thioridazine, pimozide, certain antiarrhythmics, and fluoroquinolones.

Relative: history of seizure disorder, bipolar disorder (may induce mania), urinary retention, narrow-angle glaucoma, delirium, hyperthyroidism, bradycardia (or drugs that cause bradycardia), or electrolyte disturbance (esp. K^+ or Mg^{2+}). Use caution in conjunction with other antidepressants (including MAOIs and SSRIs), other anticholinergic medications, drugs that increase plasma levels (phenothiazines, haloperidol, cimetidine), or drugs that lower seizure threshold (esp. tramadol). Use caution in elderly, children/adolescents,

Table 85.1. Tricyclic antidepressant formulations, side effects, active metabolites and plasma levels (in descending order by side effect profile).[3]

Generic name	Formulations (mg)	Maximum daily dose (mg)	Side effects						Upper limit of therapeutic plasma level (ng/mL)
			α-1 blockade	Cholinergic blockade	Dopamine blockade	Histamine blockade	Norepinephrine reuptake blockade	Serotonin reuptake blockade	
			Orthostatic hypotension	Blurred vision	EPS	Sedation	Sweating	• Diarrhea	
			Dizziness	Dry mouth	Prolactin elevation	Weight gain	Anxiety	• Nausea	
			Tachycardia	Memory loss					
				Urinary retention					
				Constipation					
Tertiary amines									
Doxepin (active metabolite: desmethyldoxepin)	Capsule: 10, 25, 50, 100, 150 oral sln: 10 mg/mL	300	++++	+++	+	++++	+	+	200
Amitriptyline (active metabolite: nortriptyline)	Tablet: 10, 25, 50, 75, 100, 150 parenteral: 10 mg/mL	300	++++	++++	+	+++	++	++	160
Clomipramine (active metabolite: desmethylclomipramine)	Capsule: 25, 50, 75	250	++++	+++	+	+++	++	+++	300
Imipramine (active metabolite: desipramine)	Tablet: 10, 25, 50 parenteral: 25 mg/2 mL	300	+++	+++	+	++	++	++	350
Secondary amines									
Nortriptyline	Capsule: 10, 25, 50, 75 Oral sln: 10 mg/5 mL	150	+++	++	+	++	+++	+/-	150
Desipramine	Tablet: 10, 25, 50, 75, 100, 150	300	++	++	+	+	++++	+/-	n/a

pregnant/nursing women, and those with renal, hepatic, or cardiac impairment.

Common doses

Doses of tricyclic antidepressants are generally lower for pain than therapeutic ranges for depression. Most tricyclics can be started at 10–25 mg and titrated 25 mg at weekly intervals to therapeutic level (typically 75 mg for pain, maximum 150 mg) [1]. Nortriptyline is typically effective at about half the dose of amitriptyline. Although not routinely recommended, plasma concentration may be measured to ensure nontoxic levels.

Oral and parenteral dosing: refer to Table 85.1 for formulations.

Potential advantages

Tricyclics are not narcotics and are not addictive. They are easily prescribed and widely available in pharmacies and hospital formularies. Less caution is needed in low analgesic doses.

Cost: inexpensive generics are widely available and often covered by insurance.

As monotherapy: may be effective for some types of pain.

As used for multimodal analgesia: often a useful analgesic adjunct to other therapeutic interventions; may also improve mood and sleep.

Potential disadvantages

Toxicity: supratherapeutic plasma concentrations (Table 85.1) can cause severe, life-threatening toxicity resulting in cardiac arrhythmia/arrest, seizures (rare), hepatic failure, paralytic ileus, and hyperthermia (both due to anticholinergic toxicity).

Drug interactions: extreme caution with concomitant MAOIs or SSRIs, cimetidine, haloperidol, or phenothiazines (all increase plasma levels). Avoid QT-prolonging or potentially proarrhythmic agents, sodium channel blocking agents such as type 1a and 1c antiarrhythmics, cardiac glycosides, cocaine, or amphetamines. Agents that precipitate bradycardia (β-blockers, clonidine, calcium channel blockers), or lower serum magnesium or potassium levels (diuretics, stimulant laxatives, parenteral amphotericin B, glucocorticoids) all may potentiate QTc prolongation. Use caution in conjunction with drugs that lower seizure threshold or have anticholinergic properties.

Adverse events, tolerability: side effects may limit tolerability (Table 85.1).

Drug-related adverse events

Common adverse events: include sedation, weight gain, dry mouth, and constipation (Table 85.1). Abrupt discontinuation should be avoided.

Serious adverse events: related to cardiac effects of QTc prolongation and drug interactions described.

Treatment of adverse events: some common side effects may resolve over time or with lower doses. In addition to supportive therapy, the mainstay of treatment for severe toxicity is serum alkalinization with sodium bicarbonate to increase protein binding and decrease QRS interval. Although no reversal agent exists, substances that may reverse cardiotoxicity are being studied.

References

1. McQuay HJ, Moore RA. Antidepressants in chronic pain. *BMJ* 1997;**314**:763–764.

2. O'Connor AB, Noyes K, Holloway RG. A cost-effectiveness comparison of desipramine, gabapentin, and pregabalin for treating postherpetic neuralgia. *J Am Geriatr Soc* 2007;**55**(8):1176–1184.

3. Adapted from Maxmen J, Ward N. *Psychotropic Drugs: Fast Facts*, 3rd ed. New York: W.W. Norton & Company, 2002, and respective drug package inserts.

86

Trazodone

JinLei Li

Generic Name: trazodone HCl

Proprietary Name: Desyrel™

Drug Class: tetracyclic antidepressant

Manufacturer: Bristol-Myers Squibb, 345 Park Ave, New York, NY; Apothecon, P.O. Box 4500, Princeton, NJ; Labopharm, 480 Armand-Frappier Blvd, LAVAL, Quebec H7V 4B4 (extended-release formula)

Chemical Structure: see Figure 86.1

Chemical Name: 2-[3-[4-(3-chlorophenyl)-1-piperazinyl]propyl]-1,2,4-triazolo[4,3-a]pyridin-3(2H)-one hydrochloride

Chemical Formula: $C_{19}H_{22}ClN_5O \cdot HCl$

Introduction

Trazodone is a tetracyclic atypical antidepressant that also provides analgesic effects at supraspinal and spinal levels in the central nervous system (CNS).

Mode of activity

Trazodone is a modulator that augments the serotonin (5-HT) system and increases the excitatory effects of this neurotransmitter. It inhibits reuptake of serotonin and induces significant changes in 5-HT presynaptic receptor [1]. It may also act as a serotonin agonist via an active metabolite. Additionally it has a minor inhibitory effect on the catecholamine system through decreasing norepinephrine uptake, alpha-1 receptor blockage, beta-receptor subsensitivity and decreased beta-receptor density. Thirdly trazodone also blocks histamine (H_1) receptors and has minor anti-cholinergic effects.

Metabolic pathways, drug clearance and elimination

Trazodone is currently available in standard and extended-release oral formula. Transdermal preparation and suppository delivery are under development for pain control. The serum concentration of standard-release trazodone tablets peaks at around 30–100 minutes, which can be significantly delayed with food for up to 2.5 hours. In blood trazodone is highly protein-bound, 85% to 95%. It is metabolized by liver extensively to an active metabolite, *m*-chlorophenylpiperazine (mCPP), through CYP3A4 (major) and CYP2D6 (minor). Trazodone metabolism is biphasic with the half-life of redistribution around 1 hour and half-life of elimination around 10–12 hours [2,3]. Trazodone is excreted primarily in urine 75% (<1% unchanged), with feces excretion accounting for about 20%. Trazodone's anti-insomnia effect may be noted within 1–3 hours following administration. The precise time to onset of its analgesic effects in patients suffering chronic pain is variable and may be delayed. Theoretically the onset of trazodone's anti-neuropathic effects may occur around the same time as that of its antidepression effects, around 1–3 weeks [3].

Indications

Trazodone was approved by the FDA in 1982 for depression, and while it is not approved for chronic pain management it has been advocated for use in multimodal analgesic regimens. In acute pain settings its ability to quickly restore a normal sleeping pattern contributes to better overall pain control. Trazodone is most effective in treating chronic neuropathic pain: its ability to inhibit serotonin and norepinephrine uptake provides measurable analgesic and mood elevation effects [3–5]. Okuda and coworkers [4] evaluated the analgesic effect of trazodone on thermal hyperalgesia in a chronic constriction injury of the sciatic nerve in rats. They also examined the effects of lesions in the descending and ascending serotonergic system upon trazodone's antihyperalgesic effects. Trazodone showed a clear dose dependency, and lesion studies suggested that the serotonergic descending pain control pathway is primarily responsible for its analgesic effect.

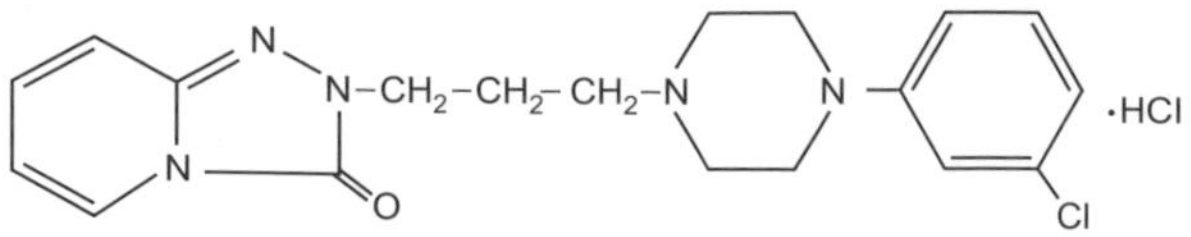

Figure 86.1.

Trazodone is effective in pain states associated with anxiety, depression, insomnia, and adrenergic hyperactivity [3]. It is also useful in settings where tricyclic antidepressants are contraindicated, not tolerated or ineffective. Ventafridda and colleagues [5] compared the analgesic effects of trazodone and amitriptyline for the treatment of chronic deafferentation pain in 45 patients with oncological peripheral nerve lesions. The therapeutic effectiveness of trazodone in terms of pain intensity, hours of sleep, hours standing and lying, mood, anxiety, and weakness was equivalent to that provided by amitripyline, although side effects were less pronounced. Trazodone 100–150 mg daily has also been shown to be effective in chest pain secondary to esophageal mobility abnormalities. In pediatrics, trazodone has also been used in children's migraine headache.

Contraindications

Absolute: patients allergic to trazodone or nefazodone or any components of the formulation.

Relative: avoid using in patients taking sodium oxybate as their central nervous system and respiratory-depressant effects are synergistic. Avoid using together with linezolid or MAOIs for the risk of serotonin syndrome. Avoid using in patients with recent suicidal ideations or attempts as trazodone may increase risk of suicide especially at the start of treatment or with dose escalation. Avoid using in the setting of a recent heart attack as trazodone increases heart rate and therefore adds to stress on the heart.

Common doses

Oral: take it after a meal or a snack to reduce the risk of dizziness and vomiting. It comes in preparations of 50, 100, 150, and 300 mg. Oral adult initial dose is 25–50 mg daily and final dose 25–150 mg daily. In general, trazodone is effective for pain control at an overall dose lower than that required for treatment of depression.

Potential advantages

As an oral antidepressant, trazodone is easy to use, with good absorption and bioavailability, well tolerated and affordable. Trazodone has little of the aminergic properties of tricyclics or monoamine oxidase inhibitors. This results in its low cardiotoxicity with almost no effect on cardiac conduction and little anticholinergic effect. Trazodone is therefore used in neuropathic pain patients when tricyclics are contraindicated, not tolerated, or ineffective, such as cardiac patients, especially patients with arrythmias, Alzheimer's, and the elderly. Trazodone is the first antidepressant that does not cause death with overdose as compared with the lethal effects of tricyclic overdose. Trazodone is available as low-cost generic preparations. The extended-release formula has just been approved by the FDA. In summary trazodone has opioid-sparing effects in chronic pain control, restores sleep patterns, has a low side-effect profile, and no death has been reported for overdose.

Potential disadvantages

Major drug interactions: trazodone interacts with MAOIs with the risk of serotonin syndrome. When switching between trazodone and an MAOI, a 2-week no-trazodone no-MAOI gap is necessary to safely stop and start treatment. Trazodone should not be stopped abruptly. Trazodone interacts with alcohol with worsening sedation. Tegretol decreases blood levels while Nizoral and Norvir increase blood levels of trazodone. Co-administration of trazodone can increase blood concentrations of digoxin and phenytoin. Trazodone may also pass into breast milk and affect a nursing baby.

Drug-related adverse events

Common/serious adverse events: dizziness, headache, sedation, nausea, xerostomia, blurred vision.

Less common adverse events: syncope, hypo/hypertension, edema, confusion, decreased concentration, diarrhea/constipation, tremor, myalgia, nasal congestion.

Rare but important events: agitation, allergic reactions, alopecia, anxiety, bradycardia/tachycardia, extrapyramidal symptoms, hepatitis, priapism (i.e. prolonged or constant penile erection that can be painful), rash, seizure, speech impairment, urinary retention, risk of suicidal ideations or attempts.

Disease-related concerns

Use cautiously in patients with cardiovascular disease especially during the acute recovery phase of MI. Possible dose adjustment in patients with hepatic or renal dysfunctions, seizure disorders, head trauma, alcoholism, schizophrenia, or bipolar manic depression. Use with caution in patients with drug abuse history.

Overdose

Symptoms vary from person to person and are also influenced by co-injection of alcohol or other sedative/psycoative medications. Overdose of trazodone may cause an increase in incidence or severity of any of the reported adverse reactions, with drowsiness and vomiting being the most common ones, followed by hypotension, breathing difficulty, seizures, priapism, and arrhythmia. There is the potential for loss of life but it has not been reported. There is no specific antidote for trazodone. Any patient suspected of having taken an overdose should be admitted to hospital as soon as possible. Acute management is geared to promote elimination and avoid further absorption such as activated charcoal, gastric lavage, and forced diuresis when indicated. Ipecac is contraindicated. In the meantime proper monitoring of cardiac, respiratory, neurological status, and NPO may be warranted. Treat symptomatically, such as IVF/dopamine/norepenephrine for hypotension, benzodiazepines/barbiturates for seizure, cyproheptadine for serotonin syndrome.

Conclusion

Trazodone provides useful analgesia for patients suffering chronic neuropathic pain, although it is not formally approved for this condition. It does not appear to offer efficacy advantages over amitriptyline and other TCAs but may provide improved tolerability.

References

1. Stoelting RK, Hillier SC. Chapter 19: Drugs used for psychopharmacologic therapy. In *Pharmacology and Physiology in Anesthetic Practice*, 4th ed. pp. 398–406.

2. Ansari A. The efficacy of newer antidepressants in the treatment of chronic pain: a review of current literature. *Harv Rev Psychiatry*: 2000;7(5):257–277.

3. Ventafridda V, et al. Antidepressants for cancer pain and other painful syndromes with deafferentation component: comparison of amitriptyline and trazodone. *Ital J Nerurol Sci* 1987;**8**:579–587.

4. Okuda K, Takanishi T, Yoshimoto K, et al. Trazodone hydrochloride attenuates thermal hyperalgesia in a chronic constriction injury rat model. *Eur Acad Anaesthesiol* 2003;**20**:409–414.

5. Ventafridda V, Caraceni A, Saita L, et al. Trazodone for deafferentation pain. Comparison with amitriptyline. *Psychopharmacology* 1988; **95**:S44–S49.

**Section 9
Chapter**

87

Antidepressants

Duloxetine

Eric S. Hsu

Generic Name: duloxetine-HCl

Proprietary Name: Cymbalta Delayed-Release Capsules for Oral Use

Manufacturer: Eli Lilly and Company, Indianapolis, IN 46285

Chemical Structure: see Figure 87.1

Chemical Name: (+)-(S)-N-methyl-γ-(1-naphthyloxy)-2 thiophenepropylamine hydrochloride

Empirical Formula: $C_{18}H_{19}NOS\cdot HCl$; molecular wt 333.88

Description

Duloxetine is a selective serotonin and norepinephrine reuptake inhibitor (SNRI). Duloxetine is available as delayed-release capsules for oral route.

Mode of activity

Proposed mechanism of action: the potentiation of serotonergic and noradrenergic activity in the CNS may attribute to the clinical efficacy.

Receptor interactions: preclinical studies have shown that duloxetine is a potent inhibitor of serotonin and norepinephrine reuptake and a less potent inhibitor of dopamine reuptake. Duloxetine has no significant affinity for dopaminergic, adrenergic, cholinergic, histaminergic, opioid, glutamate, and GABA receptors. Duloxetine does not inhibit monoamine oxidase (MAO).

Pharmacokinetics: duloxetine has an elimination half-life of about 12 hours and its pharmacokinetics is dose-proportional over the therapeutic range. Patients may reach steady-state plasma concentrations after dosing for 3 days. Elimination of duloxetine is mainly through hepatic metabolism involving two P450 isozymes, CYP1A2 and CYP2D6.

Absorption and distribution: oral duloxetine is well absorbed with maximal plasma concentrations in 6 hours. Food delays the time to reach peak concentration from 6 to 10 hours and decreases 10% of absorption. There is a 3 hour delay in absorption and a one-third increase in apparent clearance of duloxetine after an evening dose as compared to a morning dose.

Metabolism and elimination: duloxetine undergoes extensive metabolism to numerous inactive metabolites. The major biotransformation pathways for duloxetine involve oxidation of the naphthyl ring followed by conjugation and further oxidation. Both CYP1A2 and CYP2D6 catalyze the oxidation of the naphthyl ring in vitro. Most (about 70%) of the duloxetine dose appears in the urine as metabolites of duloxetine; about 20% is excreted in the feces.

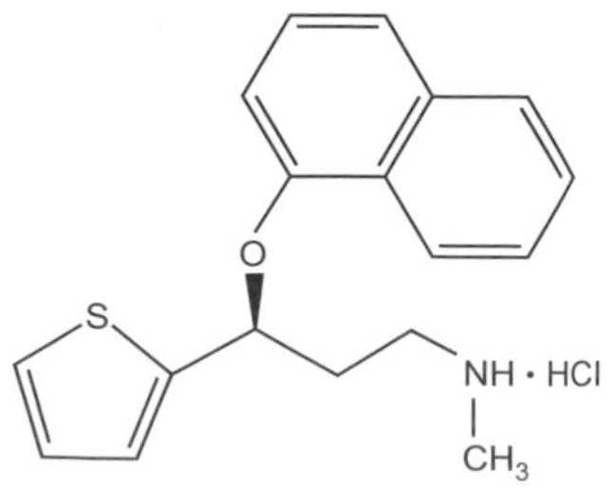

Figure 87.1.

Indications

1. Major depressive disorder
2. Generalized anxiety disorder
3. Diabetic peripheral neuropathy
4. Fibromyalgia

Contraindications

Patients taking monoamine oxidase inhibitors. The potential interactions with serotonergic drugs may include hyperthermia, rigidity, myoclonus, autonomic instability with possible rapid fluctuations of vital signs. Mental status changes may involve extreme agitation and then progress to delirium and coma resembling neuroleptic malignant syndrome.

Patients have uncontrolled narrow-angle glaucoma. There was an increased risk of mydriasis associated with use of duloxetine.

Warnings and precautions

1. Clinical worsening and suicide risk
2. Activation of mania/hypomania
3. Hepatotoxicity
4. Orthostatic hypotension and syncope
5. Effect on blood pressure
6. Serotonin syndrome or neuroleptic malignant syndrome (NMS-like reactions)
7. Seizures
8. Abnormal bleeding
9. Hyponatremia
10. Urinary hesitation and retention

Common doses

There is no standard recommendation for laboratory tests while patients take duloxetine. Patients may take duloxetine without regard to meals or fasting.

It should be swallowed whole and not chewed or crushed as this may affect the enteric coating of duloxetine.

Initial treatment

Diabetic peripheral neuropathic pain: patients may start duloxetine with 60 mg or a lower dose and gradually titrate due to the concern of common renal insufficiency in patients with diabetes.

Fibromyalgia: start with 30 mg once daily for 1 week and allow patients to adjust to duloxetine before considering increasing to 60 mg daily or higher dose.

Maintenance treatment

Diabetic peripheral neuropathic pain: the effectiveness of duloxetine must be assessed carefully based on the progress of diabetic peripheral neuropathy.

Fibromyalgia: the efficacy of duloxetine in fibromyalgia was demonstrated in placebo-controlled trials up to 12 weeks. Efficacy up to 6 months has also been documented in placebo-controlled studies after FDA approval.

Discontinuing duloxetine

A gradual reduction in the dose rather than abrupt cessation is recommended whenever possible. At least 14 days should pass between discontinuation of an MAOI and initiation of therapy with duloxetine. In addition, at least 5 days after stopping duloxetine should be allowed before switching to an MAOI.

Potential advantages

Diabetic peripheral neuropathic pain

The efficacy of duloxetine in pain management of diabetic peripheral neuropathy was recognized in two randomized, 12-week, double-blind, placebo-controlled, fixed-dose studies. These were adult patients with at least 6 months history of peripheral neuropathic pain due to diabetes.

Both studies compared duloxetine 60 mg once daily or twice daily with the placebo. Duloxetine 60 mg once or twice a day provided statistically significant improvement of endpoint mean pain scores from baseline. The proportion of patients with at least a 50% reduction in pain score was higher in the treatment group than in the placebo.

Fibromyalgia

The efficacy of duloxetine for pain management of fibromyalgia was well established in two randomized, double-blind, placebo-controlled, fixed-dose studies. These adult patients all met the American College of Rheumatology criteria for fibromyalgia (a history of widespread pain for 3 months, and pain present at 11 or more of the 18 specific tender point sites).

Both studies compared duloxetine 60 mg once daily or 120 mg daily (given in divided doses in Study 1 and as a single daily dose in Study 2) with the placebo. The treatments using duloxetine 60 mg once or twice daily resulted in statistically significant improvements of endpoint mean pain scores from baseline.

The proportion of patients with at least a 50% reduction in their pain score was higher in the treatment group than in the placebo.

In addition, those nonresponders with less than 30% pain reduction after 8 weeks of duloxetine were no more likely to meet response criteria at the end of 60 weeks of treatment even if blindly titrated to 120 mg as compared to those continued on 60 mg.

Potential disadvantages

Duloxetine may cause significant drug–drug interactions. Both liver P450 isozymes CYP1A2 and CYP2D6 are accountable for the metabolism of duloxetine. Simultaneous use with inhibitors of CYP1A2 and 2D6 resulted in higher levels of duloxetine. Duloxetine is an inhibitor of CYP1A2 and 2D6. The desipramine (a CYP2D6 substrate) level was increased by three-fold when administered together with duloxetine 120 mg/day. The concomitant use of duloxetine with other SSRIs, SNRIs, or tryptophan is not recommended due to the potential for serotonin syndrome.

Drugs that raise the gastrointestinal pH may lead to an earlier release of duloxetine. Co-administration of duloxetine with another highly protein-bound drug may cause higher free levels and potential adverse reactions.

Serotonin release by platelets plays an important role in hemostasis. Psychotropic drugs that interfere with serotonin reuptake may increase the occurrence of upper gastrointestinal bleeding with concurrent use of an NSAID or aspirin. Altered anticoagulant effects have been reported when either SSRIs or SNRIs are co-administered with warfarin. Hemostasis in warfarin therapy should be carefully monitored whenever duloxetine is initiated or discontinued.

Drug-related adverse events

The most commonly observed adverse reactions associated with duloxetine were nausea, constipation, decreased appetite, dry mouth, somnolence, and hyperhidrosis. Patients in DPNP trials also reported dizziness and asthenia.

Drug abuse and dependence

Abuse

In animal studies, duloxetine did not demonstrate any barbiturate-like (depressant) abuse potential.

While duloxetine has not been systematically studied in humans for abuse potential, there was no suggestion of any drug-seeking behavior in the clinical trials. Physicians should carefully evaluate and follow up patients with a history of drug abuse while on duloxetine.

Dependence

Duloxetine did not demonstrate dependence-producing potential in studies using a rat model.

Overdosage

Signs and symptoms

In postmarketing experience, fatal outcomes have been reported for acute overdoses, primarily with mixed overdoses, but also with duloxetine only, at doses as low as 1000 mg. Signs and symptoms of overdose on duloxetine included somnolence, coma, serotonin syndrome, seizures, syncope, tachycardia, hypotension, hypertension, and vomiting.

Management of overdose

There is no specific antidote to duloxetine, but if serotonin syndrome ensues, specific treatment (such as with cyproheptadine and/or temperature control) may be considered. In a case of acute overdose, treatment should consist of general measures employed in the management of overdose with any drug.

Clinical pearls

It is mandatory to set up a realistic goal prior to initiating pain management. Duloxetine, as an adjuvant analgesic, may contribute to pain relief gradually but not instantaneously. Previous studies have demonstrated mild to moderate pain relief in patients who responded to duloxetine treatment. The efficacy and timeline with duloxetine were quite different than analgesics such as opioids or NSAIDs that were not FDA approved for DPN and/or fibromyalgia.

It is an empirical decision whether to start with duloxetine or anti-epileptics for neuropathic pain management. Vigilant follow-up and patient education on drug–drug interactions are crucial to a successful launch of duloxetine. It is prudent to start with a low dose (20–30 mg) of duloxetine and titrate cautiously to balance the risk and benefit ratio. Duloxetine doses higher than 60 mg failed to provide any additional pain relief yet caused more adverse events and withdrawals according to previous clinical studies.

Russell et al. demonstrated that duloxetine at dosages of 60 mg/day and 120 mg/day for up to 6 months was safe and effective in the treatment of fibromyalgia with or without major depressive disorder [3]. They also provided more robust assessment efficacy of duloxetine in fibromyalgia than most previous published studies that were only for 3 months duration.

Potential synergistic effects in pain management with other FDA-approved agents such as pregabalin warrant further clinical research. It is crucial to validate the current strategy with multimodal analgesia including duloxetine to improve outcome in fibromyalgia and diabetic peripheral neuropathy.

References

1. Duloxetine (Cymbalta) Prescription Information, February 16, 2009. Eli Lilly and Company, Indianapolis, IN 46285, USA.

2. Sultan A, Gaskell H, Derry S, Moore RA. Duloxetine for painful diabetic neuropathy and fibromyalgia pain: systemic review of randomized trials. *BMC Neurology* 2008;**8**:29.

3. Russell IJ, Mease PJ, Smith TR, Kajdasz DK, Wohlreich MM, Detke MJ, Walker DJ, Chappell AS, Arnold LM. Efficacy and safety of duloxetine for treatment of fibromyalgia in patients with or without major depressive disorder: results from a 6-month, randomized, double-blind, placebo-controlled, fixed-dose trial. *Pain* 2008;**136**:432–444.

88 Milnacipran

Kristin L. Richards

Generic Name: milnacipran

Trade/Proprietary Name: Savella™

Manufacturer: Forest Pharmaceuticals, a subsidiary of Forest Laboratories, Professional Affairs Department, 13600 Shoreline Drive, St Louis, MO 63045

Drug Class: serotonin norepinephrine reuptake inhibitor (SNRI)

Chemical Structure: see Figure 88.1

Chemical Formula: $C_{15}H_{22}N_2O$; molecular wt 246.3

Introduction

Milnacipran, although relatively new on the market in the USA, has been in use in Europe since 1996. It was first approved for the treatment of major depression in France in December 1996 and is currently marketed under the brand name Ixel in over 45 countries worldwide and under the brand name Toledomin in Japan. Milnacipran has been compared to imipramine, SSRIs, TCAs, and additional antidepressant medications. When comparing milnacipran with TCAs, both are equally efficacious; however, significantly fewer side effects were experienced with milnacipran. As with other antidepressant medications, 1 to 3 weeks may elapse before significant antidepressant action becomes clinically evident. In January 2009 the US Food and Drug Administration (FDA) approved milnacipran (under the brand name Savella) for the treatment of fibromyalgia, making it the third medication approved for this purpose in the USA.

Pharmacology

Milnacipran is both a serotonin and a norepinephrine reuptake inhibitor, in a 2:1 ratio and therefore exhibits a balanced action upon both transmitters. The serotonin reuptake inhibition is likely to improve depression, while the norepinephrine reuptake inhibition is likely to be effective in treating chronic pain. Milnacipran has no direct action on opioid receptors.

Pharmacokinetics

Milnacipran is effective when given orally and has a bioavailability of 85%. Peak plasma concentrations are reached 2 hours after oral dosing and the elimination half-life of 8 hours is not changed in the elderly but is increased by significant renal disease. With a creatinine clearance of 29 mL/min the maintenance dose should be decreased by 50%, with a max of 100 mg/day. The medication should be avoided with a creatinine clearance of less than 5 mL/min.

Milnacipran is conjugated to the inactive glucuronide and is then excreted in the urine as the unchanged drug and conjugate, after which only traces of the active metabolites are found. Enzymes of the CYP class do not play a role in the metabolism of milnacipran and therefore the risk of interactions with drugs metabolized by CYP enzymes is minimal.

Adverse effects

According to the FDA, the most frequently occurring adverse reactions (≥5% and greater than placebo) were nausea, headache, constipation, dizziness, insomnia, hot flush, hyperhidrosis, vomiting, palpitations, heart rate increased, dry mouth, and hypertension. In contrast to several antidepressant medications, milnacipran does not appear to have sexual side effects. In a study of over 3000 patients, the incidence of cardiovascular and anticholinergic side effects was significantly lower compared to TCAs. Elevation of liver enzymes, without signs of symptomatic liver disease, has rarely occurred.

It is important to monitor these patients for the development of rapid mood swings to mania as this has also been seen and then dictates termination of

357

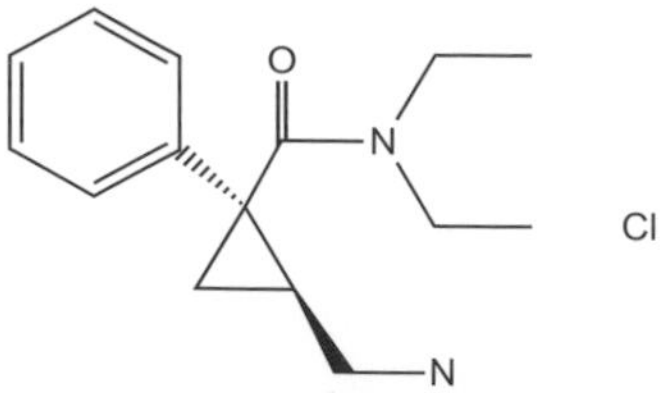

Figure 88.1.

treatment. In psychotic patients emergence of delirium has been noticed as well.

In depressed patients, milnacipran has a low incidence of sedation but improves sleep with regard to both duration and quality. In agitated patients or those with suicidal thoughts additive sedative/anxiolytic treatment is usually indicated.

Interactions

As previously discussed, milnacipran is both a serotonin and a norepinephrine reuptake inhibitor and therefore is a medication that has the potential to cause serotonin syndrome when administered with MAOIs or lithium. The development of hyperserotonergia (serotonin syndrome) can cause a potentially lethal hypertensive crisis.

Additional medication interactions include:

5-HT1 receptor agonists when taken with milnacipran can cause coronary vasoconstriction with the risk of angina pectoris and even possible myocardial infarction

Epinephrine and norepinephrine including local anesthetics with these medications – when used in patients taking milnacipran can cause a hypertensive crisis and/or cardiac arrhythmias

MDA, MDMA or other serotonergic amphetamines – hyperserotonergia, hyperthermia and potentially lethal hypertensive crisis

Clonidine – antihypertensive action of clonidine may be antagonized

Digitalis – when milnacipran is administered to patients currently taking digitalis the hemodynamic actions of the digitalis can be increased

Alcohol – no interactions known. However, as with all patients with significant alcohol abuse it is important to monitor liver function.

Contraindications

Administration of milnacipran should be avoided in the following circumstances.

As with all medications, known hypersensitivity to the medication is an absolute contraindication.

Patients under 15 years of age should not receive the medication secondary to insufficient clinical data.

Concomitant treatment with irreversible MAO inhibitors, phenelzine, (l)-deprenyl, digitalis glycosides, or 5-HT1D agonists (e.g. sumatriptan) is an absolute contraindication.

As previously stated, caution is advised when administering milnacipran in patients concurrently receiving parenteral epinephrine, norepinephrine, or with patients taking clonidine or reversible MAO-A inhibitors (moclobemide, toloxatone).

Advanced renal disease requires dosage adjustment based on creatinine clearance.

Caution should also be used in patients with benign prostatic hypertrophy, with hypertension and heart disease as well as with open-angle glaucoma.

There are insufficient clinical data regarding the administration of milnacipran in pregnancy and during lactation and therefore it should not be used in these patients.

Indications and dosage

In Europe, milnacipran is indicated for both the treatment of major depressive disorder and the management of patients with fibromyalgia. However, in the USA the only approved indication is the management of fibromyalgia.

There have been several studies regarding the most effective dosage regimen. The consensus appears to be that the recommended dose for depression is 50 mg/day (given as 25 mg 2 times daily), with a starting period of 4 days on 25 mg/day. The dose should be decreased in patients with renal disease. The recommended dose for fibromyalgia is 100 mg/day (after an initial upwards titration period) which may be increased to 200 mg/day based on the patient's response.

Clinical results: fibromyalgia

Fibromyalgia is a systemic disease affecting 2–4% of the general population in developed countries and the exact etiology and pathophysiology remain unexplained. However, the most recent studies provide increasing evidence that the pain is due to a dysfunction of pain processing within the CNS. This results in patients experiencing allodynia and hyperalgesia.

In order to establish criteria for the diagnosis the American College of Rheumatology established classification criteria in 1990; however, these criteria focus only on pain and not on the additional issues that fibromyalgia patients experience: for example, fatigue, cognitive disturbances, impaired memory, sleep abnormalities, and depression. Additionally many of these patients also experience conditions such as IBS, migraine headaches, and chronic fatigue.

The treatment of this condition has proved to be difficult and is usually accomplished with antidepressant medications. However, anticonvulsants, antispasticity, anxiolytics, sedatives, opioids, and NSAIDS have been used as well. The most effective results have been seen with antidepressants and specifically TCAs.

Placebo-controlled trials involving a total of over 2000 patients have shown milnacipran, at both 100 and 200 mg/day, to be significantly more effective than placebo in treating both pain and the broader syndrome of fibromyalgia. Additionally data show that the therapeutic effects of milnacipran were sustained for at least 1 year of therapy. Response rates with milnacipran were similar in patients with and without comorbid depression.

In closing, milnacipran, although relatively new to the market in the USA, is providing the opportunity to more effectively manage patients with fibromyalgia. These patients have historically proved to be difficult for clinicians to adequately treat and as the data continue to evolve on milnacipran hopefully more patients will have the opportunity for relief of their symptoms of not only fibromyalgia but also clinical depression.

References

1. Briley M, Prost JF, Moret C. Preclinical pharmacology of milnacipran. *Int Clin Psychopharmacol* 1996;**11**:S9–14.

2. Kasper S, Pletan Y, Solles A, Tournoux A. Comparative studies with milnacipran and tricyclic antidepressants in the treatment of patients with major depression: a summary of clinical trial results. *Int Clin Psychopharmacol* 1996;**11**(Suppl 4):35–39.

3. Lopez-Ibor J, Guelfi JD, Pletan Y, Tournoux A, Prost JF. Milnacipran and selective serotonin reuptake inhibitors in major depression. *Int Clin Psychopharmacol* 1996;**11**(Suppl 4):41–46.

4. Clauw DJ, Mease P, Palmer RH, Gendreau RM, Wang Y. Milnacipran for the treatment of fibromyalgia in adults: a 15-week, multicenter, randomized, double-blind, placebo-controlled, multiple-dose clinical trial. *Clin Ther* 2008;**30**(11):1988–2004.

5. Mease PJ, Clauw DJ, Gendreau RM, Rao SG, Kranzler J, Chen W, Palmer RH. The efficacy and safety of milnacipran for treatment of fibromyalgia. a randomized, double-blind, placebo-controlled trial. *J Rheumatol* 2009;**36**(2):398–409.

6. Moret C, Charveron M, Finberg JP, Couzinier JP, Briley M. Biochemical profile of midalcipran (F 2207), 1-phenyl-1-diethyl-aminocarbonyl-2-aminomethyl-cyclopropane (Z) hydrochloride, a potential fourth generation antidepressant drug. *Neuropharmacology* 1985;**24**(12):1211–1219.

7. Nakagawa A, Watanabe N, Omori IM, Barbui C, Cipriani A, McGuire H, Churchill R, Furukawa TA. Milnacipran versus other antidepressive agents for depression. *Cochrane Database Syst Rev* 2009;**8**(3):CD006529.

8. Papakostas GI, Fava M. A meta-analysis of clinical trials comparing milnacipran, a serotonin – norepinephrine reuptake inhibitor, with a selective serotonin reuptake inhibitor for the treatment of major depressive disorder. *Eur Neuropsychopharmacol J Eur Coll Neuropsychopharmacol* 2007;**17**(1):32–36.

9. Puozzo C, Panconi E, Deprez D. Pharmacology and pharmacokinetics of milnacipran. *Int Clin Psychopharmacol* 2002;**17**:S25–35.

Overview of muscle relaxants in pain

David A. Lindley

Unlike many categories of pharmaceutical agents, the group "muscle relaxants" has no reference to a common structure or mechanism of action. Whereas "local anesthetics" indicates a group of pharmaceutical agents with similar structure and mechanism of action, the approximately ten drugs of the "muscle relaxants" category have virtually no shared structure and no shared mechanism of action.

This chapter will present the evolution of muscle relaxants in the chronological order they appeared in the clinical setting, a brief overview of structure, mechanism of action, and efficacy. The chapter will conclude with a brief discussion of prescribing considerations as well as a more detailed description and discussion of each muscle relaxant.

Our chronology of muscle relaxants starts strangely enough in 1952 with the expectorant guaifenesin (Figure 89.1). Although this medication was marketed as an expectorant, it was associated with reports of pain relief. In fact, guaifenesin has been studied for its use in treatment of fibromyalgia. In 1957, guaifenesin was modified with a carbamate group, making a guaifenesin prodrug called methocarbamol. This drug was, and continues to be, marketed as a muscle relaxant under the brand name Robaxin.

Although some opine that guaifenesin and its prodrugs have discrete analgesic and muscle relaxant activities, the March 2008 Prescribing Information indicates the mechanism of action of methocarbamol (Figure 89.2) as a muscle relaxant "has not been established" and may be related to "general CNS depression". Of course, any drug that causes general sedation will have the secondary effect of "muscle relaxation". The package insert goes on to state that methocarbamol has "no direct action on the contractile mechanism of striated muscle, the motor end plate or the nerve fiber" [1,2].

Several other drugs to follow were also marketed as "muscle relaxants" and share the "CNS depression"

mechanism of action. Some of these drugs are marketed as "centrally acting muscle relaxants" to distinguish them from "direct muscle relaxants" [3].

Guaifensin (1952) and methocarbamol (Robaxin) (1957)

Efficacy: very limited or inconsistent data supporting efficacy for peripheral spasm.

No studies supporting evaluating efficacy in central spasticity [4].

Chlorzoxazone (Parafon Forte DSC) (1958)

Chlorzoxazone (Figure 89.3) is said to act primarily at the level of the spinal cord and subcortical areas of the brain where it inhibits multisynaptic reflex arcs involved in producing and maintaining skeletal muscle spasm of varied etiology. Some studies state the mechanism is mediated via calcium-activated potassium channels, whereas other studies state the mechanism is not mediated via potassium channels [6–8].

Efficacy: "There is very limited or inconsistent data regarding the effectiveness of [chlorzoxazone] compared to placebo in patients with musculoskeletal conditions." Not investigated for efficacy in central spasticity [4].

In 1955, meprobamate (Figure 89.4) was introduced as a "mild tranquilizer". It gained the epithet "Happy Pills" and was associated with abuse and habituation. In 1959, the drug was modified with an isopropyl group and marketed as a muscle relaxant, carisoprodol (Soma). Carisoprodol (Figure 89.5) is metabolized to meprobamate. Carisoprodol, like meprobamate, has addictive properties. Carisoprodol has been ranked number 14 of the 20 most abused mood-altering drugs in the USA [9,10].

The Essence of Analgesia and Analgesics, ed. Raymond S. Sinatra, Jonathan S. Jahr and J. Michael Watkins-Pitchford. Published by Cambridge University Press. © Cambridge University Press 2011.

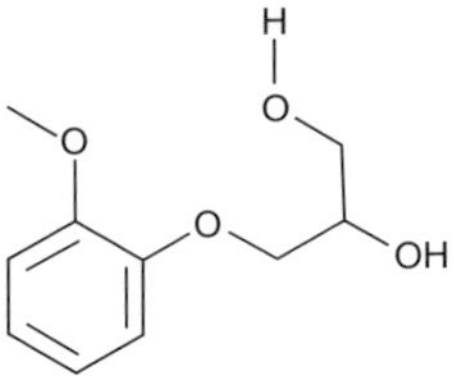

Figure 89.1.

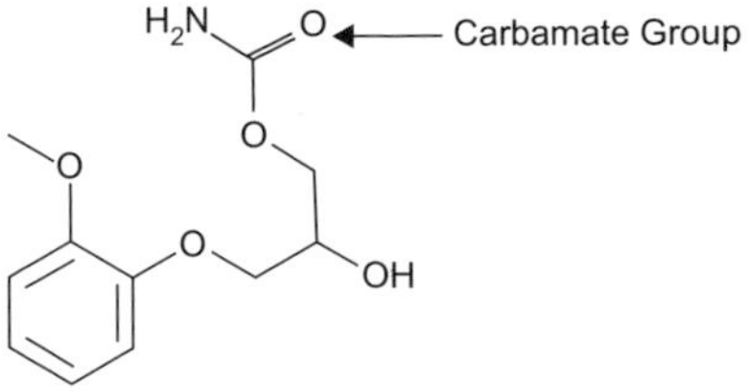

Carbamate Group — Figure 89.2.

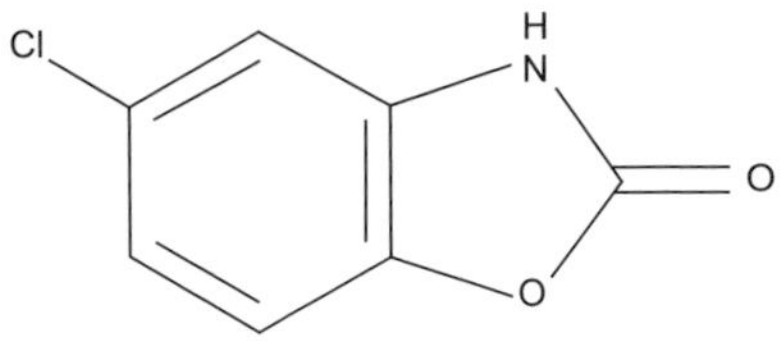

Figure 89.3.

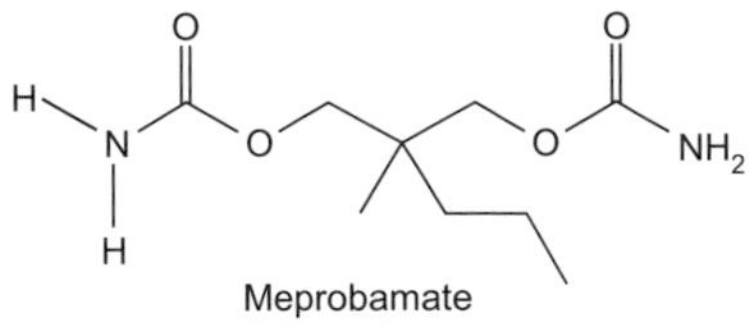

Figure 89.4.

Meprobamate
(Miltown)

Figure 89.5.

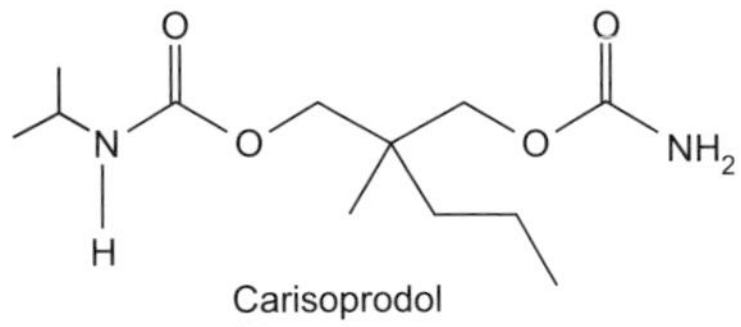

Carisoprodol
(Soma)

Carisoprodol (Soma) (1959)

Although not fully understood, the mechanism of action of carisoprodol has been attributed to the effects of the metabolite meprobamate, including inhibition of interneuronal activity at the descending reticular formation and spinal cord [9,11]. There is no direct skeletal muscle relaxation. Recent evidence indicates the mechanism of action is due to a barbiturate-like effect of both carisoprodol (parent)

and meprobamate (metabolite) at GABA-A receptors [12]. Meprobamate impairs cerebellar function prior to producing muscle relaxation [17].

Efficacy: fair evidence compared to placebo for treatment of peripheral spasm [4]. The drug is indicated for short-term use up to 3 weeks, and has not been tested for chronic use for central spasticity [4,11].

Orphenadrine (Norflex) (1959)

The next drug marketed with a muscle relaxant indication is a structural analog of diphenhydramine (Benadryl) (Figure 89.6). Consider this structural similarity when thinking of its mechanism of action and side-effect profile.

Mechanism of action

Orphenadrine does not cause direct skeletal muscle relaxation. Proposed mechanisms of action of orphenadrine include H1 receptor antagonist [5,13,14], NMDA receptor antagonist and muscarinic antagonist [5,13] activities. Recent evidence also demonstrates orphenadrine has a sodium channel blockade effect which has been attributed to the analgesic characterisics of the drug (as well as proarrhythmic and proconvulsive effects) [13].

Efficacy: orphenadrine has been shown to be superior to placebo for the treatment of pain of musculoskeletal etiology [9,15]. Orphenadrine was determined to have fair evidence compared to placebo for treatment of peripheral spasm, but not central spasticity, in another review [4].

Metaxalone (Skelaxin) (1962)
Mechanism of action

Metaxalone (Figure 89.7) has no direct relaxation effect on skeletal muscle, the motor end plate, or the nerve fiber. The mechanism of action of metaxalone may be due to general CNS depression.

Efficacy: one review found it is "difficult to determine the effectiveness of this medication in the treatment of muscle spasm", citing the paucity of studies and the poor design of available studies, such as the failure to control for physical therapy [9]. Another review found metaxalone has "very limited or inconsistent data" for treatment of peripheral spasm and no evidence for treatment of central spasticity [4].

361

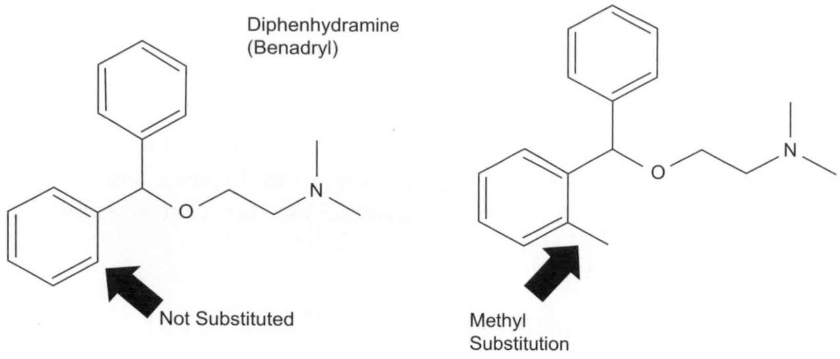

Diphenhydramine (Benadryl)

Not Substituted

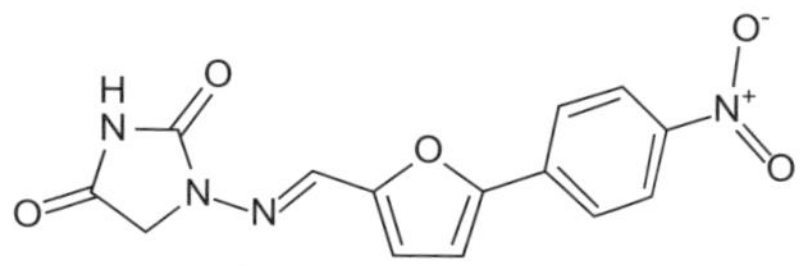

Methyl Substitution

Figure 89.6.

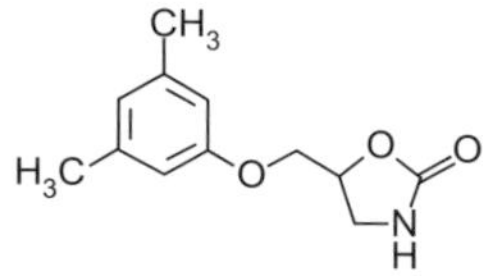

Figure 89.7.

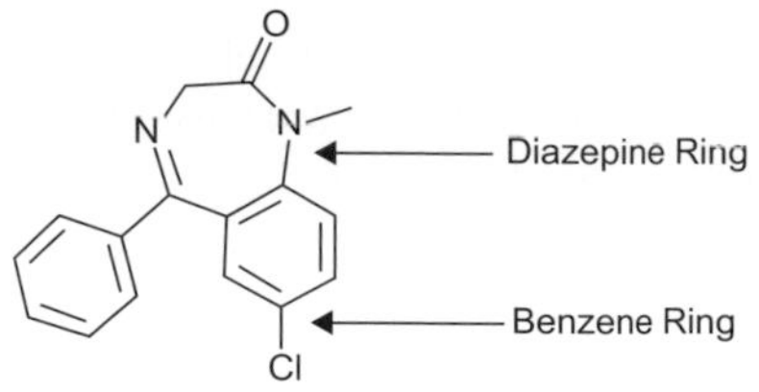

Diazepam (Valium) (1963)

Mechanism of action

Diazepam (Figure 89.8) binds to and stabilizes the GABA-A receptor in a conformation that is more sensitive to GABA binding. This increases the frequency of Cl⁻ channel opening and hyperpolarizes the cell [17,18].

Efficacy: statistically similar improvement in spasms and stiffness as dantrolene [17].

Figure 89.8.

Diazepine Ring

Benzene Ring

Dantrolene (1975) See Figure 89.9

Mechanism of action

Inhibits the ryanodine receptor complex thereby limiting its activation by calmodulin and calcium and inhibiting the voltage-dependent activation of calcium release in skeletal muscle [20].

Cyclobenzaprine (Flexeril) (Amrix) (1977)

Compare the structures of amitriptyline (Figure 89.10) and cyclobenzaprine (Figure 89.11) to see their similarities. Cyclobenzaprine has another double bond, giving it a cycloheptene ring compared to amitriptyline's cycloheptane ring.

Figure 89.9.

Mechanism of action

Tricyclic analogs, including cyclobenzaprine and amitriptyline, inhibit 5-HT$_2$ receptors in the ventral spinal cord, thereby inhibiting the tonic alpha-motorneuron excitation produced by descending serotonergic pathways from the medullary raphe to the ventral horn of the spinal cord [21]. The mechanism of action of cyclobenzaprine is independent of sedation [9].

Efficacy: fair evidence compared to placebo for treatment of peripheral spasm [4].

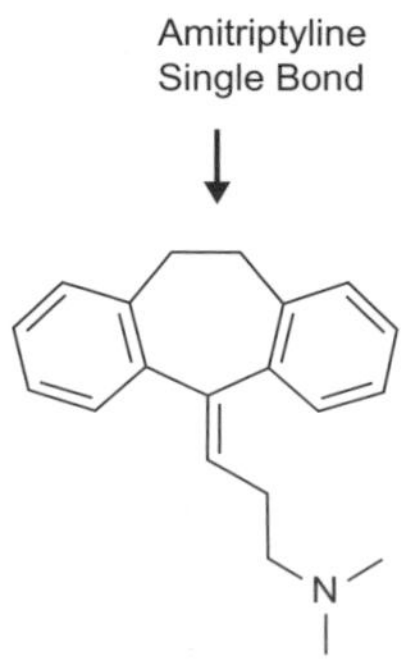

Amitriptyline Single Bond

Figure 89.10.

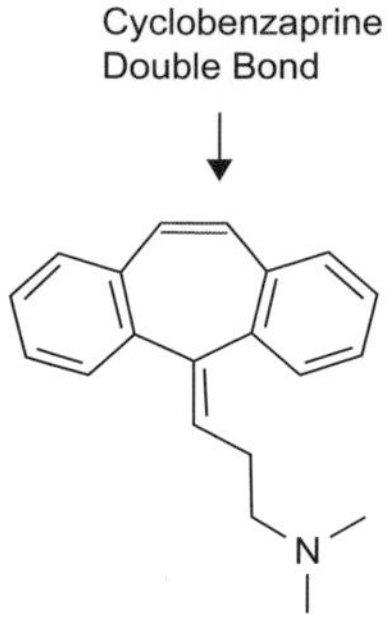

Cyclobenzaprine
Double Bond

Figure 89.11.

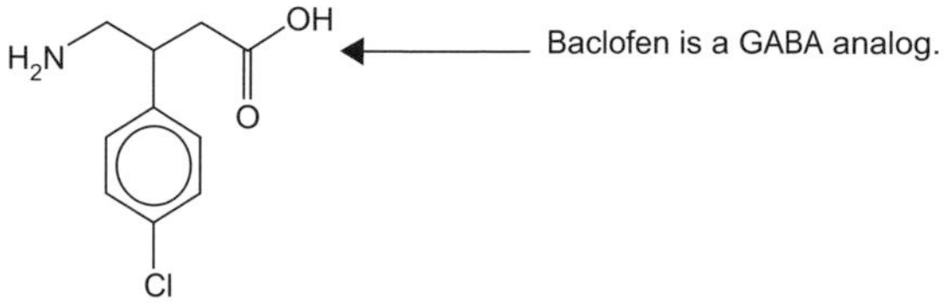

Figure 89.12.

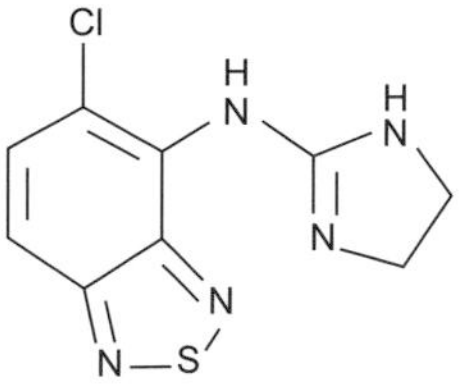

Baclofen is a GABA analog.

Figure 89.13.

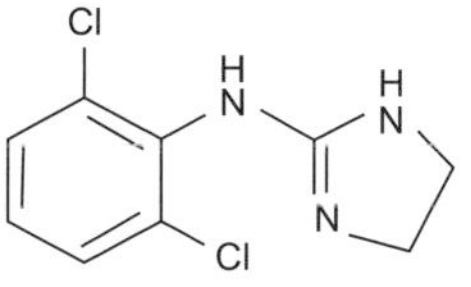

Tizanidine

Figure 89.14.

Clonidine

Baclofen (1977)

Mechanism of action

Baclofen (Figure 89.12) is a presynaptic and postsynaptic GABA-B receptor agonist. When activated, a G protein second-messenger system stimulates opening of K^+ channels, thereby hyperpolarizing the neuron [23,24].

Efficacy: fair evidence compared to placebo for central spasticity [4].

Very limited or inconsistent data for peripheral spasm [4].

Tizanidine (Zanaflex) (1996)

Structure: very similar structure to clonidine. See differences in Figures 89.13 (tizanidine) and 89.14 (clonidine).

Mechanism of action

Tizanidine and clonidine are both alpha-2 agonists. As evidenced by their differing effects on blood pressure, the specific pharmacodynamic profiles of the two drugs differ somewhat. This may be due to variation in the agonist activity at the specific alpha-2 receptor subtypes A, B, and C [26,27].

As an alpha-2 agonist, tizanidine decreases presynaptic excitatory neurotransmitter release and postsynaptic neurotransmitter effectiveness. Alpha-2 receptor agonists attenuate monosynaptic and polysynaptic reflexes in the spinal cord [25]. Tizanidine decreases excitatory neurotransmitter release and Substance P release from small sensory afferents [28]. Tizanidine decreases locus coeruleus activity, thereby modulating descending motor regulatory pathways [28]. Tizanidine decreases activity of both alpha and gamma motor neurons [28].

Efficacy: fair evidence compared to placebo for central spasticity and peripheral spasm.

Some prescribing considerations

- Know the mechanism of action of your muscle relaxant. If the patient is already taking tramadol or tapentadol as well as amitriptyline, consider your rationale for adding a third agent with serotonergic activity such as cyclobenzaprine, as well as the increased risk of serotonin syndrome. Do not use cyclobenzaprine within 2 weeks of the last dose of an MAOI. Some MAOIs include isocarboxazid (Marplan), tranylcypromine (Parnate), phenelzine (Nardil), selegiline (Eldepryl, Emsam),

- Utilize rational drug prescribing. Does the muscle relaxant have an independent mechanism of action for muscle relaxation, or does it rely on CNS depression/sedation to secondarily cause muscle relaxation?

- Does the muscle relaxant you are considering have high potential for habituation or addiction? Is your patient particularly at risk for habituation, compulsive use, or addiction?

- What is the indication for prescribing a muscle relaxant? Is it central spasticity such as from stroke, spinal cord injury, or multiple sclerosis?

Table 89.1. Compromises of liver or kidney

Drug	Caution with compromise of:
Chlorzoxazone (Parafon Forte DSC)	liver
Methocarbamol (Robaxin)	liver or kidneys
Carisoprodol (Soma)	liver or kidneys
Orphenadrine (Norflex)	liver or kidneys
Metaxalone (Skelaxin)	liver or kidneys
Diazepam (Valium)	liver
Dantrolene	liver
Cyclobenzaprine (Flexeril) (Amrix)	liver
Baclofen	kidneys
Tizanidine (Zanaflex)	liver or kidneys

Is it peripheral spasm? What is the evidence of your muscle relaxant choice for the patient's etiology?

- Are there contraindications to concomitant drug use? For instance, tizanidine is contraindicated in patients with concomitant use of CYP450 1A2 inhibitors such as fluvoxamine, amiodarone, mexiletine, propafenone, cimetidine, fluoroquinolones (ciprofloxacin, norfloxacin), rofecoxib, oral contraceptives, and ticlopidine [27].
- Consider the anticholinergic side effects of various muscle relaxants, and use caution when prescribing, especially in the elderly. For instance, methocarbamol has clinically significant anticholinergic side effects.
- Know the metabolism and clearance of your muscle relaxant choice. Does your patient have liver or kidney compromise (Table 89.1)?

References

1. Methocarbamol prescribing information, March 2008.
2. http://web.mit.edu/london/www/guai.html. Accessed July 5, 2009.
3. http://www.whocc.no/atcddd/. Accessed July 5, 2009.
4. Chou et al. Comparative efficacy and safety of skeletal muscle relaxants for spasticty and musculoskeletal conditions: a systematic review. *J Pain Symptom Manage* 2004;**28**(2);140.
5. http://www.neurotransmitter.net/muscle_drug_reference.html. Accessed July 5, 2009.
6. Chlorzoxazone Prescribing Information, August 2000, Ortho-McNeil Pharmaceutical, Inc., Raritan, NJ 08869.
7. Cao et al. Modulation of recombinant small-conductance Ca2-activated K+ channels by the muscle relaxant chlorzoxazone and structurally related compounds. *J Pharmacol Exp Ther* 2001;**296**(3):683.
8. Dong et al. Chlorzoxazone inhibits contraction of rat thoracic aorta. *Eur J Pharmacol* 2006;**545**:161.
9. Toth et al. Commonly used muscle relaxant therapies for acute low back pain: a review of carisoprodol, cyclobenzaprine hydrochloride, and metaxalone. *Clin Ther* 2004;**26**(9)1355–1367.
10. Rosenbaum R, Pagliaro LA, Pagliaro AM. *Psychologists' Psychotropic Drug Reference*. Psychology Press, 1998, p. 338.
11. Carisoprodol prescribing information, MedPointe Healthcare Inc., Somerset, NJ. 08873, Rev. 9/2007.
12. Gonzalez et al. Carisoprodol-mediated modulation of GABAA receptors: in vitro and in vivo studies. *J Pharmacol Exp Ther* 2009;**329**(2)827.
13. Desaphy J-F, et al. Involvement of voltage-gated sodium channels blockade in the analgesic effects of orphenadrine. *Pain* 2009;**142**:225–235.
14. Orphenadrine prescribing information, *1/2006*, Akorn, Inc., Buffalo Grove, IL 60089.
15. Valtonen. A controlled clinical trial of chlormezanone, orphenadrine, orphenadrine/paracetamol and placebo in the treatment of painful skeletal muscle spasms. *Ann Clin Res* 1975;**7**(2):85.
16. Meprobamate prescribing information, 2008, King Pharmaceuticals, Inc., Bristol, TN 37620.
17. Schmidt et al. Comparison of dantrolene sodium and diazepam in the treatment of spasticity. *J Neurol Neurosurg Psychiatry* 1976;**39**:350–356.
18. Valium prescribing information, 1998, Hoffmann-LA Roche Limited, Ontario.

19. Dantrolene prescribing information, 2007, Proctor & Gamble Pharmaceuticals, TM owner.

20. Fruen et al. Dantrolene inhibition of sarcoplasmic reticulum Ca2+ release by direct and specific action at skeletal muscle ryanodine receptors. *J Biol Chem* 1997;**272**(43):26965.

21. Honda et al. Tricyclic analogs cyclobenzaprine, amitriptyline and cyproheptadine inhibit the spinal reflex transmission through 5-HT2 receptors. *Eur J Pharmacol* 2003;**458**:91.

22. Day et al. Serotonin syndrome in a patient taking Lexapro and Flexeril: a case report. *Am J Emerg Med* 2008;**26**:1069.

23. Baclofen prescribing information, Upsher-Smith Laboratories, Inc., 2002.

24. Newberry et al. Direct hyperpolarizing action of baclofen on hippocampal pyramidal cells. *Nature* 1984;**308**(5958):450.

25. Tanabe et al. Spinal α_1- and α_2-adrenoreceptors mediate facilitation and inhibition of spinal motor transmission, respectively. *Japan J Pharmacol* 1990;**54**:69.

26. Zanaflex package insert. Acorda Therapeutics, Hawthorne NY, July 2006.

27. Philipp. Physiological significance of α2-adrenergic receptor subtype diversity: one receptor is not enough. *Am J Physiol Regul Integrat Compar Physiol* 2002;**283**:R287.

28. Coward. Tizanidine. Neuropharmacology and mechanism of action. *Neurology* 1994;**44**(Suppl 9):S6.

**Section 10
Chapter**

90

Muscle Relaxants

Diazepam and lorazepam

Mirjana Lovrincevic and Mark J. Lema

Generic (proprietary) Names: diazepam (Valium, Diastat)

Manufacturer: Roche Laboratories (Valium), 340 Kingsland Street, Nutley, NJ 07110–1199

Generic (proprietary) Names: lorazepam (Ativan, Temesta)

Manufacturer: Baxter Healthcare Corporation, Deerfield, IL 60015

Class: benzodiazepines (BNZs)

Chemical Structure: diazepam, see Figure 90.1; lorazepam, see Figure 90.2

Mode of activity

Major and minor sites of action: GABAA receptors in the brain and spinal cord.

Receptor interactions: benzodiazepines enhance the actions of the neurotransmitter gamma-aminobutyric acid (GABA) on its receptor by modulating the GABA system in the brain, through the presence of high-affinity binding receptors [1,2]. Interaction of benzodiazepines with GABAA receptors opens chloride ion channels, and enhances the frequency of chloride channel opening. It has been shown that in order to elicit the different effect, a different degree of GABAA receptor occupation is necessary. For instance, full agonists are able to elicit an anxiolytic or anticonvulsant effect at a low overall receptor occupation. Partial agonists, because of their lower intrinsic efficacy for enhancement of GABAergic transmission, need a higher receptor occupation to produce the same effect. However, the weak enhancement of GABAergic transmission by a partial agonist is not sufficient to induce sedative/hypnotic and muscle relaxant actions, since even full agonists need a rather high receptor

365

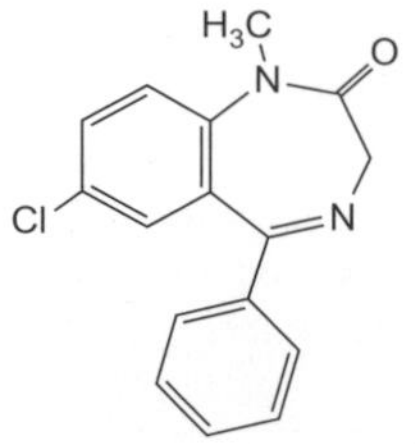

Figure 90.1. Diazepam

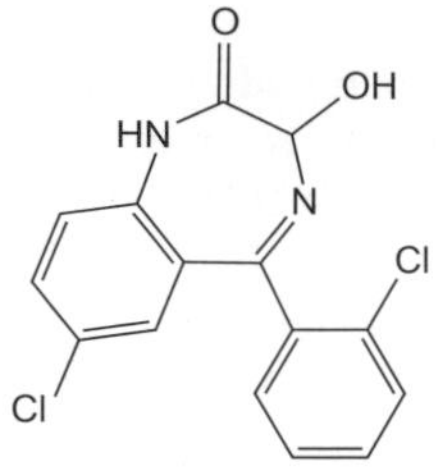

Figure 90.2. Lorazepam

occupation in order to produce these effects. As an example, the benzodiazepine agonistic receptor occupancy was found to differ among the various physiological responses in the following order: antipanic > anticonvulsion > sedation > muscle relaxation [3]. This graded response explains why only pure agonists of GABA receptors are able to display muscle relaxant properties, and why the price for that is always prominent sedation.

Metabolic pathways, drug clearance and elimination (Diazepam)

Diazepam is primarily metabolized by hepatic cytochrome enzyme responsible for S-mephenytoin hydroxylation, with very little unchanged drug eliminated in the urine [1,2]. Hepatic N-demethylation results in the formation of the active metabolite desmethyldiazepam. This metabolite is hydroxylated to form oxazepam. Another minor active metabolite is temazepam. The half-life $(t_{1/2})$ of diazepam ranges from approximately 24 hours to more than 48 hours. With chronic dosing, steady-state concentrations of diazepam are achieved between 5 days and 2 weeks. The half-life is prolonged in the elderly and in patients with cirrhosis or hepatitis.

Metabolic pathways, drug clearance and elimination (Lorazepam)

Elimination of lorazepam occurs by metabolism within the liver and renal excretion of the metabolites. Glucuronidation to form lorazepam-glucuronide is the major pathway for metabolism. Minor metabolites include a hydroxylated derivative, a quinazolinone derivative and a quinazoline carboxylic acid. Seventy to seventy-five percent of the dose is excreted as the glucuronide compound in the urine. All the metabolites of lorazepam are inactive. Lorazepam is readily and completely absorbed from the gastrointestinal tract after oral absorption. Peak plasma levels are reached at approximately 2 hours. Its half-life $(t_{1/2})$ is between 10 and 20 hours, with 14 hours often cited [2,3].

Indications (approved/non-approved)

Diazepam approved uses: treatment of anxiety, acute alcohol withdrawal, seizures and muscle spasms. Also used as a sedative/hypnotic/amnesic.

Lorazepam approved uses: treatment of anxiety, panic attacks, insomnia, chemotherapy-induced nausea and vomiting, alcohol withdrawal, treatment of seizures. Non-approved: muscle spasms.

There have been several studies assessing the effectiveness of diazepam in prevention of succinylcholine-induced myalgia after general anesthesia. While some older studies concluded that diazepam significantly reduced post-operative myalgia other randomized, controlled studies have found no such effect. Diazepam is also effective in alleviating symptoms of muscle contraction headache, but its sedation side effect precludes its routine use to treat this condition. Spasticity associated with cerebral palsy is generally treated with high doses of diazepam. Side effects, including habituation, memory impairment, and dyscoordination, are very common and often intolerable. Stiff-person syndrome, a rare neurological disorder with autoimmune features characterized by progressive, severe muscle rigidity and stiffness affecting mostly the spine and lower extremities, has been successfully treated with diazepam plus immunomodulation therapy.

Benzodiazepines are also being used in the symptomatic treatment of dystonias with prominent muscle spasms.

Contraindications

Absolute: myasthenia gravis, known allergy to BNZ, less than 6 months old, severe respiratory failure.

Relative: pregnancy (teratogenesis), acute intoxication, sleep apnea, ataxia, acute narrow-angle glaucoma.

Common doses/uses

Diazepam

Oral: 2–10 mg, 3–4 times daily for muscle spasm (up to 30 mg/day).

Tablets – 2 mg, 5 mg, 10 mg.

Capsules, time-release – 15 mg (marketed by Roche as Valrelease).

Liquid solution – 1 mg/mL in 500 mL containers and unit-dose (5 mg and 10 mg); 5 mg/mL in 30 mL dropper bottle (marketed by Roxane as Diazepam Intensol).

Parenteral: 2–10 mg IV/IM every 3–4 hours

Solution for IV/IM injection – 5 mg/mL. 2 mL ampoules and syringes; 1 mL, 2 mL, 10 mL vials; 2 mL Tel-E-Ject; also contains 40% propylene glycol, 10% ethyl alcohol, 5% sodium benzoate and benzoic acid as buffers, and 1.5% benzyl alcohol as a preservative.

Neuraxial: none.

Lorazepam

Oral: 2–6 mg/day, given in two or three divided doses.

Tablets – 0.5 mg, 1 mg, 2 mg.

Parenteral: (IM/IV) 2–6 mg/day, given in two or three divided doses.

Solution for IM/IV injection – 2 mg/mL in either 1 mL or 10 mL vials, 4 mg/mL in either 1 mL or 10 mL vials.

Neuraxial: none.

Potential advantages

Ease of use, tolerability, opioid-sparing: both drugs are available for oral as well as parenteral use. Injectable doses can cause irritation to veins and can lead to thrombophlebitis. Both drugs should be used with caution with opioids as they can enhance the opioid effects of respiratory depression and somnolence.

Cost/availabilty: both drugs come in generic form and are widely available. Since they are a schedule C-IV drug, prices can be inflated due to extra handling. Diazepam per tablet – 2 mg ($0.18), 5 mg ($0.16), 10 mg ($0.17), 2 mg solution ($0.34); injectable – 10 mL of 5 mg/mL dose ($1.84). Lorazepam per tablet – 0.5 mg ($2.50), 1 mg ($2.90), 2 mg ($4.50); injectable – per 1 mL ($3.44).

As monotherapy: these drugs are often used alone for muscle spasm and are interchangeable. Lorazepam has a longer therapeutic half-life even though diazepam metabolizes over 24 hours.

As used for multimodal analgesia: cyclobenzaprine (Flexeril), carisoprodol (Soma), oral steroids, opioids, and NSAIDs can all be used in combination therapy with caution, based on the severity and onset of symptoms.

Potential disadvantages

Toxicity: BNZs are known to cause unconsciousness, seizures, respiratory failure, and profound hypotension but are rarely lethal.

Drug interactions: sedatives/hypnotics, opioids, barbiturates, antihistamines, alcohol, neuroleptics, anticonvulsants, and SSRIs can all enhance the sedative effects of BNZs.

Drug-related adverse events

Common adverse events: sedation, dizziness, weakness, unsteadiness, irritation on injection, respiratory depression, hypoventilation (IV), hypotension.

Serious adverse events: dependency, abuse, withdrawal syndrome, respiratory failure, seizures, depression, hypersensitivity reaction.

Less common adverse events: suicidality, anaphylactoid reactions, blood dyscrasias, hepatic encephalopathy exacerbation.

Treatment of adverse events: flumazenil (Romazicon) may be of some benefit in reversing sedation or respiratory depression. Treatments for other causes are largely symptomatic and may necessitate observation in an ICU.

References

1. Duka T, Hollt V, Herz A. In vivo receptor occupation by benzodiazepines: correlation with pharmacological effect. *Brain Res* 1979;**179**:147–156.

2. Haefely W, Kyburz E, Gerecke M, Mohler H. Recent advances in the molecular pharmacology of benzodiazepine receptors and in the structure-activity relationships of their agonists and antagonists. In Testa B, ed. *Advances in Drug Research*, vol. 14. London: Academic Press, 1985, pp. 165–322.

3. Sieghart W. Pharmacology of benzodiazepine receptors: an update. *J Psychiatr Neurosci* 1994;**19**: 24–29.

Generic Name: methocarbamol

Proprietary Name: Robaxin®

Manufacturer: Baxter Healthcare Corporation, Deerfield, IL 60015

Class: muscle relaxant

Chemical Structure: see Figure 91.1

Chemical Name: 2-hydroxy-3-(2-methoxyphenoxy)propyl carbamate

---

Introduction

Methocarbamol is a central-acting muscle relaxant used to treat skeletal muscle spasms and pain related to severe muscle spasm. It is also associated with significant sedative properties.

Mode of activity

Methocarbamol's mechanism of action in humans has not been established, but may be related to general central nervous system (CNS) depression. It has no direct action on the contractile mechanism of striated muscle, the motor end plate, or the nerve fiber.

Methocarbamol is metabolized via dealkylation and hydroxylation. Conjugation of methocarbamol also is likely. Essentially all methocarbamol metabolites are eliminated in the urine. Small amounts of unchanged methocarbamol also are excreted in the urine.

In healthy volunteers, the plasma clearance of methocarbamol ranges between 0.20 and 0.80 L/h per kg, the mean plasma elimination half-life ranges between 1 and 2 hours, and the plasma protein binding ranges between 46% and 50%.

Indications (approved/non-approved)

Methocarbamol is indicated as an adjunct to rest, physical therapy, and other measures for the relief of discomfort associated with acute, painful musculoskeletal conditions, including acute back injury, acute discogenic back pain with related muscular spasm, and muscle spasm associated with severe post-operative abdominal and back pain.

There is clinical evidence which suggests that methocarbamol may have a beneficial effect in the control of the neuromuscular manifestations of tetanus. It does not, however, replace the usual management of tetanus.

Contraindications

Absolute: methocarbamol is contraindicated in patients hypersensitive to methocarbamol or to any of the tablet components.

Relative: methocarbamol may inhibit the effect of pyridostigmine bromide. Therefore, methocarbamol should be used with caution in patients with myasthenia gravis receiving anticholinesterase agents.

Safe use of methocarbamol has not been established with regard to possible adverse effects upon fetal development. Thus, methocarbamol should not be used in women who are or may become pregnant and particularly during early pregnancy unless in the judgment of the physician the potential benefits outweigh the possible hazards.

Methocarbamol may cause a color interference in certain screening tests for 5-hydroxyindoleacetic acid (5-HIAA) using nitrosonaphthol reagent and in screening tests for urinary vanillylmandelic acid (VMA) using the Gitlow method.

Common doses/uses

Methocarbamol tablets (Robaxin®) USP, 500 mg are white, round, bisected tablets, debossed with LAN over 1302, supplied in bottles of 100 and 500 tablets.

Oral dosing

500 mg tablets: adults: initial dosage: 3 tablets QID. Maintenance dosage: 2 tablets QID.

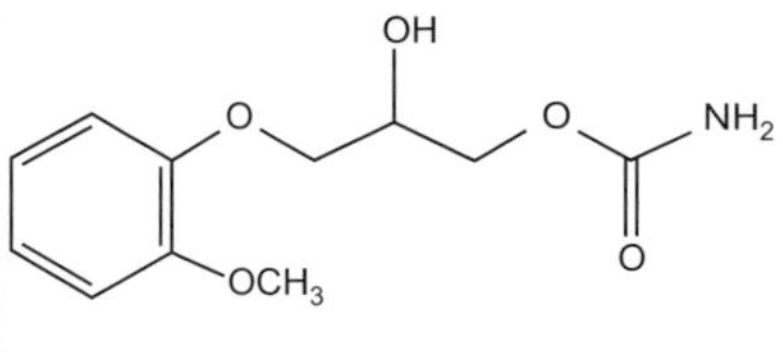

Figure 91.1.

750 mg tablets: adults: initial dosage: 2 tablets QID. Maintenance dosage: 1 tablet q4h or 2 tablets TID.

Six grams a day are recommended for the first 48 to 72 hours of treatment (for severe conditions 8 g a day may be administered). Thereafter, the dosage can be reduced to approximately 4 g a day.

Parenteral (IV/IM): adults – moderate pain: one dose of 1 g may be adequate. Ordinarily this injection need not be repeated, as the administration of the oral form will usually sustain the relief initiated by the injection.

Adults – severe pain/post-op pain: additional doses of 1 g may be repeated every 8 hours up to a maximum of 3 g/day for no more than 3 consecutive days.

Total adult parenteral dosage should not exceed 3 g/day for more than 3 consecutive days except in the treatment of tetanus. If the condition persists, a similar course may be repeated after a drug-free interval of 48 hours.

Safety and effectiveness of methocarbamol in pediatric patients below the age of 16 have not been established.

Potential advantages

Methocarbamol can be used alongside rest and physical therapy as well as combined with other medications as part of multimodal analgesia in the treatment of musculoskeletal pain. Since it may possess a general CNS depressant effect, caution is advised when used in combination with other CNS depressants.

Methocarbamol is available as a generic medication.

Potential disadvantages, drug-related adverse events

Adverse reactions reported coincident with the administration of methocarbamol include:

Generalized: anaphylactic reaction, angioneurotic edema, fever, headache

Cardiovascular system: bradycardia, flushing, hypotension, syncope, thrombophlebitis

GI system: dyspepsia, jaundice (including cholestatic jaundice), nausea and vomiting

Hematological and lymphatic system: leukopenia

Immune system: hypersensitivity reactions

Nervous system: amnesia, confusion, diplopia, dizziness or lightheadedness, drowsiness, insomnia, mild muscular incoordination, nystagmus, sedation, seizures (including grand mal), vertigo

Skin and special senses: blurred vision, conjunctivitis, nasal congestion, metallic taste, pruritus, rash, urticaria.

Limited information is available on the acute toxicity of methocarbamol. Overdose of methocarbamol has been reported in conjunction with alcohol, psychotropic drugs, or other CNS depressants and includes the following symptoms: nausea, drowsiness, blurred vision, hypotension, seizures, coma, and death.

Management of overdose includes symptomatic and supportive treatment. Supportive measures include maintenance of an adequate airway, monitoring urinary output and vital signs, and administration of intravenous fluids if necessary. The usefulness of hemodialysis in managing overdose is unknown.

Cost: average price ranges $50–$99 per 30 day supply and is generally covered by prescription drug insurance.

References

1. http://www.drugs.com/methocarbamol.htm.
2. http://www.fda.gov/downloads/Drugs/InformationOn Drugs/UCM086233.pdf. Orange Book Cumulative Supplement 05 May 2009 (Approved Drug Products with Therapeutic Equivalence Evaluations). Accessed June 18, 2009.
3. http://www.rxlist.com/methocarbamol-drug.htm.

Generic Name: cyclobenzaprine

Proprietary Name: Flexeril®

Class: central-acting muscle relaxant/anticholinergic

Manufacturer: Merck & Co. Inc., West Point, PA 19486

Chemical Name: (5H-dibenzo[a,d]cyclohepten-5-ylidene)-N,N-dimethyl-1-propanamine

Chemical Structure: see Figure 92.1

Molecular Formula: $C_{20}H_{21}N$

Introduction

Cyclobenzaprine is a central-acting muscle relaxant that is commonly used to treat pain from injury, muscle spasms, and other painful musculoskeletal conditions. It is structurally related to first-generation tricyclic antidepressants such as imipramine and amitriptyline and appears to inhibit the uptake of norepinephrine in the locus coeruleus. Tricyclic compounds with norepinephrine reuptake-inhibiting properties have been shown to exert analgesic effects in chronic nerve and muscle pain by acting primarily within the central nervous system at brainstem as opposed to spinal cord levels, although their action on the latter may contribute to their overall skeletal muscle relaxant activity. The exact mechanism of action of cyclobenzaprine is unknown.

Cyclobenzaprine is extensively metabolized by the liver via glucoronide conjugation and N-demethylation and is excreted primarily by the kidneys. Estimates of mean oral bioavailability of cyclobenzaprine range from 33% to 55%. It is highly bound to plasma proteins. Cyclobenzaprine is eliminated quite slowly, with an effective half-life of 18 hours, and has a plasma clearance of 0.7 L/min.

Indications (approved/non-approved)

Cyclobenzaprine is indicated as an adjunct to rest and physical therapy for relief of muscle spasm associated with acute, painful musculoskeletal conditions. Like other tricyclic antidepressants, it is also prescribed off-label for the treatment of fibromyalgia and as a sleep aid.

Cyclobenzaprine should be used for up to 2–3 weeks as there is lack of adequate evidence of effectiveness for more prolonged use. Generally, muscle spasm associated with acute, painful musculoskeletal conditions is of short duration and specific therapy for longer periods is seldom warranted.

Cyclobenzaprine has not been found effective in the treatment of spasticity associated with cerebral or spinal cord disease, or in children with cerebral palsy.

Contraindications

Absolute

Cyclobenzaprine is contraindicated in patients hypersensitive to cyclobenzaprine or to any of the tablet components.

Concomitant use of monoamine oxidase inhibitors (MAOIs) or within 14 days after their discontinuation is contraindicated as hyperpyretic crisis, seizures, and deaths have occurred in patients receiving cyclobenzaprine (or structurally similar tricyclic antidepressants) and MAOIs.

Cylcobenzaprine is contraindicated in the acute recovery phase of myocardial infarction, and in patients with arrhythmias, heart block or conduction disturbances, congestive heart failure, or hyperthyroidism.

Relative

Because of its atropine-like action, cyclobenzaprine should be used with caution in patients with a history of urinary retention, angle-closure glaucoma, increased intraocular pressure, and in patients taking

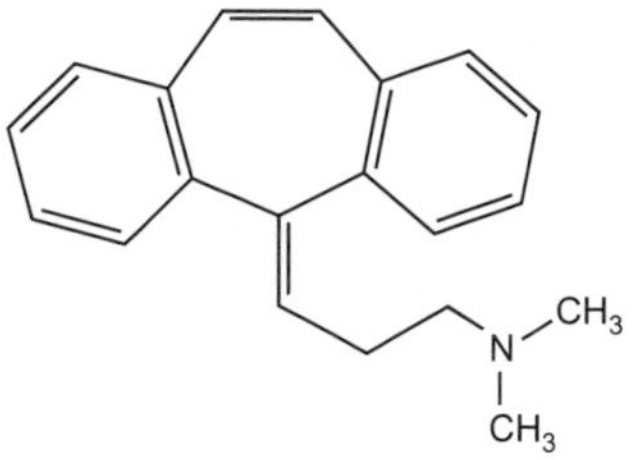

Figure 92.1.

anticholinergic medication. Cyclobenzaprine may also enhance the effects of alcohol, barbiturates, and other CNS depressants.

The plasma concentration of cyclobenzaprine is generally higher in the elderly and in patients with hepatic impairment, thus it should be used with caution in subjects with mild hepatic impairment. Due to the lack of data in subjects with more severe hepatic insufficiency, the use of cyclobenzaprine in subjects with moderate to severe impairment is not recommended.

Tricyclic antidepressants and structurally similar drugs may block the antihypertensive action of guanethidine and may enhance the seizure risk in patients taking tramadol.

Common doses/uses

Oral: Flexeril® 5 mg – adults: recommended dosage: 1 tablet TID or QID.

Based on individual patient response, the dose may be increased to 10 mg three times a day. Use of Flexeril for periods longer than 2–3 weeks is not recommended.

Less frequent dosing should be considered for hepatically impaired or elderly patients.

The safety and effectiveness of cyclobenzaprine in pediatric patients below 15 years of age and in pregnant and nursing women have not been established.

Potential advantages

Cyclobenzaprine is indicated as an adjunct to rest and physical therapy for relief of muscle spasm and it has been shown to have an opioid-sparing effect when used alongside weak and intermediate-strength painkillers such as codeine, dihydrocodeine, and hydrocodone.

Cyclobenzaprine is available as a generic medication and is relatively inexpensive.

Cost: average price is $60 per 30 tablets and is generally covered by prescription drug insurance.

Potential disadvantages, drug-related adverse events

Side effects are common and are generally dose-dependent. They include drowsiness, fatigue, dry mouth, headache, and dizziness. Other less common side effects are respiratory depression, blurred vision, pharyngitis, and decreased functionality in various muscles. A thorough medical history should be assessed prior to prescribing this medication. Patients with a medical history which includes a recent heart attack, congestive heart failure, heart rhythm problems, heart block, thyroid problems, or a substance abuse problem may not be able to take cyclobenzaprine or may require careful monitoring while undergoing drug therapy with this medication. Agitation is a common side effect observed especially in the elderly. Long-term use has been associated with vision damage.

Overdose

The most common CNS effects associated with cyclobenzaprine overdose are drowsiness and tachycardia. Less frequent manifestations include tremor, agitation, coma, ataxia, hypertension, slurred speech, confusion, dizziness, nausea, vomiting, and hallucinations. Rare but potentially critical manifestations of overdose are cardiac arrest, chest pain, cardiac dysrhythmias, severe hypotension, seizures, and neuroleptic malignant syndrome and stroke. Changes in the electrocardiogram, particularly in QRS axis or width, are clinically significant indicators of cyclobenzaprine toxicity.

Although rare, deaths may occur from overdosage, particularly with multiple drug ingestion (including opioids and alcohol). Patients should be instructed to contact the prescribing caregiver if symptoms such as severe drowsiness, fast heartbeat, slurred speech, hallucinations, chest pain, seizures, increased muscle stiffness with fever and sweating of overdose are experienced. If overdose is suspected, dosing should be discontinued immediately. As management of overdose is complex and changing, it is recommended that the physician contact the US national poison hotline at 1–800–222–1222 for current information on treatment.

Conclusion

Muscle relaxants such as cyclobenzaprine should be considered for the multimodal management of acute musculoskeletal injuries. When combined with a nonsteroidal anti-inflammatory drug and occasional doses of an opioid-acetaminophen compound, patients often experience reductions in pain and associated skeletal muscle spasm, and may also benefit from improvements in functionality. The downside of central-acting muscle relaxants is their sedating and cognitive effects, which can be particularly troublesome in elderly patients.

Cyclobenzaprine is not appropriate for children under 12 years of age. Patients who have taken an MAOI in the previous 14 days should not take this medication.

The American Food and Drug Administration rated this medication as a Pregnancy Risk Category B. This medication is not expected to cause harm or birth defects in unborn babies. It has yet to be determined whether or not Flexeril will pass into the mother's breast milk and affect a nursing baby. The prescribing physician should discuss whether the benefits outweigh the risks before prescribing this medication to a pregnant or nursing woman.

There is a risk of side effects associated with Flexeril, some of which are severe. A patient who is experiencing a serious side effect or an allergic reaction should seek immediate emergency medical attention. An allergic reaction will present with symptoms which include facial swelling, including swelling of the lips, mouth, throat, or tongue, hives, and difficulty breathing. Other serious side effects which require emergency medical attention include symptoms such as chest pain or heaviness that involves the arm, fast heart rate, uneven heart rhythm.

References

1. http://www.drugs.com/cyclobenzaprine.htm.
2. http://www.fda.gov/ucm/groups/fdagov-public/@fdagov-drugs-gen/documents/document/ucm071436.pdf (Approved Drug Products with Therapeutic Equivalence Evaluations) 29th ed. Accessed June 18, 2009.
3. http://www.rxlist.com/cyclobenzaprine-drug.htm.

Section 10 Chapter

93

Muscle Relaxants

Metaxalone

Eric S. Hsu

Generic Name: metaxalone

Proprietary Name: Skelaxin™

Distributor: King Pharmaceuticals, Inc., Bristol, TN 37620

Manufacturer: Mallinckrodt Inc., Hobart, NY 13788. Each oval, scored tablet contains 800 mg metaxalone

Chemical Structure: see Figure 93.1

Chemical Name: 5-[(3, 5-dimethylphenoxy) methyl]-2-oxazalidinone

Empirical Formula: $C_{12}H_{15}NO_3$; molecular wt 221.25

Mode of activity

In contrast to neuromuscular blocking agents used in anesthesia, there is no direct action by metaxalone on

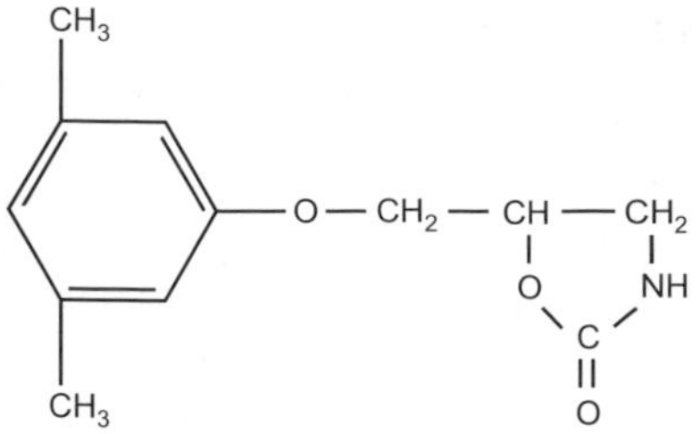

Figure 93.1.

the contractile mechanism of striated muscle, motor end plate, or the nerve fiber.

Although the exact mechanism of action of metaxalone has not been well established, it may be related to the general depression of the central nervous system in the human or modification of signals conducted through polysynaptic fibers controlling passive stretch.

Metabolic pathways, drug clearance and elimination

The potential increase in metaxalone exposure and a reduction in half-life may be attributed to the more complete absorption of metaxalone associated with a high-fat meal. The bioavailability of metaxalone under fasting conditions increases with age. Metaxalone is metabolized by the liver and excreted in the urine as some unidentified metabolites. There could be extensive distribution in various tissues according to the apparent volume of distribution and lipophilicity of metaxalone.

Hepatic cytochrome P450 enzymes CYP1A2, CYP2D6, CYP2E1, CYP3A4, CYP2C8, CYP2C9, and CYP2C19 may all contribute to the metabolism of metaxalone. However, metaxalone does not significantly inhibit or induce major CYP enzymes such as CYP1A2, CYP2D6, CYP2E1, and CYP3A4. There is a gender difference in the pharmacokinetics of metaxalone. The mean half-life is 11.1 hours in females and 7.6 hours in males. The data show the bioavailability of metaxalone is significantly higher in females than males.

Metaxalone should be prescribed with precaution in all patients with hepatic and/or renal impairment due to unknown impact of disease and dysfunction on the pharmacokinetics.

Indications

Metaxalone is a muscle relaxant for relieving pain caused by strains, sprains, and other musculoskeletal conditions. Metaxalone may be prescribed as an adjuvant to rest, physical therapy, and alternative modalities to reduce acute musculoskeletal pain. Metaxalone does not directly relax any tense skeletal muscles in human. The mode of action of metaxalone has not been clearly identified, but may be related to general CNS depression and sedation.

Contraindications

1. Known hypersensitiviy to any components of metaxalone.
2. Known tendency to drug-induced, hemolytic, or other anemias.
3. Significantly impaired renal or hepatic function.

Warnings

Metaxalone may impair mental and/or physical abilities required for performance of hazardous tasks, such as operating machinery or driving a motor vehicle. Patients must refrain from these tasks especially while taking metaxalone together with either alcohol or other CNS depressants.

Common doses

The recommended dose of metaxalone for adults and children over 12 years of age is 800 mg three to four times a day as needed.

How supplied

Skelaxin (metaxalone) is available as an 800 mg oval, scored pink tablet inscribed with 8667 on the scored side and "S" on the other. Available in bottles of 100 (NDC 60793–136–01) and in bottles of 500 (NDC 60793–136–05).

Store at controlled room temperature, between 15°C and 30°C (59°F and 86°F).

Potential advantages

Metaxalone was approved by the FDA in 1964 as an adjuvant therapy to rest, physical therapy, and other measures for relief of discomfort associated with acute painful musculoskeletal conditions. There were two double-blind studies of similar design in the mid-1960s that demonstrated the safety and efficacy of metaxalone compared to placebo. The treatment with metaxalone resulted in marked or moderate improvement of acute low back syndrome (either pain or spasm) or acute exacerbation of chronic low back disorders. Metaxalone was also found to be effective for treating acute involuntary muscle spasm in a later double-blind placebo-controlled study published by Dent et al. in 1975 [4].

Metaxalone (Skelaxin) is commonly considered as a moderately strong muscle relaxant and does not have any significant drug–drug interactions. Although cases of polydrug fatality involving metaxalone were reported, metaxalone is usually well tolerated with variable incidence of side effects.

Potential disadvantages

It is hard to interpret the previous studies on metaxalone due to many study limitations. There were only 200 patients recruited in the two mid-1960s trials that led to FDA approval. However, there was no clear description of the duration and type of back pain and treatment before enrollment. Whether there were concomitant analgesics, sedatives, hypnotics, and/or physical therapy had not been elucidated clearly. Although Dent et al. illuminated the use of associated medications before and during their trial, there were only 228 patients enrolled in the study published in 1975.

The inadequacy of accessible data and exclusion of metaxalone from the Cochrane Review could further compromise the clinical application of metaxalone in the management of acute or chronic low back pain.

The absolute bioavailability from metaxalone tablets is not known. The precise impact of a patient's age, gender, hepatic, and renal disease on the pharmacokinetics of metaxalone has not been determined yet. Skelaxin should always be used with caution particularly in the elderly and any patient with hepatic and/or renal impairment.

Drug interactions: metaxalone may augment the effects of alcohol, opioids, benzodiazepines, barbiturates, and other CNS depressants.

Drug-related adverse events

Metaxalone treatment was linked with rare instances of hepatic enzyme elevation and anemia based on a false-positive hepatic assay using the cepalin flocculation test. Serial liver function studies should be considered for close follow-up. Metaxalone may fabricate a false-positive Benedict's tests, due to an unknown reducing substance. A glucose-specific test, alternatives to urine glucose testing, will be helpful to differentiate clinical findings. Metaxalone should be administered with great care to patients with any pre-existing liver and renal disease.

Adverse reactions

The most frequent reactions to metaxalone include:

1. CNS: drowsiness, dizziness, headache, and nervousness or "irritability"
2. Digestive: nausea, vomiting, and gastrointestinal upset
3. Immune system: hypersensitivity reaction, rash with or without pruritus
4. Hematological: leukopenia, hemolytic anemia
5. Hepatobiliary: jaundice
6. Anaphylactic reactions have been reported with metaxalone.

Overdosage

Deaths by deliberate or accidental overdose have occurred with muscle relaxants including metaxalone, particularly in combination with any antidepressants and/or alcohol. When determining the LD_{50} in rats and mice, progressive sedation, hypnosis, and finally respiratory failure were noted as the dosage increased. In dogs, no LD_{50} could be determined as the higher doses produced an emetic action in 15 to 30 minutes.

Treatment: gastric lavage and supportive therapy should be initiated. Urgent consultation with a regional poison control center is highly recommended .

Clinical pearls

Metaxalone is often introduced as less sedating in comparison with other muscle relaxants such as Flexeril or Soma. However, patients should always start with only half a tablet (400 mg) and adjust dose with precaution. The full dose (800 mg) may then be considered after careful assessment of side effects and clinical improvement.

Metaxalone, like any other muscle relaxants, should be prescribed for regular usage only in the acute phase of persistent musculoskeletal spasm and pain. Metaxalone may be considered in a case of acute flare-up in patients with chronic musculoskeletal pain.

Patients need to be warned about common side effects of dizziness and drowsiness that apply to muscle relaxants including metaxalone. There is no available head-to-head comparison of muscle relaxants to establish that any one muscle relaxant is superior to another. Clinicians may select a muscle relaxant of choice based on a patient's specific need, risks and benefits ratio, drug–drug interaction, and potential risk of abuse.

References

1. Metaxalone (Skelaxin) Prescribing Information April 2008. King Pharmaceuticals, Inc., Bristol, TN 37620.

2. Toth PP, Urtis J. Commonly used muscle relaxant therapies for acute low back pain: a review of carisoprodol, cyclobenzaprine hydrochloride, and metaxalone. *Clin Ther* 2004;**26**:1355–1367.

3. Chou R, Peterson K, Helfand M. Comparative efficacy and safety of skeletal muscle relaxants for spasticity and musculoskeletal conditions: a systemic review. *J Pain Symptom Manage* 2004;**28**(2):140–175.

4. Dent RW, Ervin DK. A study of metaxalone (Skelaxin) vs. placebo in acute musculoskeletal disorders: a cooperative study. *Curr Ther Res Clin Exp* 1975;**18**:433–440.

**Section 10
Chapter**

94

Muscle Relaxants

Tizanidine

Tariq Malik

Generic Name: tizanidine

Trade/Proprietary Names: Zanaflex™ Sirdalud™, Ternelin™, Tizanidinu™

Drug Class: skeletal muscle relaxant, centrally acting

Manufacturer: Elan Pharma International, Ltd, Athlone, Ireland

Generic Manufacturers: Alpha Pharm PTY, Ltd; Barr Laboratories Inc, 223 Quaker Road Pomona, NY; Mylan Pharmaceuticals, 1500 Corporate Drive, Canonsburg, PA

Chemical Structure: see Figure 94.1

Chemical Name: 5-chloro-4-(2- imidazoline-2-ylamino)-2,1,3-benzothiodaizole hydrochloride

Formula: $C_9H_8ClN_5$ S-HCl

Introduction

Tazanidine is a centrally acting muscle relaxant prescribed for skeletal muscle spasm and associated pain. It is supplied as a white crystalline powder that is slightly soluble in water. Aqueous solubility decreases with increase in pH. It is supplied as tablets and capsules, both of which have different pharmacokinetics and are not totally bioequivalent. It was approved by the FDA in 1996 as an oral anti-spastic agent [1].

Mode of action

The exact mechanism of action of tizanidine is unknown. It acts in the CNS at different sites, both at spinal and supraspinal level, which accounts for its anti-spastic effect. Its main affect is via its alpha-2 agonism though its affect on imidazoline receptors may also play a role, as shown by reversal of its anti-spastic effects by alpha-2 antagonists such as yohimbine and idazoxan in animals [1,2].

Tazanidine acts predominantly at presynaptic level, reducing the release of the excitatory amino acids glutamate and aspartate from the presynaptic terminals of spinal cord interneurons. It may also facilitate the action of the inhibitory neurotransmitter glycine. At the supraspinal level tizanidine inhibits the facilitatory descending noradrenergic system (from the locus coeruleus) on the spinal interneurons.

Spasticity is defined as velocity-dependent increase in muscle tone which could be due to a number of different mechanisms. The pathways involved are both

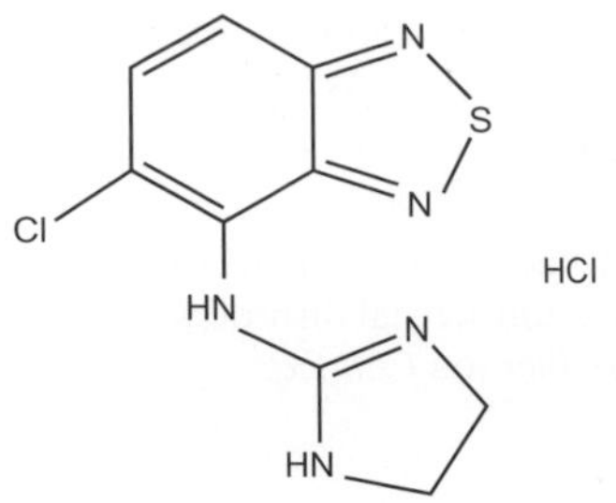

Figure 94.1.

mono- and polysynaptic at the spinal level. Tizanidine has been found to be more effective in reducing the magnitude of polysynaptic excitation vs. monosynaptic excitation, unlike baclofen, which is more effective on monosynaptic pathways [1–3].

Clinical effects

Muscle relaxation: in animal models tizanidine reduces drug-induced rigor, decerebrate rigidity and reflex muscle activity. In clinical trials it reduced muscle tone in most of the patients in a dose-dependent manner which peaked at 2–3 h and lasted for 6 h. It is a short-acting drug.

Cardiovascular effect: by virtue of its affinity for imidazoline receptors and alpha-2 receptors, tazanidine causes bradycardia, a decrease in SBP and DBP of about 7–15% from the baseline. The effect is due to central sympatholytic activity similar to clonidine, albeit of lower magnitude. Change is dose-dependent and peaks at 90–120 minutes after oral intake [1].

Antinociceptive effect: in animal models a dose-dependent analgesic activity is seen which appears to be mediated by alpha-2 receptors at the spinal level. Tizanidine attenuates the abstinence syndrome precipitated by giving nalaxone to rats addicted to morphine.

GI effects: tizanidine slows GI motility and transit time. It inhibits stimulated gastric secretion and offers some protection against drug-induced ulcers in rats.

Miscellaneous effects: the drug has shown anticonvulsant activity and hypothermic effects in animals. In one healthy volunteers study 6 mg and 12 mg doses reduced oxygen consumption from baseline by 3–8%. Mean energy consumption also decreased by 5–9% from baseline.

Pharmacokinetics

Absorption: it is rapidly absorbed with peak plasma concentration reached in 45–120 minutes. The absorption ratio is 0.53 to 0.66 but due to the extensive first-pass effect through the liver bioavailability is only 21% of the dose. Dose and plasma levels are dose-dependent over the dose range studied (2–20 mg). There is little dose–plasma level variability within the same person but significant variability between individuals. Only 30% of the drug is protein-bound.

Metabolism: 95% of the drug is metabolized by the cytochrome P450 system, primarily by the CYP1A2 isoenzyme. Metabolism is via oxidation of the imidazoline part of the molecule. There are three main metabolites and four minor identified in humans, all of which are pharmacologically inactive. Tizanidine is extensively metabolized by the liver with only 3% excreted unchanged in the urine. The drug is eliminated from the body mostly in the urine (66%) and the rest (23%) in the feces. Elimination half-life is 2–4 hours [1–3].

Renal impairment: drug clearance is reduced in patients with renal impairment (CrCl < 25 mL/min) with elimination half time increasing to 13.6 h from 2–4 h.

Tizanidine tablets vs. capsules

The capsule is a multi-particulate formulation of the drug. In different studies it has been shown that food facilitates drug uptake (both increasing bioavailability and peak drug level) when the drug is taken as a tablet but significantly impairs drug uptake when taken in capsular form. The effect is quite significant (about 22–40%) in magnitude. Sprinkling the capsule on food also increases drug absorption by 10–15%. Therefore patients should be cautioned when switching from one formulation to another or changing their intake in relation to food. Patients should be consistent in how and when they take the drug in relation to food [1].

Indications

FDA-labeled: spasticity

The efficacy of tizanidine as a muscle relaxant was established in several pivotal randomized trials [1–3]. Dosage used in these trials ranged from 18 to 36 mg per day in three daily doses. Improvement in Ashworth scale occurred by 3.9–4.7 points. Functional improvement was not significant compared to placebo. Nance et al. in 1997 [4] studied 142 MS patients in a well done study and found a high degree of inter-patient variability and found no relation between plasma level and Ashworth score. In general higher doses resulted in higher plasma levels and more side effects. The authors concluded that each patient will

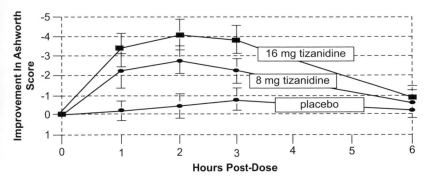

Figure 94.2. Graph shows dose dependence improvement in Ashworth score after single dose, but irrespective of dose effect wears off by 6 h.

require individual titration to the optimum dose for maximum benefit. Dosage up to 36 mg per day does not decrease any muscle strength. In double-blind comparative studies, tizanidine up to 36 mg/day improved the muscle tone comparable to baclofen 60–90 mg/day or diazepam 30 mg/day when studied in people with MS or cerebrospinal injury. The duration of treatment was about 4–8 weeks in the trials. Long-term treatment of spasticity with tizanidine for 8 to 36 months was found to be effective in controlling symptoms with minimal or no upward adjustment of dosage during that period [1,3] (Figure 94.2)

Non-FDA-labeled indications

As adjunct therapy for headache disorders and acute back pain. In many small clinical trials tizanidine has improved chronic tension headache and facial pain from TMJ, and shown transient improvement in pain of trigeminal neuralgia and low back pain. All these studies are small and short-term. Doses used in these trials were low, mostly 2 mg twice a day. It also may have a role in helping patients wean off narcotics by minimizing withdrawal symptoms.

Side effects

Most common reported side effects are fatigue, somnolence, dry mouth, dizziness, and hypotension, happening in 3–5% of patients and the most common reason to stop the medication. They are dose-dependent and peak at 2–3 h post-ingestion and clearly correlate with the peak plasma level of the medication [1–3]. Infrequent side effects are liver function abnormalities, constipation and vomiting, feeling nervous or depression, speech disorder or visual hallucination or blurred vision and UTI. Formed visual hallucinations were reported in 5/170 patients (3%) in two North American clinical trials. It happened within

6 weeks of initiation and resolved after stopping the drug but in one person it took 2 weeks for complete resolution of the symptoms.

There is no known case of drug abuse.

Drug interactions

Most of the interactions are due to its primary dependence on P450 CYP1A2 for metabolism. Any inhibition or potentiation of this isoenzyme dramatically alters the drug level and clearance from the body. Fluvoxmine and ciprofloxacin are potent inhibitors of CYP1A2. Hence giving tizanidine to patients taking any of these drugs will increase the peak level by seven to ten fold and increase half-life by three fold. This will result in a very high incidence of side effects and/or complications such as too much sedation or significant hypotension.

Acetaminophen delays the peak plasma level by 16 minutes. Alcohol increases the AUC of tizanidine by 20%, resulting in more side effects [1]. Other sedatives will have a synergistic sedative effect with tizanidine. Any CNS depressant is going to potentiate the sedative effect of tizanidine. In a study of healthy volunteers, tizanidine's half-life was 10% lower and the AUC ($0-\infty$) was 33% less in male smokers when compared to male nonsmokers. Oral contraceptives decrease clearance of the drug, resulting in a three- to four-fold higher peak level and higher AUC ($0-\infty$). Tizanidine has been known to cause severe hypotension when given to patients taking ACE inhibitors. In controlled clinical trials drug use has resulted in elevated liver enzymes ($3\times$ the baseline) in 5% of subjects. The enzyme elevation normalizes on cessation of therapy. A case of death due to liver injury has been reported. Periodic monitoring of the LFT is recommended for the first 6 months (0, 1, 3, 6 months) and periodically thereafter. Due to its extensive hepatic metabolism, the drug should be avoided or used with extreme caution in patients with liver dysfunction.

Dosing guidelines

The most effective dose for each individual is determined by dose titration due to the great inter-patient pharmacokinetic and pharmacodynamic variability. The starting dose is usually 4 mg unless the patient is elderly or has renal insufficiency (CrCl < 25 mL/min), when it is started at 2 mg. The dose is repeated every 6–8 h. The dose can be increased every 2–4 days. In clinical trials final doses ranged from 2 to 36 mg per day. The dose can be titrated up to a daily dose of 36 mg per day unless the optimal effect appears at a lower dose or side effects limit upward titration. It is given in three divided doses. No single dose should be more than 12 mg though a single dose as high as 16 mg has been studied; but such a high single dose can cause too many side effects. If a single dose is causing too much sedation or drowsiness it can be given four times a day in smaller individual doses. Frequency as often as six times per day has been suggested to overcome individual dose side effects.

Contraindications

Absolute: allergy, co-administration of ciprofloxacin, co-administration of fluvoxmine. Relative : renal failure, liver insufficiency.

Toxicology

The minimum toxic dose has not been established. An adult survived ingestion of 360 mg of tizanidine though he required intubation for loss of airway reflexes [2]. Overdose with tizanidine results in exaggerated pharmacological effects of the drug. It affects predominantly the CNS and CVS. Clinical effects include lethargy, bradycardia, hypotension, agitation, confusion, vomiting, and coma. Therapy is primarily supportive and includes use of activated charcoal for gut decontamination, support of CV with fluid, pressors and atropine for bradycardia.

Comparative standing

In general all muscle relaxants are equally efficacious. They just differ in their side-effect profile and cost.

Tizanidine is in general better tolerated by patients compared with baclofen and diazepam. In a comparative review of different muscle relaxants, Chou et al. [5] reviewed 101 trials and concluded that baclofen and tizanidine are equally effective in treating patients with spasticity, though tizanidine is more often associated with dry mouth, while baclofen causes increased weakness.

Supplied as

Zanaflex capsule: 2 mg, 4 mg, 6 mg

Zanaflex tablet: 2 mg, 4 mg

Generic oral tablet: 2 mg, 4 mg

Buccal formulation (non-commercial formulation)

Slow release formulation (Sirdalud MR 6 mg and 12 mg available in Europe).

Drug cost: Zanaflex capsules are more expensive than comparable doses of generic tizanidine [6].

Zanaflex: 2 mg (150): $266.18, 4 mg (150): $360.62, 6 mg (150): $500.58

Tizanidine capsules: 2 mg (90) $19.99, 4 mg (90): $81.99

References

1. http://tizanidine.org/.

2. Henney HR, Runyan DJ. A clinically relevant review of Tizanidine hydrochloride dose relationships to pharmacokinetics, drug safety and dose effectiveness in healthy subjects and patients. *Int J Clin Pract* 2008;**62**(2):314–324.

3. Wagstaff AJ, Bryson HM. Tizanidine: a review of its pharmacology, clinical efficacy and tolerability in the management of spasticity associated with cerebral and spinal disorders. *Drugs* 1997;**53**(3):435–452.

4. Nance PW, Sheremata WA, Lynch SG, et al. Relationship of the antispasticity effect of Tizanidine to plasma concentration in patients with multiple sclerosis. *Arch Neurol* 1997;**54**:731–736.

5. Chou, et al. *J Pain Symptom Manage* 2004;**28**(2): 141–175.

6. Cost taken from www.drugstore.com.

Generic Name: baclofen

Brand Names: Lioresal, Lioresal intrathecal

Drug Class: skeletal muscle relaxant

Manufacturers: Novartis Pharmaceuticals, East Hanover, NJ; Medtronic Neurological, Minneapolis, MN; Aligen Independent Laboratories, Jackson, WY; Allscripts Healthcare Solutions, Libertyville, IL; American Health Packaging, Columbus, OH; Auro Pharmaceutical, Phila, PA; Barr Laboratories Inc, Pomona, NY

Chemical Structure: see Figure 95.1

Chemical Name: 4-amino-3-(4-chlorophenyl) butanoic acid

Introduction

Baclofen is a centrally acting skeletal muscle relaxant that is used to treat spasticity. It is a chemical analog of gamma-aminobutyric acid (GABA), an inhibitory neurotransmitter, and is a specific agonist at GABA-B receptors.

Mode of activity

Although the exact mechanism of action is not completely known, it is thought to bind to presynaptic and postsynaptic GABA-B receptors. Baclofen works mainly at the spinal cord level to inhibit monosynaptic and polysynaptic reflexes by interfering with the release of excitatory neurotransmitters. Activity at supraspinal sites may also contribute to its clinical effect.

Metabolic pathways, drug clearance and elimination

Oral administration: baclofen is rapidly absorbed from the GI tract. Its oral bioavailability is approximately 70%. It is approximately 30% plasma protein-bound. Peak plasma concentrations occur 0.5 to 3 hours after an oral dose. Approximately 70 to 85% is excreted in the urine unchanged and about 15% is metabolized by deamination in the liver. Its elimination half-life is 2 to 4 hours in plasma. Baclofen crosses the blood–brain barrier in small amounts after an oral dose, with concentrations in CSF approximately 12% of that in plasma. Baclofen crosses the placenta and is also found in breast milk.

Intrathecal administration: plasma concentrations of intrathecally administered baclofen are thought to be low. Limited data suggest that baclofen injected into the lumbar CSF travels cephalad, producing a lumbar–cisternal baclofen concentration gradient of approximately 4:1 during continuous intrathecal infusion. CSF elimination of baclofen probably occurs by bulk flow removal of CSF and approximates CSF turnover. Its elimination half-life is approximately 1.5 hours after a 50 to 100 μg intrathecal loading dose.

Indications (approved/non-approved)

FDA-labeled indications

Baclofen is approved for the treatment of reversible spasticity and its associated pain in a variety of neurological conditions of both spinal cord and cerebral origin, such as multiple sclerosis, amyotrophic lateral sclerosis, and spinal cord injuries. It can be administered orally or intrathecally. Intrathecal baclofen is used to manage chronic intractable spasticity in patients who are unresponsive, or who have intolerable side effects, to a minimum 6 week course of oral therapy. There must be a positive response to a test dose of intrathecal baclofen prior to implantation of a continuous infusion pump. The safety and efficacy of baclofen have not been established in the pediatric population.

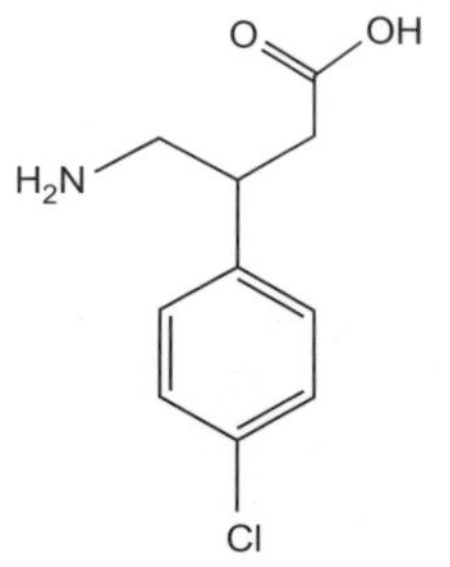

Figure 95.1.

Non-FDA-labeled indications

Oral baclofen, in daily divided doses of 15 to 80 mg, has been found to be effective in treating neuropathic pain; it has been used alone and as an adjuvant for the treatment of trigeminal neuralgia. Oral baclofen, in similar doses, has been used to treat intractable hiccups. In addition, though not a conventional analgesic itself, it may potentiate opioid analgesia. Continuous intrathecal baclofen infusion of 1 to 2 mg daily for the management of tetanus has been reported.

Contraindications

Absolute: hypersensitivity to baclofen or any component of the product.

Relative/precautions:

- Baclofen increases gastric acid secretion; use with caution in patients with a history of peptic ulcer disease.
- Baclofen may exacerbate severe psychiatric or seizure disorders. Patients with cerebrovascular disease may also tolerate baclofen poorly.
- Severe renal impairment may cause baclofen toxicity. Patients with renal insufficiency or those ungerdoing hemodialysis require a reduced dose.
- Baclofen may increase blood glucose concentrations; use with caution in patients with diabetes.
- Baclofen should be used with caution in patients who require their spasticity to maintain posture or function.
- Baclofen is considered unsafe in patients with porphyria.
- Baclofen may precipitate bronchospasm and should be used with caution in patients with respiratory impairment.
- Baclofen may cause alterations in liver function tests; monitor in patients with hepatic disease.

- The safety and efficacy of baclofen have not been established in the pediatric population.
- Small children may be unable to accommodate an implantable baclofen pump.
- Baclofen is classified as Pregnancy Category C.
- The concentrations of baclofen found in breast milk are low; the American Academy of Pediatrics considers baclofen acceptable with breast-feeding.
- Adverse effects may be more common in the elderly.
- Baclofen may enhance the effects of alcohol and other CNS depressants.

Common doses

Baclofen can be administered orally or intrathecally. Intrathecal administration is accomplished by means of an intrathecal catheter and a surgically implanted refillable pump. Intrathecal administration is often preferred in patients with severe spasticity, as very little of the oral dose actually reaches the CSF. These patients may be unresponsive to oral baclofen and/or intolerant of its side effects at high doses. While intrathecal administration may minimize side effects, it poses the risk of potentially severe CNS depression.

How supplied:

- oral tablet: 10 mg, 20 mg
- Lioresal intrathecal test solution : 0.05 mg/mL
- Lioresal intrathecal refill solution: 0.5 mg/mL, 2 mg/mL

Oral: baclofen is given in divided doses, preferably with or after food. The initial dose is 5 mg three times a day for 3 days, increased to 10 mg a day for 3 days, then titrated up in a similar manner until a therapeutic effect is obtained or a maximum daily dose of 80 mg is reached. Doses of more than 80 mg daily are usually not recommended. If there is no clinical response within 6 weeks of achieving the maximum dose, the drug should be gradually withdrawn. Elderly patients should receive lower initial doses. Patients with renal insufficiency or those undergoing hemodialysis should receive reduced doses; 5 mg daily has been recommended.

Intrathecal: before starting intrathecal baclofen,any existing anti-spastic therapy should be gradually withdrawn. Initial intrathecal test doses are given to determine clinical response. If there is a positive response, an intrathecal catheter is placed and connected to a subcutaneously implanted pump whose reservoir can be refilled by percutaneous injection. Intrathecal test doses start at 25 to 50 μg, given over at least 1 minute, and are increased by 25 μg every 24 hours until a dose of 100 μg is reached or a positive response of 4 to 8 hours is obtained. A positive response is considered a reduction in muscle spasm, passive limb movement, and/or pain relief. Patients who do not respond to a test dose of up to 100 μg are not candidates for intrathecal treatment. For those with a positive response lasting longer than 8 hours, the test dose required to produce that response is then given as a 24-hour infusion. If the response to the test dose lasted 8 hours or less, a dose equivalent to twice the test dose is given as a 24-hour infusion. Daily dosage can then be adjusted as needed. Maintenance doses range from 10 μg to 2 mg daily, depending on the cause of spasticity, with most patients requiring 300 to 800 μg daily. Most patients require a gradual increase in dose over time to maintain an optimal response (Table 95.1).

Potential advantages

Significant tolerance does not seem to occur and baclofen retains its therapeutic effects after many years of use.

Potential disadvantages

Baclofen, like other GABA agonists, can produce CNS depression. In addition, the intrathecal pump systems are complex and expensive. Like most implantantable devices they carry the risk of infection. Their subcutaneous position makes them vulnerable to damage with the potential for release of the entire baclofen dose. Inadvertent intrathecal overdose may also occur secondary to pump malfunction or dispensing errors. In approximately 5% of patients, the intrathecal route has no effect.

Drug-related adverse events

Common adverse events: drowsiness, dizziness, weakness, nausea, vomiting, constipation (intrathecal 100%).

Less common adverse events: fatigue, headache, elevated liver enzymes, elevated blood glucose, urinary retention, incontinence, euphoria, depression, paresthesias, xerostomia, taste alteration, anorexia, abdominal pain, diarrhea, constipation, respiratory depression, cardiovascular depression, chest pain, syncope, paradoxical increase in spasticity, impotence/inability to ejaculate (intrathecal), aseptic meningitis (intrathecal).

Serious adverse events

Withdrawal: abrupt discontinuation of baclofen can result in withdrawal symptoms, which may include hyperthermia, tachycardia, seizures, hallucinations, psychosis, agitation, and exaggerated rebound spasticity. In rare cases this may progress to rhabdomyolysis, multiple organ-system failure, and death. With the exception of serious adverse events, baclofen should be gradually reduced over 1 to 2 weeks before discontinuing, especially in those patients on chronic high-dose therapy. The FDA has issued a black-box warning advising against the abrupt withdrawal of intrathecal baclofen.

Toxicity: weakness, drowsiness, confusion, agitation, delirium, hallucinations, nausea and vomiting are common in mild to moderate toxicity. Respiratory depression, hypotension, bradycardia, hypotonia, hypothermia, seizures, and coma may occur in severe toxicity. Rare events include status epilepticus, rhabdomyolysis, and first-degree AV block. Oral doses of 200 mg or more and intrathecal doses of 1.5 mg or more often produce significant toxicity.

Treatment of adverse events: adverse events are often transient and dose-related. Mild side effects can

Table 95.1. Adult baclofen dosing for spasticity

Oral	5 mg PO TID; increase by 15 mg/day q 3 days to maximum dose 80 mg/day
Intrathecal test dose	25–50 μg in 1 mL intrathecal over ≥ 1 min; increase by 25 μg q24 h until maximum dose 100 μg or 4–8 h sustained clinical response. Must respond to a single bolus dose of ≤100 μg/2 mL to be a candidate for infusion pump therapy.
Initial intrathecal infusion rate	If test dose response < 8 h: initial daily dose = 2× test dose intrathecally over 24 h. If test dose response > 8 h: initial daily dose = test dose intrathecally over 24 h.
Intrathecal infusion titration	For spinal cord spasticity: after first 24 h, may increase dosage by 10–30% q24 h. For cerebral origin spasticity: after first 24 h, may increase dosage 5–15% q24h.
Intrathecal pump refill	For spinal cord spasticity: may increase daily dose by 10–40% (max) or reduce daily dose by 10–20% PRN during pump refill. For cerebral origin spasticity: may increase daily dose by 5–20% (max) or reduce daily dose by 10–20% PRN during pump refill.

generally be minimized by increasing doses gradually or controlled by a decrease in dose. Serious adverse events usually require intervention, as described below.

Withdrawal: manage withdrawal from oral baclofen by resuming the usual dose. Manage withdrawal from intrathecal baclofen by either resuming the infusion or administering by lumbar puncture. Give oral baclofen if intrathecal administration is not possible. Supplement with IV benzodiazepines if needed. Cyproheptadine may also be useful; the initial dose is 12 mg orally, then 2 mg every 2 hours as needed, to a maximum dose of 32 mg/day.

Toxicity: management of mild to moderate toxicity usually requires only supportive care. Management of severe toxicity may require more aggressive intervention. Monitor the need for airway management, including endotracheal intubation in patients with CNS depression or recurrent seizures. Treat seizures with IV benzodiazepines and barbiturates. Treat hypotension with fluids and vasopressors. Atropine may be used to treat hypotension associated with bradycardia.

For patients who have ingested more than 100 mg, and who are alert or have a protected airway, activated charcoal may be administered. Hemodialysis may be particularly useful in patients with impaired renal function. In the event of intrathecal overdose, immediately empty the remaining baclofen solution from the pump reservoir. If not contraindicated, withdraw approximately 40 mL of CSF through the access port or by lumbar puncture. Frequently monitor mental status, cardiopulmonary status, urine output, and the ability to protect the airway. Monitor CPK in patients with prolonged or recurrent seizures.

References

1. http://www.onlinedrugtest.info. July 12, 2009.

2. http://en.wikipedia.org/wiki/Baclofen. July 12, 2009.

3. MICROMEDEX® Healthcare Series: DRUGDEX® Drug Point. May 15, 2009.

4. MICROMEDEX® Healthcare Series: Martindale – The Complete Drug Reference. Copyright 2008.

5. http://www.drugs.com/mmx/apo-baclofen.html. May 19, 1999.

96

Corticosteroids: intravenous, neuraxial, and articular

Johan Raeder

Indroduction

The corticosteroids (Figure 96.1) are naturally occurring hormones in the body, with a diurnal variation in circulating levels and increased circulating levels during trauma and stress. Typically about 25–50 mg of cortisone is secreted during a normal 24 hour period. The clinical analgesic effect of stress hormones has long been acknowledged, for instance during combat situations where the pain threshold seems to be significantly elevated, possibly partly due to corticosteroids and other stress hormones. It has also been shown that animals with elevated levels of endogenous corticosteroids experience less pain than others. Potential analgesic and clinical benefits of corticosteroids are outlined in Table 96.1.

Mechanisms of action

Corticosteroids act by binding to a class of nuclear receptors (corticosteroid receptors). Upon binding to the receptor transfer (chaperone) protein, the drug–receptor complex diffuses into the nucleus of the cell and binds to DNA. Then production of proteins and enzymes with subsequent clinical effects are initiated. Traditional pharmacokinetic parameters are not appropriate for describing corticosteroid pharmacodynamics, since genetic activation is associated with significant latency to effect. For this reason, onset is typically delayed, with maximum effects observed after 3–4 hours or more. For the same reason, the duration of clinical effect is prolonged and does not correlate with plasma concentrations of drug. In general, effects on cellular processes will continue for hours to days, despite complete clearance of drug from plasma. Some direct cellular membrane effects of corticosteroids have also been suggested. The rapid membrane stabilization from glucocorticoids during anaphylactoid reactions and a study showing analgesic effect within 1 hour of administration are clinically supportive of these non-DNA mediated effects of corticosteroids.

Molecular mechanisms of corticosteroids

The family of steroid molecules includes potent hormones, necessary for normal homeostasis and growth of the human body. Basically both mineralocorticoids and glucocorticoids are subclasses of the corticosteroid family, but for analgesia and the rest of this chapter only the glucocorticoids will be discussed. The glucocorticoids have virtually no sex hormonal properties, but some of them may still have slight mineralcorticoid effects (Table 96.2) resulting in renal sodium and water retention. There are also some reports of increased blood sugar levels, especially in diabetic patients. The major effects of the glucocorticoid subclass of steroid hormones are linked with the inflammatory response; including inhibition of inflammatory gene expression and stimulation of anti-inflammatory gene expression. Important mediators include TNF inhibition and leukocyte inhibition in the peripheral injured tissue. COX-2 inhibition is seen both in the periphery, in the spinal dorsal horn and in the central nervous system. As a part of this general anti-inflammatory action, glucocorticoids also have direct effects on blood capillaries, with decreased permeability and reduced vasodilatation.

A general anti-inflammatory action may be very important for pain reduction per se, by reducing local tissue pressure and limiting the release of potent pain mediators. The glucocorticoids have also been shown to have direct effects on pain neurons and receptors. They reduce neuropeptide release, inhibit signal transmission in C fibers and stimulate the secretion of endogenous endorphins.

Clinical actions of glucocorticoids

The well-known clinical effects of glucocorticoids include anti-inflammation, anti-edema, anti-allergic and antipyrexia. Also, analgesia and antiemetic effects

383

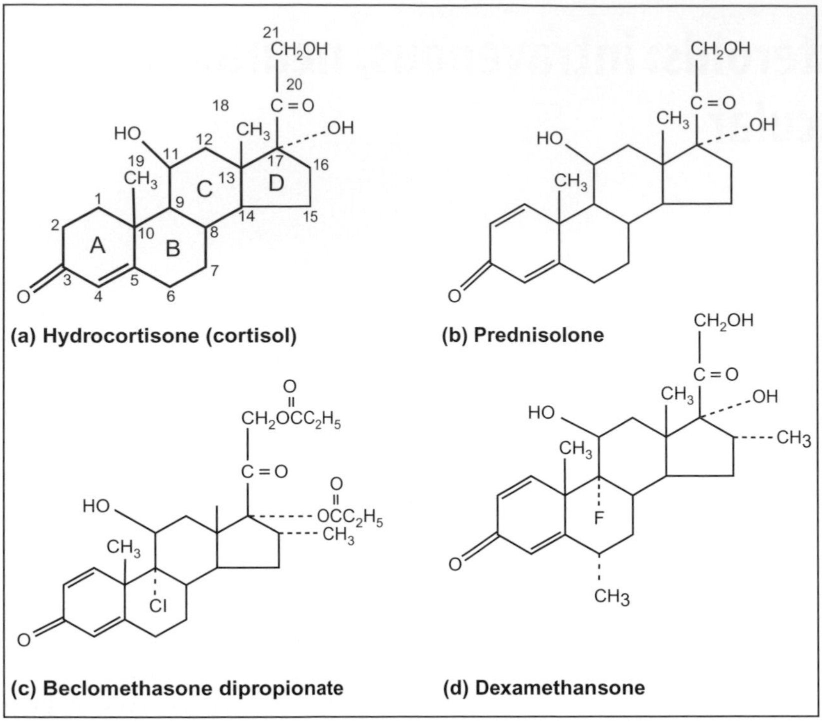

Figure 96.1. The chemical structure of glucocorticoids and other steroid hormones.

(a) Hydrocortisone (cortisol)

(b) Prednisolone

(c) Beclomethasone dipropionate

(d) Dexamethansone

Table 96.1. Clinical effects of glucocorticoid actions

Anti-inflammatory
Anti-edema
Analgesia
Antiemesis
Antipyretic
Euphoria
Increased alertness
Increased energy
Restlessness
Increased appetite

are well documented, although the mechanism especially of antiemesis is less well understood. The glucocorticoids frequently induce a slight feeling of euphoria and alertness, being documented in the post-operative setting as less sedation when these drugs are used (Table 96.1). The patient may sometimes describe a sensation of more "energy" and also increased appetite may be beneficial in this setting. On the other hand, there are also reports of restlessness, dysphoria, and even rare cases of abrupt psychosis, when glucocorti-coids are used for analgesia. Less post-operative shivering has been observed and fewer cardiac arrhythmias. Antiarrhythmic effect is only shown in some studies, whereas others have not demonstrated this effect.

With prolonged use of these drugs there is a very long list of non-beneficial effects, resulting from a generalized reduction in tissue growth, deprived cellular activation and wound healing. The clinical manifestations may be: wound rupture, non-fusion of fractures, gastric ulceration and perforation, skin vulnerability and wound formation, poor infection control. Also, hormonal side-effects may develop, such as moon-face appearance, sexual hormone dysfunction, mental disturbances, and hyperglycemia. Some adverse events associated with long-term glucocorticoid exposure are outlined in Table 96.3.

Clinical analgesic action after systemic injection

The analgesic effect of glucocorticoids has been well documented, especially in the post-operative setting. Compared with other analgesics, the onset of clinical effect is generally delayed. In this investigator's experience, no analgesic effect was evident during the first 4 hours following IV administration of 16 mg dexamethasone to patients recovering from breast surgery. This

Table 96.2. Steroid pharmocokinetic/dynamic characteristics

Drug	Half-life (hr)	Equivalent dose (mg)	Anti-inflammatory potency	Mineral corticoid potency	Na$^+$-retaining potency
Short-acting Hydrocortisone	8–12	20	1	1	1
Cortisone	8–12	25	0.8	0.8	0.8
Intermediate Prednisolone	18–36	5	4	0.8	0.8
Prednisone	18–36	5	4	0.8	0.8
Methylprednisone	18–36	4	5	0.5	0.8
Triamcinolone	18–36	4	5	0	0
Long-acting Dexamethasone	36–54	0.75	25	0	0

Endogenous cortisone production: 25–50 mg/day ≈ 1–2 mg dexamethasone. Modified from Salerno A, Hermann R. *J Bone Joint Surg* 2006;**88**:1361–1372.

Table 96.3. Steroid side effects

Dermatological	Endocrine
Skin thinning	Diabetes
Alopecia	Adrenal-pituitary insufficiency
Hirsuitism	
Acne	
Striae	
Bone	Gastrointestinal
Osteoporosis	Gastritis
Avascular necrosis	Peptic ulcer disease
	Bowel perforation
Muscle	Neuropsychiatric
Myopathy	Euphoria
	Dysphoria
Renal	Psychosis
Fluid volume shifts	Insomnia
Hyperkalemia	
Cardiovascular	Reproductive
Hypertension	Amenorrhea
Cardiomyopathy	Infertility
Immunological	
Increased risk of infection	
Herpes zoster	

correlates with previous reports of delayed onset of effect. However, there are reports of onset of post-surgical analgesia provided by 125 mg IV methylprednisolone, evident at 60 min after administration. This is in accordance with experimental and clinical evidence suggesting that glucocorticoids may have rapid and direct, non-genomic actions on cellular membranes.

The duration of analgesic effect provided by single doses of IV glucocorticoid may be prolonged for at least 3 days. The plasma elimination half-life of dexamethasone is only about 6 h, thus there seem to be ongoing drug effects for a significant period after drug clearance from the plasma. Both the slow onset and prolonged effect from a single dose may be explained by the assumed basic major effect mechanisms of glucocorticoid.

The optimal dose for glucocorticoid analgesic effect is not established, as controlled dose-finding studies have not been performed. For the antiemetic effect, a dexamethasone dose of 3–4 mg seems to be optimal, whereas for analgesia 8–16 mg seems to be necessary in adults.

Although glucocorticoids have been shown to inhibit the cyclooxygenase 2 (COX-2) enzyme system, much like NSAIDs, they also have hormonal effects and act on a variety of other enzyme systems. Thus, it is of interest to elucidate how the analgesic effect compares with other analgesics in placebo-controlled models. Paracetamol seems to have more analgesic efficacy during the first 3–4 hours after administration, whereas dexamethasone provides delayed analgesia. Patients treated with a single IV dose NSAID (i.e. ketorolac) experienced a more rapid onset of analgesia, while those treated with methylprednisolone required significantly less rescue analgesics during post-operative days 2 and 3.

An important question that must be addressed is whether or not the glucocorticoids provide measurable analgesic effects when they are administered in multimodal analgesic regimens.

In one placebo-controlled study, the analgesic effect of dexamethasone, 8 mg, was effective in addition to a regimen of local wound anesthesia, paracetamol and ketorolac. Similarly, in another study, the analgesic effect of a glucocorticoid was additive to that provided by local anesthesia, paracetamol and codeine. Several studies have shown that the specific analgesic effects of a glucocorticoid plus an NSAID or coxib is better than NSAID or coxib alone, also when paracetamol is included in the control group.

Neuraxial glucocorticoids

Neuraxial glucocorticoids are used for pain management associated with acute and chronic localized low back pain as well as radiating pain, such as with ischialgia. The concept is to benefit from the local, peripheral effect of the glucocorticoid on inflamed or edematous tissue as well as blocking some of the actions of activated cytokines and immunological mediators in the tissue structures which are believed to be involved with the etiology of the pain. Whether or how much such effect from a localized high concentration is achieved by neuraxial injection different from simple intravenous or oral systemic administration is still debated. There are some data suggesting that glucocorticoids hardly penetrate the dura and thus should not be expected to reach elevated, nonsystemic concentrations around the nerveroots. Still, other data show that efficacy may be achieved with virtually no measurable glucocorticoid in the systemic circulation. In some studies, a transforaminal technique with aid of fluoroscopy has been used, in order to ensure deposition of drug closer to the painful structures than with conventional epidural technique.

Still, with all controversies as to mode of administration, choice of drug, dose, concentration or adjuvants, there seems to be proper documentation of analgesic effect from neuraxial glucocorticoids during acute episodes of low back pain and radiating pain. The effect may be evident within a few hours and may last for 1–3 weeks and up to 3–6 months in some studies. However, the analgesic effect does not seem to be superior to placebo when evaluated beyond this timeframe, or in terms of outcome or risk of recurrence. With chronic or subacute pain, the data provide far less, but still mostly positive, evidence for analgesia

with neuraxial glucorticoids. However, the potential risks of these neuraxial injections should be noted: headache from accidental dura puncture, nerve injury, hematoma, or localized infection.

Articular glucocorticoid

As with neuraxial injections, the concept of articular injection is to provide a high concentration of drug proximal to the location of the suspected origin of pain. Although intra-articular deposition certainly will produce a high concentration inside the joint, there is still a debate as to whether this is the major relevant site for pain treatment, as much of articular pain is believed to be mediated from structures outside the joint cavity, such as tendons, connective tissue, capsules, and muscle. Also, there is a concern that high concentration of intra-articular corticosteroid may have deleterious effects on cartilage and bone, as reported in some rare cases.

The joints most commonly studied for intra-articular glucocorticoid injection include the knee joint and the shoulder joint. In recent meta-analyses of knee joint injections, there was a significant analgesic effect of corticosteroids during the first week, lasting for 3–4 weeks in many patients, but not beyond. Similar effect and profile have been demonstrated for subacromial and other joint injections. No significant deleterious effects on cartilage or bone have been demonstrated after single injections in prospective studies. The injections seem to be more efficacious in patients with joint effusion or flares.

Other clinical effects and side effects

Glucocorticoids may also have beneficial effects on minimizing nausea and vomiting, and improving alertness, appetite, and mood. Potential adverse effects include hyperglycemia, flushing, restlessness, impaired wound healing, gastrointestinal ulceration, and increased infection risk. Increased alertness has also been described, which may be beneficial in a post-operative setting with more rapid clearheaded recovery and discharge. Adverse effects are unlikely following single-dose administration, but may increase with repeated doses.

In a meta-analysis of adverse effects after single-dose administration, no significant side effects were demonstrated in the 17 studies of 941 patients receiving dexamethasone. Even more impressive is the absence of side effects revealed in the meta-analyses of a much higher dose of mehylprednisolone (i.e. 15–30 mg/kg) used for chest-trauma care. In more than 2000 patients from 51 single studies, the only significant effect found was an improvement of pulmonary function with glucocorticoid. However, there have been intermittent reports of psychotic reactions after a single, high-dose administration of glucocorticoids. Also, in studies of dexamethasone 5–15 mg, a 20–40% non-dose-dependent increase in post-operative blood sugar has been noted.

Conclusion: glucocorticoids for analgesic injection

The glucocorticoids have analgesic effect with delayed onset of 1–4 h and prolonged duration for at least 1–3 days after a single IV dose. The analgesic peak potency seems to be comparable to the effects provided by optimal doses of NSAIDs and paracetamol. The combination of a glucocorticoid plus NSAIDs provides additive anti-inflammatory effects and analgesia. In addition, the glucocorticoids may offer a safe and useful substitute for patients with known contraindications to NSAIDs (asthma, allergy, renal failure, bleeding tendency).

For injection of glucocorticoids into neuraxial and joint structures, there seems to be the best analgesic effect with acute pain, lasting for some weeks; whereas the documentation of benefit declines with the increasing chronicity of pain and when observations beyond 2–3 months are done.

There seems to be minor difference in the effect of different glucocorticoids, although few comparative studies on equipotent doses of different drugs have been done. Still, for injection into delicate structures such as joints and peri-neuraxial tissue, there is a debate about which drug, formulation, and particle size is optimal.

References

1. Raeder J, Dahl V. Clinical application of glucocorticoids, anti-neuropathics and other analgesic adjuvants for acute pain management. In Sinatra R et al., eds. *Acute Pain Management*. Cambridge University Press, 2009, pp. 377–390.

2. Salerno A, Hermann R. Efficacy and safety of steroid use for post-operative pain relief. Update and review of the medical literature. *J Bone Joint Surg Am* 2006;**88**:1361–1372.

3. Abdi S, Datta S, Trescot AM, et al. Epidural steroids in the management of chronic spinal pain: a systematic review. *Pain Physician* 2007;**10**:185–212.

4. Arroll B, Goodyear-Smith F. Corticosteroid injections for painful shoulder: a meta-analysis. *Br J Gen Pract* 2005;**55**:224–228.

5. Bellamy N, Campbell J, Robinson V, et al. Intraarticular corticosteroid for treatment of osteoarthritis of the knee. *Cochrane Database Syst Rev* 2005;CD005328.

6. Gruson KI, Ruchelsman DE, Zuckerman JD. Subacromial corticosteroid injections. *J Shoulder Elbow Surg* 2008;**17**:118S–130S.

7. Staal JB, de Bie RA, de Vet HC, et al. Injection therapy for subacute and chronic low back pain: an updated Cochrane review. *Spine* (*Phila Pa* 1976) **2009**;34:49–59.

8. Stafford MA, Peng P, Hill DA. Sciatica: a review of history, epidemiology, pathogenesis, and the role of epidural steroid injection in management. *Br J Anaesth* 2007;**99**:461–73.

Oral corticosteroids

Kianusch Kiai and David Burbulys

Numerous preparations are available including:

Generic Name: dexamethasone

Chemical Name: 9α-fluoro-11β,17α,21-trihydroxy-16α-methylpregna-1,4-diene-3,20-dione

Proprietary Names: Decadron®, DexPak®, Maxidex®, Baycadron®, Ozurdex® and several others in the USA and other countries

Manufacturers: Merck and several others in the USA and other countries

Class: corticosteroid, adrenal glucocorticoid, synthetic glucocorticoid

Generic Name: prednisone

Chemical Name: 17α,21-dihydroxypregna-1,4-diene-3,11,20-trione

Proprietary Names: Deltasone®, Deltacortisone®, Deltadehydrocortisone®, Orasone®, Prednisone® and several others in the USA and other countries

Manufacturers: Bristol-Myers-Squibb, Merck, Novartis, Pharmacia & Upjohn and several others in the USA and other countries

Class: corticosteroid, adrenal glucocorticoid, synthetic glucocorticoid

Chemical Structure: dexamethasone, see Figure 97.1; prednisone, see Figure 97.2

Mode of activity

Oral corticosteroids have many properties which may be beneficial in acute and chronic pain relief. They are principally anti-inflammatory or immunosuppressant agents that are derived from adrenal steroids and have primarily glucocorticoid activity with limited or no mineralocorticoid activity.

At the molecular level, unbound glucocorticoids easily cross the cell membrane and bind to specific cytoplasmic receptors. This modifies transcription and protein synthesis of many enzyme systems to achieve the drug's goal. These include stabilizing leukocyte lysosomal membranes, preventing the release of destructive acid hydrolases from leukocytes, reducing leukocyte adhesion to capillary endothelium, inhibiting macrophage accumulation in inflamed areas, reducing capillary wall permeability and edema formation, antagonizing histamine activity and the release of kinins from substrates, reducing the inflammatory response to bacterial endotoxins and cell-wall components, reducing the release of cytokines, reducing activity and volume of the lymphatic system producing lymphocytopenia, decreasing the activity of tissue to antigen–antibody complexes and depressing immunoglobulin and complement concentrations and passage of immune complexes through basement membranes.

The anti-inflammatory actions are thought to involve phospholipase A_2 inhibitory proteins. These, in turn, control many of the mediators of inflammation such as prostaglandins and leukotrienes by inhibiting the release of the precursor molecule arachidonic acid. This reduction in inflammation, edema, and tumor burden is especially beneficial in reducing bone pain, neuropathic pain from infiltration or compression of structures, spinal cord compression, pain from bowel obstruction or organ capsule distention, pain from lymphedema, and headache pain associated with increased intracranial pressure.

In addition to these anti-inflammatory and immunosuppressive activities of pain control, oral corticosteroids have several other properties that make them useful as multipurpose adjuvant analgesics, especially in patients with pain associated with chronic disease or cancer. The mechanisms of these effects are less well worked out but corticosteroids also stimulate the erythroid cells of bone marrow and prolong the survival time of erythrocytes and platelets. They promote gluconeogenesis and protein catabolism. They reduce chemotherapy-induced nausea and vomiting, and alleviate dyspnea, effusion

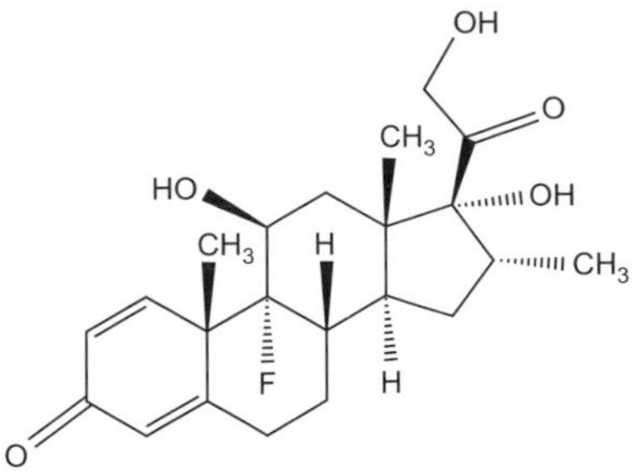

Figure 97.1.

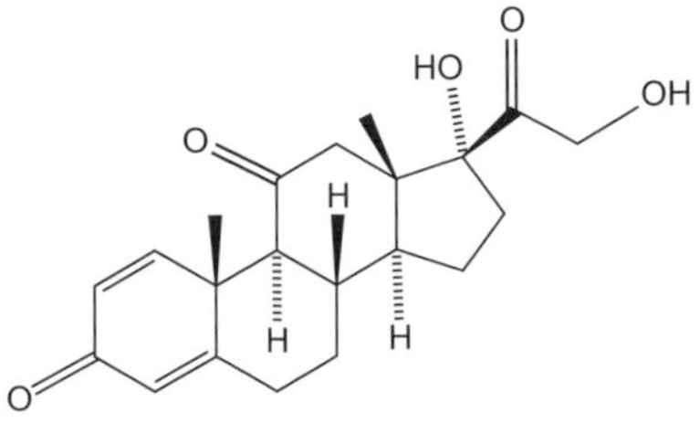

Figure 97.2.

or hypercalcemia, stimulate appetite and improve malaise and mood, and lead to a sense of well-being.

Corticosteroids have also been shown to have use as an adjunctive treatment for acute post-operative neuropathic pain in several animal studies. This most probably involves inhibiting the production of proinflammatory cytokines secreted at or near the site of nerve injury and reducing the development and maintenance of central sensitization and neuropathic pain. Further research is needed, however, in this area.

Prednisone and dexamethasone are rapidly absorbed across the GI mucosa following oral administration. Peak effects are observed in 1–2 hours. The circulating drugs bind extensively to plasma albumen and transcortin. Unbound drug is quickly distributed into the kidneys, intestine, skin, liver, and muscle where dexamethasone has its active effects. Prednisone undergoes hepatic metabolism to its active metabolite, prednisolone, prior to redistribution to the tissues for its effects. Both drugs are further metabolized by the liver to inactive compounds which are then excreted in the urine. Prednisone has a plasma half-life of approximately 1 hour but has a biological half-life of 18–36 hours. Dexamethasone has a biological half-life of 2–3 days. Corticosteroids are well distributed into breast milk and easily cross the placenta.

Indications

FDA-approved uses

Oral corticosteroids have several FDA-approved indications; none of which is for primary pain management.

There are several, though, which may be considered adjuvant analgesia uses. These include treating:

- cerebral edema associated with primary or metastatic brain tumor, craniotomy or head injury
- hypercalcemia of malignancy
- inflammatory disorders of the musculoskeletal system
- palliative management of leukemia and lymphoma.

Off-label uses

Several studies have suggested that oral corticosteroids may also have benefit in the direct or adjuvant relief of acute or chronic pain associated with:

- headache (migraine, cluster, acute mountain sickness)
- cancer (leukemia, lymphoma, myeloma)
- complications of cancer (edema, inflammation, effusions, treatment complications, hollow viscous obstruction, solid organ capsule distension, nausea and vomiting, loss of appetite, and depressed mood)
- post-operative nausea and vomiting
- AIDS wasting syndrome and cachexia
- various inflammatory, infectious or autoimmune disorders.

Contraindications

Absolute: hypersensitivity to the drug or any other component of the product. Active or suspected ocular or periocular infection (herpes simplex keratitis, vaccinia, varicella, mycobacterial disease or fungal infection), systemic fungal infections, advanced glaucoma or concurrent administration of live vaccines in patients receiving immunosuppressive doses.

Relative: active or latent peptic ulcer disease, recent intestinal anastomoses, nonspecific ulcerative colitis (increased risk of perforation), diabetes, adrenocortical insufficiency (may persist for months after discontinuing therapy), active or latent tuberculosis, cerebral malaria, chicken pox, measles, latent amebiasis or strongyloides infection, inactivated viral or bacterial vaccines where antibody response may not be induced, cirrhosis, congestive heart failure, renal failure or hypertension (increased risk of sodium retention, edema and potassium loss), hypokalemia or hypocalcemia, emotional instability or psychotic tendencies, hypothyroidism, growth retardation in infants and children, myasthenia gravis (risk of acute myopathy), optic neuritis, osteoporosis, pregnancy, breast feeding, birth control (may reduce effectiveness), and recent myocardial infarction (may increase risk of wall rupture).

Common doses and uses

Oral corticosteroids are generally administered in either a high- or low-dose regimen depending on the indication. A high-dose regimen of dexamethasone, up to 80–100 mg/day in four divided doses, is often used for spinal cord compression or an acute episode of severe pain that cannot be reduced with opioids. For prevention of chemotherapy-induced nausea and vomiting, 20 mg of dexamethasone is often given followed by 8 mg twice a day for 3 days. A 10 mg loading dose, followed by 4 mg every 6 hours, is often used for acute cerebral edema due to primary or metastatic brain tumor. These doses are generally tapered rapidly over a few days once the symptoms improve or other therapy is instituted. Lower-dose regimens of 2–4 mg once or twice a day of dexamethasone may be used for patients with advanced cancer who continue to have moderate pain despite optimal dosing of opioid drugs. Similar dosing may also be beneficial for intractable nausea and vomiting or to improve appetite and malaise. Five mg of prednisone is equivalent to 0.75 mg of dexamethasone. Because the therapeutic effects of corticosteroids are of longer duration than the metabolic effects, intermittent treatment (every other day) may allow the metabolic rhythm of the body to become re-established while maintaining the therapeutic value.

Potential advantages

As part of multimodal analgesia they are a useful adjunctive agent to relieve pain through their anti-inflammatory and immunosuppressant properties. This is especially beneficial for pain associated with arthritis or other chronic inflammatory processes, cancer, AIDS, and other chronic painful disease states. In addition to modulating pain, they have the added benefit of reducing swelling, edema, effusions, and inflammation and improving appetite, controlling nausea and vomiting, and promoting a sense of general well-being. They are easily prescribed, inexpensive, non-addictive, widely available, and in oral formulation.

Potential disadvantages

Side effects

Mineralocorticoid adverse effects include hypertension, sodium and water retention, potassium and calcium depletion, hypokalemic alkalosis, edema and potentially congestive heart failure in susceptible individuals. Glucocortocorticoid adverse effects include mobilization of calcium and phosphorus leading to osteoporosis and spontaneous fractures, avascular necrosis of bone, muscle wasting, hyperglycemia, peptic ulceration, lypolysis and fat redistribution, hirsutism, bruising, striae, acne, thromboembolic complications, impaired tissue repair and delayed wound healing, impaired immune function and increased susceptibility to infection, masking and early dissemination of infection, skin thinning, the development of glaucoma and cataracts, mental and neurological disturbances, and secondary adrenocortical insufficiency which may persist for months or years.

Drug interactions

Corticosteroids interact with many drugs and classes including amphotericin B (may worsen severe hypokalemia), hepatic P450 enzyme inducers (increases metabolism of corticosteroids), antacids (decreases bioavailability), digoxin (increases digoxin toxicity due to hypokalemia), diuretics (increases diuretic effects, worsens hypokalemia), insulin and other oral hypoglycemic agents (corticosteroids worsen glucose intolerance), NSAIDS (increased risk of GI bleeding), and vaccines (increases risk of disseminated infection with live virus and reduces effectiveness of attenuated or killed vaccines).

Drug-related adverse events

There are no commonly reported specific drug-related adverse effects with oral corticosteroids, but there are numerous significant effects and side effects (listed above), many of which may be life-threatening.

References

1. DynaMed®, EBSCO Publishing. Dexamethasone, 2009.
2. DynaMed®, EBSCO Publishing. Prednisone, 2009.
3. Micromedex®Healthcare Series, DrugDex® Evaluations, Martindale – The Complete Drug Reference, and Posindex®, Tompson Healthcare. Dexamethasone, 2009.
4. Micromedex®Healthcare Series, DrugDex® Evaluations, Martindale – The Complete Drug Reference, and Posindex®, Tompson Healthcare. Prednisone, 2009.
5. Knotkova H, Pappagallo M. Adjuvant analgesics. *Anesthesiol Clin North Am* 2007;**27**:775–786.
6. Lussier D, Huskey A, Portenoy R. Adjuvant analgesics in cancer pain management. *Oncologist* 2004;**9**:571–591.

Antihistamines

98

Sharon Lin

Antihistamines

First-generation H1 antihistamines

Generic Name (proprietary name): chlorpheniramine (Aller-chlor®, Ahist™, Chlor-Trimeton®), diphenhydramine hydrochloride (Benadryl®), hydroxyzine (Vistaril®)
Manufacturer: Pfizer Inc., New York, NY
Generic Name (proprietary name): promethazine (Phenergan®)
Manufacturer: Baxter Healthcare, Deerfield, IL

Second-generation H1 antihistamines

Generic Name (proprietary name): acrivastine (Semprex®-D)
Manufacturer: UCB Pharma, Inc., Smyrna, GA
Generic Name (proprietary name): cetirizine (Zyrtec®), desloratadine (Clarinex®)
Manufacturer: Schering-Plough, Kenilworth, NJ
Generic Name (proprietary name): fexofenadine (Allegra®)
Manufacturer: Sanofi-Aventis U.S. LLC, Bridgewater, NJ
Generic Name (proprietary name): levocetirizine (Xyzal®)
Manufacturer: UCB Pharma, Inc., Smyrna, GA; Sanofi-Aventis U.S., LLC, Bridgewater, NJ
Generic Name (proprietary name): loratadine (Claritin®, Alavert™)
Manufacturer: Shering-Plough HealthCare Products Inc. Division of Merck & Co., Inc.,1 Merck Dr, Whitehouse Station, NJ

H2 antihistamines

Generic Name (proprietary name): cimetidine (Tagamet®), famotidine (Pepcid®)
Manufacturer: Merck & Co., Inc., Whitehouse Station, NJ
Generic Name (proprietary name): nizatidine (Axid®), ranitidine (Zantac®)
Manufacturer: GlaxoSmithKline, Philadelphia, PA
Chemical Structure: diphenhydramine hydrochloride, see Figure 98.1; fexofenadine hydrochloride, see Figure 98.2

Description

More than 40 H1 antihistamines are available and are among the most widely used medications. The most common use of antihistamines is to suppress allergic inflammation in the mucous membranes and other body organs, preventing symptoms such as itching, congestion, rhinorrhea, tearing, sneezing, flushing, and urticaria. Antihistamine medications have also been used for antiemetic effects, as a peri-operative sedative, and for the treatment of insomnia. With the beneficial anti-inflammatory effects, antihistamines have been utilized as an adjunct agent to promote analgesia in patients with an inflammatory component to pain (post-surgical or infectious etiology). First-generation H1 antihistamines cross the blood–brain barrier and are seldom the drugs of choice due to sedation, while second-generation H1 antihistamines do not cross the blood–brain barrier to any appreciable extent and are popular because they are less sedating. H2 antihistamines are used primarily to inhibit gastric acid secretion in patients with gastroesophageal reflux disease, dyspepsia, or peptic ulcer disease.

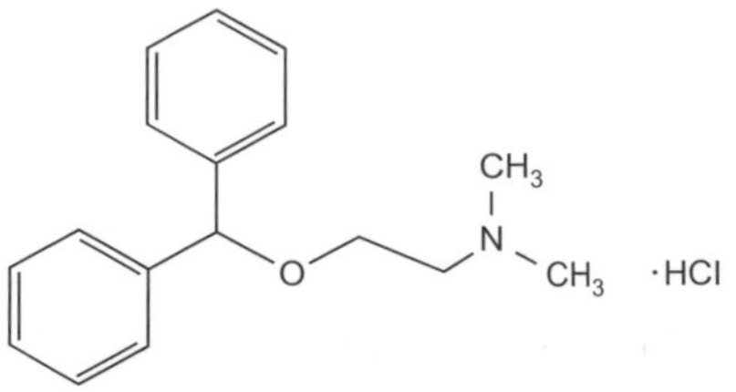

Figure 98.1.

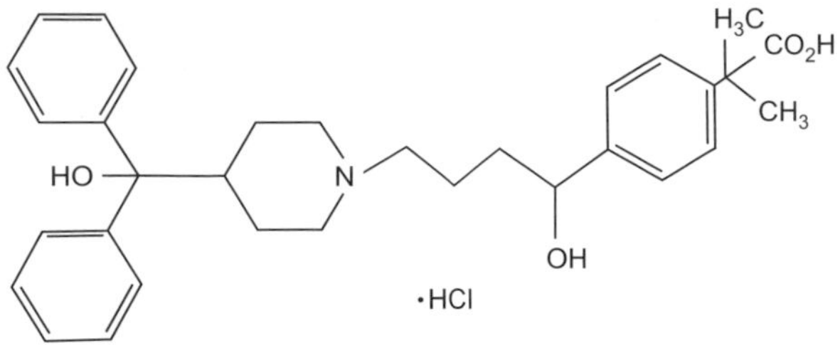

Figure 98.2.

Mode of activity

Major and minor sites of action: the major sites of action include the H1 and H2 receptors, which are widely expressed throughout the body. The H1 receptors are expressed in neurons, smooth muscle of airways, and vasculature, while H2 receptors are primarily expressed in gastric mucosa parietal cells, smooth muscle, and cardiac cells. Although H3 and H4 receptors have been discovered in histaminergic neurons and bone marrow, respectively, currently there are no inverse agonists available for clinical use.

Receptor interactions

Antihistamines are classified as inverse agonists, which bind and stabilize the inactive form of the histamine receptor. H1 antihistamines act on endothelial cells to decrease postcapillary venule permeability and leakage of plasma protein, decreasing the size of wheal and flare response. The effect of H1 antihistamines in airway smooth muscle histamine receptors is bronchodilatation. In the central nervous system, first-generation H1 antihistamines cross the blood–brain barrier and bind with the H1 receptors, resulting in sedation and antiemetic effects via blockade of the histaminergic signal from the vestibular nucleus to the vomiting center in the medulla. As second-generation H1 antihistamines do not significantly penetrate the blood–brain barrier and are highly specific for the H1 receptor, they are non-sedating and without significant side effects. H1 antihistamines also interact with muscarinic receptors, alpha-adrenergic receptors, serotonin receptors, and cardiac ion channels, resulting in decreased inflammatory mediator release. H2 antihistamines bind H2 receptors in the gastric parietal cells, inhibiting acid secretion and decreasing vascular permeability.

Metabolic pathways

The onset of action of most second-generation oral antihistamines is within 1–3 hours, with peak serum levels in 2–3 hours and dosing once to twice daily. Antihistamines are absorbed well orally due to the liposolubility of these molecules, facilitating their bioavailability. The typical elimination half-life of H1 antihistamines ranges from 2 hours for acrivastine to 27 hours for desloratadine. The residual effects of H1 antihistamines may persist for days after discontinuation of the drug. If allergen skin tests are to be performed, most H1 antihistamines need to be discontinued 5–6 days prior to testing. Second-generation H1 antihistamines are extensively metabolized by the hepatic cytochrome P450 (CYP450) system and are largely excreted unchanged in the urine and feces.

Indications (approved/non-approved)

Surgical acute pain: oral and parenteral doses of antihistamines are used as an adjunct to decrease inflammation to promote analgesia. Following noxious stimulation, an inflammatory response occurs and locally released neurotransmitters such as substance P and tachykinins promote vasodilatation and histamine release from blood cells. Additional histamine is released in response to tissue damage and activation of mast cells. Antihistamines in combination with opioids have been found to provide superior pain relief compared to equivalent doses of opioids alone, therefore antihistamines may have an opioid-sparing effect. However, one study found no difference in pain relief with a single dose of terfenadine (withdrawn by FDA in 1997) after oral surgery.

Medical pain: H1 antihistamines appear to be effective in treating renal colic pain, one of the most severe forms of pain. The mechanism involves the inhibition of renal vasodilatation in the occluded ureter, the inhibition of prostaglandin release, and prevention of spontaneous urethral contractions. H2 receptor antagonists are used for the treatment and maintenance of gastroesophageal reflux disease, peptic ulcer disease, and dyspepsia.

Chronic non-malignancy pain: antihistamines may be helpful in patients with myofascial pain, as one of the possible mechanisms of pain is believed to be associated with stimulation of H1 receptors on sensory nerve terminals resulting in arterial vasodilatation and increased capillary permeability.

Cancer pain: currently, there is no well-defined role for H1 antihistamines in treating cancer pain.

Contraindications

Absolute: hypersensitivity or documented severe allergic reaction.

Relative: patients with hepatic or renal dysfunction may require dose adjustment.

Common doses

See Tables 98.1–98.3.

Potential advantages

Ease of use, tolerability: second-generation H1 antihistamines are better tolerated by patients compared to first-generation H1 antihistamines because they are less sedating and have fewer side effects. Although there is no pharmacological tolerance to antihistamines, some first-generation H1 antihistamines have been drugs of abuse.

Table 98.1. First-generation H1 antihistamines

Drug	Dose	Preparations	Duration of action	Common adverse reactions	Considerations
Chlorpheniramine (Aller-chlor®, Ahist™, Chlor-Trimeton®)	4 mg PO q4h-q6h or sustained release 8–12 mg PO q8h-q12h, maximal oral dose 24 mg/day; 5–40 mg IM, IV or SC as a single dose, maximum parenteral dose 40 mg/day	4 mg (Aller-Chlor®), 12 mg (Ahist™, Chlor-Trimeton®), SR 8 mg and 12 mg tablets (PO); 10 mg/mL (IV)	3–6 hours	Cardiac dysrhythmias, constipation, drowsiness, dizziness, epigastric discomfort, hypotension, increased bronchial secretions, urinary retention, somnolence	No specific advantages, available without prescription
Diphenhydramine hydrochloride (Benadryl®)	25–50 mg PO q4h-q6h, maximal oral dose 300 mg/day; 10–50 mg IV/ IM or IV q2h-q3h, maximal parenteral dose 400 mg/day	25 mg, 50 mg tablets (PO); 50 mg/mL (IV)	4–6 hours	Dizziness, drowsiness, photosensitivity, paradoxical excitement, tachycardia, thickened bronchial secretions, urinary retention	Most sedating antihistamine, useful for insomnia, available without prescription
Hydroxyzine (Vistaril®)	25 mg PO TID-QID; 25–100 mg IM q4–6h	10 mg, 25 mg, 50 mg tablets (PO); 50 mg/mL (IM)	4–6 hours	Agitation, drowsiness, dizziness, dry mouth, weakness	IV route not recommended due to digital gangrene, possible psychological effects of withdrawal, requires prescription
Cyproheptadine (generic)	4 mg PO TID- QID, maximal dose 0.5 mg/kg per day	4 mg tablets (PO)	6–9 hours	Abdominal discomfort, dry mouth diarrhea, nausea, rash, urticaria, photosensitivity, weight gain	Serotonin antagonist, requires prescription
Promethazine (Phenergan®)	6.25–12.5 mg PO QD; 12.5–25 mg IV q4h-q6h	12.5 mg, 25 mg, 50 mg tablets (PO); 25 mg/mL (IV)	4–6 hours	Drowsiness, dermatitis, photosensitivity, somnolence	Effective antiemetic and adjunct for post-operative pain, requires prescription

Table 98.2. Second-generation H1 antihistamines

Drug	Dose	Preparations	Duration of action	Common adverse reactions	Considerations
Acrivastine (Semprex®-D)	8 mg acrivastine one tablet PO TID, maximal dose 4 tablets/day	8 mg acrivastine/ 60 mg pseudoephedrine tablets (PO)	12 hours	Blurred vision, dizziness, dry mouth, excitability, headache, hypertension, palpitations, somnolence, thickened bronchial secretions	Usually combined with pseudoephedrine; relatively non-sedating, requires prescription
Cetirizine (Zyrtec®)	5–10 mg PO QD	5 mg, 10 mg tablets (PO)	24 hours	Abdominal pain, diarrhea, dizziness, drowsiness, headache, dry mouth, nausea	Once-daily dosing, favorable side-effect profile, relatively non-sedating, available without prescription, expensive
Desloratadine (Clarinex®)	5 mg PO QD	5 mg tablets (PO)	24 hours	Dry mouth, dizziness, dyspepsia, headache, myalgia, nausea, somnolence	Once daily dosing, relatively non-sedating, requires prescription
Fexofenadine (Allegra®)	60 mg PO BID or 180mg PO QD	30 mg, 60 mg, 180 mg tablets (PO)	12–24 hours	Diarrhea, dizziness, dyspepsia, headache, myalgia, somnolence	Relatively non-sedating, favorable side-effect profile, expensive, requires prescription
Levocetirizine (Xyzal®)	5 mg PO QD	5 mg tablets (PO)	32 hours	Dry mouth, epistaxis, nasopharyngitis, somnolence, weakness	Active *R*-enantiomer of cetirizine with higher affinity for H1 receptor, unclear clinical relevance, relatively non-sedating, requires prescription
Loratadine (Claritin®, Alavert™)	10 mg PO QD	10 mg tablets (PO)	24–48 hours	Abdominal pain, diarrhea, drowsiness, headache, dry mouth, paradoxical excitement	Relatively non-sedating, favorable side-effect profile, available without prescription

Cost: inexpensive over-the-counter formulations are available for both H1 antihistamines and H2 antihistamines. Second-generation H1 antihistamines are generally more expensive than first-generation and may not be covered by insurance carriers due to the availability of over-the-counter formulations.

Availability: over-the-counter and prescription antihistamines are available in virtually all pharmacies.

As monotherapy: while H1 antihistamines have the potential to decrease opioid requirement and enhance analgesia, these medications are rarely used as monotherapy.

As used for multimodal analgesia: H1 antihistamines have been reported to decrease morphine and acetaminophen requirement for post-operative pain. When H1 antihistamines are given in combination

Table 98.3. H2 antihistamines

Drug	Dose	Preparations	Duration of action	Common adverse reactions	Considerations
Cimetidine (Tagamet®)	300 mg PO QID;300 mg IV/IM q6h-q8h, maximal oral and IV dose is 2400 mg/day	200 mg, 300 mg, 400 mg, 800 mg tablets (PO); 150 mg/mL (IV/ IM)	4–8 hours (PO), 4–5 hours (IV)	Confusion, diarrhea, dizziness, elevated LFTs, gynecomastia, headache, drowsiness, nausea, rash	May cause confusion in geriatric patients, multiple drug interactions due to hepatic microsomal enzyme inhibition (CYP3A4, CYP2D6), some formulations require prescription
Famotidine (Pepcid®)	20 mg PO BID; 20 mg IV BID	10 mg, 20 mg, 40 mg tablets (PO); 10 mg/mL (IV)	9–12 hours (PO); 10–12 hours (IV)	Constipation, diarrhea dizziness, headache	More potent than cimetidine and ranitidine, requires prescription
Nizatidine (Axid®)	150 mg PO BID	75 mg tablets (PO)	10 hours	Abdominal pain, agitation, constipation, dizziness, dyspepsia, elevated LFTs, headache, nausea, somnolence	Highest bioavailability, least hepatic metabolism, available without prescription
Ranitidine (Zantac®)	150 mg PO BID; 50 mg IV/IM q6h-q8h	75 mg, 150 mg, 300 mg tablets (PO); 25 mg/mL (IV)	4–12 hours (PO); 6–8 hours (IV)	Diarrhea, dizziness, dry mouth, constipation, headache, myalgias, nausea, rash, vertigo	Useful for patients unresponsive to cimetidine, available without prescription

with opioids, there is higher analgesic efficacy compared to equivalent doses of opioids alone.

Potential disadvantages

Toxicity: H1 antihistamines exert effects on cardiac ion channels independently of the H1 receptor, resulting in prolonged QT intervals. Terfenadine (Seldane) and astemizole (Hismanal), first-generation H1 antihistamines which have been withdrawn by the FDA and replaced by second-generation H1 antihistamines, inhibit the potassium rectifier currents resulting in slower repolarization and rarely ventricular arrhythmias such as torsades de pointes. Diphenhydramine and other first-generation H1 antihistamines may result in supraventricular arrhythmias, and dose-related QT prolongation and sinus tachycardia. There have been no reported cardiotoxic effects of second-generation H1 antihistamines. Patients at increased risk of cardiotoxicity include patients with organic heart disease, cardiac arrhythmias, or electrolyte imbalance (hypocalcemia, hypokalemia, hypomagnesemia). The effects of H1 antihistamines on alpha-adrenergic receptors may result in hypotension, dizziness, and reflex tachycardia. Large doses of antihistamines may cause seizure activity; however, it has been suggested that H1 receptors are clustered around epileptogenic foci in the brain and inhibit generalized seizure activity. H2 antihistamines may result in rare renal or hepatotoxicity, polymyositis, interstitial nephritis, or myelosuppression with thrombocytopenia, anemia and neutropenia. H2 antihistamines are associated with confusion, restlessness, somnolence, agitation, headaches, and dizziness. Rapid infusion of a H2 antihistamine may result in sinus bradycardia, hypotension, prolonged QT interval, AV block, and cardiac arrest.

Drug interactions

Concomitant use of drugs or alcohol with CNS depressant effects may increase the risk of adverse reactions with H1 antihistamines. H2 antihistamines have numerous effects including increasing the metabolism of drugs metabolized by CYP2B6, decreasing the absorption of antifungal medications, increasing the serum concentration of fentanyl via CYP3A4 inhibition, and decreasing the metabolism of selective serotonin reuptake inhibitors (SSRIs), amiodarone, anticonvulsants, benzodiazepines, and carvedilol.

Drug-related adverse events

Common adverse events

First-generation H1 antihistamines commonly result in sedation and impaired cognitive and psychomotor performance due to decreased CNS neurotransmission. Some first-generation H1 antihistamines have been associated with accidental or intentional overdose and have been drugs of abuse. Second-generation H1 antihistamines are less sedating and have few toxic effects in the setting of overdose. The effects on muscarinic receptors

may cause urinary retention, sinus tachycardia and dry eyes, dry mouth, constipation, diplopia, and hypotension. The effects on both the H1 receptor and the serotonin receptor may stimulate appetite and weight gain.

Treatment of adverse events

There is no specific antidote for antihistamine overdose. The treatment is primarily supportive therapy. Activated charcoal, cardiovascular monitoring when appropriate, and benzodiazepines for convulsions may be used to treat antihistamine overdose.

References

1. Simons FE. Advances in H1-antihistamines. *N Engl J Med* 2004;**351**(21):2203–2217.

2. Yilmaz E, Ertan B, Deniz T, et al. Histamine 1 receptor antagonist in symptomatic treatment of renal colic accompanied by nausea: two birds with one stone? *Urology* 2009;**73**(1):32–36.

3. Micromedex® Healthcare Series, DrugDex® Evaluations.

4. Berthold CW, Dionne RA. Clinical evaluation of H1-receptor and H2-receptor antagonists for acute postoperative pain. *J Clin Pharmacol* 1993;**33**:944–948.

5. Simons FE. H1-antihistamines: more relevant than ever in the treatment of allergic disorders. *J Allergy Clin Immunol* 2003;**112**(4):S42–S52.

Section 11 Chapter

99

Adjuvant Analgesics and Antiemetics

Parenteral antiemetics

Zhuang T. Fang

Nausea and vomiting are common side effects of opioids and volatile anesthetics. Opioid use is identified as one of the four major anesthetic risk factors (female gender, non-smoker, history of PONV and post-operative opioids) for post-operative nausea and vomiting (PONV). It is estimated as many as one-third of

patients who receive opioids for post-operative pain will experience nausea and vomiting. PONV can lead to significant morbidity; including dehydration and electrolyte abnormality, damage to wound closure, prolonged hospital stay or unanticipated hospital admission following ambulatory surgery, aspiration

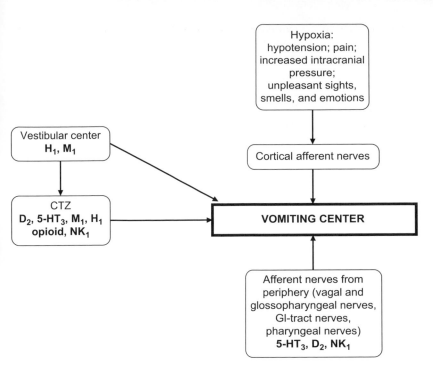

Figure 99.1. Pathways and neurotransmitters involved in post-operative nausea and vomiting. (With permission from Am J Health-Syst Pharm, 2005.)

pneumonia, and patient dissatisfaction. Prevention and treatment of PONV is an important part of the practice of modern anesthesia.

The precise mechanisms of nausea and vomiting are not clearly delineated. However, several receptors, including serotonin type 3 (5-hydroxytryptamine [5H-T$_3$]), dopamine type 2 (D$_2$), acetylcholine, histamine, and substance P have been identified in the chemoreceptor trigger zone (CTZ), nuclei tractus solitarii (NTS) and gastrointestinal (GI) tract. All are thought to play important roles in the afferent and efferent neurological process of nausea and vomiting. Activation of these receptors can lead to nausea and vomiting by delaying gastric emptying peripherally, and increasing emetic signaling at the CTZ and the vomiting center centrally (Figure 99.1). Opioid-induced nausea and vomiting (OINV) has not been studied alone extensively due to the challenge in separating nausea and vomiting induced by opioids per se from that caused by PONV, chemotherapy, or radiation. OINV may be due to the direct effects on the CTZ and vomiting center, decrease of pyloric tone leading to the delayed gastric emptying as well as the enhanced vestibular sensitivity. The experience of nausea and vomiting from all the causes (PONV, OINV, chemotherapy, radiation, etc.) may involve multiple receptors. Physiologically, vomiting is a reflex mediated by both the autonomic and somatic nervous systems and coordinated by the vomiting center in the brainstem. The dorsal and ventral respiratory groups are also involved in the process by regulating the phrenic nerve, leading to contraction of the diaphragm during vomiting. Drugs that are designed to inhibit these receptors significantly reduce post-operative and opioid-induced nausea and vomiting.

Ondansetron is the most popular drug currently used in the treatment and prevention of PONV. Ondansetron inhibits 5H-T$_3$ receptors in the CTZ as well as the GI tract. It is most efficacious when given immediately before the end of surgery for the prophylaxis of PONV. It is more effective in preventing vomiting than nausea. When used alone, ondansetron is superior to conventional antiemetic agents, such as droperidol and metoclopramide, in the prevention of PONV with minimal adverse effects. In certain surgical procedures where PONV must be avoided, including retinal, brain, head and neck, gastrointestinal and facial plastic surgeries, ondansetron is the drug of choice. An oral form of ondansetron is also available, but it is more commonly prescribed for the treatment of nausea and vomiting caused by chemotherapy or radiation therapy. Although it is not a common practice, 8 to 16 mg oral ondansetron given 1 hour before the induction of general anesthesia can significantly reduce the incidence of PONV in high-risk patients.

Although used extensively for the past several decades, droperidol and metoclopramide are less commonly used today because of their potential severe adverse effects, the black-box warning from the FDA for both drugs, and the comparable price of the generic ondansetron. Possible prolongation of the QT interval leading to torsade de pointes following droperidol use and tardive dyskinesia associated with metoclopramide use limit their use. However, there is little evidence to show that antiemetic doses (0.625 to 1.25 mg) of droperidol trigger this potentially fatal dysrhythmia. On the other hand, the tardive dyskinesia is usually associated with chronic (>3 months) use of metoclopramide for certain medical conditions, such as diabetic gastroparesis and symptomatic gastroesophageal reflux disease (GERD). Because of these concerns, both drugs should be reserved for patients who do not respond to or cannot tolerate other treatments. Both droperidol and metoclopramide are mainly the antagonists of D_2 receptors. Droperidol is

Table 99.1. General information

Agents	Ondansetron	Droperidol	Metoclopramide
Generic Name	Ondansetron	Droperidol	Metoclopramide
Chemical name	9-Methyl-3-[(2-methylimidazol-1-yl)methyl]-2,3-dihydro-1H-carbazol-4-one	3-[1-[4-(4-Fluorophenyl)-4-oxobutyl]-3,6-dihydro-2H-pyridin-4-yl]-1H-benzimidazol-2-one	4-Amino-5-chloro-N-(2-diethylaminoethyl)-2-methoxybenzamide
Proprietary name	Zofran	Droleptan	Reglan
Manufacturer and address	Baxter, One Baxter Parkway, Deerfield, IL 60015–4625	American Regent, Inc., One Luitpold Drive, P.O. Box 9001, Shirley, NY 11967	Hospira, Inc., 275 North Field Drive, Dept. 051M, Bldg. H1–2S, Lake Forest, IL 60045
Class	$5HT_3$ antagonist	Dopamine 2 antagonist	Dopamine 2 antagonist and GI stimulant

Table 99.2. Pharmacology

Agents	Ondansetron	Droperidol	Metoclopramide
Major site of action	Chemoreceptor trigger zone	Chemoreceptor trigger zone	Gastrointestinal tract
Minor site of action	Gastrointestinal tract	Gastrointestinal tract	Chemoreceptor trigger zone
Receptor interactions	Ondansetron is a selective serotonin 5-HT_3 receptor antagonist. It blocks 5-HT_3 receptors in the central CTZ and peripheral vagus nerve resulting in the reduction of vomiting reflex	Droperidol strongly antagonizes the effect of dopaminergic D_2 receptors in the CTZ and weakly antagonizes the cholinergic action leading to ganglionic blockage and reduction of afferent pathway of nausea and vomiting	It inhibits peripheral dopamine D_2 receptors resulting in increased GI motility and tone. Its antagonism of the central D_2 receptors raises the threshold of activity in the CTZ and decreases the sensitivity of visceral nerves supplying afferents to the vomiting center. It also antagonizes 5-HT_3 receptors at high dose
Metabolic pathways, drug clearance and elimination	Ondansetron is 70–76% protein-bound. It is metabolized by the hepatic cytochrome P450 and excreted in the urine and feces. Less than 10% of the dose is unchanged in the urine. Its half-life is 5.7 hours	Droperidol is 90% protein-bound. Its volume of distribution is 2.5 L/kg. Droperidol is extensively metabolized in the liver. 75% of the metabolites are excreted in the urine with 22% in the feces. Its elimination half-life is about 2 hours	Metoclopramide is 10–20% protein-bound. Its volume of distribution is 2–3.5 L/kg. Metoclopramide is mainly metabolized in the liver and its major metabolite is sulfate derivative; 80% of metoclopramide is excreted in the urine and 20% of that is unchanged. Its elimination half-life is 2.5–5 hours

Table 99.3. Clinical use of the agents

Agents	Ondansetron	Droperidol	Metoclopramide
Indications	Post-operative and chemotherapy-induced nausea and vomiting	Nausea and vomiting in surgical and diagnostic procedures; hiccups	Gastroesophageal reflux disease (GERD), PONV
Contraindications	Known hypersensitivity to the drug	Known hypersensitivity to the drug; known or suspected QT prolongation	Known hypersensitivity; patients receiving other drugs which may cause EPSs; epileptics; GI tract obstruction, perforation or hemorrhage; pheochromocytoma
Doses/uses (IV)	4 mg, IV	0.625–1.25 mg IV	10 mg, slow IV
Potential advantages	It is a most effective and safe drug for the prophylaxis and/or prevention of PONV. More effective for vomiting than nausea. Its side effects are mild. It is easy to administer and tolerated well	It is effective in the treatment of PONV. More effective in nausea than vomiting	It is easy to administer and tolerated well. It is effective if nausea and vomiting is due to gastric stasis
Potential disadvantages	Although it is a concern, no sufficient data to support dose adjustment in patients receiving P450 inducer or inhibitor	FDA black-box warning for QT prolongation and torsade de pointes. It can cause oversedation in patients receiving opioids. It can also cause hypotension and neuroleptic effects	FDA black-box warning for EPSs in chronic users. It can also cause neuroleptic effects
Toxicity	May lead to low blood pressure and fainting, sudden blindness and severe constipation	May cause extrapyramidal reactions (EPSs) and abnormalities of liver function tests	May cause EPSs and increase in prolactin production
Drug interactions	See additional information	See additional information	See additional information
Cost	$0.29 per vial of 4 mg	$0.76 per vial of 5 mg	$0.36 per vial of 10 mg
Drug-related adverse events	Headache, constipation, elevated liver enzymes and short-lasting QT prolongation, which is transient and usually self eliminated	Sedation, dizziness, anxiety, hypotension, QT prolongation and EPSs	Drowsiness, diarrhea and EPSs
Treatment of adverse events	Closely monitoring and supportive measure	Patients receiving droperidol should be monitored by EKG for 2 to 3 hours. If torsades de pointes should occur, ACLS protocol should start immediately	Slow IV push and administration of anxiolytics might reduce the incidence of EPSs. EPSs can also be prevented and treated by diphenhydramine and benzodiazepam

more effective in women than men. A small dose (0.625–1.25 mg) of droperidol and short term use of metoclopramide is still safe in carefully selected and monitored patients when the use of these drugs is indicated (i.e. treatment failure with ondansetron and/or dexamethasone). An oral form of metoclopramide is also available, but rarely used in the prophylaxis or the treatment of PONV or OINV.

In high-risk patients for PONV, combinations of drugs from different classes (5-HT$_3$ antagonists, anti-dopaminergics, anticholinergics, antihistamines and steroids) given peri-operatively are more effective, and therefore recommended. The antiemetic effect from the combination of ondansetron and droperidol is superior to the single use of either drug. It was estimated that the frequency of PONV in patients who carried all four risk factors decreased from 80% without antiemetics to 59%, 44% and 32% and 24% when one, two, three or four drugs (ondansetron, dexamethasone, droperidol and propofol) were administrated, respectively. However, patients receiving combined therapy could potentially face "combined" side effects as well. Acute cardiac dysrhythmia associated with the simultaneous or close administration of ondansetron and metoclopramide has been reported. For low-risk patients, it is not recommended to treat PONV prophylactically since the gain in benefit (the number needed to treat is about 40) does not outweigh the expense and risk of treatment. The efficacy of antiemetic treatment critically depends on surgical patients' baseline risk.

Post-operative pain is one of the major stressors leading to patients' discomfort and morbidity. Opioid analgesia, administered by the intravenous (bolus injection or patient controlled analgesia [PCA]), oral, intramuscular, or epidural routes, is the main stream of management for surgical patients' pain control. However, the opioid-induced nausea and vomiting may limit their usefulness. IV ondansetron (4 mg) was very effective in the treatment of nausea and vomiting in patients who underwent surgery with regional anesthesia (spinal, epidural, plexus, or peripheral nerve blocks) and required opioids (by IV or epidural injection) for pain post-operatively. It provided not only a 6-hour period free of nausea and vomiting but also significant reduction of nausea and vomiting in the 24-hour period compared to the placebo group. The addition of droperidol to the PCA with morphine in a dose of 0.017–0.17 mg droperidol/mg of morphine prevented nausea or vomiting in one in every three patients, with only an infrequent incidence of excessive drowsiness or extrapyramidal reactions. On the other hand, mixing metoclopramide with morphine for the use of PCA had insignificant effectiveness in reducing nausea and vomiting. However, the prokinetic effect of metoclopramide could be useful if patients' nausea and vomiting is partially caused by the delay of gastric emptying from opioid use, by enhancing pyloric and lower esophageal sphincter tone, especially after the failure of other antiemetic treatment. Special caution should be exercised in patients who undergo bowel surgery (due to obstruction, perforation, or hemorrhage) since the stimulation of gastrointestinal motility from metoclopramide could potentially lead to the rupture of the bowel anastomosis.

General information, pharmacology, and clinical use of the three drugs are summarized in Tables 99.1–99.3.

Additional information

Drug interaction with ondansetron

Potent P450 inducers, including phenytoin, rifampicin, and carbamazepine, can significantly increase the clearance and decrease the blood concentration of ondansetron. However, there are not sufficient data to support dosage adjustment for patients taking these drugs.

Ondansetron may be associated with an increase in patient-controlled administration of tramadol.

Drug interaction with droperidol

CNS depressant drugs, including barbiturates, benzodiazepines, opioids, and general anesthetics, can increase or potentiate the sedative effect of droperidol.

Drug interaction of metoclopramide

Absorption of digoxin in the stomach may be diminished. Absorption of oral medication (e.g. acetaminophen, levodopa, tetracycline, and ethanol) in the small bowel may be increased. Insulin dosage may require adjustment because the action of metoclopramide will influence the delivery of food to the intestines and thus the rate of absorption. Metoclopramide increases the effect of succinylcholine and the serum levels of cyclosporine.

References

1. Gan TJ, Meyer TA, Apfel CC, et al. Society for Ambulatory Anesthesia guidelines for the management of postoperative nausea and vomiting (special article). *Anesth Analg* 2007;**105**:1615–1628.

2. Golembiewski J, Chernin E, Chopra T. Prevention and treatment of postoperative nausea and vomiting. *Am J Health Syst Pharm* 2005;**62**:1247–1260.

3. Domino KB, Anderson EA, Polissar NK, et al. Comparative efficacy and safety of ondansetron, droperidol, and metoclopramide for preventing postoperative nausea and vomiting: a meta-analysis. *Anesth Analg* 1999;**88**:1370–1379.

4. Rung GW, Claybon L, Hord A, et al. The intravenous ondansetron for postsurgical opioid-induced nausea and vomiting. *Anesth Analg* 1997;**84**:832–838.

5. Apfel CC, Korttila K, et al. A factorial trial of six interventions for the prevention of postoperative nausea and vomiting. *NEJM* 2004;**350**(24):2441–2451.

100

Oral antiemetics – aprepitant

Philip F. Morway

Aprepitant, a new class of antiemetics known as neurokin-1 (NK-1) receptor antagonists, was developed and marketed by Merck & Co. under the brand name Emend. It was initially approved in March of 2003 by the US Food and Drug Administration (FDA) as an oral medication for use in the prevention of acute and delayed chemotherapy-induced nausea and vomiting (CINV). By July of 2006 the FDA amended its initial recommendation to include aprepitant for use in the prevention of post-operative nausea and vomiting (PONV). In January of 2008, Merk & Co applied for and gained FDA approval for the use fosaprepitant, trade name Ivemend, an intravenously administered prodrug of aprepitant.

Chemical Structure: aprepitant, see Figure 100.1; fosaprepitant, see Figure 100.2
Systematic (IUPAC) Names: aprepitant: 5-([[(2R,3S)-2-((R)-1-[3,5-bis(trifluoromethyl)phenyl] ethoxy)-3-(4-fluorophenyl)morpholino] methyl)1H-1,2,4-triazol-3(2H)-one; fosaprepitant: [3-{[(2R,3S)-2-[(1R)-1-[3,5-bis (trifluoromethyl)phenyl]ethoxy]-3-(4-fluorophenyl)morpholin-4-yl]methyl}-5-oxo-2H-1,2,4-triazol-1-yl]phosphonic acid

Description

Aprepitant is the first member of this new class of antiemetic drugs which is a potent, selective, CNS-penetrant oral nonpeptide antagonist of the NK1 receptor. NK1 receptors are located throughout the GI tract, by way of vagal afferents, and the central nervous system. When stimulated by the neurotransmitter substance P, the vomiting reflex may be directly initiated. Like other antiemetic agents which exert their effects by blocking the action of specific neurotransmitters, aprepitant exerts its antiemetic effect by blocking the action of substance P on the NK1 receptor.

The study and development of aprepitant was initially focused on obtaining a more effective treatment for CINV. Following the administration of cytotoxic chemotherapeutic agents, such as cisplatin, more than 80% of patients experience chemotherapy-induced emesis, which appears to consist of both an acute and a delayed phase. Prior to the use of aprepitant the acute phase emesis responded well to 5-HT3 antagonists while the delayed phase was poorly controlled. With the advent of the NK1 receptor antagonist aprepitant, both the acute and delayed phase of CINV are well controlled. The control of the delayed phase of CINV may be due in part to the prolonged elimination half-life exhibited by aprepitant (9 to 13 hours compared to the elimination half-life of 3.8 to 4 hours for ondansetron, a $5HT_3$ receptor antagonist).

One of the fundamental features of aprepitant, and a major advantage it has over other chemotherapy-induced side-effect treatments, is that while it successfully antagonises the NK1 receptors it has very little affinity over other receptors such as serotonin, dopamine, and corticosteroids. It is estimated that aprepitant is at least 3000 times more selective of NK1 receptors compared to the other well-known neurotransmitter antagonists.

Mode of action

The mechanism of action of aprepitant is to block the neurotransmitter substance P from stimulating the NK1 receptor, thereby disrupting the vomiting reflex. NK1 receptors are located throughout both the central and peripheral nervous systems. Within the CNS, the majority of NK1 receptors are located within the medulla oblongata, most notably in the area postrema (AP) and in the nucleus tractus solitarius (NTS). These regions of the brainstem along with the dorsal motor vagal nucleus (DMVN) comprise what is referred to as the "vomiting center". In the PNS the NK1 receptors involved in promoting emesis are located within the vagal afferent fibers which originate in the GI tract and migrate directly to the

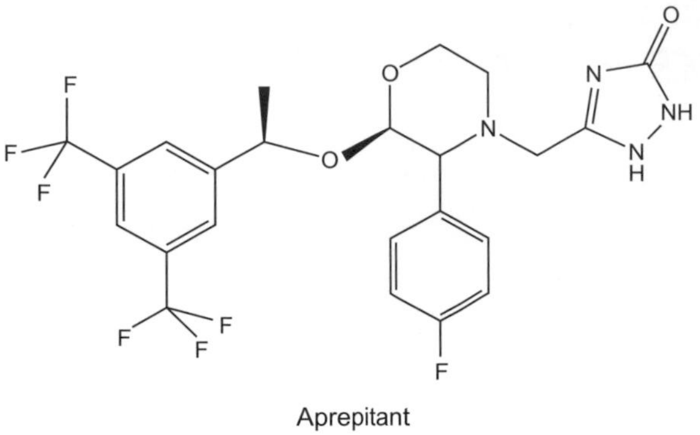

Aprepitant

Figure 100.1.

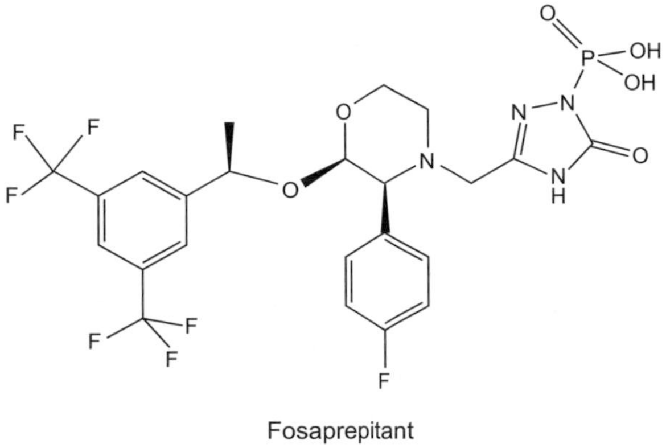

Fosaprepitant

Figure 100.2.

vomiting center in the medulla. The neurotransmitter substance P can be found in high concentrations within the vomiting center of the CNS, the gastrointestinal vagal afferent fibers of the PNS as well as stored in the enterochromaffin cells of the gastric mucosa.

The release of substance P can be elicited by the administration of certain cytotoxic agents used in chemotherapy as well as various anesthetic agents. Following the release of substance P within the CNS, the NK-1 receptors of the vomiting center can be directly stimulated, initiating the vomiting reflex. The vagal afferents of the GI tract can also be stimulated by substance P when it is released from the enterochromaffin cells of the GI tract following their destruction by these cytotoxic agents.

The use of aprepitant has also been shown to increase the activity of the 5-HT3 receptor antagonist ondansetron and the corticosteroid dexamethasone, which are also used to prevent the acute phase of CINV caused by chemotherapy.

Pharmacokinetic data

Summary:

Drug is absorbed orally with a t_{max} of 4 hours

Bioavailability 60–65%

Protein binding > 95%

Volume of distribution (Vdss) – 70 L in humans

Half-life 9–13 hours

Metabolism – hepatic, mostly mediated by CYP3A4

Minor metabolism by CYP1A2 and CYP2C19

In healthy young adults, aprepitant accounts for approximately 24% of the radioactivity in plasma over 72 hours following a single oral 300-mg dose of [14C] aprepitant, indicating a substantial presence of metabolites in the plasma. Seven metabolites of aprepitant, which are only weakly active, have been identified in human plasma.

Indications (approved/non-approved)

Aprepitant, in combination with other antiemetic agents, is indicated for the prevention of acute and delayed nausea and vomiting associated with initial and repeat courses of highly emetogenic cancer chemotherapy including high-dose cisplatin, and the prevention of nausea and vomiting associated with initial and repeat courses of moderately emetogenic cancer chemotherapy.

Aprepitant is indicated for the prevention of postoperative nausea and vomiting.

Contraindications

Absolute: aprepitant is contraindicated in patients who are hypersensitive to any component of the product. Aprepitant is a weak-to-moderate (dose-dependent) cytochrome P450 isoenzyme 3A4 (CYP3A4) inhibitor. Aprepitant should not be used concurrently with pimozide, terfenadine, astemizole, or cisapride. Dose-dependent inhibition of CYP3A4 by aprepitant could result in elevated plasma concentrations of these drugs, potentially causing serious or life-threatening ventricular arrhythmias.

Precautions and drug interactions

Precautions

1. Aprepitant is a dose-dependent inhibitor of CYP3A4, and should be used with caution in

patients receiving concomitant medications that are primarily metabolized through CYP3A4.

2. Moderate inhibition of CYP3A4 by aprepitant, 125 mg/80 mg regimen, could result in elevated plasma concentrations of these concomitant medications.

3. Weak inhibition of CYP3A4 by a single 40 mg dose of aprepitant is not expected to alter the plasma concentrations of concomitant medications that are primarily metabolized through CYP3A4 to a clinically significant degree.

4. When aprepitant is used concomitantly with another CYP3A4 inhibitor, aprepitant plasma concentrations can also be elevated

Drug interactions

Effects of aprepitant on:

1. Corticosteroids: noted an increase in plasma levels of dexamethasone or methylprednisolone when given concurrently with aprepitant. Corticosteroids are substrates for CYP3A4 and the inhibition of this enzyme by high-dose aprepitant leads to raised plasma levels of corticosteroids.

2. Benzodiazepines: midazolam is also metabolized by the isoenzyme CYP3A4, which when inhibited by high-dose aprepitant will lead to an increase in plasma levels for any given dose.

3. Warfarin: decrease in plasma levels of warfarin are seen due to the induction of the metabolic enzyme CYP2C9 by concomitant administration of aprepitant

4. Oral contraceptives: the co-administration of aprepitant may reduce the efficacy of hormonal contraceptives during and for 28 days after administration of the last dose of aprepitant. Alternative or backup methods of contraception should be used during treatment with aprepitant and for 1 month following the last dose of aprepitant.

Effects of drugs on aprepitant:

1. Ketoconazole, a strong inhibitor of CYP3A4, increases the effective half-life of aprepitant three fold.

2. Rifampin, a strong CYP3A4 inducer, effectively decreases the effective half-life of aprepitant three fold.

3. Diltiazem effectively doubles aprepitant's half-life while simultaneously decreasing its own efficacy.

4. Paroxetine, when given simultaneously with aprepitant, effectively decreases both agents' effective half-life.

Common doses

For the prevention of post-operative nausea and vomiting, 40 mg of aprepitant is given orally 3 hours prior to the induction of anesthesia.

When used for the treatment of chemotherapy-induced nausea and vomiting, aprepitant is given over 3 days as part of a combination antiemetic regimen that also includes a $5HT_3$ antagonist as well as a corticosteroid. The recommended dose is 125 mg orally 1 hour before chemotherapy on day 1 and 80 mg orally each morning on days 2 and 3.

Fosaprepitant, a prodrug of aprepitant, is rapidly converted in hepatic and extrahepatic tissues to aprepitant. When used for the treatment of CINV, 115 mg of fosaprepitant reconstituted in normal saline should be administered over 15 minutes 1 hour prior to chemotherapy. It has been determined that 115 mg of injectable fosaprepitant is equivalent to 125 mg of oral aprepitant.

To date, intravenous dosing has not been established for the prevention of PONV.

Potential advantages

A combined analysis of the two studies demonstrates that both aprepitant doses (40 and 125 mg) improved protection against nausea and vomiting and reduced the need for rescue therapy, compared with ondansetron. The 40 mg aprepitant dose also was found to be superior to ondansetron for the prevention of nausea, vomiting, and the need to use rescue therapy in the same patient.

Cost: the cost of one unit 40 mg dose of aprepitant used for the prevention of PONV is $47.84, whereas the cost for a 3-day course of aprepitant for use in the treatment of CINV (total dosage given over 3 days equals 285 mg of aprepitant) is approximately $250.00.

Currently, the most expensive drug for chemotherapy-induced nausea and vomiting is aprepitant since the generic version of ondansetron became available in 2007. A 4 mg dose of ondansetron may now cost the patient less than $20.00. The addition of aprepitant to this standard regimen increases the cost of antiemetic therapy more than 30 times but can increase the quality of life by reducing vomiting and nausea and decreasing the costs of additional antiemetics for rescue therapy.

Monotherapy: as noted above, for the treatment of PONV, aprepitant when used as a single antiemetic agent was superior to ondansetron in preventing nausea and vomiting as well as decreasing the need for rescue therapy.

Multimodal therapy: the addition of aprepitant to the combined ondansetron and dexamethasone regimen demonstrated a decrease in both the acute and delayed phases of chemotherapy-induced emesis.

Potential disadvantages

Toxicity: specific information regarding the toxicity of aprepitant has not been fully investigated. Single doses of up to 600 mg of aprepitant are well tolerated by healthy subjects with no subjective or objective side effects noted. This is also seen when 375 mg of aprepitant was administered daily for up to 42 days. Drowsiness and headache were reported in one patient who ingested 1440 mg of aprepitant. In the event of overdose, aprepitant should be discontinued and supportive treatment provided. Due to the antiemetic effect of aprepitant, drug-induced emesis may not be effective. Aprepitant cannot be removed by hemodialysis.

Drug-related adverse events

The results of various clinical trials indicated that the incidence of adverse events was similar in the aprepitant group compared with the group which received only standard regimen of ondansetron and dexamethasone. The most commonly observed side effects with aprepitant treatment were asthenia, hiccups, diarrhea, gastritis, elevation in liver function tests, and dizziness. There are also reports of thrombocytopenia and dehydration.

References

1. Roila F, Fatigoni S. New antiemetic drugs. *Ann Oncol* 2006;(supplement 2):96–100.

2. Girish C, Manikandan S. *Indian J Cancer* 2007;**44**: 5–30.

3. Sood M, et al. Aprepitant in PONV. *Clin Pharmacol* 2007;**23**(4):395–398.

4. Gan T, et al. A randomized, double-blind comparison of the NK1-antagonist, aprepitant, versus ondansetron for the prevention of postoperative nausea and vomiting. *Anesth Analg* 2007;**104**:1082–1089.

5. Aprepitant Oral: AHFS detailed monograph. Aprepitant/Fosaprepitant Dimeglumine http://cme.medscape.com/druginfo/monograph. Class Antiemetics, miscellaneous (56:22.92).

6. Product information: Aprepitant capsules (Emend–Merk) 2006.

101

Transdermal scopolamine

Joe C. Hong

Generic Name: transdermal scopolamine
Proprietary Name: Transderm Scop™
Class: antiemetic, antimuscarinic
Manufacturer: ALZA Corporation, Mountain View, CA; distributed by Norvartis Consumer Health, Inc., Parsippany, NJ
Chemical Structure: see Figure 101.1
Chemical Name: 9-methyl-3-oxa-9-azatricyclo [3.3.1.02,4]non-7-yl ester
Chemical Formula: $C_{17}H_{21}NO_4$; molecular wt 303.3

Introduction

Transdermal scopolamine is a muscarinic receptor antagonist used for the prevention of post-operative nausea and vomiting. It is supplied as a circular adhesive patch (0.2 mm thick and 2.5 cm²) applied to the post-auricular skin. Each patch contains 1.5 mg of the belladonna alkaloid programmed to continuously release in vivo approximately 1.0 mg over 72 hours. The patch consists of four distinctive layers. Going from visible surface to the surface adherent to the skin, these layers are: (1) backing layer; (2) drug reservoir of scopolamine; (3) microporous polypropylene membrane that controls the rate of scopolamine delivery; (4) adhesive contact surface with the skin.

Mode of activity

Major site of action: muscarinic-type acetylcholine receptors in the chemoreceptor trigger zone. In terms of nausea and vomiting prophylaxis, scopolamine is a competitive inhibitor of muscarinic acetylcholine receptors in the chemoreceptor trigger zone which communicates with the emetic center within the reticular formation of the brainstem. Outside the chemoreceptor trigger zone, scopolamine is also a competitive inhibitor at postganglionic muscarinic receptors in the parasympathetic nervous system. Antagonism of the parasympathetics is responsible for anticholinergic symptoms such as inhibition of salivation and perspiration, decreased gastrointestinal secretions and motility, drowsiness, mydriasis, and tachycardia.

Absorption and metabolism: circulating plasma levels of the percutaneously absorbed scopolamine are detected within 4 hours after applying the patch. Due to the tertiary amine structure of scopolamine (non-ionized), it readily crosses the blood–brain barrier as well as the placenta.

Scopolamine is extensively metabolized hepatically by the cytochrome P450 system. Less than 10% of the total transdermal dose is excreted in the urine as the parent compound or metabolites. The elimination half-life of scopolamine is 4.8 hours.

Indications

Transdermal scopolamine has current FDA indication only for the prevention of nausea and vomiting associated with motion sickness and recovery from anesthesia and surgery in adults. There is currently no FDA approval for use in the pediatric setting. A single 1.5 mg transdermal scopolamine patch should only be applied to the hairless area of the skin overlying the mastoid process. Only one patch should be worn at any time. The patch should not be cut or altered in any way as this will disrupt the delivery process.

In the peri-operative setting, the manufacturer currently recommends applying a single patch onto the post-auricular area the evening prior to the scheduled surgery. Alternatively, the patch can also be applied at least 4 hours before the antiemetic effect is required. In the obstetrics setting, the manufacturer recommends applying the patch 1 hour prior to cesarean

405

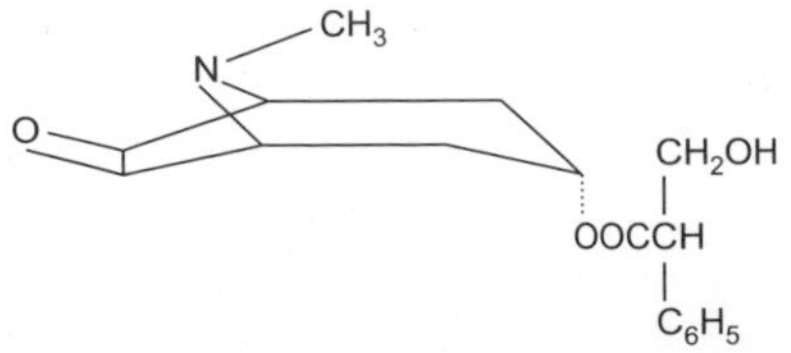

Figure 101.1.

$$CH_3$$

$$CH_2OH$$
$$OOCCH$$
$$C_6H_5$$

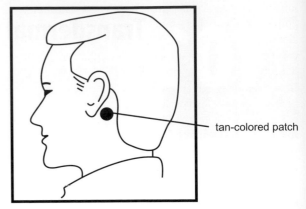

Figure 101.2. Placement of the transdermal scopolamine patch.

tan-colored patch

section to minimize exposure of the newborn baby to the drug. The patch may be safely removed 24 hours after surgery.

Contraindications

Absolute: transdermal scopolamine is absolutely contraindicated in patients with documented hypersensitivity to scopolamine or belladonna alkaloids. Hypersensitivity to the inactive components within the delivery system, which includes mineral oil and polyisobutylene, is also contraindicated. Patients with angle-closure (narrow-angle) glaucoma, myasthenia gravis, and intestinal bowel obstruction should not receive scopolamine. Patients scheduled for MRIs should have the patch removed as the aluminized backing may cause burn injury.

Relative: transdermal scopolamine may cause mydriasis leading to an increase in intraocular pressure in patients with chronic open-angle (wide-angle) glaucoma and should be used with caution. Patients with known liver or kidney dysfunction should use scopolamine patch with caution. Patients with history of psychosis or seizures should also avoid transdermal scopolamine.

Common doses

General: transdermal scopolamine is only available as a 1.5 mg patch designed to deliver approximately 1.0 mg of scopolamine over a 72 hour period. The patch must not be ingested, cut, divided, or altered in any way as this will disrupt the delivery system.

Peri-operative use: transdermal scopolamine can be applied to the post-auricular skin either the evening prior to scheduled surgery or 4 hours prior to the time of the desired antiemetic effect (Figure 101.2). In the obstetric setting, the patch should be applied 1 hour prior to delivery by cesarean section to minimize exposure to the newborn. The patch should be kept in place for 24 hours following surgery, at which time it should be removed and discarded.

Motion sickness: transdermal scopolamine should be applied 4 hours prior to the time of the desired antiemetic effect. The patch may be left on for up to 72

hours as needed to prevent motion sickness. Should therapy be needed for greater than 72 hours, the initial patch must be removed prior to the application of a new patch.

Potential advantages

Transdermal scopolamine has multiple advantages over its parenteral compound. The ability to deliver scopolamine transdermally results in needle-free administration and therefore a less-invasive therapy as well as improved safety for the healthcare provider. Blood concentration of transdermal scopolamine also tends to remain at or above the defined therapeutic level over time compared to the variable plasma concentrations with high peaks and low troughs with parenteral scopolamine. The lower continuous dose of transdermal scopolamine also minimizes the dose-dependent antimuscarinic side effects. Lastly, transdermal scopolamine provides a much longer duration of action (up to 72 hours) compared to 4 hours with parenteral scopolamine. Ambulatory patients therefore can continue to receive post-operative nausea and vomiting prevention from hospital to home.

Potential disadvantages

Common adverse events: common adverse events of transdermal scopolamine are related to its antimuscarinic effects outside the chemoreceptor trigger zone. The most common side effects are dryness of the mouth followed by drowsiness, dizziness, and transient impairment of eye accommodation resulting in blurred vision and dilatation of the pupils.

Serious adverse events: rare but serious adverse events of transdermal scopolamine are also antimuscarinic in nature. Signs and symptoms of severe antimuscarinic toxicity include lethargy, somnolence, coma, confusion, agitation, hallucination, convulsion, decreased GI motility, urinary retention, tachycardia, hypotension, and supraventricular arrhythmias. Scopolamine should therefore be used with caution in patients with suspected bowel obstruction, urinary bladder neck obstruction, history of seizures, or psychosis. Because scopolamine relies mostly on hepatic metabolism and to a lesser extent renal elimination, it should be used with caution in the elderly or patients with known or suspected liver or kidney dysfunction due to the increased likelihood of drug accumulation.

Drug-related adverse events

Drug interactions: because of the CNS depressant effect of transdermal scopolamine, caution needs to be excercised if the patient is concomitantly taking other CNS depressants such as alcohol, benzodiazepines, antihistamines, and opioid-based pain medications. The concomitant use of opioids may also increase the risk of decreased gastric motility and delayed gastric emptying.

Treatment of adverse events: in the presence of excess antimuscarinic side effects, the scopolamine patch must immediately be removed. Simple removal of the patch should resolve most cases of toxicity. However, in the setting of serious antimuscarinic toxicity, the patient must be continuously monitored and vital signs taken regularly. Continuous EKG monitoring is recommended as well as establishing intravenous access. Physostigmine may be titrated as needed to offset the antimuscarinic effects of scopolamine toxicity.

References

1. Kotelko DM, et al. Transdermal scopolaine decreases nausea and vomiting following cesarean section in patients receiving epidural morphine. *Anesthesiology* 1989;**71**:675–678.

2. Gan TJ, et al. Society for Ambulatory Anesthesia guidelines for the management of postoperative nausea and vomiting. *Anesth Analg* 2007;**105**(6): 1615–1628.

3. Clissold SP, et al. Transdermal hyoscine (scopolamine): a prelimary review of its pharmacodynamic properties and therapeutic efficacy. *Drugs* 1985;**29**:189–207.

4. Cronin CM, et al. Transdermal scopolamine in motion sickness. *Pharmacotherapy* 1982;**2**:29–31.

5. Transderm Scopolamine (package insert). Deerfield, IL: Baxter Healthcare Corporation; 2003.

Section 11
Chapter

102

Adjuvant Analgesics and Antiemetics

Topical capsaicin

Jure Marijic

Chemical Structure: see Figure 102.1

Description

Capsaicin is the main ingredient in the "hot" chili peppers that produces a hot, burning sensation when peppers are ingested and irritates eyes when they are exposed to the substance. Capsaicin is also the active ingredient in a number of creams that are marketed as over-the-counter remedies for topical pain control, "pepper spray" used by police for crowd control or individuals for self-defense, as well as more recently in some nasal decongestant and sinus medications.

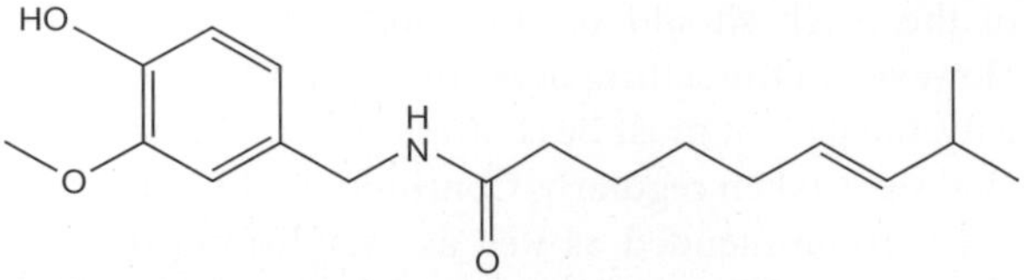

Figure 102.1.

Table 102.1. Commonest indications for capsaicin

Post-herpetic neuralgia
Pain in osteoarthritis
Diabetic neuropathy pain
Nondiabetic chronic polyneuropathy
Stump pain
Painful neuroma
Trigeminal neuralgia
Primary headaches
Pain from cancer infiltrating skin
Pain in oral mucositis
Postmastectomy pain syndrome

Mode of activity and pharmacology

Capsaicin is used topically for symptomatic relief of pain. Unlike other pain medications that decrease inflammation (NSAIDs) or prevent transmission (local anesthetics) and perception of pain (narcotics), capsaicin works on a special type of nociceptors at the origin of the pain signal. Capsaicin activates the capsaicin or vaniloid 1 receptor, which is a special type of temperature-sensitive transient receptor potential (TRP) non-selective ion channel (TTRP1). Capsaicin also induces release of substance P, which is responsible for runny nose, watery eyes, sweating, and gastric juice production. Capsaicin also releases endorphins; however, it appears that this does not play a major role in pain relief by capsaicin.

Pain relief by capsaicin is not immediate. In fact it usually takes several days to several weeks to get pain relief. Patients with arthritis can typically expect relief after 1–2 weeks of treatment, while with patients with neuralgias it may take twice as long (2–4 weeks). Patients with head and neck neuralgias may have to apply capsaicin for a much longer period of time to get pain relief. For this group of patients it may take over 6 weeks to get pain relief. The long time needed for capsaicin-induced pain relief appears to be due to the fact that capsaicin attenuates pain by producing neuroplastic changes in medullar dorsal horn and spinal cord nociceptive neurons.

In addition to its analgesic effect capsaicin has many other beneficial effects including a nasal decongestant effect, a topical anti-inflammatory effect and even an effect on cancer cell growth and death, cardiovascular disease, asthma, and bacterial infections.

How to use capsaicin in pain management

Capsaicin is used topically for symptomatic relief of pain. The medicine is applied to the painful area and gently rubbed in. Capsaicin is applied topically three or four times daily. It should be applied on clean dry skin and should not be used if skin is damaged, irritated, or infected. If capsaicin is used for treatment of pain associated with herpes zoster it should not be used until herpetic lesions have healed over. Care should be taken not to get capsaicin into the patient's eyes since it will cause pain and irritation. Therefore it is recommended to wash hands with soap and warm water after applying capsaicin to remove any medication from the hands and prevent eye irritation. A problem arises when the targets of treatment are hands and hand joints. In that case it is recommended not to wash the hands for as long as possible and at a minimum 30 minutes. In patients with painful osteoarthritis addition of glyceryl trinitrate enhances the analgesic effect of capsaicin. The mechanism of this enhancement is not clear. In certain patients with post-herpetic neuralgia (PHN) great symptomatic relief can be obtained from topical capsaicin; however, only 20% of patients get significant relief. Despite the lack of dramatic effect several pain societies still recommend topical capsaicin in treatment of PHN. Other indications for use of capsaicin include painful diabetic neuropathy and HIV-associated distal sensory neuropathy.

Capsaicin is available from many manufacturers and in many different concentrations ranging from 0.025 to 0.1%. A new experimental patch containing 8% capsaicin has been shown in two studies to be more effective than regular-dose (0.04%) capsaicin in treatment of post-herpetic neuralgia.

Capsaicin is not recommended for children younger than 2 years. For children 2 years or older topical capsaicin is believed to work in a similar way as for adults; however, caution should be used and this medicine should be used only under the supervision of a pediatric pain specialist. When used in the geriatric population its effectiveness, safety profile, and complications are believed to be similar to those in the adult population although there are no specific studies comparing different age groups (Table 102.1).

Side effects

When capsaicin is first applied to skin a warm stinging and sometimes burning sensation is felt by a majority of patients. With time (usually 2–4 weeks or in some patients longer) this sensation is diminished and most of the time completely disappears (tolerance). It seems that the higher the dose and the shorter the interval between applications of capsaicin the faster is the disappearance of the local sensations. Bathing in warm water, heat, humidity, and sweating will increase the sensation or may lead to reappearance of symptoms after they have disappeared. Since very little capsaicin is absorbed systemically there is little chance of interaction with systemically administered medication or a systemic effect of capsaicin. As preparations with higher concentrations (up to 8%) of capsaicin become available there is an increasing chance of systemic effects and interaction with other medications.

Bioavailability after topical administration of capsaicin is very low. The blood capsaicin levels are much lower than after ingestion of peppers and are not sufficient to produce systemic effects.

Potential advantages

Capsaicin is a natural product (extract from hot peppers) that is easy to use, delivered directly to the site of pain, with minimal systemic absorption and very low risk of toxicity and drug–drug interactions. There is also no need to titrate the dosage.

Potential disadvantages

Capsaicin is seldom effective in conditions associated with moderate to severe pain when used alone. Studies show no significant difference between capsaicin and placebo when used as a sole analgesic in cases of PHN or other causes of neuropathic pain.

Contraindications

The only known absolute contraindication is allergy to capsaicin. Capsaicin should not be used if skin is damaged, irritated, or infected.

References

1. Pittler MH, Ernst E. Complementary therapies for neuropathic and neuralgic pain. *Clin J Pain* 2008;**24**:731–733.

2. Caterina MJ, Leffler A, Malmberg AB, Martin WJ, Trafton J, Petersen-Zeitz KR, Koltzenburg M, Basbaum AI, Julius D. Impaired nociception and pain sensation in mice lacking the capsaicin receptor. *Science* 2000;**288**:241–242.

3. Honda K, Kitagawa J, Sessle BJ, Kondo M, Tsuboi Y, Yonehara Y, Iwata K. Mechanisms involved in an increment of multimodal excitability of medullary and upper cervical dorsal horn neurons following cutaneous capsaicin treatment. *Mol Pain* 2008;**4**:59.

4. Backonja M, Wallace MS, Blonsky ER, Cutler BJ, Malan P Jr, Rauck R, Tobias J. NGX-4010, a high-concentration capsaicin patch, for the treatment of postherpetic neuralgia: a randomised, double-blind study. *Lancet Neurol* 2008;**7**: 1106–1112.

5. Knotkova H, Pappagallo M, Szallasi A. Capsaicin (TRPV1 agonist) therapy for pain relief: farewell or revival? *Clin J Pain* 2008;**24**:142–154.

Topical salicylates

Jeremy M. Wong

Generic Name: methyl salicylate

Chemical Name: methyl O-hydroxybenzoate

Proprietary Formulations: Oil of wintergreen (98%), Icy Hot Extra Strength Cream (30%), Bayer Muscle Joint Pain Relief Cream (30%), Muscle Rub Extra Strength Cream (30%), Ben-Gay Extra Strength Cream (30%), Tiger Balm Liniment (28%), Ben-Gay Original Cream (18.3%), Pain Bust-R II Ointment (17%), Thera-Gesic Cream (15%), Banalg Hospital Strength Lotion (4.9%), asian herbal remedies (15–67%)

Generic Name: trolamine salicylate

Chemical Name: 2-(bis(2-hydroxyethyl)amino) ethanol; 2-hydroxybenzoic acid

Proprietary Formulations: Aspercreme Cream (10%), Myoflex Cream (10%), Mobisyl Crème (10%), Sportscreme Pain Relieving Rub (10%)

Generic Name: diethylamine salicylate

Chemical Name: diethylazanium; 2-hydroxy-benzoate

Proprietary Formulations: Algesal (10%)

Manufacturers: Pfizer, Chattem, Bayer, B F Ascher & Co., others

Class: external analgesic

Chemical Structure: methyl salicylate, see Figure 103.1; trolamine salicylate, see Figure 103.2

Mode of activity

Salicylate can be applied to the skin as un-ionized salicylic acid (normally for its keratolytic activity), as a salicylate salt (most commonly trolamine salicylate), as esters such as methyl salicylate and, rarely, as aspirin. In the form most often used in topical products, salicylates work primarily as rubefacients. Rubefacients are compounds that work by counter-irritation, causing skin irritation, local vasodilatation, and a feeling of warmth when applied to the skin surrounding soft tissue injuries. With this surface stimulation, an analgesic effect is achieved by masking the perception of pain. This is in contrast to topical NSAIDs (such as topical diclofenac), which act by inhibiting cyclooxygenase enzymes responsible for development of inflammatory processes.

Like topical NSAIDs, topical salicylates permeate the skin and are absorbed to a depth of 3–4 mm. The effect of rubefacients is thought to be due to the activation of Aβ fibers, which modulate pain signals transmitted by C fibers to the dorsal horn of the spinal cord. This prevents pain signals reaching the brain. The action of rubbing the skin also increases the penetration of rubefacient into the skin, disperses local tissue pain mediators, and results in the activation of Aβ fibers, thus enhancing the analgesic effect of rubefacients.

As well as being counter-irritants, salicylate compounds are hydrolyzed in the dermal and subcutaneous tissues to salicylic acid and have an anti-inflammatory action, although the exact mechanism of action of topical salicylates is still unclear. Salicylates may interfere with the activity of transcription factors and kinases involved in inflammatory processes, but do not appear to work through COX inhibition. In fact, data suggest that salicylates are approximately 100-fold less potent as inhibitors of COX-2 relative to ASA.

The salicylate compounds used topically share with aspirin the common metabolic breakdown product, free salicylate (see section on aspirin earlier in this text), which is primarily responsible for the toxicity observed. On average, 12–20% of the dose of methyl salicylate is absorbed through the skin. Methyl salicylate is readily hydrolyzed to salicylate, although some methyl salicylate is found in blood. Some unchanged methyl salicylate is excreted in urine as hydrolysis is relatively slow in humans.

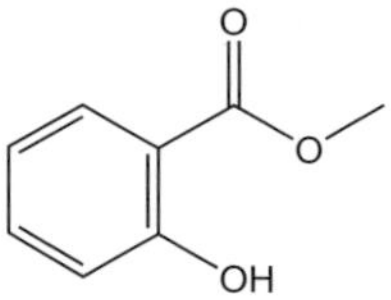

Figure 103.1.

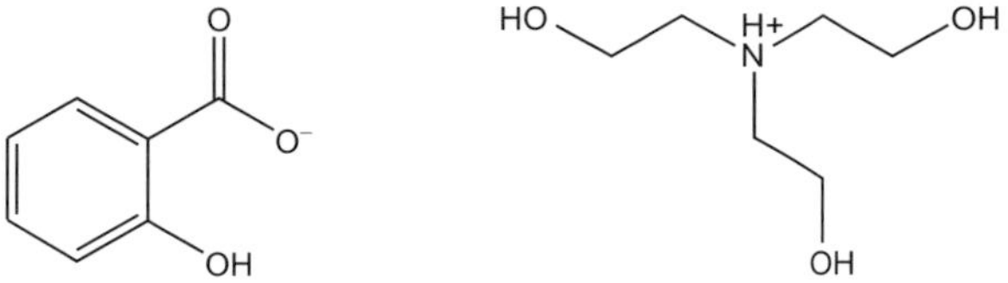

Figure 103.2.

Absorption of methyl salicylate from the skin depends on the pharmaceutical formulation (i.e. the type and quantity of vehicle), the area covered, the time and site of application, skin blood flow, temperature, and hydration, but in all cases studied the absorption of salicylate has been incomplete. For example, when creams and an ointment containing methyl salicylate were applied to 50 cm² areas of the forearm, only 12–20% of the methyl salicylate was absorbed over a 10-hour period, even though the skin was covered. The plasma levels of salicylate were low, at less than 10 mg/l. Nevertheless, substantial amounts of methyl salicylate are absorbed when applied to large areas of skin, especially when covered.

In contrast, percutaneous absorption of a salicylate salt (i.e. trolamine salicylate) is only about 1%, and the concentrations in the dermis and subcutaneous tissue are much lower than after application of methyl salicylate.

Aspirin is slowly absorbed from the skin. Very low levels of ASA are found in the blood after topical application (about 2 μM), but still sufficient to reduce prostaglandin synthesis in the GI tract with consequent gastric damage.

Diffusion of salicylate salts from skin into synovial fluid has only been studied in the knee, where the concentrations are too low for significant anti-inflammatory effect. Direct diffusion from skin into the synovial fluid appears insignificant, although these agents may still be effective for soft tissue rheumatism, which is frequently superficial.

Indications (approved/non-approved)

Indicated for the temporary relief of minor aches and pains of muscles, tendons, and joints such as those associated with strains, arthritis, simple backache, sprains, etc.

Acute surgical pain: topical salicylates are not often used for the treatment of acute surgical pain as they should not be applied to broken skin nor should they be covered with a dressing. These compounds can also potentially contribute to bleeding as evidence suggests they can interfere with platelet aggregation (see below).

Medical pain and chronic non-malignancy pain: efficacy estimates for rubefacients are unreliable because, while there are numerous case reports of efficacy of topical salicylates for the treatment of both acute and chronic pain, there is a lack of good clinical trials. The trials that have been performed are limited by number, size, quality, and validity. The only systematic review available of rubefacients containing salicylates concluded, from the limited information available, that these agents may be efficacious in acute pain and moderately to poorly efficacious in chronic arthritic and rheumatic pain. In acute conditions, the number needed to treat was 2.1 for at least 50% pain relief compared with placebo at 7 days. For chronic conditions, the number needed to treat for topical salicylate compared with placebo was 5.3. Of note, however, high-validity trials of chronic pain showed significantly less analgesic effect than low-validity trials. Interestingly, while it is thought that topical analgesics owe much of their efficacy to rubbing during application, a high placebo response rate has not been observed in the available clinical studies.

Although further study is needed, topical aspirin (local aspirin applied in a suitable solvent) has been found in some studies to be as effective as lidocaine for the treatment of post-herpetic neuralgia, with over 70% of patients responding to both treatments. In these studies, significantly more pain relief was provided by topical aspirin as compared to oral aspirin. The local levels of acetylsalicylate were 80–100-fold higher than after oral aspirin and circulating levels much lower.

Cancer pain: topical salicylates are unlikely to be beneficial for the treatment of anything other than localized cancer pain as the area of application must be limited to avoid toxicity.

Contraindications

Absolute: allergy to salicylate or sensitivity to any of its components.

Relative: patients with preexisting coagulation abnormalities (or taking warfarin) should use topical salicylates cautiously. Because of the risk of systemic absorption, also consider contraindications to aspirin.

Common doses/uses

Topical preparations should only be used externally on the skin. The compound is applied liberally to the painful area and massaged until absorbed. The total number of applications is recommended not to exceed three or four applications per day. The product should not be used on irritated or broken skin, and not covered with a tight bandage or used with a heating pad as this may cause skin damage. Use near the eyes or mucous membranes is advised against, and hands should be washed thoroughly after applying.

Potential advantages

Rubefacients can be used as adjuvants to oral analgesic therapy, support bandages, rest, ice, and compression, and may be useful in patients who cannot tolerate oral analgesics. They are often used in combination with massage therapy, with the rubbing action also contributing to the local heat and rubefacient effect. Depending on the type of compounds used, either a "warm" or "cold" sensation can be produced after topical administration. These compounds are easy to use, relatively inexpensive, available over the counter, well-tolerated by most, and may be efficacious for treatment of acute pain.

Potential disadvantages

If ingested or used improperly, there is a risk of salicylate toxicity. Evidence exists that topical salicylates can impair coagulation, by impairing platelet aggregation as well as by potentiating the warfarin effect. There is a small risk of local irritant or allergic contact dermatitis, as well as anaphylaxis. Topical salicylates have questionable efficacy, especially for the treatment of chronic pain conditions.

Drug-related adverse events

Contact dermatitis or anaphylaxis can occur from local application. Absorption through the skin is increased by large areas of application, repeated application, exercise, heat, broken skin, or covering the area with a bandage, and is higher with methyl salicylate preparations.

Systemic salicylate toxicity is possible with excess percutaneous absorption or after oral ingestion. The signs and symptoms of salicylate intoxication are related to local irritation of the GI tract (after oral ingestion), direct stimulation of the CNS respiratory center, stimulation of the metabolic rate, disturbance of carbohydrate and lipid metabolism, and interference with hemostasis. Typical GI symptoms of acute ingestion include vomiting, abdominal pain, and occasional hematemesis. Symptoms of acute systemic toxicity include hyperpnea, tachypnea, tinnitus, deafness, hyperpyrexia, diaphoresis, lethargy, confusion, coma, and seizures. Complications of salicylate poisoning include dehydration, electrolyte disturbances, mixed and complex acid–base disturbances, gastrointestinal ulcers, hepatitis, cerebral edema, CSF glucopenia, and noncardiogenic pulmonary edema. Salicylates rarely produce spontaneous hemorrhage, but even topically applied salicylates can impair platelet function and potentiate the effect of warfarin by inhibiting the vitamin K-dependent synthesis of factors VII, IX, and X. Symptoms of chronic salicylate poisoning are similar to those of acute poisoning, but GI symptoms may be less pronounced, patients appear more severely ill, and CNS symptoms may be more prominent. These findings can include agitation, confusion, slurred speech, hallucinations, seizures, and coma.

If skin irritation occurs, use of the product should be stopped and the skin washed thoroughly with soap and water. Professional advice should be obtained for ingestion of topical salicylate products, or immediate medical care for evidence of systemic toxicity. Emesis should not be induced for ingestion of salicylates, but activated charcoal may be helpful. Supportive care may be required, including intubation and ventilation, treatment of acid–base and electrolyte abnormalities, anticonvulsants, and vasopressors.

For ocular exposure, the eye(s) should be irrigated with room-temperature tap water for 15 minutes. If after irrigation the patient is having pain, decreased visual acuity, or persistent irritation, referral for an ophthalmological examination is indicated.

References

1. Rainsford KD. *Aspirin and Related Drugs*. Illustrated. Boca Raton: CRC Press, 2004.

2. Mason et al. Systematic review of efficacy of topical rubefacients containing salicylates for the treatment of acute and chronic pain. *BMJ* 2004;**328**; 995.

3. Altman et al. Topical therapy for osteoarthritis: clinical and pharmacologic perspectives. *Postgrad Med* 2009;**121**(2):139–147.

4. Chyka PA, et al. Salicylate poisoning: an evidence-based consensus guideline for out-of-hospital management. *Clin Toxicol* 2007;**45**:95–131.

5. Davis JE. Are one or two dangerous? Methyl salicylate exposure in toddlers. *J Emerg Med* 2007;**32**(1):63–69.

Adjuvant Analgesics and Antiemetics

Pamidronate

Rex Cheng and Zoreh Steffens

Class: analgesic agent

Generic Name: pamidronate, pamidronate disodium

Proprietary Name: Aredia

Manufacturer: Bedford Laboratories, Bedford, OH; several other manufacturers produce generic version of this medication

Chemical Structure: see Figure 104.1

Description

Aredia, pamidronate disodium (APD), is a bone-resorption inhibitor used to treat hypercalcemia associated with malignancy and osteolytic bone lesions associated with multiple myeloma, metastatic breast cancer, and moderate to severe Paget's disease of bone. Aredia, a member of the group of chemical compounds known as bisphosphonates, is an analog of pyrophosphate. Pamidronate disodium is designated chemically as phosphonic acid (3-amino-1-hydroxypropylidene) bis-, disodium salt, pentahydrate, (APD).

Pamidronate disodium is a white powder with inactive ingredients mannitol, USP, and phosphoric acid (for adjustment to pH 6.5 prior to lyophilization).

Pamidronate is not metabolized and is exclusively eliminated by renal excretion.

Mode of activity

Pamidronate disodium is a bisphosphonate which binds irreversibly to hydroxyapatite in bone. It is a strong inhibitor of bone resorption, reducing osteoclast or osteoclast precursor activity. Bisphosphonates inhibit bone resorption by selective adsorption to mineral surfaces and subsequent internalization by bone-resorbing osteoclasts.

Indications (approved/non-approved)

Pamidronate is one of the first drugs that has been proven to reduce the incidence of skeletal complications of metastatic breast cancer and prostate cancer. It also relieves bone pain caused by metastatic bone lesions. Other indications include treatment of osteolytic bone lesions of multiple myeloma, moderate-to-severe hypercalcemia of malignancy, and moderate-to-severe bone lesions due to Paget's disease.

Non-approved uses include treatment of pediatric osteoporosis and treatment of osteogenesis imperfecta. It has also been used to treat refractory pain of lumbar degenerative spinal stenosis.

Contraindications

Absolute: hypersensitivity to pamidronate, other bisphosphonates or any component of the formulation.

Relative: avoid use during pregnancy, breast-feeding or if conception is planned. Use caution when using in renally impaired patients.

Common doses

Pamidronate is poorly absorbed following oral administration, therefore IV treatment is preferred. Dilute prior to administration and infuse over at least 2 hours. Dosing intervals vary by treatment protocol.

Pamidronate is available in two doses:

Vials – 30 mg – each contains 30 mg of sterile, lyophilized pamidronate disodium and 470 mg of mannitol, USP

Vials – 90 mg – each contains 90 mg of sterile, lyophilized pamidronate disodium and 375 mg of mannitol, USP.

Due to the risk of deterioration of renal function, which may progress to renal failure, single doses of Pamidronate should not exceed 90 mg.

413

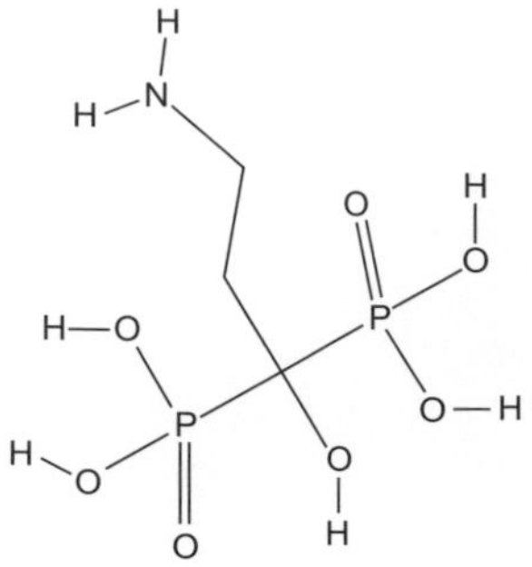

Figure 104.1.

Dosing should be adjusted for use in the elderly and in patients with renal impairment.

Potential advantages

Pamidronate has been shown to decrease pain associated with bone resorption of Paget's disease. Reductions of 30–50% in analgesic requirements have been documented with use of pamidronate in bone metastasis patients.

Skeletal complications, including pathological fractures, the need for radiation to bone or bone surgery, spinal cord compression, and hypercalcemia have been reduced in patients receiving pamidronate.

Potential disadvantages

Pamidronate has several drug interactions. Aminoglycosides may result in enhanced hypocalcemia. NSAIDs may enhance GI and nephrotoxicity. Phosphate supplements may enhance hypocalcemia. Thalidomide may result in increased nephrotoxicity.

Pamidronate may interfere with diagnostic imaging agents such as technetium-99m-diphosphonate in bone scans.

Drug-related adverse events

Central nervous system: fatigue, fever, headache, insomnia, somnolence, psychosis, seizure

Endocrine and metabolic: hypophosphatemia, hypokalemia/hyperkalemia, hypomagnesemia, hypocalcemia, hypernatremia, hypothyroidism

Cardiovascular: atrial fibrillation/flutter, hypertension/hypotension, syncope, tachycardia, CHF, edema, anaphylactic shock

Gastrointestinal: nausea, vomiting, anorexia, abdominal pain, dyspepsia, constipation, gastrointestinal bleeding, diarrhea, stomatitis

Genitourinary: UTI

Hematological: anemia, granulocytopenia, leucopenia, neutropenia, thrombocytopenia

Local: infusion site reaction

Neuromuscular and skeletal: weakness, myalgia, arthralgia, osteonecrosis of the jaw, back pain, bone pain

Renal: increased serum creatinine, uremia, acute renal failure

Respiratory: dyspnea, cough, URI, sinusitis, rales, pleural effusion, rhinitis, ARDS, bronchospasm

References

1. Katzung BG. *Basic & Clinical Pharmacology*, 10th ed. New York: McGraw-Hill.

2. McPhee SJ, Papdakis MA. *Current Medical Diagnosis & Treatment*. New York: McGraw-Hill, 2009.

3. Clezardin P, Gligorov J, Delma, P. Mechanisms of action of bisphosphonates on tumor cells and prospects for use in the treatment of malignant osteolysis. *Joint Bone Spine* 2000;**67**(1): 22–29.

Adjuvant Analgesics and Antiemetics

Ziconotide

Sunil J. Panchal

Generic Name: ziconotide

Trade/Proprietary Name: Prialt™

Drug Class: conopeptide analgesic

Manufacturer: Elan Pharmaceuticals, South San Francisco, CA 94080

Chemical Structure: see Figure 105.1

Chemical Formula: $C_{102}H_{172}N_{36}O_{32}S_7$; molecular Wt 2639; ziconotide is a 25 amino acid, polybasic peptide containing three disulfide bridges

Introduction

Ziconotide is a synthetic equivalent of a naturally occurring conopeptide found in the piscivorous marine snail, *Conus magus*. Ziconotide binds to N-type voltage-gated calcium channels located on the primary nociceptive (Aβ and C) afferent nerves in the superficial layers (Rexed laminae I and II) of the dorsal horn in the spinal cord. It was approved for use in the USA in 2004 for control of severe chronic pain.

Mode of activity

The exact mechanism of action of ziconotide has not been established in humans. Results in animals suggest that its binding blocks N-type voltage-gated calcium channels on the spinal terminals of primary afferent noxious fibers. Blockade of these channels inhibits the release of glutamate, substance P and other excitatory neurotransmitters from the central terminals of primary noxious fibers, and suppression of second-order spinal cell depolarization.

Metabolism

Ziconotide is cleaved by endopeptidases and exopeptidases at multiple sites on the peptide. Following passage from the CSF into the systemic circulation during continuous IT administration, ziconotide is expected to be susceptible to proteolytic cleavage by various peptidases/proteases present in most organs (e.g. kidney, liver, lung, muscle, etc.), and thus readily degraded to peptide fragments and their individual constituent free amino acids. Human and animal CSF and blood exhibit minimal hydrolytic activity toward ziconotide in vitro. The biological activity of the various expected proteolytic degradation products of ziconotide has not been assessed.

Elimination

Minimal amounts of ziconotide (< 1%) were recovered in human urine following IV infusion. The terminal half-life of ziconotide in CSF after an IT administration was around 4.6 hours (range 2.9–6.5 hours). Mean CSF clearance (CL) of ziconotide approximates adult human CSF turnover rate (0.3–0.4 mL/min).

Indications (approved/non-approved)

Approved indication: ziconotide intrathecal infusion is indicated for the management of severe chronic pain in patients for whom intrathecal therapy is warranted, and who are intolerant of or refractory to other treatment, such as systemic analgesics, adjunctive therapies, or intrathecal morphine.

Contraindications

Contraindications: Prialt is contraindicated in patients with a known hypersensitivity to ziconotide or any of its formulation components and in patients with any other concomitant treatment or medical condition that would render intrathecal administration hazardous. Patients with a preexisting history of psychosis should not be treated with ziconotide. Contraindications to the use of intrathecal analgesia include conditions such as the presence of infection at the microinfusion injection site, uncontrolled bleeding diathesis, and spinal canal obstruction that impairs circulation of CSF.

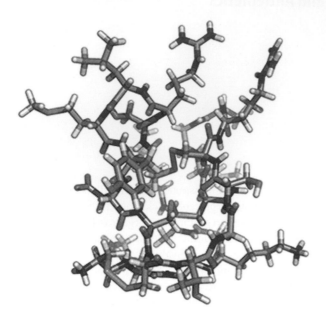

H–Cys—Lys—Gly — Lys

Ala — Gly

Cys   Lys

Cys   Asp - Tyr

H₂N— Cys

Thr   Cys —— Ser –Arg –Leu-Met

Lys   Gly – Ser

Gly – Ser –Arg – Cys

Figure 105.1.

Common doses

Ziconotide is approved as a neuraxial (intrathecal) analgesic for chronic pain. It is not approved for postoperative analgesia or for labor and delivery analgesia. The manufacturer recommends that intrathecal ziconotide should be initiated at no more than 2.4 µg/day (0.1 µg/h) and titrated to patient response. Doses may be titrated upward by up to 2.4 µg/day (0.1 µg/h) at intervals of no more than two or three times per week, up to a recommended maximum of 19.2 µg/day (0.8 µg/h) by day 21. Dose increases in increments of less than 2.4 µg/day (0.1 µg/h) and increases in dose less frequently than two or three times per week may be used. However, at a consensus conference of 30 international experts in intrathecal therapy, a majority recommended that therapy be initiated at 0.5 µg/ day, and slowly titrated in 0.5 µg increments every 1–2

weeks. This recommendation to be more conservative was based on concerns of reducing the risk of adverse events and improving patient tolerability.

Availability: available for purchase from the manufacturer for injection into an intrathecal pump reservoir by a physician or designee.

Cost: approximately $7.00 per microgram.

Potential advantages

Ziconotide provides powerful and prolonged analgesia for patients suffering chronic intractable pain that is poorly responsive to conventional opioid and nonopioid analgesics. An important advantage of ziconotide is the avoidance of opioid-induced adverse events such as GI issues, pruritus, decreased testosterone levels, opioid-induced hyperalgesia, as well as behavioral issues.

Potential disadvantages

Toxicity: elevation of serum creatine kinase (CK-MM). In clinical studies (mostly open label), 40% of patients had serum creatine kinase (CK) levels above the upper limit of normal (ULN), and 11% had CK levels that were three times the ULN or more. In cases where CK was fractionated, only the muscle isoenzyme (MM) was elevated. The time to occurrence was sporadic, but the greatest incidence of CK elevation was during the first 2 months of treatment. Elevated CKs were more often seen in males, in patients who were being treated with antidepressants or anti-epileptics, and in patients treated with intrathecal morphine. Most patients who experienced elevations in CK, even for prolonged periods of time, did not have limiting side effects. However, one case of symptomatic myopathy with EMG findings and two cases of acute renal failure associated with rhabdomyolysis and extreme CK elevations (17 000–27 000 IU/L) have been reported. It is recommended that physicians monitor serum CK in patients undergoing treatment with ziconotide periodically.

Drug interactions

Formal PK drug–drug interaction studies have not been performed with Prialt. As ziconotide is a peptide, it is expected to be completely degraded by endopeptidases and exopeptidases (Phase I hydrolytic enzymes) widely located throughout the body, and not by other Phase I biotransformation processes (including the cytochrome P450 system) or by Phase

II conjugation reactions. Thus, intrathecal administration, low plasma ziconotide concentrations, and metabolism by ubiquitous peptidases make metabolic interactions of other drugs with ziconotide unlikely. Further, as ziconotide is not highly bound in plasma (approximately 50%) and has low plasma exposure following IT administration, clinically relevant plasma protein displacement reactions involving ziconotide and co-administered medications are unlikely.

Adverse events

Ziconotide has been associated with CNS-related adverse events, including psychiatric symptoms, cognitive impairment, and decreased alertness/unresponsiveness. The dose should be reduced or discontinued if signs or symptoms of cognitive impairment develop, but other contributing causes should also be considered. Some patients have become unresponsive or stuporous while receiving ziconotide.

Adverse reactions: the most frequently reported adverse events (25%) in the 1254 patients (662 patient years) in clinical trials were dizziness, nausea, confusional state, and nystagmus. Serious adverse events and discontinuation of ziconotide for adverse events are less frequent when the drug is slowly titrated.

Drug-related adverse events

Common/serious adverse events: dizziness, nausea, confusional state, and nystagmus.

Less common adverse events: vertigo, blurred vision, diarrhea, nausea, vomiting, asthenia, abnormal gait, pyrexia, rigors, sinusitis, anorexia, muscle spasms, pain in limb, amnesia, ataxia, dizziness, dysarthria, dysgeusia, headache, memory impairment, nystagmus, somnolence, tremor, anxiety, confusional state, insomnia, urinary retention, pruritus, sweating.

At less than 2% in the clinical investigations: acute renal failure, atrial fibrillation, cerebrovascular accident, sepsis, meningitis, psychotic disorder, suicidal ideation, respiratory distress, rhabdomyolysis, electrocardiogram abnormal, stupor, loss of consciousness, incoherent, clonic convulsion and grand mal convulsion. Rare instances of fatal pneumonia aspiration and suicide attempt were reported (<1%).

Treatment of adverse events: there is not an antagonist available for ziconotide. For mild adverse events, the clinician may either monitor the patient to see whether there is improvement with time, or reduce the dose. For severe adverse events, it is recommended that the delivery of ziconotide be discontinued, and that the drug is completely removed from the intrathecal pump by aspirating and rinsing the reservoir with preservative-free saline, as well as aspirating the pump's side port, to remove drug from the intrathecal catheter. The clinician will need to provide supportive care until the adverse effects stop, which may take up to several days.

References

1. Product insert, revised 10/08.

2. Deer T, Krames E, Hassenbusch S, Burton A, Caraway D, Dupen S, Eisenach J, Erdek M, Grigsby E, Kim P, Levy R, McDowell G, Mekhail N, Panchal SJ, Prager J, Rauck R, Saulino M, Sitzman T, Staats P, Stanton-Hicks M, Stearns L, Willis KD, Witt W, Follett K, Huntoon M, Liem L, Rathmell J, Wallace M, Buchser E, Cousins M, Ver Donck A. Polyanalgesic Consensus Conference 2007: Recommendations for the management of pain by intrathecal (intraspinal) drug delivery: report of an interdisciplinary expert panel. *Neuromodulation* 2007;**10**(4):300–328.

Methylnaltrexone

Kathleen Ji Park, Anthony DePlato and Jill Zafar

Generic Name: methylnaltrexone bromide

Trade/Proprietary Name: Relistor™

Drug Class: peripheral μ-opioid-receptor antagonist

Manufacturer: Wyeth Corporation, Madison, NJ

Chemical Name: (R)-N-(cyclopropylmethyl)nor-oxymorphone methobromide

Chemical Structure: see Figure 106.1

Description

Methylnaltrexone is a peripherally acting mu-opioid-receptor antagonist. It is a quaternary ammonium derivative of naltrexone that binds selectively to peripheral mu opioid receptors. Due to its low lipid solubility and an addition of a polar methyl group, methylnaltrexone cannot cross the blood–brain barrier, in contrast to naltrexone, a central-acting, uncharged, opioid antagonist. Methylnaltrexone exerts peripheral blockade of mu opioid receptors in the gastrointestinal tract, and it is used to relieve the gastrointestinal-related adverse effects of opioids while maintaining centrally based analgesia. The drug was FDA-approved in April 2008 for administration via subcutaneous injection in the treatment of patients who develop opioid-induced constipation with advanced illnesses. Unlike naltrexone, methylnaltrexone does not induce opioid withdrawal.

Mode of activity

Major and minor sites of action: methylnaltrexone is a peripheral opioid-receptor antagonist. It is also a partial agonist at mu, delta, and kappa opioid receptors.

Receptor interactions: the primary effects of methylnaltrexone are mediated by antagonism of mu opioid receptors in the gastrointestinal tract. These receptors are primarily concentrated in neural cells and terminal endings located in the myenteric plexus. Oral, parenteral and, to a lesser degree, neuraxial opioids bind to and activate these receptors. Neurons within the myenteric plexus are stimulated, resulting in constriction of circular smooth muscle, decreased secretion, decreased gastrointestinal motility, and delayed transit time (Figure 106.2). Methylnaltrexone blocks these opioid receptor mediated effects.

Metabolic pathways: following subcutaneous injection, the drug is absorbed rapidly and reaches peak plasma concentration after about 30 minutes with a half-life of 8 hours. Up to 15% of the drug is protein-bound. Methylnaltrexone undergoes metabolism to multiple compounds. The most frequent metabolite is methyl-6-naltrexol (5%). N-Demethylation of methylnaltrexone to produce naltrexone is not significant. Up to 85% of the drug is excreted unchanged in the urine or feces.

Indications (approved)

Methylnaltrexone is FDA-approved for subcutaneous injection in the treatment of opioid-induced constipation in patients with advanced illness who are receiving palliative care and are insufficiently responding to laxative therapy.

Indications (non-approved)

Multiple clinical trials are currently under way to investigate methylnaltrexone, orally or subcutaneously, in healthy chronic pain patients as a treatment for constipation and opioid-induced bowel dysfunction. Intravenous methylnaltrexone is being investigated to treat and prevent post-operative ileus; however, the drug has not yet received approval for these indications. Chronic use of methylnaltrexone for greater than 4 months has not been studied.

Contraindications

Absolute contraindications: methylnaltrexone is absolutely contraindicated in known or suspected

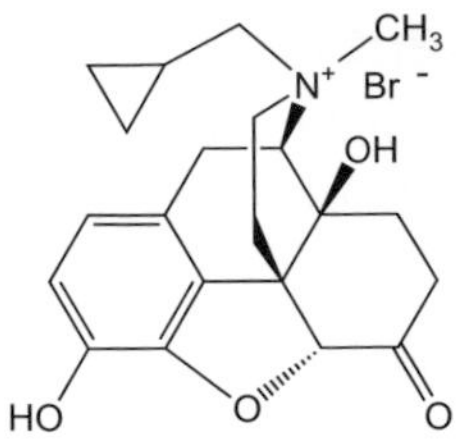

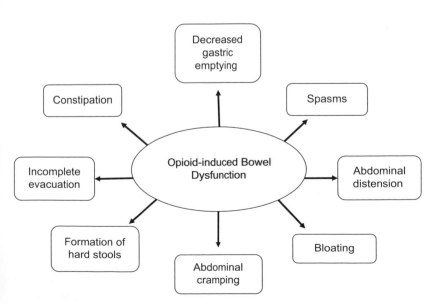

Figure 106.1.

mechanical gastrointestinal obstruction and in patients with severe allergic reaction to methylnaltrexone.

Relative contraindications: the drug is listed as a Pregnancy Category B drug. It is unknown whether the drug is secreted via lactation. The drug has not been studied in patients with end-stage renal disease or severe hepatic dysfunction.

Methylnaltrexone should be used with caution in patients with recent histories of bowel surgery, colonoscopy, colon cancer, or active diverticulitis.

Common dosage

Adult doses are adjusted according to body weight and are administered subcutaneously in the upper arm, thigh, or abdomen. The typical dosing schedule is every other day as needed. The maximum dose is once a day. Usual dosing is 8 mg for patients between 38 and 61 kg and 12 mg for patients between 62 and 114 kg. For weights outside the previously described ranges, dosing is calculated as 0.15 mg/kg.

Elderly dosing is the same as adult dosing.
Pediatric dosing is currently unavailable.

No dosing adjustment is required in mild to moderate renal impairment. For severe renal impairment with creatinine clearance of less than 30 mL/minute, the recommended dosing is 50% of normal adult dose. Patients with end-stage renal disease have not been studied.

No dosing adjustment is needed for patients with mild to moderate hepatic dysfunction. Severe hepatic impairment has not been studied with respect to methylnaltrexone.

Potential advantages

Methylnaltrexone is a drug that is well tolerated and offers a treatment in relieving opioid-induced constipation. It was found to be effective in causing laxation in almost 50% of patients within 4 hours after one dose (Figure 106.3). The drug does not affect central analgesia or precipitate opioid withdrawal. There are no known significant drug interactions with methylnaltrexone. Patients can easily and safely administer self-injections. Methylnaltrexone can improve patients' symptoms and possibly their quality of life.

Finally, caregivers must recognize that, unlike nonselective antagonists, methynaltrexone will not reverse excessive sedation, respiratory depression, and other symptoms associated with central opioid toxicity.

Potential disadvantages

The toxicity of the drug is low, with less than 1% of patients suffering from life-threatening complications. Cost may be an issue to patients as there is no generic

Figure 106.2. Opioid-induced bowel dysfunction (OBD). Opioids increase intestinal fluid absorption, inhibit intestinal secretions and peristalsis, and block propulsive movements in the colon. Constipation and other symptoms associated with OBD occur in 15–90% of cancer patients and may be more distressful and debilitating than pain. Tolerance rarely develops to these symptoms and traditional therapy including stimulants, lubricants, and bulk laxatives may not be effective.

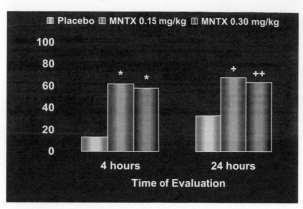

Figure 106.3. Patients with advanced illness and opioid-induced constipation who experienced laxation within 4 and 24 hours after receiving methylnaltrexone or placebo. *$P < 0.0001$ vs. placebo; +$P < 0.0004$ vs. placebo, ++$P < 0.0014$ vs. placebo With permission from: Thomas J, et al. *J Clin Oncol.* ASCO Meeting Proceedings 2005;23(16S):abstract 8003.

alternative to the brand name methylnaltrexone Relistor™. Methylnaltrexone is new to the market, and clinical trials are still under way to investigate its efficacy and safety in other clinical settings.

Drug-related adverse events

Serious reaction is severe diarrhea and common reactions are abdominal pain, flatulence, dizziness, nausea and vomiting.

Treatment of adverse events

Patients who are suffering from severe persistent diarrhea, as well as other known adverse reactions, are advised to discontinue methylnaltrexone and immediately notify the prescribing healthcare worker.

References

1. Thomas J, et al. Methylnaltrexone for opioid-induced constipation in advanced illness. *N Engl J Med* 2008;**358**:2332–2343.

2. Relistor subcutaneous injection package insert. Wyeth 2008. http://www.wyeth.com/hcp/relistor/prescribing-information.

3. Viscusi E, et al. Peripherally acting mu-opioid receptor antagonists and postoperative ileus: mechanisms of action and clinical applicability. *Anesth Analg* 2009;**108**:1811–1822.

Section 11
Chapter

107

Adjuvant Analgesics and Antiemetics

Alvimopan

Victor A. Filadora II and Sidney Allison

Victor A. Filadora II and Sidney Allison

Generic Name: alvimopan
Trade Name: Entereg™
Drug Class: peripheral opioid antagonist
Manufacturer: Adolor Corporation, Exton, PA 19341–1127
Chemical Structure: see Figure 107.1
Chemical Name: [[2(S)-[[4(R)-(3-hydroxyphenyl)-3(R),4-dimethyl-1-piperidinyl]methyl]-1-oxo-3-phenylpropyl]amino]acetic acid dihydrate
Chemical Formula: $C_{25}H_{32}N_2O_4 \cdot 2H_2O$; molecular wt 460.6

Description

Alvimopan is a peripheral μ opioid receptor antagonist. It was first synthesized at Lilly Research Laboratories, and introduced in May 2008 by Adolor Corporation and GlaxoSmithKline under the brand name Entereg. Its indication is to accelerate upper and lower gastrointestinal recovery time following partial large or small bowel resection surgery with primary anastomosis. It is the first pharmacotherapy approved by the US FDA for this application [1–3].

Alvimopan's activity is peripherally restricted because at physiological pH, its large zwitterionic

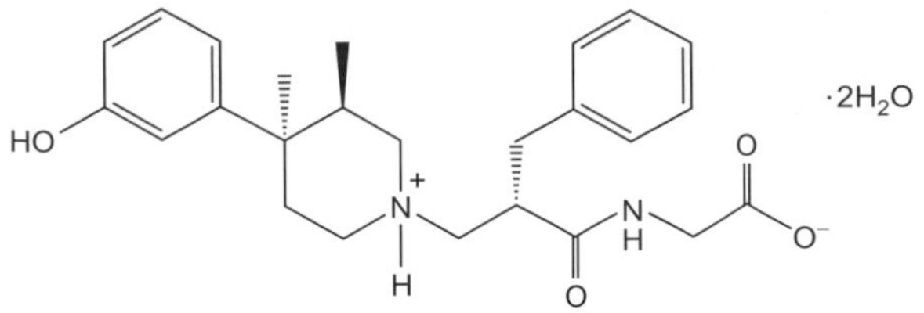

Figure 107.1.

form and polarity limit gastrointestinal absorption and prevent passage through the blood–brain barrier. It competitively antagonizes the effects of morphine on gastrointestinal contractility without reversing the central analgesic effects of μ opioid agonists [1,2]. No dosage adjustments are required in patients with co-administration of morphine or acid blockers. Patients with recent exposure to opioids are more sensitive to μ opioid receptor antagonists. This sensitivity is limited to gastrointestinal tract discomfort, which may include abdominal pain, nausea and vomiting, and diarrhea.

Mode of activity

As an opioid antagonist, alvimopan interacts selectively with gastrointestinal μ opioid receptors with no central nervous system activity. It has not shown affinity for non-opioid receptors such as adrenergic, dopaminergic, histaminergic, GABAergic, or cholinergic receptors [1,2,4].

Metabolic pathways

After multiple oral doses, the mean terminal-phase half-life of alvimopan ranges from 10 to 17 hours. It is absorbed systemically and its oral bioavailability in humans is estimated at only 6%. After 5 days of oral administration of alvimopan 12 mg twice daily, its mean peak plasma concentration is 10.98 ± 6.43 ng/mL with a time to reach this peak concentration of 1.5 to 3 hours. Alvimopan is converted to its active metabolite, ADL 08–0011, via amide hydrolysis as a product of intestinal flora activity, not by hepatic metabolism. After 36 hours of standard dosing of alvimopan, the mean peak plasma concentration of the metabolite is 35.73 ± 35.29 ng/mL. Cytochrome P450 isoenzyme metabolism, glucuronidation, and sulfation are not involved in alvimopan metabolism [1].

Alvimopan does not affect concomitant administration of acid blockers or antibiotics. The plasma concentrations of metabolite, however, are lower in patients receiving acid blockers and pre-operative oral antibiotics. Since the metabolite is not required for efficacy of alvimopan, no dosage adjustments are required.

Alvimopan does not affect co-administration of morphine and its metabolite, morphone-6-glucuronide, when morphine is intravenously administered. No dosage adjustments of intravenous morphine are necessary.

Excretion pathways

The primary elimination pathway of alvimopan is via biliary secretion, with renal excretion accounting for approximately 35% of its clearance. Alvimopan's metabolites undergo systemic absorption and first-order elimination. These metabolites and other glucuronidated conjugates are eliminated unchanged in the feces and urine.

Indications (approved/non-approved)

Alvimopan is indicated to prevent post-operative ileus by accelerating the time to upper and lower gastrointestinal recovery following partial large or small bowel resection surgery with primary anastomosis [1,2].

Contraindications

Alvimopan is contraindicated in patients who have taken opioids for more than 7 consecutive days immediately prior to taking alvimopan.

Common doses

Capsule: 12 mg. For short-term use in hospitals that have registered in and successfully met all of the requirements for EASE (En>

Capsule: 12 mg. For short-term use in hospitals that have registered in and successfully met all of the requirements for EASE (Entereg® Access Support and Education) program.

Adult: a maximum of 15 doses is indicated. The first dose of 12 mg is administered orally between 30 minutes and 5 hours prior to surgery. Subsequent dosage is 12 mg twice daily after surgery for a maximum of 7 days or until discharge.

Administration of alvimopan to patients receiving more than three doses of an opioid a week prior to surgery was not studied in the post-operative ileus clinical trials and should be closely monitored.

Geriatric use: although the bioavailability and oral clearance of alvimopan decrease with age, this has minor clinical significance. Therefore, no dosage adjustment based on increased age is necessary.

421

Pediatric use: safety and effectiveness in children have not been established.

Hepatic impairment: although there is a potential for higher plasma concentration of alvimopan in patients with mild-to-moderate hepatic impairment, no dosage adjustment is necessary. A high alvimopan or metabolite level, however, may cause possible adverse effects, such as diarrhea, gastrointestinal pain, and cramping. These patients should be closely monitored for these effects. If adverse events occur, discontinue administration of alvimopan.

Alvimopan is not recommended for use in patients with severe hepatic impairment.

Renal impairment: although no dosage adjustment is necessary in patients with mild-to-severe renal impairment, those with severe renal impairment should be closely monitored for possible adverse effects, such as diarrhea, gastrointestinal pain, and cramping. These effects could indicate high alvimopan or metabolite levels. Discontinue alvimopan if adverse events occur.

Alvimopan has not been studied in patients with end-stage renal disease and is not recommended for use in these patients.

Bowel obstruction: patients undergoing surgery for correction of complete bowel obstruction are not recommended for administration with alvimopan.

Potential advantages

Alvimopan has low systemic absorption and limited ability to enter the central nervous system. Since it is peripherally restricted, it does not reduce the pain relief of therapeutic opioids. As a result, patients may have pain control and improved bowel motility.

Because alvimopan reverses the adverse effects of opioids on the gastrointestinal tract, it accelerates gastrointestinal recovery in patients following colorectal or small-bowel resection surgery. This potentially improves patient comfort while reducing healthcare expenditure due to extended hospitalization.

Alvimopan also has no known potential for dependence or abuse.

Potential disadvantages

Toxicity

Intravenous administration of alvimopan up to 10 mg/kg per day in female mice (about 3.4 to 6.8 times the recommended human oral dose) did not produce adverse effects on fertility and reproductive performance.

Oral administration of alvimopan at 4000 mg/kg per day for 104 weeks in female mice (about 674 times the recommended human dose) increased incidences of fibroma, skin fibrosarcoma and sarcoma, and osteoma/osteosarcoma. In rats, however, oral administration of alvimopan up to 500 mg/kg per day for 104 weeks (about 166 times the recommended human dose) did not produce any tumor [1,2].

In the Ames test, mouse lymphoma cell (L5178Y/TK$^{+/-}$) forward mutation test, Chinese Hamster Ovary (CHO) cell chromosome aberration test, and mouse micronucleus test, alvimopan was not found genotoxic. Its metabolite was negative in the Ames test, CHO cell chromosome aberration test, and mouse micronucleus test.

Drug interactions

Alvimopan can be co-administered with morphine or acid blockers without dosage adjustments.

Drug-related adverse events

Although alvimopan is generally well tolerated, its most common side effects include nausea, vomiting, abdominal distention, constipation, dyspepsia, and flatulence.

Patients with long-term or intermittent opioid therapy, including any opioid use a week prior to administration of alvimopan, could be more sensitive to its adverse effects. These effects, such as abdominal pain, nausea and vomiting, as well as diarrhea, are limited to the gastrointestinal tract.

No causal relationship between alvimopan and myocardial infarctions has been established. In a 12-month study of patients treated with opioids for chronic pain, incidences of myocardial infarctions in patients treated with alvimopan 0.5 mg twice daily were reported to be higher than those treated with placebo. The majority of myocardial infarctions occurred between 1 and 4 months after the first treatment of alvimopan.

Patients with severe hepatic impairment are not recommended for treatment with alvimopan. The plasma level of drug was found to be potentially 10-fold higher than in a healthy control volunteer. No studies have been established for alvimopan administration in patients with severe hepatic impairment.

Other adverse reactions that were reported in nine worldwide placebo-controlled alvimopan trials in 1650 patients include anemia, hypokalemia, back pain, and urinary retention. Although hypokalemia was more common with bowel resection patients, it was less frequent in the overall surgical population [1,4].

Treatment of adverse events

No specific antidote has been indicated for overdosage with alvimopan. Patients should be managed with appropriate supportive therapy.

References

1. Bream-Rouwenhorst HR, Cantrell MA. Alvimopan for postoperative ileus. *Am J Health-System Pharm* 2009;**66**:1267–1277.

2. Delaney CP, Yasothan U, Kirkpatrick P. Alvimopan. *Nature Rev* 2008;**7**:727–728.

3. Ludwig K, Enker WE, Delaney CP, Wolff BG, Du W, Fort JG, Cherubini M, Cucinotta J, Techner L. Gastrointestinal tract recovery in patients undergoing bowel resection. *Arch Surg* 2008;**143**(11):1098–1105.

4. Udeh E, Goldman M. Alvimopan. *Formulary* 2005;**40**:176–183.

Overview: novel targets for new analgesics

Ian W. Rodger and Peter G. Lacouture

Introduction

Novel targets for new analgesics may be described in several different ways. One could consider new applications for existing compounds including route of administration (nasal, pulmonary, transdermal, intraosseous, etc.) or delivery technologies (extended-release, iontophoresis, etc.). Many of these new approaches, or products, are discussed in the chapters that follow, including the TRP channel blockers (Chapter 128), the cannabinoid agonists (Chapters 125 and 126), and the NMDA-receptor antagonists (neramexane, Chapter 129). In addition, chapters preceding this section describe relatively new targets including μ agonists (tapentadol, Chapters 31 and 115), NMDA antagonists (Section 6), α-adrenergic receptor agonists (clonidine, Chapter 81; dexmeditomidine, Chapter 83), calcium channel blockers ($\alpha_2\delta$-subunit antagonists, Chapter 70), and some biological products such as ziconotide (Chapter 105).

This overview will not revisit the above topics in detail, but will place them in an appropriate perspective as future targets. Many of these targets have been identified previously. However, recent emerging information on mechanisms of action continues to shed new light on novel areas for analgesic development. Novel targets can be discussed as mechanism-based or as chemical (drug)-based. The chapters that follow in this section of the textbook are drug-based discussions, so this introductory chapter will focus on mechanism-based principles. The objective of this chapter is to provide a scientific foundation for modification or repurposing of existing drugs as well as identifying pathways for new drug therapies.

This overview has been divided into four families; ion channels, enzymes, receptors, and cytokines. Where appropriate each targeted family has been subdivided into members that reflect the mechanistic theme.

While the basis of this chapter is highly scientific and clinical, we would be remiss if, at the outset, we did not examine the future development of any of these novel therapies based on commercial considerations. Table 108.1 presents one perspective on the potential sales for these new treatments projected from 2018 to 2023.

In both of these time segments, the growth factor modulators and the CGRP antagonists show the greatest economic return (estimates in excess of $1 billion/year). It is also worth noting that all of these targets show meaningful growth over the 5 year period reviewed. The groups showing at least a doubling of sales include the cannabinoid modulators, the ion channel modulators, the CGRP antagonists and the cytokine modulators

Ion channel families
Acid-sensing ion channels (ASICs)

Acid-sensing ion channels are a family of transmembrane-spanning proteins that form ion channels in nociceptors that are uniquely sensitive to the action of H^+ ions (see Figure 108.1). Thus, any reduction in the pH (increase in H^+) of tissues, such as that which occurs during inflammation, will cause activation of ASICs leading to a reduction in the excitation threshold of the nociceptor and enhanced sensory nerve activation. The growing awareness of the importance of ASICs in regulating sensory nerve activation is currently the subject of intense research investigation. However, to date, there are no selective agents that have the selectivity of action necessary for them to assume the status of clinical candidates.

Transient receptor potential (TRP) channels

Arguably one of the most interesting targets in the past decade has been the family known as the transient receptor potential (TRP) channels (Figure 108.1). They compose a superfamily of ion channels that play important roles in the transmission

The Essence of Analgesia and Analgesics, ed. Raymond S. Sinatra, Jonathan S. Jahr and J. Michael Watkins-Pitchford. Published by Cambridge University Press. © Cambridge University Press 2011.

Table 108.1.

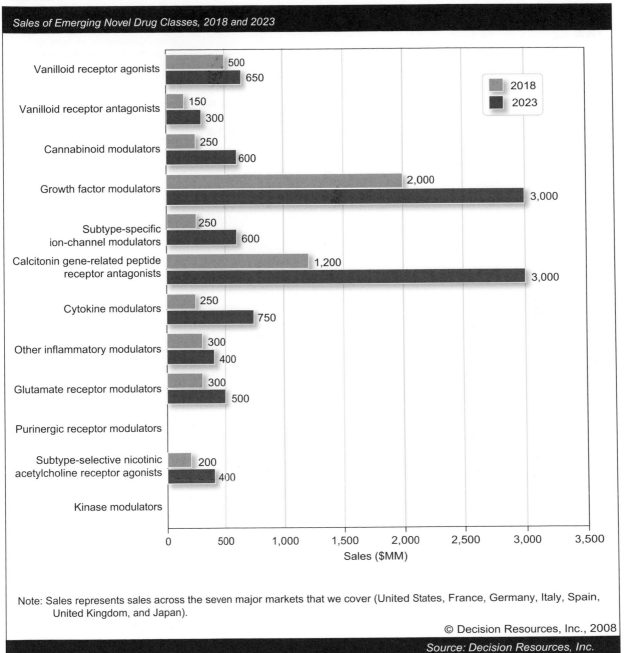

Sales of Emerging Novel Drug Classes, 2018 and 2023

Legend: 2018, 2023

Drug Class	2018	2023
Vanilloid receptor agonists	500	650
Vanilloid receptor antagonists	150	300
Cannabinoid modulators	250	600
Growth factor modulators	2,000	3,000
Subtype-specific ion-channel modulators	250	600
Calcitonin gene-related peptide receptor antagonists	1,200	3,000
Cytokine modulators	250	750
Other inflammatory modulators	300	400
Glutamate receptor modulators	300	500
Purinergic receptor modulators		
Subtype-selective nicotinic acetylcholine receptor agonists	200	400
Kinase modulators		

Sales ($MM)

Note: Sales represents sales across the seven major markets that we cover (United States, France, Germany, Italy, Spain, United Kingdom, and Japan).

© Decision Resources, Inc., 2008

Source: Decision Resources, Inc.

of sensory input through the nerve cell. They are strictly cationic channels (admitting Na⁺, K⁺ and Ca^{2+}) and frequently nonselective in that they will permit entry of more than one cation. These channels, expressed in primary afferent fibers, are of interest because they are involved in the transduction of noxious stimuli. The principal interest in these channels has focused on TRPV1 (Chapters 96 and 128). While the majority of research has focused on antagonists of TRPV1 there is certain interest in low molecular weight agonists that desensitize the cationic channel. Both approaches have been shown to be effective in neuropathic and inflammatory pain states

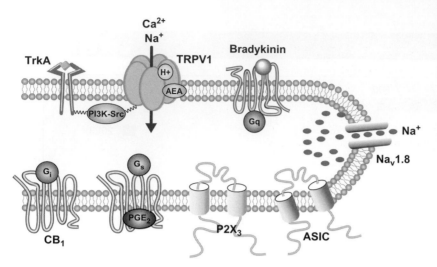

Figure 108.1. Diagrammatic representation of the nociceptor (adapted from Julius and Basbaum, 2001 [8]). The elements shown in the figure that are known to modulate the nociceptors in an excitatory manner are tyrosine kinase A (TrkA), the receptor for nerve growth factor, the transient receptor potential channel (TRP) V_1, bradykinin receptor(s), the tetrodotoxin-resistant, sensory neuron-specific Na^+ channel ($Na_v1.8$), the acid-sensing ion channels (ASIC), the adenosine P_2X_3 receptor, and prostaglandin (PG)E_2 receptors. Inhibitory modulation of the nociceptor is achievable via stimulation of the cannabinoid type 1 receptors (CB_1).

Sodium (Na^+) channels

Peripheral nociceptors are the sensory anatomical detectors of painful stimuli. The nociceptors transduce the initial stimuli by creating action potentials that are largely a consequence of the entry of sodium ions (Na^+) into the neuron. There are several types of voltage-gated Na^+ channels that can be classified according to their sensitivity to tetrodotoxin (TTX) and their primary structure. A variety of Na^+ channels are involved in regulating nociceptor excitability. They are the TTX-sensitive $Na_v1.3$ and 1.7 channels and the TTX-insensitive $Na_v1.8$ and 1.9 channels. However, it is the latter two sodium channels that are of particular importance. While both these TTX-resistant channels are present in the nociceptor membrane the $Na_v1.8$ sub-type is of greatest interest (Figure 108.1). These channels are primarily expressed in slow-conducting sensory C fibers. $Na_v1.8$ channel opening leads directly to the generation of action potentials that pass up through the dorsal root ganglion to the dorsal horn of the spinal cord. Furthermore, the expression and biological properties of these $Na_v1.8$ channels can be modulated by ongoing nociceptor activity and further enhanced by inflammatory events or injury occurring locally. The $Na_v1.8$ channel is solely responsible for the detection of pain induced by noxious cold.

There has been a concerted effort to identify drugs that selectively block the $Na_v1.8$ and/or $Na_v1.9$ channels. To date, however, there is but one report of such a selective blocker, A-803467. A-803467 is more than 100-fold more selective for the human $Na_v1.8$ expressed in recombinant cell lines compared with other Na_v channels (1.2, 1.3, 1.5, and 1.7). It is highly effective in animal models of both inflammatory and neuropathic pain. The effects of A-803467 are dose-dependent and reversible and, in contrast to classical sodium channel blockers such as the local anesthetics (see Section 5), the ability to block the $Na_v1.8$ current was not frequency-dependent. Interestingly, while A-803467 was highly effective in the different chronic pain models it was ineffective in blocking acute pain, suggesting that this $Na_v1.8$ may not be involved in physiological nociception

Calcium (Ca^{2+}) channels

Ca^{2+} entry into the presynaptic terminal of the primary sensory neuron is essential for the release of the neurotransmitters necessary for conveying the wave of excitation upwards to the central nervous system. In the dorsal horn this is achieved via the opening of specific N-type, voltage-gated Ca^{2+} channels that have been designated $Ca_v2.2$ (Figure 108.2). Given the importance of this channel there has been significant effort directed towards the discovery of antagonists of $Ca_v2.2$. A key consideration in targeting $Ca_v2.2$ is to design a molecule that would inhibit Ca^{2+} entry during conditions in which the primary sensory neuron is firing rapidly, as is the case in painful conditions, as opposed to the lower-frequency discharge that occurs under normal, physiological conditions. In essence, what one seeks is a so-called "use-dependent" inhibitor of $Ca_v2.2$. Today there are both preclinical and clinical data to support the involvement of the $Ca_v2.2$ channels since inhibition of this channel is associated with analgesic effects in both chronic and neuropathic pain syndromes.

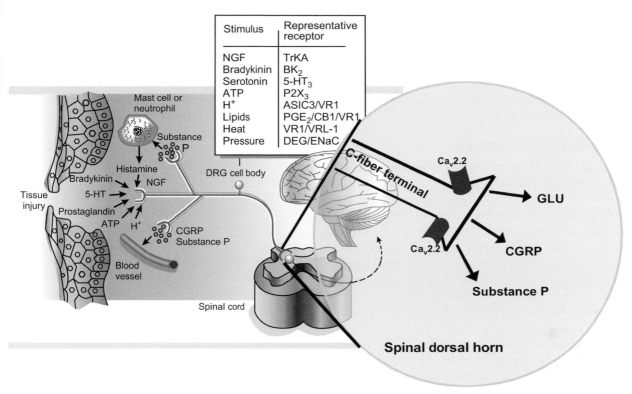

Stimulus	Representative receptor
NGF	TrKA
Bradykinin	BK_2
Serotonin	$5\text{-}HT_3$
ATP	$P2X_3$
H^+	ASIC3/VR1
Lipids	PGE_2/CB1/VR1
Heat	VR1/VRL-1
Pressure	DEG/ENaC

Figure 108.2. Schematic representation of events occurring after tissue injury leading ultimately to the perception of pain. The initial injury releases a chemical "soup" that alters the peripheral nociceptors to enhance their sensitivity to stimuli by lowering their threshold for stimulation. This "soup" contains growth factors, lipids, H^+, ATP, and a host of humoral mediators including cytokines. The end result is enhanced firing of the sensory neuron sending impulses via the dorsal root ganglion to the dorsal horn of the spinal cord. Neurochemical transmission at this junction is achieved via Ca^{2+} entry through $Ca_v2.2$ channels and the release of glutamate, substance P, and CGRP. (Adapted from Julius and Basbaum, 2001 [8].)

The $Ca_v2.2$ channel, like all ion channels, is composed of numerous subunits. A critical component of the $Ca_v2.2$ is the $\alpha_2\delta$-subunit (see Chapter 70), which is known to be up-regulated in animal models of neuropathic pain and it is this subunit that is the proposed target of the GABA analogs gabapentin and pregabalin (see Chapters 71 and 72). Additionally, gabapentin has also been shown to down-regulate channel expression as well as conformationally altering the channel structure. Both these compounds are used for the treatment of chronic pain syndromes although their side-effect profile is poorer than one would have anticipated. In all likelihood this is a consequence of the $\alpha_2\delta$ subunit not being the exclusive province of the $Ca_v2.2$ channel, with it being expressed in a wide variety of other voltage-gated Ca^{2+} channels. A gabapentin prodrug, XP13512 (GSK), is currently in phase II clinical development.

The small-molecule approach of Neuromed led to the discovery of NMED 160, which showed selective,

use-dependent inhibition of $Ca_v2.2$ in a wide range of animal pain models. Beyond the developments mentioned above, this compound provides substantial validation of the approach to targeting $Ca_v2.2$ as a novel mechanism for providing analgesic efficacy. This compound, renamed MK-6721, has been studied in a phase II clinical trial but is not regarded as a candidate for further clinical development. An alternative approach to generation of small-molecule, selective inhibitors of $Ca_v2.2$ has been based upon the key structural features of cone snail ω-conotoxins. The snail conopeptide, ziconotide (Prialt from Elan/Eisai; see Chapter 105) is an example of this approach. This peptide (which has to be administered intrathecally) has been shown in several clinical studies to have substantial analgesic efficacy in both chronic and severe pain states even in patients who were unresponsive to morphine. The downside to ziconotide is that either by intrathecal or systemic routes of administration it is associated with orthostatic hypotension and a litany of neurological side effects.

Notwithstanding some of the developmental difficulties the $Ca_v2.2$ channel remains a viable and attractive target for novel analgesic drugs that would have therapeutic benefit in both inflammatory and neuropathic pain conditions

Potassium (K⁺) channels

Clearly, the cationic pathways of the sodium and calcium channels are the most well-recognized and have been explored to a greater degree than any other channels of this type. However, there is evidence that in certain conditions, modulation of the K⁺ channel may have merit as a therapeutic agent. A less well-known member (at least for pain) of this ion channel family of the potassium channel modulators is KCNQ (Kv7). Five sub-groups of this channel exist. Four family members (KCNQ2–5) are primarily associated with the nervous system but KCNQ2/3 are most relevant in relation to neuropathic pain. What is fascinating is that while nerve injury increases expression of certain Na⁺ channels the exact opposite occurs with K⁺ channels. Thus, decreased expression of K⁺ channels occurs after injury in both A and C fibers, contributing to an exaggerated sensory response.

Retigabine (Valeant) has been explored in this area and in particular the KCNQ2/3 channel. Retigabine is classified as a potassium channel activator. It is structurally similar to the analgesic flupirtine developed by Asta Medica. These products have been targeted for acute, neuropathic, and migraine pain.

While the potassium channel modulation may play an important role in the future of pain management particularly in neuropathic states, this potential has yet to be realized. The existing family representative (flupirtine) has shown limited utility and currently research and interest in this area is somewhat low

Chloride (Cl⁻) channels

Chloride channels represent the only anionic channel of interest for analgesic development. These channels often play an important role in neural excitability and therefore are important in the roles of several neurotransmitters including GABA and glycine. Hyperpolarization of the post-synaptic cell body leads to a less excitable nerve fiber and the resultant loss of sensory transmission through select fibers. Through several cascading events, interactions at the Cl⁻ channel result in a hyperpolarization by the inward rush of Cl⁻.

Therefore, the enhanced movement of Cl⁻ into the neural cell results in hyperpolarization and decreased excitability of the membrane while the cancellation of Cl⁻ movement into the cell results in an increase in nerve membrane excitability. Thus molecules which enhance chloride movement into the sensory nerve will potentially demonstrate analgesic activity. These channels also play important roles with respect to the neurotrophins (see BDNF receptors) and the nonsteroidal anti-inflammatory analgesic drugs (see mPGES-1 below).

At the present time, targets for analgesic potential have not been realized. However, their role in modulating neural membrane excitability makes them a promising target for future development. Specific chloride channel modulators in development for the treatment of pain are not known but are often contributors to action of other transmitters such as GABA and glycine.

Enzyme families

Microsomal prostaglandin E synthase-1 (mPGES-1)

Prostaglandins (PGs), in particular PGE_2, have long been known as pivotal mediators of inflammation and the pain associated with inflammatory events (see Figure 108.2). PGE_2 is the product of the cyclooxygenase (COX) pathways, both COX-1 and COX-2. Drugs that inhibit these pathways in a nonselective fashion have been available for some time. These are the so-called nonsteroidal anti-inflammatory drugs (NSAIDs) (see Section 4). Within this class of drugs there are those that are nonselective for the cyclooxygenase enzymes COX-1 and COX-2, typified by ibuprofen and naproxen, and those that are selective inhibitors of COX-2, typified by celecoxib and etoricoxib. Both nonselective and selective NSAIDs are highly effective at reducing pain and inflammation but, not surprisingly, only in those settings where there is a PG-dependent mechanism involved. Thus, at best, they have limited efficacy in neuropathic pain conditions. A further complication is that NSAIDs have a side-effect profile that is less than desirable. The nonselective agents, through COX-1 inhibition, cause gastrointestinal complications and fluid retention. The selective COX-2 inhibitors cause fluid retention and have been associated with potentially serious cardiovascular side effects when used for extended periods of time.

In an attempt to obviate the cardiovascular side effects of the selective COX-2 inhibitors attention has been directed towards inhibition of prostaglandin biosynthesis at a point further down the pathway leading to PGE_2. COX-2 is responsible for the conversion of arachidonic acid to the cyclic endoperoxides and ultimately to a variety of prostanoids (thromboxane, PGD, PGE, and prostacyclin). It has been postulated that a component of the cardiovascular side effects of selective COX-2 inhibition is a consequence of the reduction in the formation of the vascularly protective substance prostacyclin. To circumvent this effect attention has been focused on the biosynthetic step that occurs after COX-2, namely the conversion of the cyclic endoperoxides by microsomal PGE synthase-1 (mPGES-1) to PGE_2. The rationale underlying this approach is that by allowing the formation of the cyclic endoperoxides some of that substrate can be converted to prostacyclin thereby allowing for the vascular benefits to remain unaffected. Such a targeted approach to inhibit the formation of PGE_2 at the mPGES-1 step is an attractive way of creating analgesic and anti-inflammatory agents that have the undeniable efficacy of NSAIDs but with much diminished cardiovascular risk profiles. Currently there are no candidate molecules in clinical development but several companies have significant preclinical programs underway

Kinase modulators

The kinase family of enzymes participates in many pathways contributing to the modulation of pain responses. Many of these roles are described in the neurotrophin family (see Neurotrophin receptors) and in the actions of GABA and glycine. They are ubiquitous enzymes acting in many different cells. However, their particular activity in neural sensory cells is highly relevant to analgesic development.

One group of compounds that is of particular interest for future development is the p38 kinase inhibitors. This group is particularly interesting because of the extensive research that has described them as a potential treatment focused on inflammatory pain mechanisms. P38 kinase has long been known to play an important role in inflammation especially in joint-related pathologies. Briefly, these kinases are thought to exhibit their therapeutic benefit by inhibiting many of the pro-inflammatory cytokines such as TNFα, IL-6 and IL-1β (see Cytokine family). BMS has advanced a candidate as an orally active inhibitor targeted for the treatment of rheumatoid arthritis. BIRB-796 (Boehringer-Ingelheim) has also advanced in the clinic, but very few data are available. VX-745 (Vertex) was dropped from development on toxicity grounds; however, VX-702 has advanced to patient trials.

While activity after the turn of the century has markedly increased in this area, no lead candidates have made significant progress in the clinic. Many have been discontinued after demonstrating hepatotoxicity and CNS effects characterized as dysphoria. It does, however, remain an important target for the future in inflammatory pain as better selectivity, potency, and oral activity are identified. The hope is that somewhere in this family of compounds a specific disease-modifying product for immune-based pathologies such as RA will develop

Nitric oxide synthase

Nitric oxide synthase (NOS) is an enzyme that produces nitric oxide from arginine. Nitric oxide is then utilized in the communication between neurons, in effects on the immune system, and in contributing to vasodilatation. There are three known important isoforms; endothelial NOS (eNOS), neuronal NOS (nNOS), and inducible NOS (iNOS). iNOS plays a role in immune and inflammatory responses, while nNOS is an important modulator of pain and neuronal sensitization. Several compounds have been advanced by Neuraxon in this arena. NXN-188, a selective nNOS inhibitor and 5HT agonist, devoid of cardiovascular side effects, is targeted for migraine headache. Since iNOS plays an important role in inflammation and nNOS plays a role in central sensitization, the development of a dual inhibitor of iNOS and nNOS may be found in the near future. Early testing in headache is promising for this family and a possible beneficial role in neuropathic pain is evolving. In addition, a potential role in poorly managed visceral pain has merit. Juxtaposed to compounds decreasing the production of nitric oxide is AZD-3582/HCT-3012 (Naproxcinod), which acts as a nitric oxide donor. However, this product has focused on the beneficial actions of nitric oxide to reduce severe cardiovascular (stroke/heart attack) and possibly gastrointestinal toxicities

Receptor families

Purinoceptors

Receptors preferentially activated by adenosine triphosphate (ATP) are termed purinoceptors. There are two distinct classes of purinoceptor that have been designated P2X and P2Y. In the context of pain mechanisms and analgesic control of pain, the P2X receptors are the ones that have been most studied. Two particular sub-types of the P2X receptor are worthy of mention; $P2X_3$ and $P2X_4$.

$P2X_3$ receptors

The purine $P2X_3$ receptor is a specific sub-type of ATP-gated ion channel which is found on peripheral nociceptors (Figure 108.1). While its role in modulating the peripheral nociceptor is not clearly understood, it has been suggested that it may well be the receptor that is responsive to pressure or tissue deformation/distension/damage. The rationale underlying this thesis is that ATP is released by these types of stimuli and because small-diameter C fibers express the $P2X_3$ receptor for which ATP is the natural ligand. Some support for this notion comes from experiments where filling and stretching of the urinary bladder is known to cause the release of ATP from the stratified columnar epithelial cells and activation of $P2X_3$ to induce bladder emptying. Thus, the release of ATP could be regarded as a signal that enables immediate detection by nociceptors of tissue damage or distension. While there is considerable interest in this potential therapeutic target there are no molecules that are currently in clinical development.

$P2X_4$ receptors

Microglia have long been known for their specific homeostatic scavenging functions within the central nervous system. However, it has been recognized that they, along with satellite cells, play a much wider role. For example, nerve injury activates microglia in the spinal cord and these cells are implicated in the induction of neuropathic pain. Until relatively recently, however, it was not known whether activated microglia were a cause or a consequence of the altered pain states. It is now recognized that they are a contributing factor. In injured and certain inflammatory states microglia are stimulated by the local release of ATP in the spinal cord that acts upon the purinoceptor, $P2X_4$. This action induces the formation, and release, of a small neuronal modulating protein termed brain-derived neurotrophic factor (BDNF) from the microglia. BDNF, in turn, diffuses from the microglia to exert its effect (see Neurotrophin receptors) predominantly on the post-synaptic cell in the dorsal horn of the spinal cord. The end result is the disinhibition of the GABA-ergic and glycinergic control of synaptic function. The fact that today BDNF is recognized to play a pivotal role in the development of neuropathic pain states makes the $P2X_4$ receptor a fascinating target for novel analgesics since blockade at this point would impede the induction and release of BDNF.

Adenosine receptor agonists/antagonists

Adenosine receptors are found throughout the body and mediate a number of biological functions. Adenosine has an important role in the function of nerve cells, it has a role in cell proliferation, and it acts as a signal of inflammation. Basically, there are four adenosine receptors, A1, A2a and b, and A3. These receptors are linked to G protein-coupled receptors and the complex functions that they orchestrate. A1 receptors are closely linked to cardiac function, A3 is inextricably linked to cell growth and cell death and A2b is probably linked to airway function. However, it is the A2a receptor that is a major driver of inflammatory events by sensing excessive tissue inflammation and enhancing neural communications.

A2a receptors have defined roles in Parkinson's disease, schizophrenia, pain states, and possibly Alzheimer's disease, and A2a agonists are in clinical trials as anti-inflammatory agents. However, interestingly, A1a agonists are in clinical trials for neuropathic pain. In fact, recent evidence suggests that two A1 receptor agonists (GR79236 and GR190178) have potential as treatments for migraine headache via effects on CGRP. Hence the roles and activities of these adenosine agonists have far-reaching effects.

There are few compounds in development as adenosine agonists. However, two such compounds have advanced to the clinic. GW-493838 (GSK) has been examined as an adenosine agonist and has advanced to phase 2 trials in neuropathic pain. Also T-62 (King Pharmaceutical) has begun early studies with a similar agonist for neuropathic pain. It is also of interest to note that while the A2a agonists have attracted the most attention for pain, an A2b antagonist has advanced as an enhancer for opioid analgesia. Clearly, the success of future candidates will require further development and understanding of these ubiquitous receptors with broad actions

Bradykinin receptors

Bradykinin has long been recognized as one of the G protein-coupled receptors that can modulate both pain and inflammation (see Figures 108.1 and 108.2). Two receptor types have been described: B1 and B2. The B2 receptor is expressed constitutively in a wide variety of tissues including nociceptive neurons whereas the B1 receptor lies dormant. In inflammatory states the B1 receptor is induced/activated and can generate both pain and inflammation. Stimulation of the bradykinin receptor leads to activation of a phosphoinositide signaling pathway, the release of intracellular calcium ions, and activation of a kinase system. This ultimately opens TRPV1 channels in the sensory nerve membranes, so enhancing nociception.

While the potential role of bradykinin antagonists is significant, years of research have not been able to adequately define the type of bradykinin receptor that is responsible for pain and inflammation in humans. A B2 antagonist (HOE140; Icatibant) was evaluated clinically but failed to alleviate acute pain. To date there is no B1 antagonist and a clear clinical candidate for B2 is not on the horizon. Nevertheless, the proven involvement of bradykinin in inflammatory pain renders an antagonist of the relevant B-receptor a worthwhile target.

Calcitonin gene-related peptide (CGRP) receptors

CGRP is one of a family of substances believed to play a meaningful role in the condition referred to as "neurogenic inflammation". This peptide is released from the terminals of primary sensory neurons in almost all tissues with particular density in perivascular, dorsal root, vagal, and trigeminal ganglia (Figure 108.2). Sensory nerve stimulation, subsequent extravasation, and vasodilatation, which are all considered part of the migraine attack, were initially thought to be inhibited by neurokinin receptor (NK1) antagonists. However, since these blockers failed to change the direction of these painful conditions, CGRP antagonists were tested and found to block the neurogenic vasodilatation and the subsequent migraine headache. In addition, it has been suggested that CGRP antagonists could play a role in other painful conditions as well as opioid-induced tolerance and dependence.

CGRP exerts a number of effects in the human body, but one of the most significant is its role in arterial vasodilatation (see Figure 108.2). Sensory nerve fibers that contain CGRP innervate small arteries and have the ability to control vasomotor activity. CGRP also causes vascular relaxation through a nitric oxide pathway (see Nitric oxide synthase) affecting vascular smooth muscle. In a migraine attack, vasodilatation in the intra-cranial and extra-cranial arteries is believed to cause the headache phase of migraine. Neurogenic inflammation mediated by activation of the trigeminal C fibers known to trigger migraines is completely abolished by CGRP antagonists. Furthermore, this effect has also been seen with cluster headaches. It is of interest to note that the existing anti-migraine treatments (ergot, triptans) inhibit CGRP release.

Early discovery of a peptide antagonist showed promise in animal models, but it had poor penetration through the blood–brain barrier because of its peptide nature. Shortly thereafter, telcagepant (MK-0974 from Merck) was shown to be orally active and effective in relieving headache. Key to success in this area will be the design of a molecule which can be administered by convenient routes (oral, sub-lingual, intranasal) providing a rapid onset of action. BMS-694153 could be just such a molecule in that it is potent, water-soluble, has good intranasal bioavailability and favorable toxicology.

Glutamates receptor agonists/antagonists

The excitatory neurotransmitter glutamate (Figure 108.2) has a variety of family members that have been evaluated as targets for analgesic development especially in the initiation and maintenance of neuropathic pain resulting from central injury (spinal cord), peripheral injury (PDN, radiculopathy), and inflammatory injury (arthritis).

There is added excitement around this neurotransmitter family because they have been suggested to be involved in three significant problems with pain – hyperalgesia, allodynia, and spontaneous pain generation. Furthermore, glutamatergic signaling is involved in the process of central sensitization. Glutamate receptors are classified into ionotropic and metabotropic receptors. Generally, glutamate, NMDA, AMPA and kainate-selective agonists are pro-nociceptive, while metabotropic glutamate attenuates pain. Therefore, antagonists of NMDA, AMPA and kainate as well as agonists of metabotropic glutamate are potentially analgesic.

Ionotropic receptors

NMDA

NMDA antagonists are probably the most recognized glutamate modulators. In animal models, these molecules have shown significant activity as analgesics, but have also shown concerning side effects and therefore have a weak therapeutic index. Ketamine is a specific dissociative anesthetic which acts through NMDA pathways but has poor efficacy and a myriad side effects including hallucinations and sedation. MK801 (dizocipine) showed similar short-comings, but did lead to the development of a lower affinity channel blocker such as memantidine (see Chapter 77), which has shown limited success in the clinic. However, antagonists of the NMDA sub-types (NR1 and NR2) have been evaluated to enhance efficacy and reduce toxicity with this class of compounds. These compounds are directed at the strychnine-insensitive glycine$_B$ regulatory site of the NMDA channel. One specific NR1-glycine antagonist (GV196771), however, has not shown meaningful pain relief with reduced side effects probably due to inadequate penetration into the CNS. Another candidate (NR2B) has been suggested to have very specific sensory distribution and therefore a target for specific antagonist development. Many of these compounds that interact through NR1 and 2 have been evaluated in ischemic stroke and cognition, but there is possible activity in neuropathic pain exemplified by RGH896 (Gideon Richter), EV101 (Evotec), and CP101606 (Pfizer).

AMPA

AMPA receptors are a family of proteins that line sodium ion channels expressed in the brain, spinal cord, dorsal root, and periphery. These receptors transmit both sensory and nociceptive stimuli. Transmission mediated by AMPA is believed to play an important role in wind-up and central plasticity. Thus, it is an important component in persistent pain states. Antagonists of the AMPA receptor have significant analgesic potential; however, the well-known side effects of ataxia and sedation have hampered their development.

Torrey-Pines has advanced the development of a specific AMPA-kinase antagonist (NGX426/tezampanel) for pain. However, poor bioavailability (it has only been evaluated as an injectable) and several side effects are problematic. Development of an orally active prodrug have, however, resurrected interest in this compound. NS-1209 (NeuroSearch) has also advanced into Phase 1 clinical trials.

Kainate receptors

This receptor family is very similar to NMDA and AMPA. These receptors are largely distributed in both the central and peripheral nervous systems. They are localized in dendrites, postsynaptic membranes, nerve fibers, and synapses. They generally play an excitatory role in the postsynaptic membrane of excitatory neurons. They can also modulate GABA release from inhibitory neurons and also sensory ganglia within the dorsal horn.

The focus of several compounds in development has focused on the GLU$_{k5}$ subunit. LY382884 has been advanced as a treatment for peripheral neuropathy and LY 466195 for migraine; however, neither has gone deep into the clinic.

Metabotropic receptors

This sub-family of glutamate receptors has been extensively researched. The receptors are separated into three groups: Group I includes mGluR1 and 5 and their variants; Group II includes mGluR2 and 3; and Group III includes mGluR4, 6, 7, and 8. Group I receptors generally couple G protein receptors, while Groups II and III generally couple with adenyl cyclase.

In particular, mGluR1 and 5 have shown promise in the modulation of central excitability in chronic pain, but minimal effects in acute pain. Activation of mGluR1 receptors plays a critical role in the induction and maintenance of central sensitization induced by inflammation. Therefore, antagonists of these pathways are targets for persistent inflammatory pain. LY367385, a specific antagonist has been shown to have analgesic effects in multiple models of inflammatory pain which is apparently mediated by both central and peripheral targets. Further studies have also suggested a role in attenuating persistent neuropathic pain. Peripheral mGluR5 receptors have been suggested to modify pain and several antagonists (MPEP and SIB 1747) have shown activity in animal models of neuropathic pain. ADX10059 and ADX4861 (Addex) have proven clinically effective in both migraine and fibromyalgia and AZD2066 and

AZD9272 (Astra Zeneca) are in phase 1 and 2 clinical trials.

mGluR2 and 3 have been evaluated for their effects on pain transmission. There is emerging information that suggests that these pathways and receptors are involved in the central sensitization in the dorsal horn and spinal cord. mGluR2 is located in sensory nerves and believed to play an important role in reversing allodynia whereas mGluR3 is located in several sites in the brain as well as in the spinal dorsal horn after nerve injury. Several agonists, LY379268, LY354740 and LV389795, have been shown to support the development of persistent pain following inflammatory reactions. Furthermore, antagonists of these mGluR2/4 receptors have shown reversal or prevention of these outcomes. While there is significant analgesic potential with antagonists of these receptors clinical development is very slow.

Nicotinic receptor agonists/antagonists

Neuronal nicotinic receptors (NNRs) have been investigated for years as part of the very complex ligand-gated ion channel family. Basically, there are five subunit proteins that form this channel expressing both α and β sites. While the definition of these units and binding sites continues to evolve, their potential role in pain modulation has garnered significant interest, particularly with regard to neuropathic states. Models of chronic pain secondary to nerve injury have demonstrated an overexpression of several of these subunits. Interestingly, both agonists and antagonists of these NNRs have been evaluated for therapeutic potential.

Abbott developed one of the early agonists (ABT-594), which was a selective agonist of subunits α4 and β2 demonstrating anti-nociceptive activity, but not acceptable tolerability. ABT-894 was subsequently advanced as a candidate and has shown significant potential. TC-6499 (GSK/Targacept), classified as a neuronal nicotinic receptor agonist, has also advanced into the clinic. On the antagonist side, ACV-1 (Metabolic Pharmaceuticals), which was discovered from the Australian marine cone snail, has entered phase 1 trials for neuropathic pain. While its effectiveness in neuropathic pain models is well-defined, it may also be effective in certain inflammatory pain states. The seemingly paradoxical effect of this antagonist is believed to be based on the different NNR subtypes. Significant interest in this conopeptide exists because it appears to have no effect on motor coordination, can be delivered subcutaneously or by inhalation, and possibly demonstrates the ability to assist in the repair of damaged nerves.

Cannabinoid receptors

There are two cannabinoid receptors of interest to pain: CB-1 and CB-2. Their present development for analgesia is described in Chapters 125 (general agonists) and 126 (peripheral agonists). The significant interest in these receptors is driven by the finding that the CB receptor is found in both the central and peripheral nervous systems. Essentially, it is the CB-1 receptor which has been defined as the target for future development (see Figures 108.1 and 108.2). The earliest agonist candidate (THC) demonstrated analgesic effectiveness in neuropathic pain, but widespread nonspecific binding of CB-1 and CB-2 resulted in distressing side effects.

At least three candidates have since been advanced in the clinic. One of the first (Sativa, GW Pharma) was approved as a nasal spray for MS pain and allodynia. KDS2000 (Kadmus Pharma) has advanced their candidate into patients with PDN and PHN using a topical formulation. Astra Zeneca has also made significant progress with a selective CB-2 agonist (AZD 1940).

Neurotrophin receptors

Neurotrophins are a family of related proteins that contain the following family members: nerve growth factor (NGF), brain-derived neurotrophic factor (BDNF), neurotrophin-3 (NT-3), and NT-4/5. All neurotrophins are synthesized as proforms that are cleaved to release the active, mature forms. Each neurotrophin binds with high affinity to one of the tyrosine receptor kinase (trk) family of transmembrane receptors; NGF to trkA, BDNF and NT-4/5 to trkB and NT-3 to trkC. The neurotrophins all act on trks that are expressed on sensory nerve terminals, the end result being enhanced sensitivity of the nociceptors. The two neurotrophins that have been most intimately linked to both injury-induced nociceptive and neuropathic pain are NGF and BDNF.

NGF

NGF is one of the most intensively studied of the neurotrophins. Its increased expression and release is a hallmark event associated with injury and a wide variety of inflammatory conditions. It is intimately involved in modulation of peripheral nociceptors (Figures 108.1 and 108.2). Once NGF activates its receptor, trkA, it turns on the phosphoinositide 3-kinase (PI3K)-src kinase signaling pathway leading to the phosphorylation of intracellular $TRPV_1$ stores which ultimately leads to their enhanced insertion into the nociceptor membrane. The upshot is a marked reduction in the threshold of stimulation of the $TRPV_1$ complex and consequent enhanced nociceptor activation. Furthermore, NGF activation of trkA significantly influences several other nociceptor modulating systems notably $P2X_3$ and bradykinin receptors, acid-sensing ion channels (ASICs) and the TTX-insensitive $Na_v1.8$ channels. By virtue of trkA phosphorylation all of these systems markedly enhance nociceptor sensitivity to provoking stimuli.

Few NGF/TrkA antagonists/inhibitors have been reported to date. However, the therapeutic concept of blocking NGF's actions has been established through use of the humanized anti-NGF monoclonal antibodies RN624 (Tanezumab; Pfizer) and AMG403(Amgen). Additionally, in rodent models of chronic pain the NGF antagonist ALE-0540 has shown anti-allodynic properties. Also, several antibodies to NGF from Sanofi-Aventis/Regeneron and Abbott/PanGenetics (PG110) have entered clinical trials.

BDNF

The receptor for BDNF is trkB, which is located in close proximity to both the GABA and glycine receptor, chloride ion (Cl^-) channel complexes on the post synaptic cell body of the second order sensory neurons in the dorsal horn of the spinal cord. Once activated trkB phosphorylates the GABA and glycine complexes in such a manner that the normal inward movement of Cl^- (which hyperpolarizes the membrane) is reversed. The outward movement of Cl^- creates a depolarized membrane and sensitization of the cell. Thus, BDNF from the activated microglia is capable of disrupting the very necessary inhibitory actions of both GABA and glycine that are normally released from the descending interneurons. It has been suggested that this action of BDNF may well be a critical component of the spinal "wind-up" phenomenon that can convert acute pain into more chronic, possibly even neuropathic, pain.

BDNF has also been linked with a direct effect on neuronal excitability as well as enhancement of NMDA receptor activation, both mediated via trkB phosphorylation.

At the present time there are no molecules that selectively interfere with the action of BDNF at its trkB receptor site. However, the realization that microglia, and BDNF in particular, have an important role to play in the development of chronic and neuropathic pain states makes them a very logical target for novel analgesic agents.

Cytokine family

There are several members of the family of cytokines that play important roles in the inflammatory responses in the central and peripheral nervous systems. Certain cytokines when secreted following injury to the spinal cord, the dorsal root ganglion (DRG), or other injured nerves lead to pain generated from abnormal spontaneous activity in the injured nerve or in compressed or inflamed DRGs. These cytokines are small proteins secreted by cells that control communication among cells. The subgroups include lymphokines, monokines, chemokines, and interleukins. The network and interactions of cytokines are extremely complicated, but the family members associated with inflammatory pain seem to be largely limited to IL-1β, IL-6, and TNFα.

IL-1β

This cytokine is released primarily by monocytes and macrophages as well as fibroblasts and endothelial cells during injury or inflammation. Nearly a decade ago it was discovered that IL-1β was expressed in nociceptive DRG neurons. It is expressed after peripheral crush injuries and CNS trauma (microglia and astrocytes). Following injection into the body this cytokine produces hyperalgesia and is found to increase the production of substance P and PGE2 in a number of neural cells. Administration of a specific receptor blocker (IL-1ra) has been shown to prevent or attenuate cytokine-mediated hyperalgesia and mechanical allodynia.

AV-411 (Ibudilast), manufactured by Avigen, is currently in clinical trials for pain associated with diabetic neuropathy. It has been described as an IL-1β and IL-6 inhibitor as well as a cytokine glial attenuator.

IL-6

This cytokine has been shown to play a central role in the neuronal reaction following nerve injury. It is closely involved with microglial and astrocytic activation and neuropeptide expression. There is significant information that indicates that IL-6 is intimately connected to the development of neuropathic pain after peripheral nerve injury. Also, intrathecal administration of IL-6 induces tactile allodynia and thermal hyperalgesia in rats.

Antagonism of IL-6 by AV-411 is currently under investigation (see IL-1β above). In addition, Sanofi-Aventis/Regeneron have advanced a humanized antibody for RA into the clinic.

TNFα

This cytokine has a long history of involvement in a number of inflammatory pain pathways. TNFα receptors are present in numerous tissues including neurons and glia. It has been shown to play important roles in both inflammatory and neuropathic hyperalgesia. In animals, intraplantar injection of complete Freund's adjuvant results in significant release of TNFα with a resultant hyperalgesia. This effect is delayed by the administration of an anti-TNFα antiserum.

As with all of the cytokine proinflammatory proteins, their effects can be prevented or reversed by specific antibodies; however, they can also be managed by the anti-inflammatory cytokines. These cytokines can be utilized for future analgesic properties. For instance, the cytokine IL-10 has been shown to antagonize the inflammatory properties of IL-1, IL-6, and TNFα. In addition, IL-10 can up-regulate anti-inflammatory cytokines such as IL-4, IL-11, and IL-13 or down-regulate the production of IL-1, IL-6, and TNFα. Direct administration of IL-10 has been shown to reduce peripheral neuritis, spinal cord excitotoxicity, and other peripheral nerve dysfunction. Similarly, IL-4 has been shown to exhibit antihyperalgesic effects in neuropathic pain. All of this work has been conducted in animal models, but it does leave an open door for commercial development. Interestingly, minocycline, a tetracycline derivative, inhibits IL-1β converting enzyme and NO up-regulation. It prevents glial cell proliferation and activation of p38 kinase.

The promise of genetics

Probably the most significant novel targets for the future are those driven by genetic variability to pain. It is this variability that has generated the hopes for personalized medicines in the future. Unfortunately, these targets are probably the furthest off. The thrust for the present and future growth of pain genetics rests at two levels. The first is to understand the genetic basis of the pathophysiology of acute and chronic pain and the resultant differences in pain sensitivity and variability and the second is how to effectively "control" these players. Currently most of the interest in this area is describing genes that code for specific pain-related pathways. Certain genes related to insensitivities to pain have been found to encode for specific voltage-gated sodium channels and neurotrophin tyrosine-kinase receptors. Also, genes defining sodium channels (SCN1A) and calcium channels (CACNL1A4) in migraine sufferers have been identified. Furthermore, genes encoding for opioid receptors (OPRM1), ion channels (TRPV1), bioamines and nitric oxide (GHC1), adrenergic and dopaminergic transmission (COMT 472), and endogenous signaling lipids (FAAH) have been described. However, study designs, heterogeneity, sample sizes, phenotype complexities, and statistical approaches have weaknesses that must be addressed before the value of genetic intervention can be fully appreciated

Additional target considerations

It is impossible in a chapter of this nature to cover all the novel targets that are being pursued with the intention of developing novel analgesics. Thus, in Table 108.2 we have provided a list of several novel drugs that are in different phases of commercial development, the mechanism(s) that are being targeted and anticipated clinical indication.

Concluding remarks

Today we have a far greater understanding of how pain is perceived and how that perception can be modulated, both up and down. We understand far more about the humoral and neurochemical mechanisms that occur at both peripheral and central sites within the nervous system. As a consequence of the assembly of all this new knowledge there is clear evidence that points us at ion channels, receptors,

Table 108.2. Additional targets

Drug	Company	Mechanism	Phase	Indication
AGN-199981	Allergan	α 2b-Adrenergic agonist	Phase 2	Neuropathic pain
Bicifadine	DOV	5-HT, NA reuptake inhibitor, glutamate antagonist	Phase 2	Neuropathic pain
Desvenlafaxine	Wyeth	5-HT, NA reuptake inhibitor	Phase 3	PDN
Radaxafine	GSK	NA, dopamine reuptake inhibitor	Phase 1	Neuropathic pain
Reboxetine	Pfizer	Selective NA reuptake inhibitor	Phase 2	PHN
Lacosamide	Schwarz	Amino acid anticonvulsant, Nav blocker	Phase 3	Neuropathic pain
Ralfinamide	Newron	Na and Ca channel blocker	Phase 2b	Neuropathic pain
IP-751	Manhattan Pharmaceuticals	Cannabinoid derivative; TNF antagonist; LO inhibitor; IL antagonist	Phase 2	Spinal and nerve injury pain
XPI3512	GSK / Xenoport	Pro-gabapentin	Phase 2	Neuropathic pain
NGD8243	Merck / Neurogen	TRPV1 antagonist	Phase 2	Post-op dental
GRC-6211	Lilly / Glenmark	TRPV1 antagonist	Phase 2	Neuropathic pain, osteoarthritis
AZDI386	AstraZeneca	TRPV1 antagonist	Phase 1	Unknown

enzymes, and cytokines that have the potential to be targets for novel, effective analgesics. Throughout this chapter we have attempted to tease out some of the most attractive of these novel targets, ones which hold the promise that, through selective intervention at these specific points, therapeutic modalities may result that could revolutionize the management of the most intractable pain states.

References

1. Rodger IW. Analgesic targets: today and tomorrow. *Inflammopharmacology* 2009;**17**:151–161.

2. Dray A. Neuropathic pain: emerging treatments. *Br J Anaesth* 2008;**101**:48–58.

3. Rice ASC, Hill GG. New treatments for neuropathic pain. *Annu Rev Med* 2006;**57**:535–551.

4. Bevan S, Andersson DA. TRP channel antagonists for pain – opportunities beyond TRPV1. *Curr Opin Invest Drugs* 2009;**10**:655–663.

5. Bleakman D, Alt A, Nisenbaum ES. Glutamate receptors and pain. *Semin Cell Dev Biol* 2006;**17**:592–604.

6. Pezet S, McMahon SB. Neurotrophins: mediators and modulators of pain. *Annu Rev Neurosci* 2006;**29**:507–538.

7. Fields RD. New culprits in chronic pain. *Sci Am* 2009;**301**:50–57.

8. Julius D, Basbaum AI. Molecular mechanisms of nociception. *Nature* 2001;**413**:203–210. Figure 108.3. Figure reproduced from Fields (2009) [7] with permission.

109

Intranasal morphine

Denis V. Snegovskikh

Generic Name: intranasal morphine (morphine mesylate/chitosan)

Trade Name: Rylomine™

Drug Class: opioid analgesic

Manufacturer: Javelin Pharmaceuticals, 125 Cambridge Park Drive Cambridge, MA 02140; Javelin was recently acquired by Hospira, Lake Forest, IL

Chemical Structure: see Figure 109.1

Chemical Name: (5α,6α)-7,8-didehydro-4,5-epoxy-17-methyl morphinian-3,6-diol

Chemical Formula: $C_{17}H_{19}NO_3$; molecular wt 285.34

Introduction

Intranasal (IN) morphine (Rylomine™) is a patient-controlled nasal spray that delivers a single, metered dose of Morphine. Rylomine™ is currently in phase 3 clinical development and may have use as a rapid-acting analgesic in both acute and chronic pain settings.

Description

Intranasal morphine provides rapid analgesic onset (comparable to IV) together with a simple and non-invasive way to control moderate to severe pain. It consists of a combination of active ingredient morphine mesylate and ChiSys delivery system. ChiSys is based on the use of chitosan to evenly disperse and improve morphine absorption through the nasal mucosa.

Chitosan is a cationic linear polysaccharide, composed of two monosaccharides: *N*-acetyl-d-glucosamine and d-glucosamine linked together by glucosidic bonds [2]. Chitosan is obtained from partial deacetylation of chitin, which originates from shells of crustaceans (e.g. crabs and prawns) and forms positively charged salts when dissolved in inorganic and organic acids [2,11]. Glutamate salt of chitosan with a mean molecular weight of around 200 kDa and a degree of deacetylation of 80–90% is used for nasal delivery of drugs [2].

Mode of activity

Oral formulations of morphine are associated with slow and variable onset of action, and provide unreliable analgesia in patients recovering from surgery. Clinicians often rely on injectable or IV-PCA morphine to ensure rapid and effective pain relief. Injection of morphine often requires professional assistance or hospitalization. Therefore, alternative formulations of morphine that are easy to administer by a patient or caregiver and deliver rapid onset of action may provide significant medical benefits. Morphine is a hydrophilic molecule that has very low bioavailability when administered intranasally (about 10% compared with IV administration) [2]. Limiting factors of nasal absorption are the polar nature of molecules [5], drastic changes in pH of local environment, and the presence of the enzymatic system [8,9]. Mucociliary clearance mechanism is another very important limiting factor that significantly decreases the amount of time during which morphine is available for absorption [10]. Chitosan can significantly improve transmucosal absorption of morphine through different mechanisms:

Positively charged chitosan reacts with negatively charged sialic acid residues of mucin of nasal mucus (bioadhesive mechanism) [1]. As a result of this strong interaction with nasal mucus layer and epithelial cells, chitosan formulation slows

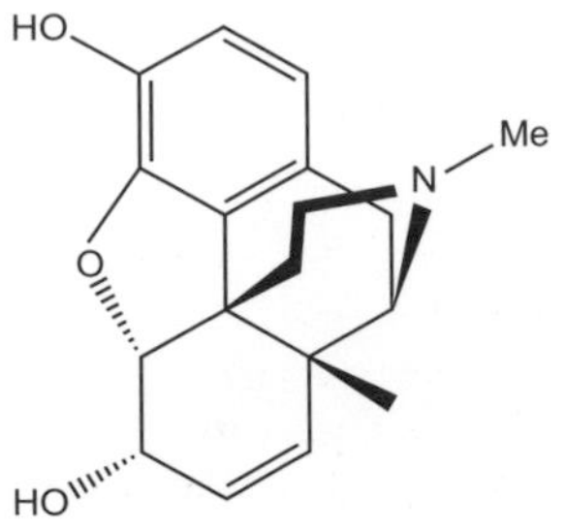

Figure 109.1.

clearance of morphine by the mucociliary system, providing a longer time for drug transport across the nasal membrane [2].

In Caco-2 cell culture studies chitosan opened transiently the tight junctions between cells, which enables hydrophilic drug to pass through the membrane by the paracellular route [2].

Median time to peak concentration (t_{max}) after intranasal administration of morphine/chitosan combination is 13–27 min and dose-dependent absolute bioavailability is 60% to 83% (oral immediate-release morphine: t_{max} 1 hour and absolute bioavailability 25% to 35%) [3].

The pharmacokinetic profile of intranasal morphine is similar to that of IV morphine with respect to plasma concentration of the drug and its metabolites [2]. Morphine plasma levels typically associated with analgesic efficacy (20–40 ng/mL) are attained as early as 5–10 minutes following intranasal administration [4]. Christensen et al. in a study of 225 post-surgical dental patients (third molar extraction) found that efficacy profile (onset, level of analgesia, and duration of effect) of intranasal morphine 15 mg was similar to that of IV morphine 7.5 mg. Analgesic superiority of IN morphine 15 mg over placebo was evident 5 minutes after administration and persisted for 6 hours [5]. The duration of analgesic effect (time to rescue medication) in that study was 3–4 hours, similar in IN and IV groups. Stoker et al. in a study of 187 post-surgical patients found that IN morphine showed a significant linear dose response, and that a 3.75 mg dose was not efficacious and a 30 mg dose caused excessive adverse events typical of systemically administered opioids (nausea, vomiting, hypotension and oxygen desaturation) [3].

The metabolite profile obtained after IN administration of the chitosan-morphine combination and IV morphine was essentially identical (M3G about 85%

and M6G about 15%). The level of both morphine-3-glucoronide and morphine-6-glucoronide were only about 25% of that found after oral administration of morphine [2].

After administration of IN morphine every 6 hours for 7 days the pharmacokinetics of morphine and its metabolites were linear within each dose. Mean plasma concentrations of morphine on day 7 were comparable to those on day 1, indicating no significant accumulation. Steady-state plasma concentrations of morphine, M6G and M3G were reached after 48 to 72 hours of dosing [6].

Each nostril can hold only 150–200 μL of administered drug. It requires approximately 15 minutes for the drug to clear the nasal passages. So attempting to introduce additional drug will result in the drug either being swallowed or dripping out of the nose [3,7].

Indications

Proposed indications for IN morphine are acute moderate-to-severe pain, including post-operative pain (orthopedic [3], dental [5]) and breakthrough pain in cancer and chronic non-cancer pain patients.

Contraindications

Proposed contraindication to IN morphine are similar to those for IV morphine.

No study was done on patients with acute upper respiratory tract infection, allergic rhinitis, or chronic nasal congestion.

Doses

A single-spray unit dose device delivers 7.5 mg of morphine mesylate intranasally in a 0.1 mL metered dose. Based upon the results of the trial of IN morphine for post-operative pain control in orthopedic patients [3] the following doses can be recommended:

7.5 mg every 1–2 hours

15 mg every 2–3 hours

A 7.5 mg dose was better tolerated, but had inferior efficacy [3].

A second metered dose cannot be given earlier than 15 minutes after the first dose [7].

Potential advantages

1. Rapid onset, comparable to IV morphine pharmacokinetics.

2. Non-invasive, simple way of administration. No need for dedicated equipment and specialized support.
3. Avoids GI metabolism, fewer GI side effects, lower level of metabolites.
4. Safe, no significant accumulation after 1 week of use, single-dose device limits abuse potential.

Potential disadvantages

Currently is in phase 3 clinical development in the USA; not approved by FDA.

Limited experience. Nasal administration may be associated with irritation and congestion, and epistaxis.

Drug-related adverse events

Local adverse events

Dysgeusia (transient bitter taste), rhinitis, rhinorrhea and nasal and throat discomfort, mostly mild to moderate in intensity [3].

Severity of symptoms is dose-dependent [2,3]. The majority of symptoms occur at 5 and 15 minutes post-dose, with few reported by 1 hour after IN dosing [3].

Systemic opioid-related adverse events

Similar to those seen with IV morphine, including oxygen desaturation, nausea, vomiting, dizziness, and hypotension. Oxygen desaturation after a single dose (that was corrected with oxygen via nasal canula) happened only after a 30 mg dose. All other symptoms were mostly mild in intensity and showed a dose-dependent pattern [3].

In the study of post-surgical dental patients who were otherwise healthy, doses of IN morphine of 7.5–15 mg did not cause any changes in respiratory rate or blood pressure. Only a mild transient decrease in oxygen saturation relative to baseline was observed. No patients required oxygen therapy [5].

References

1. Illium L, Dodane V, Iqbal K. *Drug Deliv Technonol* 2002;2(2):40–43.

2. Illum L, Watts P, et al. Intranasal delivery of morphine. *J Pharmacol Exp Ther* 2002;**301**:391–400.

3. Stoker DG, et al. Analgesic efficacy and safety of morphine-chitosan nasal solution in patients with moderate-to-severe pain following orthopedic surgery. *Pain Med* 2008;**9**:3–12.

4. Fisher A, Green G, et al. *A Phase I Absorption Study of Intranasal Morphine in Normal Volunteers*. Javelin Pharmaceuticals, Inc.

5. Christensen KS, et al. The analgesic efficacy and safety of novel intranasal morphine formulation (morphine plus chitosan), immediate release oral morphine, intravenous morphine and placebo in a postsurgical dental pain model. *Pain Med* 2008; **107**(6):2018–2024.

6. Albin R, Green G, et al. *A Phase I Single- and Multiple-Dose Pharmacokinetic Study of Intranasal Morphine in Healthy Volunteers*. Javelin Pharmaceuticals, Inc.

7. Sheckler MT, et al. *Nasal Delivery of Analgesics*. 2005. Available at: http://www.ondrugdelivery.com/publications/NASAL%20FINAL%20Lo-res.pdf.

8. Hussain A, Faraj J, et el. Hydrolysis of leucine enkephalin in the nasal cavity of the rat– a possible factor in the low bioavailability of nasally administered peptides. *Biochem Biophys Res Commun* 1985;**133**:923–928.

9. Lee VH. Enzymatic barriers to peptide and protein absorption. *Crit Rev Ther Drug Carrier Syst* 1988:**5**: 69–97.

10. Schipper NG, Verhoef JC, Merkus FW. The nasal mucociliary clearance: relevance to nasal drug delivery. *Pharm Res* 1991;**8**:807–814.

11. Muzzarelli RAA. Chitin. In Muzzarelli RAA, ed. *Natural Chelating Polymers: Alginic Acid, Chitin and Chitosan*. New York: Pergamon Press, 1973, pp. 83–252.

110

Intranasal ketamine

Daniel B. Carr and Ryan Lanier

> **Generic Name:** ketamine hydrochloride (for intranasal administration)
>
> **Brand Name:** Ereska®
>
> **Drug Class:** central-acting analgesic, NMDA antagonist
>
> **Manufacturer:** Javelin Pharmaceuticals, Inc., Cambridge, MA; Javelin was recently acquired by Hospira, Lake Forest, IL
>
> **Chemical Structure:** see Figure 110.1
>
> **Molecular Formula:** $C_{13}H_{16}ClNO[HCl]$

Description

Javelin Pharmaceuticals, Inc. (Cambridge, MA) has conducted late-stage clinical trials evaluating Ereska (intranasal [IN] ketamine HCl 150 mg/mL) as a sole analgesic agent for acute pain and cancer break-through pain (BTP) in patients on chronic opioid therapy. Ereska is an aqueous solution of 15% w/v ketamine hydrochloride (equivalent to 13% w/v ketamine base), with an antimicrobial preservative. It is administered using a "bi-dose" nasal delivery device that delivers two sprays per device (one spray in each nostril, 90 seconds between sprays) for a total unit dose of 0.2 mL or 30 mg of ketamine hydrochloride (equivalent to 26 mg ketamine base) (Figure 110.2).

Mode of activity

Ketamine is a rapid-acting dissociative anesthetic first approved 40 years ago for animals and humans, and in continuous use since. At anesthetic doses (several mg/kg) it produces a cataleptic state with nystagmus and intact corneal and light reflexes, and maintenance of ventilatory drive as well as blood pressure even in hypovolemic subjects [1]. The latter properties make it a potentially attractive alternative to morphine or other opioids in civilian emergency, mass casualty, or military settings. Soon after ketamine's introduction into clinical practice it was observed that analgesia often persists long after its anesthetic effects subside, and can be achieved in awake subjects given subanesthetic doses (0.25–0.5 mg/kg). More recent investigations have indicated that plasma ketamine concentrations in the range of 50–150 ng/mL are analgesic and also potentiate opioid analgesia with little or no psychological effects [2]. For additional information, please refer to the chapter on injectable ketamine.

The physiology of the nasal mucosa makes it an ideal environment for rapid, non-invasive delivery of systemic drugs. Its large surface area, uniform temperature, vascularity, and high permeability facilitate rapid and predictable absorption of drugs into the bloodstream. A number of drugs in current clinical use are effective when administered IN. To provide analgesia by delivering subanesthetic doses of ketamine via the IN route requires a suitable drug formulation and metered dose delivery system. Using such a system, clinical trials of intranasal ketamine have demonstrated that close to half of a 30 mg IN dose is bioavailable. Once absorbed into the bloodstream, ketamine is rapidly distributed into brain and other highly perfused tissues, in which it may reach levels 4- to 5-fold higher than plasma. The initial distribution phase from plasma to peripheral tissues occurs with a half-life of 7–11 minutes. The plasma half-life is between 2 and 3 hours. Norketamine is the primary active metabolite of ketamine, and produces effects similar to those of ketamine although with only about 1/5 to 1/3 the potency of the parent compound.

Ketamine, a non-opioid, inhibits the excitatory effects of the endogenous excitatory amino acid neurotransmitter glutamate upon the NMDA receptor. The NMDA receptor plays a key role in the development of sensitization, hyperalgesia, and tolerance to the analgesic effects of opioids, as well as in certain preclinical models of neurotoxicity. We have demonstrated that

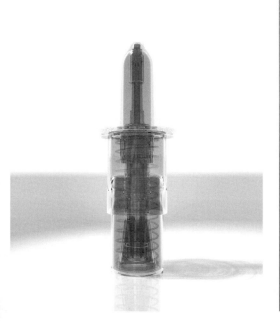

Figure 110.1.

our proprietary formulation can minimize or avert neurotoxicity observed in animal models in response to various NMDA receptor antagonists including conventionally formulated ketamine. The pharmacology and analgesic mechanisms of ketamine, the indications and contraindications for the approved injectable formulation, and its potential for neurotoxicity are reviewed elsewhere in this volume. Novel, intriguing mechanisms of ketamine's actions currently under exploration include anti-inflammatory properties as well as acute, beneficial effects upon CNS systems that regulate mood.

Indications/contraindications

Substantial published literature ranging from cases and case series through meta-analyses of randomized controlled trials describes the parenteral administration of subanesthetic doses of ketamine to provide analgesia in patients with acute pain such as burn pain, chronic pain such as neuropathic pain, and cancer-related pain as both a stand-alone analgesic as well as an adjuvant to opioids [5].

Since our intranasal ketamine product candidate delivers subanesthetic doses, "emergence reactions" observed in some patients following general anesthesia with high doses of injectable ketamine are not expected nor have been observed in clinical studies to date. Indeed, the Side Effects Rating Scale for Dissociative Anesthetics, an instrument used to characterize dissociative effects (fatigue, dizziness, nausea, headache, feeling of unreality, change in hearing, change in vision, mood change, generalized discomfort, and hallucination), has been applied during the early clinical development of IN ketamine. Most subjects reported no dissociative effects post-dosing and of those who did, the majority were weak or modest in severity. Local nasal effects of IN ketamine have likewise been mild and transient. On the other hand, caution should be used whenever ketamine or any other scheduled drug is administered via any route to patients with a history of substance abuse.

Efficacy and safety

At anesthetic or analgesic doses, ketamine has a wide margin of safety and has little impact upon cardiovascular and respiratory function even in physiologically compromised populations. Preservation, even stimulation, of blood pressure and pulse rate are seen with high doses of ketamine; such changes are minimal when very low doses are given. This pattern contrasts with the hypotension and/or bradycardia often seen

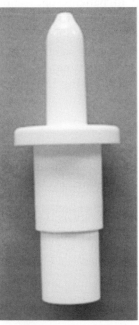

Figure 110.2. Bi-Dose Nasal Spray System™ prototypes for ketamine nasal delivery.

441

with exposure to volatile anesthetizing agents, barbiturates, benzodiazepines, and opioids. Ketamine is effective for alleviating pain refractory to opioids, such as acute or chronic neuropathic pain, and compared with opioids its use is less likely to be associated with issues of tolerance and physical dependence. The clinical literature on multimodal analgesia indicates that besides NSAIDs, only ketamine is proven to decrease pain intensity while simultaneously reducing the requirement for opioids sufficiently to decrease opioid-related side effects.

The bi-dose delivery system for our intransal ketamine product candidate provides non-invasive (i.e. needle-free) administration compared to IV or IM injections, via a rugged, simple to use device that can be patient-administered if necessary. Each disposable device delivers a total of 30 mg ketamine with well-characterized, predictable pharmacokinetics. This approach to delivering subanesthetic doses of ketamine may be particularly advantageous in emergency situations where convenience, speed of drug delivery/onset, and avoidance of accidental needle sticks in healthcare providers are desirable. In addition, our intranasal ketamine product candidate was formulated to minimize neurotoxicity, a question that has been raised regarding the differently formulated ketamine product currently approved for anesthesia.

Our intranasal ketamine product candidate is being developed for the management of acute moderate to severe pain, as well as BTP in patients on chronic opioid therapy. Pilot studies in both of these pain models, using the exploratory formulation of Ereska, have yielded encouraging results for safety and efficacy. A randomized, double-blind, single-dose parallel study [3] tested 10, 30 and 50 mg IN doses in 40 patients with acute post-operative pain following surgical removal of 2–4 impacted third molars (see Table 110.1). Dose-dependent analgesia, statistically superior to placebo, was observed over a 3-hour period. Analgesia was rapid (< 10 minutes) and meaningful pain relief was achieved within 15 minutes of the 50 mg dose. Safety was evaluated through adverse event reporting, vital signs, pulse oximetry, nasal assessments, and a standard dissociative side effects questionnaire. The majority of adverse events were mild/weak and transient. No untoward effects were observed on vital signs, pulse oximetry, and nasal examination. At the doses tested, no significant dissociative effects were evident using the Side Effects Rating Scale for Dissociative Anesthetics. Comparing results from this study and a separate study of morphine analgesia in the same molar extraction model, we estimated that 30 mg of IN ketamine had approximately the same analgesic effect as 5 mg IV morphine (Table 110.1).

A second exploratory study [4] found encouraging results in 20 patients with BTP chronically treated with opioids (> 60 mg/day of morphine or equivalent). Each patient had two BTP episodes at least 48 hours apart treated in a double-blind fashion with IN ketamine or placebo in a randomized, crossover design. Patients reported significantly greater declines in BTP pain intensity with IN ketamine than IN placebo ($P < 0.0001$), with pain relief evident within 10 minutes of dosing and persisting during the full 60 minutes of post-dose observation. Table 110.2 shows other key findings of this study. Repeated IN dosing has been shown to be feasible in our more recent unpublished clinical trials, although acute IN drug dosing is limited by the absorptive capacity of the nasal mucosa (acutely, about 400 μL).

Table 110.1. Intranasal ketamine for acute pain after extraction of impacted molars: TOTPAR scores across 1 and 3 hours (with permission from reference 3)

	TOTPAR1 (VAS)	TOTPAR3 (VAS)
Placebo	8.5 + 8.1	10.8 + 10.4
IN ketamine 10 mg	24.3 + 27.3	91.6 +109.1
IN ketamine 30 mg	24.4 + 26.3	61.7 + 71.0
IN ketamine 50 mg	46.0 + 28.4	122.3 + 97.7

All values reported as mean ± SD. VAS, visual analog scale.
For TOTPAR1, intergroup differences were significant ($P = 0.013$ by ANOVA). The 50 mg dose separated from placebo ($P < 0.01$ by Dunnett's, Tukey's, and Duncan's tests).
For TOTPAR3, intergroup differences were significant ($P = 0.028$ by ANOVA). The 10 and 50 mg doses separated from placebo ($P < 0.05$ by Duncan's test).

Table 110.2. Intranasal ketamine decreased breakthrough pain in 20 patients on chronic (>6 weeks) opioid therapy (with permission from reference 4)

Endpoint	IN ketamine	IN placebo	
Pain intensity decrease (mean + SD)	2.65 + 1.87	0.81 + 1.01	$P < 0.0001$
≥40% decrease in pain intensity	45%	5%	$P = 0.0078$
Rescue medication use during testing session	0%	35%	$P = 0.0135$
Pain intensity assessed using a 0–10 numerical scale			

In summary, subanesthetic doses of ketamine are now used increasingly in anesthesia practice as part of multimodal regimens for acute pain, as well as add-on therapy in selected patients with chronic pain. Our intranasal ketamine product candidate provides a simple, non-invasive alternative to the present invasive (IM, IV) methods of systemic administration of low-dose ketamine, and has the potential to make this agent available on a broader scale. However, it is still under development and the final assessment of its benefits and risks will await completion and integration of the results of its entire clinical investigative program.

Acknowledgments

The clinical studies described herein were supported in part by a contract from the United States Department of Defense (DAMD 17–00-1–1712; acute pain) and a grant from the NIH/NCI (1-R43-CA-86630–01; breakthrough pain).

References

1. White PF, Way WL, Trevor AJ. Ketamine – its pharmacology and therapeutic uses. *Anesthesiology* 1982;**56**:119–136.

2. Tucker AP, Kim YI, Nadeson R, Goodchild CS. Investigation of the potentiation of the analgesic effects of fentanyl by ketamine in humans: a double-blinded, randomized, placebo controlled crossover study of experimental pain. *BioMed Central Anesthesiol* 2005;**5**:2.

3. Christensen K, Rogers E, Green GA, Hamilton DA, Mermelstein F, Liao E, Wright C, Carr DB. Safety and efficacy of intranasal ketamine for acute postoperative pain. *Acute Pain* 2007;**9**:183–192.

4. Carr DB, Goudas LC, Denman WT, et al. Safety and efficacy of intranasal ketamine for the treatment of breakthrough pain in patients with chronic pain: a randomized, double-blind, placebo-controlled, crossover study. *Pain* 2004;**108**:17–27.

5. Visser E, Schug SA. The role of ketamine in pain management. *Biomed Pharmacol* 2006;**60**:341–348.

111

Inhaled fentanyl

Dana Oprea

Generic Name: inhaled (transpulmonary) fentanyl

Proprietary Name: AeroLEF™; Fentanyl TAIFUN®

Class: opioid analgesic

Manufacturers: YM Biosciences, 5045 Orbitor Drive, Building 11, Suite 400, Mississauga, Ontario; Akela Pharma Inc (Formally LAB Pharma), 11501 Domain Drive, Suite 130 Austin, TX 78758

Chemical Structure: see Figure 111.1

Chemical Name: N-phenyl-N-(1-(2-phenylethyl)-4-piperidinyl) propanamide

Chemical Formula: $C_{22}H_{28}N_2O$; molecular wt 336.4

Introduction

Fentanyl is a synthetic opioid analgesic, introduced in the 1950s, that has enhanced analgesic activity and potency and fewer adverse effects compared with morphine or meperidine. Structurally related to meperidine, fentanyl gained wide popularity as an intra-operative anesthetic adjunct as well as an effective analgesic for the management of acute and chronic pain.

Description

Fentanyl is highly lipophillic, has a rapid onset of action, and does not release histamine. It has a dose-dependent duration of action, with small bolus doses providing 30 minutes of pain relief and large boluses and continuous infusions providing highly extended durations of activity. Fentanyl is 100 to 300 times more potent than morphine, allowing a low therapeutic blood concentration of approximately 0.6 to 3 ng/mL for analgesia [1]. Given its stable cardiovascular profile, fentanyl became popular in many settings including critically ill patients. Its high lipid solubility and a pattern of rapid and extensive redistribution make it an ideal agent to be delivered through alternate routes other than the traditional intravenous or intramuscular ones. Alternative delivery methods include transdermal, buccal, intranasal, and sublingual administration for maintenance and breakthrough management of chronic pain. A new method of fentanyl administration, termed inhaled or transpulmonary administration, may offer the benefits of extremely rapid onset, convenience, and reliability for acute pain and sudden onset breakthrough pain in chronic pain settings.

Pharmacokinetics of inhaled fentanyl

Higgins et al. [2] assessed the effects of three concentrations of inhaled nebulized fentanyl citrate solution given for post-operative pain relief. Among the 30 studied patients, the patients inhaling a more concentrated solution of fentanyl citrate over 9 minutes showed a moderate analgesic response within 5 min of inhalation. In this study inhaled fentanyl did not prove more effective than the other parenteral formulations. Inhalation of 300 µg of fentanyl from the nebulizer produced a peak concentration of 0.4 ng/mL at 2 min and a plateau concentration of 0.1 ng/mL at 15 min, while with inhalation of 100 µg, blood levels remained stable at 0.02 ng/mL.

Another small study assessed the effectiveness of fentanyl delivered by aerosol for post-operative analgesia. The seven patients receiving 300 pg of inhaled fentanyl had a significant improvement versus patients receiving 100 pg. There were no adverse effects such as respiratory depression, bronchospasm, nausea or drowsiness reported in this study [3].

Mather et al. [4] also studied the use of aerosolized pulmonary fentanyl in healthy volunteers using SmartMist™. In this study, plasma concentrations from SmartMist™ were similar to those from the intravenous injection, with a bioavailability averaging ~100% within 5 minutes of delivery.

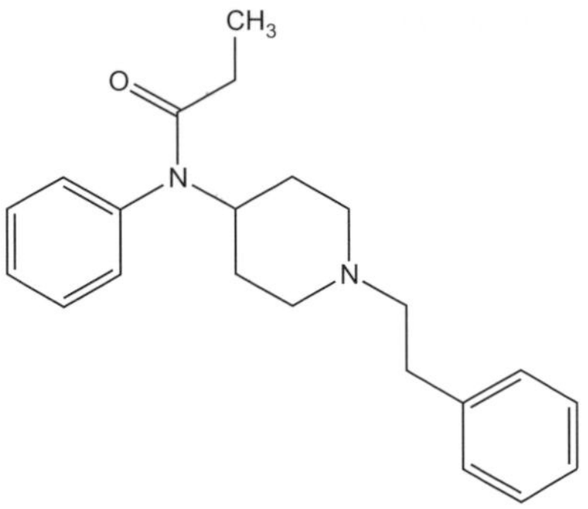

Figure 111.1.

Based on these prior studies, a liposome-encapsulated drug carrier system has been developed in order to overcome fentanyl's short duration of action. Liposomes are microscopic vesicles composed of an aqueous compartment surrounded by a phospholipid bilayer that acts as a permeable barrier to entrap molecules. Incorporation of a drug within a liposome provides a controlled, sustained release system.

In Hung's preliminary study [5] comparing nebulizer and intravenous administration of fentanyl, delivery of 2000 μg of a nebulized mixture of free (50%) and liposomal-encapsulated (50%) fentanyl (FLEF) to volunteers resulted in a peak plasma concentration of 1.15 ng/mL at 22 min. One important feature of the FLEF was that the plasma concentration decreased slowly after the single 2000 μg dose. At 8 and 24 h after inhalation, fentanyl concentration values were 0.25 ± 0.14 ng/mL and 0.12 ± 0.16 ng/mL, respectively (Figure 111.2).

In a subsequent study by the same author, five doses of 4000 μg FLEF were administered at 12-h intervals. The time to reach the peak concentration after each administration ranged from 12.5 to 19.2 min and the fentanyl concentration was maintained within the analgesic therapeutic concentration (0.6–3 ng/mL). The bioavailability of inhaled FLEF is 12–20%, which is consistent with the bioavailability of most drugs administered via the pulmonary system (10–20%).

Two inhaled fentanyl preparations are currently under investigation. AeroLEF™ is mixture of free and liposome-encapsulated fentanyl delivered through breath-actuated nebulizers. It is designed to rapidly achieve therapeutic concentrations through absorption of the free component, followed by release of fentanyl from liposomes and continued pulmonary absorption to extend the duration of action. Inhalation of small doses of free fentanyl in AeroLEF™

provides very rapid increases in plasma concentrations and appropriate therapeutic plasma concentrations (0.5 to 2 ng/mL) are achieved during inhalation dosing (Figure 111.3). Fentanyl TAIFUN® is a fast-acting fentanyl formulation delivered using the TAIFUN® dry powder inhaler platform.

Indications

Acute pain

AeroLEF™ has been specifically designed by YM Biosciences to provide rapid and extended analgesia. It is currently in development for the treatment of moderate to severe acute pain. AeroLEF™ is an investigational drug in late-stage clinical development and has already undergone phase I and phase II trials. During the phase I trial, ten healthy, non-smoking, opiate-naive volunteers received an intravenous (IV) dose of 200 μg fentanyl in the first arm of the study and a 3 mL dosage of AeroLEF™ (500 μg/mL) delivered by the AeroEclipse® breath-actuated nebulizer in a subsequent arm of the study with a washout period separated by at least 1 week.

Following the initiation of AeroLEF™ inhalation, plasma concentrations of fentanyl rapidly entered the therapeutic range within minutes, with the majority of subjects attaining maximum plasma concentrations in ≤ 10 minutes.

Administration of 1500 μg of AeroLEF™ and 200 μg of IV fentanyl achieved similar fentanyl concentrations; the achievement of maximal concentration of fentanyl within the dosing period allows subjects to safely administer therapeutic doses of fentanyl with AeroLEF™ and offers the potential for the patient to individualize the consumed dose of AeroLEF™ matched to their perception of meaningful analgesia during dosing.

Preliminary data from an eight-center, two-part phase IIb open label study suggests that AeroLEF™ is superior to placebo for providing post-operative pain relief in opioid-naive patients following orthopedic surgery. AeroLEF™ met the primary endpoint of the study, showing a statistically significant difference in SPRID4 (sum of combined changes in pain relief and pain intensity reported over the first 4 hours following initiation of dosing) from placebo.

A median time of onset of effective analgesia of 9.0 to 23.4 minutes was seen in patients with moderate to severe pain following a range of orthopedic surgeries across eight different clinical trial sites.

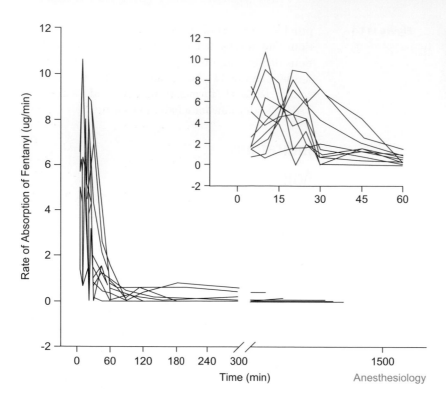

Figure 111.2. Rate of absorption of fentanyl after inhalation of the mixture of free and liposome-encapsulated fentanyl. (With permission from Hung OR, Whynot SC, Varvel JR, Shafer SL, Mezei M. *Anesthesiology.* **83**(2):277–284, August 1995.) [5]

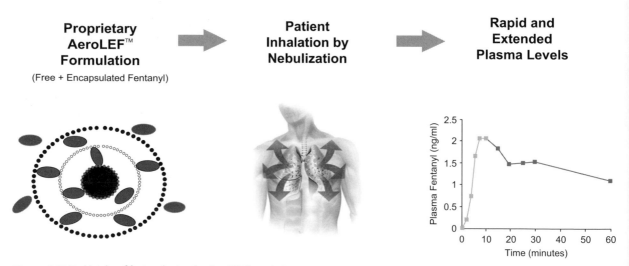

Figure 111.3. Uptake of fentanyl using the AeroLEF formulation.

Achievement of effective analgesia was the reason for stopping AeroLEF™ dosing in 88% of treated pain episodes.

A two-center, open-label study of 19 patients who had undergone anterior cruciate ligament surgery reported that 18 out of 19 subjects (95%) had reported a decrease in pain intensity at the end of dosing. Patients were allowed access to up to two nebulizers, each containing a 3 mL dosage of AeroLEF™ (500 µg/mL). AeroLEF™ self-administration achieved plasma fentanyl concentrations within the normal therapeutic range. The free fentanyl led rapidly to analgesic effects (mean time of 5 minutes) and liposomal fentanyl allowed for long-lasting analgesia in most patients (mean time of 3.7 hours).

Breakthrough cancer pain

Fentanyl TAIFUN® was developed for treatment of breakthrough cancer pain. When compared with other dosage forms used for the treatment of breakthrough pain, the inhalation route offers greater convenience and a more rapid onset of pain relief.

The results support clinical efficacy already at the lowest dose of 100 µg and a trend of dose-response relationship. The safety of Fentanyl TAIFUN® was similar to that of placebo, with the exception of an increase in mild to moderate somnolence. The TAIFUN metered inhaler is depicted in Figure 111.4.

The multi-centered, randomized, double-blind, placebo-controlled, parallel group trial of 122 cancer patients on maintenance opioid therapy was undertaken to establish formal dose-response data of Fentanyl TAIFUN®. The primary variables were the time to significant pain relief and the degree of pain relief. Fentanyl TAIFUN® was administered at doses of 100, 200, and 400 µg per dose during two episodes of breakthrough pain with rescue medication available upon request.

The time to significant pain relief was achieved on average in 7.8 to 11.6 minutes, depending on the dose. The difference from placebo was statistically significant with the 100 µg and 400 µg doses of Fentanyl TAIFUN®. Similarly, the degree of pain relief measured as the Sum of Pain Intensity Difference (SPID) was significantly better with Fentanyl TAIFUN® compared to placebo.

Preliminary data suggest positive results from the open-label arm of its Fentanyl TAIFUN® phase IIb clinical trial. The results from 24 patients demonstrated successful dose titration resulting in effective control of breakthrough pain episodes.

All 24 patients were successfully titrated to a dose of 400 µg or less. From these first 24 patients, nine patients titrated to 100 µg, ten patients titrated to 200 µg and only five patients titrated to 400 µg. The patients experienced significant pain relief in 95% of the pain episodes treated. The estimate of the median time to significant pain relief was 7 minutes. Based on the interim adverse event data, Fentanyl TAIFUN® doses have been well tolerated and adverse events recorded were in accordance with previously disclosed Fentanyl TAIFUN® clinical trial data, therefore suggesting high tolerability of Fentanyl TAIFUN® in opioid-tolerant cancer patients.

The phase III trials are ongoing.

Potential advantages

Inhaled fentanyl offers certain advantages:

(1) simple and non-invasive route of administration;
(2) rapid onset of analgesia from rapid pulmonary absorption of free fentanyl;
(3) extended analgesia from continued release of liposome entrapped fentanyl (AeroLEF™);
(4) personalized, self-titratable dosing.

In addition, the problems inherent in delivering analgesia to a patient with difficult intravenous access, to a patient who would not need an intravenous line except to receive pain medication, or in the out-of-hospital setting make the idea of having an effective inhaled analgesic very attractive. Inhaled fentanyl may also be able to be given more quickly than intravenous analgesia and the equipment costs of nebulizers compare favorably with the cost of the supplies needed for intravenous administration. Inhaled fentanyl also proved to be beneficial in the pediatric population, where it is easy to administer and does not cause additional pain or distress to the child.

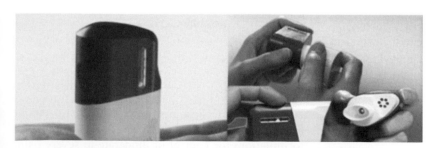

Figure 111.4. The TAIFUN metered-dose intrapulmonary fentanyl inhaler.

Dyspnea, which occurs in 70% of terminally ill cancer patients, may be significantly improved by inhaled nebulized fentanyl citrate, as well as the respiratory rate and oxygen saturation.

Potential disadvantages

Inhaling medications has certain limitations. Patients may find nebulizers cumbersome, noisy, and time-consuming and some dislike the face mask. Nebulization is also an inefficient way of administering drugs, although the dose can be increased (200 mg fentanyl citrate can be delivered in 4 mL of solution).

Side effects

Fentanyl inhalation does not cause any clinically significant adverse events and is comparable to intravenous fentanyl in terms of safety, tolerance, and preservation of pulmonary function.

Subjects reported feelings of sedation, relaxation, difficulty concentrating, tiredness, lightheadedness, vagueness, mild disorientation, heaviness in limbs, mental slowness, and pruritus after both routes of fentanyl administration: these side effects are typical of fentanyl. After the intrapulmonary route, there are reports of an unpleasant taste in the mouth and dryness of the mouth. Both side effects and subjective effects increased as the dose increased.

References

1. Peng PW, Sandler AN. A review of the use of fentanyl analgesia in the management of acute pain in adults. *Anesthesiology* 1999;**90**(2):576–599.

2. Higgins MJ, Asbury AJ, Brodie MJ. Inhaled nebulised fentanyl for postoperative analgesia. *Anaesthesia* 1991;**46**(11):973–976.

3. Worsley MH, MacLeod AD, Brodie MJ, Asbury AJ, Clark C. Inhaled fentanyl as a method of analgesia. *Anaesthesia* 1990;**45**(6):449–451.

4. Mather LE, Woodhouse A, Ward ME, Farr SJ, Rubsamen RA, Eltherington LG. Pulmonary administration of aerosolised fentanyl: pharmacokinetic analysis of systemic delivery. *Br J Clin Pharmacol* 1998;**46**(1):37–43.

5. Hung OR, Whynot SC, Varvel JR, Shafer SL, Mezei M. Pharmacokinetics of inhaled liposome-encapsulated fentanyl. *Anesthesiology* 1995;**83**(2):277–284.

Section 12 Chapter

112

New and Emerging Analgesics

Hydromorphone extended-release

Ira Whitten

Generic Name: hydromorphone extended release (ER)

Proprietary/Trade Names: Pallidone™, Exalgo™

Drug Class: opioid analgesic, class II

Manufacturers: Purdue Pharma Inc, 1 Stamford Forum, Stamford, CT; Neuromed™ Pharmaceuticals Inc; Covidien (a division of Mallinckrodt) 15 Hampshire Street, Mansfield, MA 02048

Chemical Structure: see Figure 112.1

Chemical Name: 4,5α-epoxy-3-hydroxy-17 methylmorphinan-6-one hydrochloride

Chemical Formula: $C_{17}H_{19}NO_3$; molecular wt 321

Introduction

Hydromorphone is a potent semi-synthetic opioid analgesic that is available in oral, rectal, and parenteral formulations for control of moderate to severe pain.

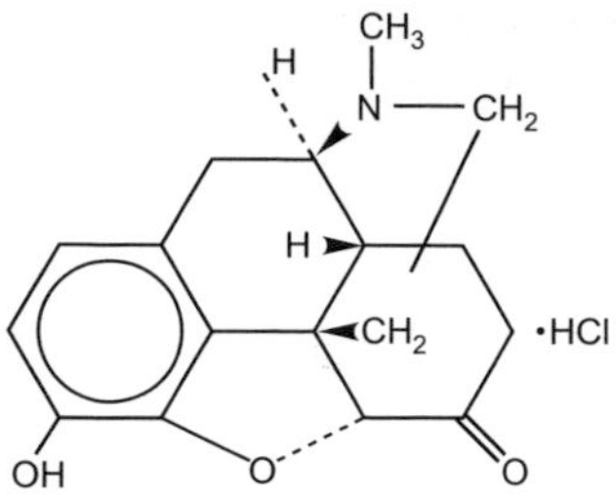

Figure 112.1.

It is prescribed as an analgesic for both acute postoperative pain and for chronic pain. Refer to chapter for additional information regarding use of immediate release preparations in pain medicine.

Mode of action

Hydromorphone binds to μ opioid receptors in the central nervous system to produce dose-dependent analgesia. Binding at μ receptors is also responsible for many of its its side effects including euphoria, pruritus, nausea, decreased GI motility, and constipation. Respiratory depression, the most troubling adverse event associated with hydromorphone, can be reversed with opioid antagonists such as naloxone.

Hydromorphone is similar in structure to morphine, yet it has higher lipid solubility and four to six times greater oral and parenteral analgesic potency. Hydromorphone has been available for many years in an oral immediate-release (IR) formulation for the treatment of acute and chronic pain, yet this form requires repeated dosing throughout a 24 hour period. Immediate-release oral formulations of hydromorphone have high oral bioavailability (62%), an onset of effect within 30 minutes and a peak effect within 1 hour of ingestion. Hydromorphone is 20% protein-bound and its respective plasma and tissue distribution half-lives are 1.3 and 14.7 minutes. Hydromorphone is primarily metabolized in the liver by conjugation to form the metabolites hydromorphone-3-glucoronide, dihydroiosmorphine, and dihydromorphine. Excretion of the drug occurs via the kidneys, where approximately 13% is excreted as the unchanged parent compound and 22–51% as conjugated hydromorphone metabolites. Total body clearance is 1.66 L/min, resulting in an elimination half-life that is 2.5 hours for the oral immediate-release formulation, which necessitates repeated administration every 4–6 hours [1–3].

Recently two new formulations of extended-release hydromorphone, Palladone™ and Exalgo™, have been developed for the treatment of chronic pain in opioid-tolerant patients. Extended-release hydromorphone may offer dosing convenience over IR preparations, and a more potent alternative to extended-release morphine and oxycodone.

Extended-release hydromorphone formulations

Two formulations of extended-release hydromorphone have been evaluated and filed for FDA approval in the USA. These formulations have been marketed under the names Palladone™, manufactured by Purdue Pharma Inc., and Exalgo™, produced by Neuromed Pharmaceuticals Inc. Palladone was initially approved for sale in the USA in 2004, but was voluntarily withdrawn from the market due to safety concerns. Exalgo is currently in the final stages of FDA approval as a once-daily administered analgesic for the management of chronic pain.

Palladone™ capsules are formulated using a controlled-release melt extrusion technology combining hydromorphone HCl with polymers to form pellets, which are then loaded into gelatin capsules. The capsules are designed to provide uniform, controlled release of hydromorphone over a 24 hour period and are produced in 12, 16, 24, and 32 mg dosages. Pharmacokinetic studies of Palladone demonstrated that a steady-state level is reached in 2 to 3 days and the formulation has an elimination half-life of approximately 18.6 hours.

In clinical trials, Palladone™ dosages were shown to be equivalent to cumulative dosages of immediate-release hydromorphone. When a 12 mg dose Palladone capsule given every 24 hours was compared to a 3 mg dose of immediate-release hydromorphone given every 6 hours the two drug formulations were found to be equivalent and Palladone showed lower steady-state peak levels, higher trough levels, and a reduction in plasma level fluctuation (Figure 112.2) [3]. The distribution pharmacokinetics following administration of Palladone show a biphasic level of drug in which there is a rapid plasma peak of drug followed by a prolonged broad second peak at therapeutic levels. The advantage to this form of dosing over immediate-release hydromorphone is that this extended-release formulation achieves a prolonged steady therapeutic level without the peak and trough effects of 6 hour dosing.

Palladone was initially approved by the FDA in 2004 for use in opioid-tolerant patients who required

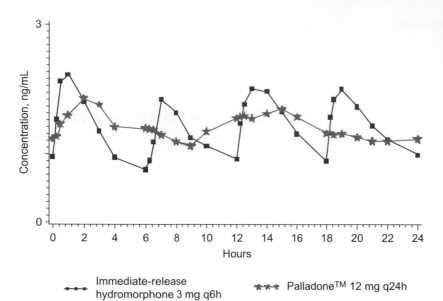

Figure 112.2. The pharmacokinetic profile of Palladone™ shows that at steady-state this formulation provides a constant therapeutic level of drug with less pronounced peak and trough levels compared to immediate-release hydromorphone.

Immediate-release hydromorphone 3 mg q6h

Palladone™ 12 mg q24h

prolonged therapy for chronic pain. Subsequent research by the manufacturer showed that when Palladone is combined with alcohol in vitro there is increased breakdown of the capsules resulting in rapid release of the hydromorphone salt. It was proposed that if this were to occur in patients that this "dose dumping" could lead to respiratory depression and death [6]. A subsequent study in healthy volunteers showed that when this extended-release formulation was taken with a solution of 40% alcohol there was on average a 5.5-fold maximum systemic exposure [7]. While no ethanol-related overdose events were found to have occurred in post-marketing surveillance, the manufacturer voluntarily withdrew the medication from the market. It is unclear at this time whether Palladone will be modified, reapproved, or remarketed.

Exalgo™ is an extended-release formulation of hydromorphone HCl manufactured by Covidien in conjunction with Neuromed Pharmaceuticals. This preparation is currently in the final stages of FDA approval for sale in the USA. Exalgo employs the OROS® push-pill™ oral osmotic delivery system to accurately deliver hydromorphone at a constant rate over a 24 hour period. Osmotic delivery of hydromorphone has been shown to deliver consistent amounts of drug over a 24 hour period and to achieve steady-state drug levels within 48 hours of initial dosing. Exalgo™ will be available in 8, 16, 32, and 64 mg dosages for once-daily administration.

A study comparing the conversion of morphine sulfate to OROS® ER hydromorphone in patients with chronic cancer pain showed that patients were able to successfully convert from morphine to hydromorphone over a short time period and that the long-acting formulation provided adequate 24 hour pain relief with lower overall pain scores [8]. Patients were easily converted using a morphine-to-hydromorphone conversion ratio of 5:1, and without prior conversion to immediate-release hydromorphone. Follow-up studies also demonstrated ease of conversion, safety, and efficacy of extended-release hydromorphone in the treatment of non-malignant chronic pain [8,9]. Exalgo™, like Palladone™, provides stable plasma concentrations with less fluctuation in drug level compared to immediate-release formulations that are dosed every 4–6 hours [8–9]. The pharmacokinetic profile of the OROS® push-pill™ hydromorphone formulation has also been shown to be independent of whether the patient takes the medication with food or not [10]. Initial studies of OROS® hydromorphone show that taking this medication with alcohol has only a minimal effect on drug release and no "dose dumping" was observed in volunteers [11]. With the approval of Exalgo™, practitioners will have a true once-daily medication for the treatment of chronic pain with less danger of rapid drug release.

Indications

The Exalgo™ formulation of hydromorphone ER is proceeding toward FDA approval for the treatment of moderate to severe chronic pain in opioid-tolerant patients. Extended- release hydromorphone may be indicated for the treatment of chronic pain secondary to cancer, back pain, osteoarthritis, and other medical conditions [3–10].

Studies of patient medication compliance have shown that complex administration schedules or use of a medication requiring repeated dosing throughout the day significantly decreases the level of patient compliance. The advantage of extended-release hydromorphone over immediate-release hydromorphone is the convenience of once-daily dosing compared to repeated dosing every 4–6 hours. Extended release hydromorphone also offers the ability to achieve a prolonged therapeutic level of drug while avoiding fluctuations in plasma/CNS concentrations. This may reduce the incidence of adverse events seen with peak plasma levels and avoid increasing pain noted with trough levels [3,4].

Contraindications

This medication is absolutely contraindicated in patients who have a hypersensitivity or allergy to hydromorphone or other opioids. Hydromorphone is relatively contraindicated in those with acute or severe asthma or COPD, conditions in which there is decreased ventilatory function, intracranial lesions or conditions associated with increased ICP, known or suspected paralytic ileus, or conditions resulting in respiratory depression or impairment. Patients with severe renal and/or hepatic impairment should be closely monitored for signs of respiratory depression as severe organ dysfunction may lead to poor drug metabolism and increase drug levels [3].

Adverse effects

The adverse effects of extended-release hydromorphone are similar to other opioid medications; with constipation, nausea, vomiting, pruritus, and urticaria being common. Other possible side effects include confusion, somnolence, euphoria, and respiratory depression. Respiratory depression is the most dangerous side effect of hydromorphone as it may result in hypoxia, coma, and death. Hydromophone should be used with caution in patients taking other CNS depressant medications. High doses of hydromorphone can result in the accumulation of neuroexcitatory metabolites which may cause seizures and myoclonus. One advantage over morphine is that hepatic metabolites of hydromorphone have minimal analgesic or respiratory depressant activity.

Extended-release hydromorphone, like other opioid-based medications, has a strong risk of physical dependence and abuse. In this regard the FDA labels hydromorphone as a Category C [3].

This medication should only be used in opioid-tolerant patients for the treatment of moderate to severe chronic pain. Patients must be instructed not to crush or adulterate the preparation as this could lead to acute toxicity.

References

1. Barash PG, ed. *Clinical Anesthesia*, 6th ed. Philadelphia: Lippincott Williams & Wilkins, 2005, pp. 465–497.

2. Weinstein SM. A new extended release formulation (OROS®) of hydromorphone in the management of pain. *Ther Clin Risk Manage* 2009;**5** 75–80.

3. Palladone medication guide. www.purduepharma.com.

4. Drover DR, Angst MS, Valle M, Ramaswamy B, Naidu S, Stanski DR, Verotta D. Input characteristics and bioavailability after administration of immediate and a new extended-release formulation of hydromorphone in healthy volunteers. *Anesthesiology* 2002;**97**(4):827–36.

5. Angst MS, Drover DR, Lotsch J, et al. Pharmacodynamics of orally administered sustained-release hydromorphone in humans. *Anesthesiology* 2001;**94**(1):63–73.

6. FDA alert: Alcohol-Palladone™ Interaction; www.fda.gov.

7. Walden M, Nicholls FA, Smith KJ. The effect of ethanol on the release of opioids from oral prolonged-release preparations. *Drug Dev Industr Pharm* 2007;**33**:1101–1111.

8. Vashi V, Harris S, El-Tahtawy A, Wu D, Cipriano A. Clinical pharmacology and pharmacokinetics of once-daily hydromorphone hydrochloride extended-release capsules. *J Clin Pharmacol* 2005;**45**(5):547–554.

9. Palangio M, Northfelt DW, Portenoy RK, Brookoff D, Doyle RT Jr, Dornseif BE, Damask MC. Dose conversion and titration with a novel, once daily, OROS osmotic technology, extended-release formulation in the treatment of chronic malignant or nonmalignant pain. *J Pain Symptom Manage* 2002;**23**(5):355–368.

10. Sathyan G, Xu E, Thipphawong J, Gupta SK. Pharmacokinetic profile of a 24-hour controlled-release OROS® formulation of hydromorphone in the presence and absence of food. *BMC Clin Pharmacol* 2007;**7**:2.

11. Sathyan G, Sivakumar K, Thipphawong J. Pharmacokinetic profile of a 24-hour controlled-release OROS formulation of hydromorphone in the presence of alcohol. *Curr Med Res Opin* 2008;**24**(1):297–305.

113

Hydrocodone extended-release

Thomas Wong

Generic Name: hydrocodone bitartrate/acetaminophen (HC/APAP)

Trade Name: Vicodin™ Controlled Release, Vicodin CR™

Drug Class: opioid analgesic

Manufacturer: Abbott Laboratories, Abbott Park, IL

Chemical Structure of hydrocodone: see Figure 113.1

Chemical Name: 4,5α-epoxy-3-methoxy-17-methylmorphinan-6-one

Chemical Formula: $C_{18}H_{21}NO_3$; molecular wt 299.3

Introduction

Hydrocodone is a well-recognized opioid analgesic, widely prescribed for acute and chronic pain management. It is a semi-synthetic opioid analgesic derived from codeine and thebaine that was synthesized in Germany in 1920 and approved by the FDA in 1943. Hydrocodone and compounds containing hydrocodone have become the most frequently prescribed opioids in the USA [1,2]. Reasons for its popularity include high efficacy, patient tolerability, low cost, and less controlled schedule III labeling.

Description

While primarily employed as an analgesic, hydromorphone is an excellent cough suppressant and is associated with less histamine release and pruritus than codeine. Hydrocodone is only available for oral administration, as either a tablet, capsule, or syrup formulation, and is usually combined with acetaminophen or ibuprofen. Standard immediate-release tablets provide 4–6 h of analgesia for patients with moderate to moderately severe pain. A new, controlled-release formulation that contains acetaminophen is pending FDA approval and has an extended 12 hour duration of effect [2–4].

Mode of activity

Major and minor sites of action: hydrocodone activates supraspinal and spinal opioid receptors. It has agonistic effects at mu, kappa, and delta subtypes and provides dose-dependent analgesia, euphoria, reduced GI motility, and respiratory depression. Its effects can be reversed by naloxone.

Hydrocodone has a half-life of 3.8 hours, peak effect at 1.3 hours, and a duration of 4.6 hours. It is metabolized by the liver and excreted primarily in urine. Hydrocodone is oxidized to hydromorphone by cytochrome P450 2D6. The extended-release formulation has measurably different pharmacokinetics: following a single dose of 1, 2 or 3 HC/APAP CR tablet(s), the mean maximum plasma concentration (C_{max}) ranged from 13.3 to 36.8 ng/mL for HC and 2.01 to 6.68 ng/mL for APAP. The mean time to reach C_{max} (T_{max}) was 6.0–6.7 hours for HC and 1.1–1.3 hours for APAP. Following twice-daily dosing of 2 HC/APAP CR tablets for 3 days, steady-state HC/APAP concentrations were attained by 24 hours [3,4]. The mean C_{max} on day 3 was 37.0 ng/mL for HC and 4.96 ng/mL for APAP. Systemic exposures of HC and APAP demonstrated a dose-proportional increase from one to three tablets. Steady-state concentrations were reached by 24 hours with minimal accumulation following twice-daily administration. Thus, it can be taken every 12 hours [4].

Indications

The extended-release formulation has been submitted for consideration and is pending FDA approval. The new preparation will offer a more prolonged and uniform duration of activity; however, like

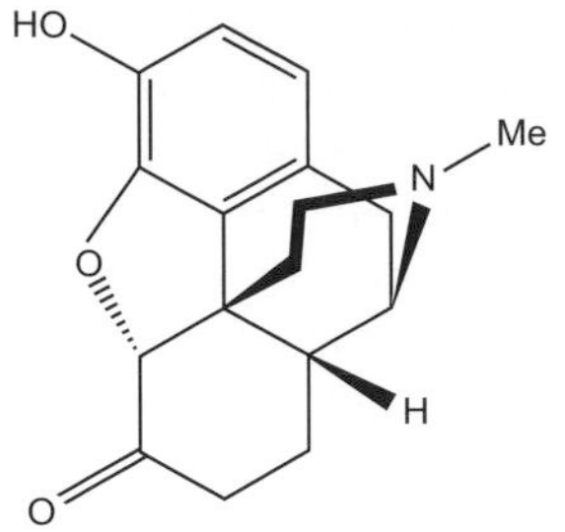

Figure 113.1.

other sustained-release opioids it will probably be approved as a more controlled schedule II narcotic, which may influence its prescription and use. The new drug application for Vicodin CR™ contains confidential information and at this time it remains unclear whether it will be approved as a schedule II or III analgesic.

Surgical acute pain: dosing will be based on investigational trials and guidance from the FDA. The efficacy and safety of controlled-release hydrocodone 15 mg/acetaminophen 500 mg (HC/APAP CR) was recently evaluated in patients recovering from bunionectomy [5]. Two hundred and twelve subjects were randomized to receive either one HC/APAP CR tablet plus placebo ($n = 70$), two HC/APAP CR tablets ($n = 70$), or two placebo tablets ($n = 72$) upon onset of moderate or severe pain following surgery. Subjects were treated for 3 days; however, the primary endpoint was the sum of pain relief over the first 12 hours. Patients treated with HC/APAP CR experienced statistically significant improvement in all efficacy variables (Table 113.1). One or two tablets of controlled-release HC 15 mg/APAP 500 mg provided significantly better pain relief for acute bunionectomy pain than placebo tablets. Two tablets provided consistently superior relief to one tablet. Time to perceptible pain relief was < 40 minutes. As might be expected, the incidence of adverse events was significantly higher for subjects receiving HC/APAP CR versus placebo. The most common adverse events were nausea, vomiting, headache, dizziness, somnolence, pruritus, and pain.

Chronic low back pain

The efficacy of HC/APAP extended-release was assessed in patients with moderate to severe chronic low back pain in a double-blind, placebo-controlled trial [6]. At the end of the open-label titration period, 511 patients entered the 12-week double-blind portion of the study and were randomized to receive one tablet of HC/APAP extended release, two tablets HC/APAP extended release, or placebo twice daily. The primary efficacy endpoint was measured as change in patients' assessments of pain intensity based on a visual analog scale, and compared to baseline. Back pain intensity was significantly lower in patients receiving either one or two tablets taken twice daily of HC/APAP extended release compared to those taking placebo (8.6, two tablets, $P = 0.001$; 13.3, one tablet, $P = 0.002$ versus 22.2, placebo). The most common adverse events in any treatment group were nausea, constipation, diarrhea, and headache. In the two-tablet HC/APAP controlled release group, 53% of patients reported adverse events, as compared to 44% in the one-tablet group [6].

Medical pain

Hydrocodone/acetaminophen may be used to treat moderate to moderately severe pain with greater convenience and possibly better patient compliance since it is dosed twice a day (q12 hours) instead of the usual 3–6 hours. The long-term efficacy of extended-release hydrocodone/acetaminophen was evaluated for osteoarthritic pain management [7]. Pain and quality of life were assessed using Brief Pain Inventory (BPI), Work Productivity and Activity Impairment (WPAI), and SF-36 questionnaires that occurred at baseline,

Table 113.1. HC/APAP CR bunionectomy trial efficacy results

Group minutes	TOTPAR score mean (SE)	Perceived pain relief (n (%))	Meaningful pain relief (n (%))	Time to rescue medication (min)
Placebo (n = 72)	2.2 (0.98)	28/70 (40%)	11/70 (16%)	101
One tablet HC/APAP CR (n = 70)	6.4 (0.99)[a]	52 (74%)[a]	28 (40%)[a]	131[a]
Two tablets HC/APAP CR (n = 70)	13.3 (1.00) [a,b]	60 (86%)[a]	45 (64%)[a,b]	251[a,b]

[a]$P < 0.01$ vs. placebo, [b]$P < 0.01$ vs. one tablet. With permission from- Desjardins P, Diamond E, Clark F. Treatment of acute pain with 12-hour controlled-release hydrocodone-acetaminophen tablets following bunionectomy: a randomized, double-blind, placebo-controlled study. The American Academy of Pain Medicine Annual Meeting, 23rd Annual Meeting, February 7–10, 2007, New Orleans, LA.

weeks 24 and 56 [7]. Patients treated with (HC/APAP CR) showed improvement in all BPI pain assessments at each evaluation period. Patients had less sleep interference (decreased ~40–50%) and less interference in walking ability due to pain (decreased ~30–40%) from baseline to weeks 4, 12, 24, 40, and 56. Overall impairment due to health decreased 17.5% at week 24 and 15.8% at week 56. The most commonly reported treatment-emergent AEs (10% of patients) were constipation, nausea, headache, and somnolence. The incidence and prevalence of these common AEs generally decreased over time. One hundred and twenty-four (29%) patients discontinued due to AE(s). The most common AEs that led to discontinuation were nausea, somnolence, constipation, dizziness, vomiting, headache, and fatigue

Chronic cancer pain

Hydrocodone/acetaminophen CR™ has not been approved but may be used to relieve moderate to moderately severe malignancy-related pain. It may be useful for control of both somatic and visceral pain symptoms.

Contraindications

Absolute: history of previous severe allergic reaction to hydrocodone or acetaminophen. Relative: head injury, increased intracranial pressure, elderly patient, severe liver or renal impairment, acute abdominal conditions, hypothyroidism, Addison's disease, prostatic hypertrophy, urethral stricture, history of drug abuse, and patients with respiratory depression [8].

Common doses/uses

Controlled-release HC/APAP is only formulated as an oral preparation containing a standard dose of hydromorphone 15 mg and acetaminophen 500 mg, to be administered every 12 hours. Phase 3 study data indicate that 12-hour dosing provided effective pain relief for patients with moderate to severe acute and chronic pain. The drug should not be crushed or tampered with as that will change the pharmacokinetics of the extended-release hydrocodone. At this time, the manufacturer has not disclosed whether HC/APAP CR will be manufactured in a tamper-resistant formulation.

Potential advantages

Ease of use, tolerability, and efficacy: this new controlled-release formulation of hydrocodone offers the promise of greater analgesic uniformity and a more extended duration of effect than that provided by immediate release formulations. As monotherapy HC/APAP CR can be used for management of moderate to moderately severe pain. As used for multimodal analgesia HC/APAP CR can be combined with other immediate-release opioids and adjuvant analgesics for pain control.

Cost: N/A.

Availability: pending FDA approval possibly in 2010.

Potential disadvantages

Toxicity: limited by acetaminophen (not to exceed 4 g acetaminophen total dose per day), and potential for hydrocodone overdose.

Diversion and abuse: similar to other CR opioids, 12 h CR dose may be adulterated for immediate use. Abuse or excessive use is also associated with the risk of acetaminophen overdose.

Drug interactions: other narcotics, antihistamines, benzodiazepines, antipsychotics, antianxiety agents, or other CNS depressants. Use of MAO inhibitors or tricyclic antidepressants can increase the effect of hydrocodone. It is not recommended for pediatric use; Pregnancy Category C [1,2,8].

Drug-related adverse events

The most common side effects are lightheadedness, dizziness, drowsiness, nausea, vomiting, headache, and constipation [1,2,8]. Other side effects listed by system include:

CNS: agitation, dependency, CNS depression, lethargy, restlessness, sedation

Cardiovascular: bradycardia, orthostatic hypotension, palpitations, tachycardia

Gastrointestinal: nausea, vomiting, anorexia, constipation, paralytic ileus, biliary spasm, cholestatic jaundice

Genitourinary: urinary retention

Respiratory: respiratory depression, respiratory paralysis

Dermatological: flushing, rash, urticaria, pruritus.

Treatment of adverse events

Tratment of adverse events is similar to that employed for other opioid agonists: naloxone for reversal of respiratory depression, stool softeners, laxatives or peripheral antagonists for constipation, and ondansetron, metoclopramide, and other antiemetics for nausea and vomiting [1,2,8].

References

1. *Physician Desk Reference*, 63rd ed. Physician Desk Reference Inc., 2009.

2. Medline Plus, www.nlm.nih.gov – U.S. National Library of Medicine.

3. www.accessdata.fda.gov – FDA database for approved drugs.

4. Klein CE, Liu W, Qian JX, et al. Pharmacokinetics of 12-hour controlled-release hydrocodone and acetaminophen tablets in healthy subjects following single- and multiple-dose(s). The American Academy of Pain Medicine Annual Meeting, 23rd Annual Meeting, February 7–10, 2007, New Orleans, LA.

5. Desjardins P, Diamond E, Clark F. Treatment of acute pain with 12-hour controlled-release hydrocodone-acetaminophen tablets following bunionectomy: A randomized, double-blind, placebo-controlled study. The American Academy of Pain Medicine Annual Meeting, 23rd Annual Meeting, February 7–10, 2007, New Orleans, LA.

6. Hitt E. Efficacy and safety evaluation of 12 weeks extended-release hydrocodone/acetaminophen treatment in patients with chronic low back pain by prior opioid use. American Academy of Pain Medicine, 2008.

7. Webster D, Herrington D, Corser BC, et al. Effects of 12-hour, extended-release hydrocodone/acetaminophen on pain-related physical function, work productivity, and sleep quality: a 56-week, open-label study AAPM annual meeting, 2008, poster #194.

8. Ellsworth et al. *Mosby's Drug Consult*. Elsevier, 2002.

Section 12
Chapter

114

New and Emerging Analgesics

Iontophoretic transdermal fentanyl

Craig T. Hartrick

Generic Name: iontophoretic transdermal fentanyl delivery system

Trade/Proprietary Name: IONSYS™

Drug Class: opioid analgesic, schedule II

Manufacturer: Ortho-McNeil Pharmaceuticals, Inc., Raritan, NJ

Chemical Structure: see Figure 114.1

Chemical Name: propanamide, *N*-phenyl-*N*-[1-(2-phenylethyl)-4-piperidinyl]monohydrochloride

Introduction

The analgesic effects of fentanyl are predominately mediated via μ_1 opioid receptor activity. The historical development of fentanyl and its continuous transdermal delivery are discussed elsewhere in this text (Section 2). The iontophoretic delivery of on-demand aliquots of fentanyl (originally called E-Trans), however, is a novel patient-activated system that employs iontophoresis to rapidly deliver drug into the subcutaneous circulatory system.

Mode of action

While patient-controlled intravenous delivery of opioids has often been a standard therapy for moderate-severe acute pain management, this needleless system allows for rapid delivery of drug across intact skin, without the need for an intravenous line or pump (Figure 114.2). Using iontophoresis, an imperceptible current generates an electric field that repulses the

455

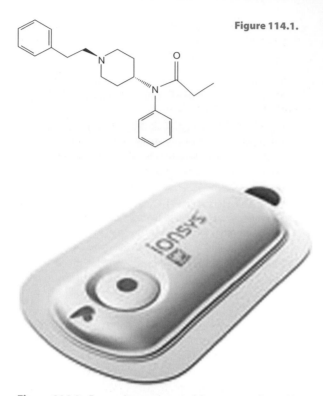

Figure 114.1.

Figure 114.2. Fentanyl iontophoretic delivery system (Ionsys™).

positively charged drug from a reservoir at the anode, forcing it through the dermis. Drug is also transported by electro-osmotic bulk flow of the solvent. Each system contains fentanyl HCl 10.8 mg in a hydrogel composed of cetylpyridinium chloride, citric acid, polacrilin, polyvinyl alcohol, sodium citrate, sodium chloride, sodium hydroxide, and purified water.

Dosing: the system is attached to the intact hairless skin of the chest or upper outer arm. When a patient activates the system by depressing a button on its surface twice within 3 seconds, a 3-V lithium battery generates a current density of 62 microamperes/cm² in the skin beneath the system. This current results in the delivery of a fixed dose of fentanyl (40 µg; equivalent to 44.4 µg fentanyl HCl) proportional to the current applied (170 microamperes). The delivery takes place over a 10-minute lock-out period, during which time the system cannot be reactivated. Blood levels of fentanyl continue to increase for 5 minutes after completion of each 10-minute dosing period. There is minimal passive drug delivery from the system; clinically significant drug delivery requires activation.

Approximately 40% of an administered dose is absorbed in the first hour of therapy; however, the system reaches near 100% efficiency after 10 hours of use.

A brief audible tone sounds and a light-emitting diode (LED) illuminates continuously during drug delivery. If the system becomes dislodged, losing effective skin contact, the LED flashes and a 20-second audible tone is produced. Depressing the button only once results in a single flash for each five successful drug deliveries, thus providing an estimate of drug consumption. The system remains active for up to 24 hours or 80 delivered doses.

The metabolism of fentanyl, as discussed in Section 2, is characterized primarily by phase 1 *N*-dealkylation to norfentanyl and other inactive metabolites via the cytochrome P450 enzyme CYP3A4. Since nearly 40% of all drugs that undergo phase 1 metabolism are substrates, inhibitors, or inducers of CYP3A4, there is considerable potential for drug–drug interaction. The patient-controlled self-administration inherent in this system, however, mitigates the clinical significance of potential interactions considerably. Rising or falling blood levels should be met with decreasing or increasing patient attempts, respectively.

Indications

Iontophoretic transdermal fentanyl (fentanyl ITS) was FDA-approved for short-term management of acute post-operative pain in hospitalized adults. The system is intended to be a patient-controlled method for maintenance of analgesia. Titration of a loading dose with opioids to an acceptable analgesic level prior to initiation of the system is recommended. Moreover, since the current (and hence the dose) are not adjustable, this system is most appropriate for opioid-naive patients and should not be preferred for opioid-tolerant subjects or those requiring a basal infusion.

Contraindications

As with all patient-controlled systems and devices, the patient must be capable of understanding how and when to use the system. Consequently it is not appropriate in patients with altered levels of consciousness or impaired cognition. The system has not been adequately studied in pediatric patients. Fentanyl is highly lipid-soluble. It crosses the placenta to the fetus in pregnancy and is excreted in breast milk.

Caution should be exercised in administering any potent opioid, such as fentanyl, in subjects with sleep apnea, severe hepatic dysfunction, head injuries, or conditions associated with increased intracranial pressure, or in patients with impending respiratory failure.

Potential advantages

Barriers to effective analgesia in acute pain management include pharmacokinetic, pharmacodynamic, logistic, economic, and technical equipment-related challenges. Rapid-acting, lipophilic agents with relatively short duration allow easier titration to effect without inducing prolonged adverse effects commonly associated with opioids. A pooled analysis by Viscusi et al. of three large randomized controlled trials ($n = 1941$) comparing fentanyl ITS to intravenous patient-controlled (ivPCA) morphine demonstrated comparable analgesia with both modalities. A meta-analysis examining adverse events by Hartrick ($n = 2597$) conservatively demonstrated that, compared to IV-PCA morphine, fentanyl ITS subjects were significantly less likely to discontinue therapy due to an adverse event (odds ratio [OR]: 1.5; 95% CI: 1.01–2.25, $P = 0.046$), had less pruritus (OR: 1.8; 95% CI: 1.3–2.4, $P = 0.001$), and, when the fixed-effects model was applied (Mantel Haenszel), less nausea (OR: 1.2; 95% CI: 1.01–1.4, $P = 0.034$) and less somnolence (OR: 1.9; 95% CI: 1.03–3.4, $P = 0.04$).

Hospital care, by its nature, is labor-intensive. Therapies requiring extra nursing and pharmacy personnel time present substantial barriers to care not only for the patients involved, but also for other patients whose care may be compromised due to time constraints imposed by the increased burden on the staff. A survey examining nursing time reported significantly less time associated with fentanyl ITS therapy compared to IV-PCA morphine. They estimated an average saving of nearly 70 minutes of nursing time alone for each patient, with most of the additional time involved in set-up and discontinuation procedures. These procedures also can lead to programming errors, resulting in accidental overdose and even death. This has been a topic of ISMP (Institute of Safe Medication Practices) Alerts; over 120 serious errors were reported to the US FDA in the past 10 years, with undoubtedly many more remaining unreported. IONSYS™ eliminates programming and therefore programming errors. It also eliminates the costs associated with actual pump purchase, maintenance, and repair.

Patient and nursing satisfaction is high with fentanyl ITS. Patients find the system convenient with no bulky pump limiting their movement and rehabilitation efforts. This is especially important after major orthopedic surgery. With respect to ease of care (EOC), patients following total joint replacement reported significantly better overall EOC compared to IV-PCA morphine (43 vs. 27%; $P < 0.001$) and better move-ment (97 vs. 71%; $P < 0.001$). Physical therapists (83 vs. 55%; $P < 0.001$) and nurses (80 vs. 55%; $P < 0.001$) likewise rated the fentanyl ITS superior for EOC. A pooled analysis ($n = 1305$) examining nursing time-efficiency and convenience confirmed these findings in post-operative patients following major orthopedic surgery, abdominal, and pelvic surgery.

Both personnel and technical issues can contribute to lapses in analgesic coverage: analgesic gaps. System-related events leading to significant analgesic gaps were compared in patients receiving fentanyl ITS with patients receiving IV-PCA morphine ($n = 1305$). Fentanyl ITS patients had fewer analgesic gaps (6 vs. 12; $P < 0.001$), shorter analgesia gaps (15 vs. 20 min.), and faster resolution of analgesic gaps (11 vs. 20 min.) compared with IV-PCA morphine.

Potential disadvantages

While the fixed-dose system eliminates errors, it also eliminates flexibility. The lack of programmability and the lack of a basal infusion mode may make fentanyl ITS unsuitable for use in many opioid-tolerant individuals. Moreover, the current design only allows an estimation of the actual number of doses administered (within five). Detailed history cannot be obtained from the system to determine the number and timing of attempts relative to deliveries.

At the end of service of the system (24 hours, or 80 doses), even if the maximal allowed drug was delivered, there is still considerable drug remaining in the reservoir. Disposal of the system requires disassembly by the pharmacist. The bottom housing containing the hydrogel reservoirs must be removed from the top housing, which contains the electronics and battery, for proper waste disposal and drug destruction according to local policy.

Skin reactions, including hypersensitivity, redness, and even prolonged hyperpigmentation, especially in dark-skinned individuals, are potential problems with transdermal systems. Failure of adherence of the system to the skin is an unusual but potential disadvantage. The skin should be clipped if necessary (not shaved) to improve adherence in hirsute patients.

Currently the principal disadvantage of fentanyl ITS is availability. Despite initial European Commission approval in January 2006 and FDA approval in May 2006, IONSYS™ is not currently being produced due to technical problems. It is likely that some design modifications will be made prior to launch that may include improved features for recording the number and timing of successful drug delivery attempts.

457

References

1. Viscusi ER, Siccardi M, Damaraju CV, Hewitt DJ, Kershaw P. The safety and efficacy of fentanyl iontophoretic transdermal system compared with morphine intravenous patient-controlled analgesia for postoperative pain management: an analysis of pooled data from three randomized, active-controlled clinical trials. *Anesth Analg* 2007;**105**(5):1428–1436.

2. Hartrick CT. Patient-controlled transdermal iontophoretic fentanyl system as an alternative to intravenous morphine PCA: review and meta-analysis. *Future Neurol* 2007;**2**(6):621–627.

3. Hartrick CT, Bourne MH, Gargiulo K, Damaraju V, Vallow S, Hewitt DJ. Fentanyl iontophoretic transdermal system for acute pain management after orthopedic surgery: a comparative study with morphine intravenous patient-controlled analgesia. *Reg Anesth Pain Med* 2006;**31**:546–554.

4. Lindley P, Pestano CR, Gargiulo K. Comparison of postoperative pain management using two patient-controlled analgesia methods: nursing perspective. *J Adv Nurs* 2009;**65**(7):1370–1380.

5. Panchal SJ, Damaraju CV, Nelson WW, Hewitt DJ, Schein JR. System-related events and analgesic gaps during postoperative pain management with the fentanyl iontophoretic transdermal system and morphine intravenous patient-controlled analgesia. *Anesth Analg* 2007;**105**(5):1437–1441.

Section 12 Chapter

115

New and Emerging Analgesics

Tapentadol ER

Raymond S. Sinatra

Generic Name: tapentadol extended-release

Trade Name: not yet named; possibly Nucynta ER™

Drug Class: opioid analgesic, class II; central-acting analgesic

Manufacturer: PriCara, Division of Ortho-McNeil-Janssen Pharmaceuticals, Inc., Raritan, NJ 08869

Chemical Name: 3-[(1*R*,2*R*)-3-(dimethylamino)-1-ethyl-2-methylpropyl]phenol monohydrochloride

Chemical Structure: see Figure 115.1

Chemical Formula: $C_{14}H_{23}NO \cdot HCl$

Description

Tapentadol is a novel schedule II central-acting analgesic. It was initially formulated as an immediate-release preparation and approved in 2008 for moderate to severe acute pain. Tapentadol immediate-release, Nucynta®, is marketed as 50, 75, and 100 mg tablets and provides analgesia (primary efficacy endpoint) comparable to 10–15 mg of immediate-release oxycodone. A sustained-duration oral formulation named Tapentadol ER is in late-stage development for chronic pain and the results of clinical trials, including four phase III pivotal trials, have been submitted to the FDA for approval.

Mode of activity

Tapentadol has dual effects in suppressing pain transmission, combining μ opioid receptor (MOR) agonism as well as norepinephrine reuptake inhibition. (The

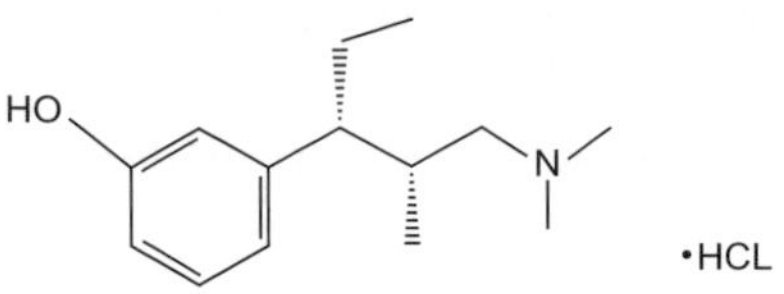

Figure 115.1.

(pharmacology of tapentadol is discussed in Chapter 31.) Tapentadol has higher binding affinity for the norepinephrine (NE) transporter than tramadol, although it is associated with limited inhibition of serotonin reuptake [1–3]. Analgesia provided by NE reuptake inhibition may augment the effect provided by mu receptor agonism and contributes a proportion of tapentadol's overall analgesic effect. In animal studies, tapentadol provided 1/3 to 1/2 the analgesic potency of morphine despite having 18 times less affinity for the mu receptor [2,3]. Tapentadol exists as a single active enantiomer [1–3] and is metabolized mainly by O-glucuronidation; its principal metabolite is inactive, having no affinity for MOR or the NE transporter. As the analgesic activity of tapentadol resides with the parent molecule, no enzymes are needed to convert it to an active metabolite (as is the case with tramadol and codeine).

Tapentadol ER was specifically developed for the management of moderate to severe chronic pain. The controlled-release formulation provides the convenience and analgesic uniformity associated with twice per day dosing. Tapentadol's analgesic efficacy is comparable to a classic extended-release opioid, oxycodone CR. Based on several large-scale clinical trials, tapentadol ER is associated with better gastrointestinal tolerability than oxycodone CR, and there is some evidence that it may have a broader spectrum of efficacy, particularly in patients with neuropathic pain. It is anticipated that tapentadol ER will be released as a schedule II opioid analgesic. In an attempt to limit abuse, tapentadol ER will be formulated as a tamper-resistant tablet that cannot be easily adulterated. The tablet is designed to provide a high degree of mechanical resistance, such as to crushing or chewing [4].

Indications

Tapentadol ER has yet to gain FDA approval. Johnson & Johnson has submitted a New Drug Application (NDA) to the FDA for tapentadol (ER) as an oral analgesic for the management of moderate to severe chronic pain in patients 18 years of age or older. The FDA submission is based on a clinical development program that included phase 3 double-blind, randomized, active- and placebo-controlled studies that evaluated its efficacy and safety for moderate to severe pain in patients with chronic osteoarthritis and low back pain, and diabetic peripheral neuropathic pain. Tapentadol ER has also been evaluated in a 1-year, active-control open-label phase 3 safety trial.

Clinical investigations

Osteoarthritis

In a randomized, double-blind investigation, the efficacy and safety of tapentadol ER were compared with placebo and oxycodone CR for the treatment of moderate to severe osteoarthritic (OA) knee pain [5]. Following a 3-week titration phase, patients were randomized to receive adjusted doses of tapentadol ER (100 to 250 mg), oxycodone CR (20 to 50 mg), or placebo twice daily (BID) over a 12-week maintenance period. Primary efficacy endpoints were the change from baseline average pain intensity at week 12. Data from 1023 patients who received at least one dose of study drug were analyzed. Treatment with tapentadol ER resulted in significant reductions in average pain intensity compared with placebo over the entire maintenance period. In contrast, oxycodone CR failed to achieve a clinically relevant decrease in mean pain intensity over 12 weeks compared with placebo. During the 15 weeks of treatment, discontinuations due to AEs occurred in 6.5% of patients treated with placebo, 19.2% with tapentadol ER, and 43.0% of patients with oxycodone CR. These findings suggest that tapentadol ER is effective for relief of osteoarthritic pain and may improve patient compliance because it is associated with lower incidences of AEs leading to treatment discontinuation.

Chronic low back pain

The safety and efficacy of tapentadol ER were evaluated in 958 patients presenting with chronic low back pain (CLBP) [6]. In blinded-randomized fashion, patients with moderate-severe pain were titrated drugs over 3 weeks to achieve effective and tolerable BID dose of tapentadol ER (100–250 mg), oxycodone HCl controlled-release (CR; 20–50 mg), or placebo, and then maintained at that dose for 12 weeks. Additional dose adjustments were allowed to maintain an optimal balance of efficacy and tolerability. Pain intensity was measured twice daily on an 11 pt NRS (0 = no pain; 10 = pain as bad as you can imagine). Efficacy was measured as change from baseline in average pain intensity at week 12 of the maintenance phase of the trial. Two hundred and thirty-five patients in the tapentadol ER group and 199 patients in the oxycodone CR group entered the 12-week maintenance period. During this time interval, the average 24 h dose for tapentadol ER was 400 mg, and the oxycodone CR dose was 80 mg. Patients treated with tapentadol ER reported significantly greater reductions in average pain intensity than patients treated with placebo at week 12 and for the overall 12-week maintenance period. Patients treated with tapentadol ER and oxycodone CR reported a greater reduction in pain intensity than patients treated with placebo. A higher percentage of patients completed the 15-week treatment period with tapentadol ER (54.1%) than with oxycodone CR (43.3%), mainly because of the lower rate of discontinuation due to GI adverse events (16.7% with tapentadol ER vs 32.3% with oxycodone CR). The authors concluded that tapentadol ER (100–250 mg BID) relieved moderate to severe chronic low back pain more effectively than placebo, and with fewer adverse event-related discontinuations than oxycodone HCl CR (20–50 mg BID) [6].

Diabetic neuropathy pain

The efficacy of tapentadol ER in managing moderate to severe chronic pain was also evaluated in patients with diabetic peripheral neuropathy [7,8]. A recent phase III randomized-withdrawal trial evaluated diabetic patients aged 18 years or older with a diagnosis of moderate-severe painful diabetic peripheral neuropathy and symptoms for a minimum of 6 months [7].

During the 3-week open-label period, patients were titrated to an optimal dose of tapentadol ER (100 to 250 mg) twice daily. The majority of these patients (79.4%) had a pain intensity rating >= 6 on the 11-point NRS.

Patients were then advanced to a double-blind phase of the trial which consisted of a 12-week maintenance period, during which time patients study medication. A total of 588 patients who received tapentadol ER in the open-label period had a mean decrease in pain intensity from 7.3 (standard deviation, SD = 1.43), or severe pain, to 3.5 (SD = 1.89), or mild pain, during open-label treatment. During the double-blind period, the tapentadol ER group had an average pain intensity that remained relatively constant, while the placebo group had a pain intensity that increased in severity ($P < 0.001$).

Table 115.1. Long-term Safety Trial: Treatment-related adverse events

Event	Tapentadol ER (n = 894)	Oxycodone CR (n = 223)
Constipation	202 (22.6)	86 (38.6)
Nausea	162 (18.1)	74 (33.2)
Vomiting	63 (7.0)	30 (13.5)
Dry mouth	81 (9.1)	10 (4.5)
Diarrhea	71 (7.9)	12 (5.4)
Dizziness	132 (14.8)	43 (19.3)
Somnolence	133 (14.9)	25 (11.2)
Headache	119 (13.3)	17 (7.6)
Fatigue	87 (9.7)	23 (10.3)
Pruritus	48 (5.4)	23 (10.3)

Values represent numbers of patients reporting an event and percentages of patients evaluated. From: Lange C, Lange R, Kuperwasser B, et al. Long-term safety of controlled, adjustable doses of tapentadol extended release and oxycodone controlled release: results of a randomized, open-label, phase 3, 1-year trial in patients with chronic low back or osteoarthritis pain. Tenth Annual EULAR Congress, Poster number SAT-0481, June 2009, Copenhagen, Denmark.

During the open-label treatment phase, 20.1% of patients experienced the onset of one or more treatment-emergent adverse events that led to discontinuation from the study. Following advancement to the double blind phase, only 11.2% of patients in the tapentadol ER group and 5.7% of patients in the placebo group discontinued due to treatment-emergent adverse events. In the open-label phase, gastrointestinal related adverse events led to discontinuation in 10% of patients [7].

Long-term safety in patients with chronic pain

The long-term safety and efficacy of tapentadol ER were evaluated in a large randomized open-label trial of patients with chronic pain (low back and osteoarthritis) [8]. Patients (1117) were randomized in a 4:1 ratio to receive twice-daily doses of tapentadol ER 50 mg or oxycodone CR 10 mg for the first 3 days, after which the dose was increased to tapentadol 100 mg BID or oxycodone 20 mg BID for the next 4 days. Patients were maintained on these analgesics for the next 51 weeks, although dose escalations or reductions were permitted. Use of acetaminophen was allowed during the study at doses of up to 1000 mg/day for no more than 7 consecutive days and no more than 14 out of 30 days. Over the 1-year study interval, reductions in average pain intensity scores and mean total daily analgesic doses were stable in both active groups. Patients treated with tapentadol ER reported a lower overall incidence of gastrointestinal treatment-related adverse events such as nausea, vomiting, and constipation (Table 115.1). A lower percentage of patients treated with tapentadol ER experienced nausea, vomiting, constipation, or pruritus; however, a greater number reported headache. Treatment-related adverse events led to discontinuation in 22% of patients in the tapentadol ER group and in 36.8% of patients in the oxycodone CR group.

Contraindications

1. Tapentadol ER, like other opioids, may be associated with significant respiratory depression, and should not be administered to patients with acute or severe bronchial asthma or hypercapnia in unmonitored settings or in the absence of resuscitative equipment.
2. Paralytic ileus (proven or suspected).
3. Patients who are receiving monoamine oxidase (MAO) inhibitors or who have taken them within the last 14 days due to potential additive effects on norepinephrine levels which may result in adverse cardiovascular events [1,3].

Warnings

Patients are at risk of developing serotonin syndrome. The development of a potentially life-threatening serotonin syndrome may occur with use of SNRI products, including tapentadol, particularly with concomitant use of serotonergic drugs such as SSRIs, SNRIs, TCAs, MAOIs, and triptans, and with drugs which impair metabolism of serotonin (including MAOIs). This may occur at the recommended dose. Serotonin syndrome may include mental-status changes (e.g. agitation, hallucinations, coma), autonomic instability (e.g. tachycardia, labile blood pressure, hyperthermia), and neuromuscular aberrations (e.g. hyperreflexia, incoordination). Since tapentadol has effects on norepinephrine reuptake, patients may experience a monoamine syndrome of poorly characterized irritability and agitation that resembles serotonin syndrome but is not associated with major complications [1,3].

Common doses

To be determined. In phase III tapentadol ER trials, dosing ranged from 100 to 250 mg twice daily. No dosage adjustment is needed in mild or moderate renal impairment. Tapentadol may be provided to opioid-dependent patients [10].

Potential advantages

1. Unlike tramadol, tapentadol is an active molecule, it is not a prodrug and does not have to be converted into an active form [1–3].
2. Tapentadol is metabolized by hepatic glucoronidation, which is usually not saturable. There is less individual variability because there is no interaction with CYP-450, CYP-2D-6 enzyme-based metabolism.
3. Nephrotoxicity or hepatotoxicity has not been reported.
4. Better gastrointestinal tolerability than oxycodone CR, specifically, less nausea and vomiting and constipation in the osteoarthritis and CLBP efficacy trials and 1-year safety trial [6,8,10].
5. The lower incidence of adverse events and greater tolerability of tapentadol ER compared to controlled-release opioids may provide a reason to prescribe this preparation. Better tolerability may result in a lower discontinuation rate, and greater patient compliance with analgesic dosing. These advantages may lead to improved analgesic effectiveness and greater patient satisfaction with therapy.

Potential disadvantages

Risk of opioid-induced respiratory depression, nausea, vomiting, and constipation. Risk of monoamine excitability and possible serotonin syndrome. Tapentadol should not be used during breast feeding. Like other extended-duration opioids, the cost of tapentadol ER will probably be higher than immediate-release opioid analgesics.

Drug-related adverse events

Tapentadol has an abuse potential similar to other potent opioid agonists and is subject to criminal diversion. It is unclear whether the tamper-resistant ER preparation will limit diversion, adulteration, and abuse. Abrupt discontinuation of tapentadol IR after 90 days of continuous treatment was associated with mild to moderate withdrawal symptoms in only 17% of patients [10].

Conclusion

Based on phase III clinical trials, tapentadol ER may offer an advance over standard CR opioid preparations

461

in that it offers better tolerability that may reduce discontinuation of therapy and improve pain intensity. Initial trials demonstrating efficacy in neuropathic pain suggests that tapentadol's dual analgesic effects may provide a broader analgesic spectrum than typical opioid analgesics.

References

1. Micromedex® Healthcare Series, DrugDex® Evaluations, Thompson Healthcare. 2009.

2. Tzschentke TM, Christoph T, Ko B, et al. (1 R,2 R)-3-(3-Dimethylamino-1-ethyl-2-methyl-propyl)-phenol hydrochloride (tapentadol hcl): a novel -opioid receptor agonist/norepinephrine reuptake inhibitor with broad-spectrum analgesic properties. *J Pharmacol Exp Ther* 2007;**323**(1): 265–276.

3. Guay D. Is Tapentadol an advance on Tramadol? *Consult Pharm* 2009;**24**;833–839.

4. http://www.jnjpharmarnd.com/jnjpharmarnd/news_release_12012009.html.

5. Afilalo M, Kuperwasser B, Kelly K, et al. Efficacy and safety of tapentadol extended release (ER) for chronic pain due to osteoarthritis of the knee: results of a phase III study. Poster presented at the 5th World Congress of the World Institute of Pain (WIP); March 13–16, 2009; New York, New York, USA. *Pain Practice* 2009;**9**(s1):159. [Abstract PB237].

6. Buynak R, Shapiro D, Okamoto A, et al. Efficacy and safety of tapentadol extended-release for chronic low back pain: results of a randomized, double-blind, placebo- and active-controlled phase III study. Poster presented at the 28th Annual Scientific Meeting of the American Pain Society (APS); May 7–9, 2009; San Diego, California, USA. *J Pain* 2009;**10**(4 Suppl. 1):S50. [Poster #301]

7. Etropolski M, Shapiro D, Okamoto A, et al. Efficacy and safety of tapentadol extended release (ER) for diabetic peripheral neuropathic pain: results of a randomized-withdrawal, double-blind, placebo-controlled phase III Study. Poster presented at the 61st Annual Meeting of the American Academy of Neurology (AAN); April 25–May 2, 2009; Seattle, Washington, USA. [Abstract P05.047]

8. Shapiro D. Efficacy and tolerability of tapentadol extended release for diabetic peripheral neuropathic pain: results of a randomized-withdrawal, double-blind, placebo-controlled phase III Study. [Abstract 113] AAPM annual meeting Feb 2010, San Antonio.

9. Lange C, Lange R, Kuperwasser B, et al. Long-term safety of controlled, adjustable doses of tapentadol extended release and oxycodone controlled release: results of a randomized, open-label, phase 3, 1–year trial in patients with chronic low back or osteoarthritis pain. Tenth Annual EULAR Congress, Poster number SAT-0481, June 2009, Copenhagen, Denmark.

10. Hale M, Upmalis D, Okamato A, et al. Tolerability of tapentadol immediate release in patients with lower back pain or osteoarthritis of the hip or knee over 90 days: a randomized, double-blind study. *Curr Med Res Opin* 2009;**25**(5):1095–1104.

116

Tamper-resistant opioids

Christopher Gharibo and Fleurise Montecillo

Generic Names: tamper-resistant oxycodone, extended-release; tamper-resistant morphine, extended-release

Trade/Proprietary Names: Remoxy™, Acurox™ Embeda™

Drug Class: opioid analgesic

Manufacturers: King Pharmaceuticals, 501 Fifth Street, Bristol, TN 37620;

Acura Pharmaceuticals, Inc., 616 N. North Court, Palatine, IL 60067; Purdue Pharma, Stamford, CT

Introduction

Physicians generally have always been mindful of potential for abuse and diversion when including opioids in a patient's analgesic plan. Prescription drugs are the second most commonly abused drugs in the USA, second only to marijuana. Of these prescription drugs of abuse, opioids make up the largest component. There is growing concern over the increasing role prescription opioids play among the first-time drug abusers. For example, studies of illicit drug use among American teenagers found that new abuse of prescription opioids from 1992 to 2003 increased over 500%. Illicit drug use includes diversion of the prescribed opioid to anyone other than the patient to whom the drugs were prescribed, and often includes friends or family members of patients with legitimate prescriptions [1].

The most common form of casual abuse includes excessive self-dosing of a prescribed drug for non-analgesic purposes. Other methods of abuse include crushing pills and snorting them, dissolving pills in alcohol and drinking the mixture or solubilizing the opioids into an injectable form. Although it may seem snorting or injection of prescription opioids would be a more common practice among intravenous drug abusers seeking euphoria, a study of prescription opioid use among street drug users in New York City found intravenous injection, inhaling, or snorting an opioid to be an extremely rare practice. Indeed, most prescription opioids are orally ingested when abused, even among street drug users and those seeking purely euphoric effects [2].

It should also be noted that a large number of prescription opioid abusers have chronic pain conditions which often necessitated legitimate opioid prescriptions before their abusive or addictive behavior developed. Other street drug users relied on prescription opioids to mitigate withdrawal symptoms from other illicit drugs such as heroin. Physician responsibility in combating prescription opioid abuse should therefore include an appropriate multi disciplinary plan of care, a multi-mechanistic analgesic plan, careful monitoring and documentation of opioid therapy, outcome monitoring and documentation as well as vigilant screening of patients for mental health issues and addictive behavior including use of urine toxicology screens [2,3].

Tamper-resistance

Recent advances to aid in combating abuse of prescription opioids have included the development of tamper-resistant formulations that contain one or more engineered strategies to mitigate euphoria and combat illicit use when the opioid is consumed in a greater amount than prescribed, crushed, snorted, or injected (Figure 116.1). The goal of such analgesics is to be able to deliver reliable pain relief to patients, while discouraging inappropriate use. Currently, the products that are close to filing or have filed a (NDA) New Drug Application with the FDA are limited in their approach and only address

Abuse Deterrent Design

Figure 116.1.

Hard-to-crush capsule

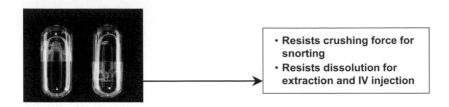

- **Resists crushing force for snorting**
- **Resists dissolution for extraction and IV injection**

Gel-cap with inextricable abusable active drug

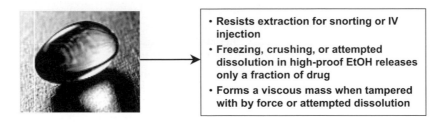

- **Resists extraction for snorting or IV injection**
- **Freezing, crushing, or attempted dissolution in high-proof EtOH releases only a fraction of drug**
- **Forms a viscous mass when tampered with by force or attempted dissolution**

a certain type or a limited range of abusive behavior. However, it is predicted that the next 5 to 10 years will yield the development of a spectrum of such agents that combine multiple tamper-resistant technologies that protect against different types of abuse into one product.

There are six potential approaches to tamper-resistance, and ideally these strategies may be combined to provide a more effective tamper-resistance that would address the different types of abuse modes present in the community.

1. Controlled delivery devices – the opioid is contained in a robust dispenser that delivers the programmed dose at a fixed interval. This type of device would not prevent hoarding and would be subject to physical breakage of the container.
2. Physical barrier – the physical properties of the pill demonstrate stability in the most demanding physical environments. For example, an opioid

pill that is uncrushable and undissolvable in extreme environments and in various solvents over a prolonged period of time (e.g. Remoxy™, EDACS) (Figure 116.1).

3. Prodrug formulation – initially inactive opioid formulation that requires activation by the gastrointestinal milieu (e.g. cleaving by digestive enzymes) or hepatic metabolism to deliver analgesic or euphoric effect, rendering snorting or injection of the prodrug form without effect.
4. Aversive component – opioids containing aversive dosages at clinically insignificant amounts such that unpleasant effects are experienced only in the event of overdosing or inappropriate delivery (e.g., Acurox™).
5. Dual mechanism – molecule(s) with dual mechanism of action that activates the opioid receptors as well as a second stimulatory CNS mechanism (e.g. norepinephrine reuptake

inhibitors) that offsets the opioid-induced CNS euphoria (e.g. tramadol).

6. Sequestered antagonist – arguably the most robust approach, an embedded reversal agent is only released upon tampering with the product (e.g. Embeda™).

Some drug formulations are specifically designed to resist crushing or dissolving, therefore providing a physical barrier to inappropriately snorting or injecting. Remoxy™ and Purdue's modified OxyContin™ represent two examples of this approach that are currently under investigation. Unlike the currently supplied OxyContin™, these preparations resist dissolution in alcohol or water in the short term, and resist extreme crushing or freeze fragmentation.

Remoxy™ is an abuse-resistant oxycodone preparation based on patented ORADUR™ technology. ORADUR™ is a high-viscosity gel cap designed to gradually dissolve in the GI tract and deliver oxycodone over 12 hours. Remoxy™ efficacy was evaluated in a pivotal randomized, placebo-controlled, double-blind phase III study in 412 patients with moderate to severe chronic pain due to osteoarthritis of the hip or knee taking 10–80 mg q12h or placebo for 12 weeks after initial titration. As expected, Remoxy™ was superior to placebo for decrease in pain intensity scores, quality of analgesia and global assessment ($P < 0.01$). A separate phase III study of Remoxy™ for moderate to severe chronic osteoarthritis patients over a 4 week period produced similar results with superior functional improvement vs. placebo on the WOMAC Osteoarthritis Index pain subscale ($P = 0.015$), stiffness subscale ($P = 0.040$), and total score ($P = 0.045$). In a head-to-head clinical comparison, these phase III trials have been accepted by the FDA and the product is currently undergoing nonclinical stability testing in common solvents before resubmission, which is anticipated in 2010. In studies performed to date, the comparator, OxyContin, released over 200% more drug than Remoxy™ when placed in high-proof alcohol. In a chewing study, OxyContin released 170% more drug than Remoxy™ during the first hour of the studies (when abusers presumably expect to get high). Purdue Pharma are also evaluating abuse-resistant technology for extended-release oxycodone. The new formulation is designed to have resistance to extraction and adulteration.

Extruded Deterrence of Abusable Controlled Substances (EDACS™) is a patent-pending physical-barrier technology being developed by Akela Pharmaceuticals. EDACS utilizes a hardened hot-melt extruded matrix to deliver drugs in a difficult to adulterate form. The extruded matrix containing dispersed drug can be shaped into hardened tablets that are water-insoluble, slightly soluble in ethanol, nonfriable, and noncompressable. The tablets are very difficult to crush for inhalation and do not allow for dissolution and injection. EDACS is being positioned as an abuse-deterrent technology that could be combined with existing, proven opioids. Using an EDACS matrix would presumably result in extended duration of pain relief with the added benefit of a more controlled slow-release delivery of the drug that is much more difficult to circumvent.

OROS™ is a patented technology designed for 24 hour drug delivery of drugs such as methylphenidate and calcium channel blockers. The system involves a patented system that requires the osmotically active core to come in contact with gastric water before delivering medication at a constant rate over 24 hours. This technology has also been combined with hydromorphone, and these formulations are currently being studied in chronic pain models. Studies investigating OROS hydromorphone for the treatment of cancer pain have suggest that it is a safe option for chronic cancer pain, and possibly more effective than extended-release morphine. Study subjects taking this formulation with varied alcohol concentrations exhibited only minimally increased plasma levels of hydromorphone, suggesting that the OROS technology can maintain its delivery rate and integrity even with alcohol-related dose dumping attempts.

Other extended-release opioid formulations undergoing clinical trials also provide a physical barrier to abusive drug dumping. Tramadol, a selective opioid receptor agonist, is available in formulations that are difficult to crush and resist alcohol extraction, such as Tramadol ER, and Tridural extended-release tablets. DETERx technology has been used to develop a sustained-release oral oxycodone formulation also known as COL-003 that when ingested and crushed results in the same plasma profile as if it had been swallowed as intended. Rexista is a 24 hour formulation of oxycodone that resists crushing and resists extraction by alcohol.

AcuroxTM is a gel cap preparation of intermediate-release oxycodone with niacin and a mucosal irritant. The pill's gel structure makes it difficult to dissolve or crush, and the integrated mucosal irritant discourages snorting, inhaling, or intravenous delivery. However, when ingested, the product is metabolized by the liver so that no irritation occurs during intended oral use. The niacin dose contained in Acurox produces no symptoms when dosed appropriately, but excessive oral intake of the pill will also lead to increased serum levels of niacin, triggering unpleasant symptoms typical of excessive niacin intake, including flushing, sweats, and headache. Further studies are needed to support the idea that the unpleasant effects of niacin are a sufficient deterrent against purposeful overdosing, as some contend that these side effects do not effectively counteract potential euphoric effects of the opioid. Critics of the Acurox formulation also cite easy strategies that abusers could use to mitigate the unpleasant effects of niacin, such as aspirin premedication and a large meal.

A more robust strategy for abuse deterrence includes preparations of instant or extended-release opioid formulations combined with antagonists such as naltrexone in their core. Tampering with such a formulation, such as crushing or dissolving it in a solvent, releases the antagonist, substantially limiting the analgesic and euphoric potential of the opioid, as well as its street value, to discourage attempts at purposeful overdosing and misuse. However, such an approach does not address the casual abuser who simply takes a dose greater than prescribed by their physician. EMBEDA™ is a product by King Pharmaceuticals that utilizes the agonist-antagonist approach. EMBEDA™ combines extended-release morphine with a naloxone core that is discussed in a separate chapter in this textbook.

The main challenge for tamper-resistant formulations has been in proving to the Federal Drug Administration that they truly provide an effective barrier against misuse as well as convincing the regulators that availability of such formulations will not create a false sense of security for the physicians leading to their increased utilization. FDA is understandably concerned about physician misperceptions that may develop. Physician education is paramount and these products are possibly tamper-resistant and there is no existing or pipeline product that is tamper-proof.

Prescription opioid abuse is a serious issue that requires a range of simultaneous strategies for prevention, detection, and treatment. Strategies to deter inappropriate use of prescription opioids are under development, and include inclusion of aversive components, sequestered antagonists, mechanism-based strategies, prodrug forms, formulations that serve as physical barriers to tampering, and controlled delivery devices. Tamper-resistant opioid formulations are not tamper-proof. They are not a panacea for abuse, but merely a small step towards maximizing patient safety and discouraging illicit use. Ultimately, the physician must bear in mind that there is no formulation that can withstand the determination of a truly desperate addict, and careful clinical vigilance is required of any patient whose pain management strategy includes the use of prescription opioids.

References

1. Manchikanti L. Prescription drug abuse. *Pain Physician* 2006;**9**:287–321.

2. Davis WR, Johnson BD. Prescription opioid use, misuse, and diversion among street drug users in New York City. *Drug and Alcohol Depend* 2008;**92**:267–276.

3. Rosenblum A, Parrino M, et al. Prescription opioid abuse among enrollees into methadone maintenance treatment. *Drug and Alcohol Depend* 2007;**90**:64–71.

117

Novel sustained-release analgesics

Danielle Perret and Michael M. Kim

Hydromorphone OROS® technology

Generic Name: hydromorphone extended-release

Proprietary Name: Jurnista™ (OROS® Push-Pull technology)

Drug Class: opioid analgesic

Manufacturer: ALZA Corporation, Mountain View, CA, USA

Chemical Structure: see Figure 117.1

Chemical Name: 4,5-α-epoxy-3-hydroxy-17-methyl morphinan-6-one

Subcutaneous extended-release sufentanil

Generic Name: sufentanil extended-release

Proprietary Name: Chronogesic™

Drug Class: opioid analgesic

Manufacturer: DURECT Corporation, Cupertino, CA

Chemical Structure: see Figure 117.2

Chemical Name: N-[4-(methoxymethyl)-1-(2-thiophen-2-ylethyl) -4-piperidyl]-N-phenyl-propanamide

Transdermal extended-release sufentanil

Generic Name: sufentanil extended-release

Proprietary Name: TRANSDUR™

Drug Class: opioid analgesic

Manufacturer: DURECT Corporation, Cupertino, CA

Chemical structure: see Figure 117.3

Chemical name: N-[4-(methoxymethyl)-1-(2-thiophen-2-ylethyl) -4-piperidyl]-N-phenyl-propanamide

Introduction

There are a variety of new and emerging analgesic options that offer the promise of prolonged and highly uniform analgesia. On the forefront of research is new sustained-release analgesic technology. Several sustained-release formulations have already been discussed such as inhaled aerosolized liposome-encapsulated fentanyl, iontophoretic transdermal fentanyl, extended-release hydrocodone, tamper-proof oxycodone and even transdermal local anesthetics. In this chapter we focus on the technology behind three new emerging sustained-release opioid formulations: extended-release hydromorphone using the OROS® system and two sufentanil formulations including DUROS® implant technology and TRANSDUR® transdermal technology.

Hydromorphone OROS® technology

Mode of activity

Hydromorphone is a semi-synthetic mu opioid analgesic having major and minor sites of action at spinal and supraspinal opioid receptors. It is widely prescribed for pain management in patients with moderate to severe acute and chronic pain. Hydromorphone is extensively metabolized by the liver and its inactive metabolite is primarily excreted in urine [1].

How it works

OROS® hydromorphone utilizes the patented Push-Pull osmotic pump technology which provides a steady and continuous release of drug over 24 hours, thus providing consistent drug plasma levels and

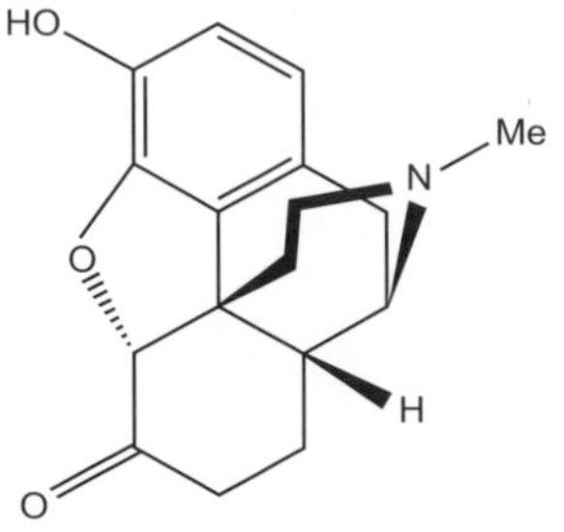

Figure 117.1.

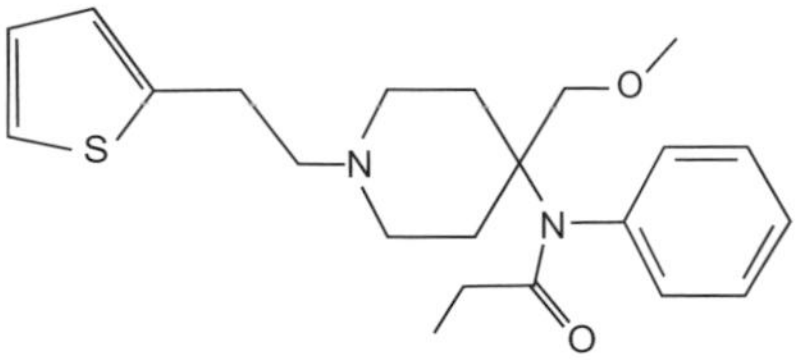

Figure 117.2.

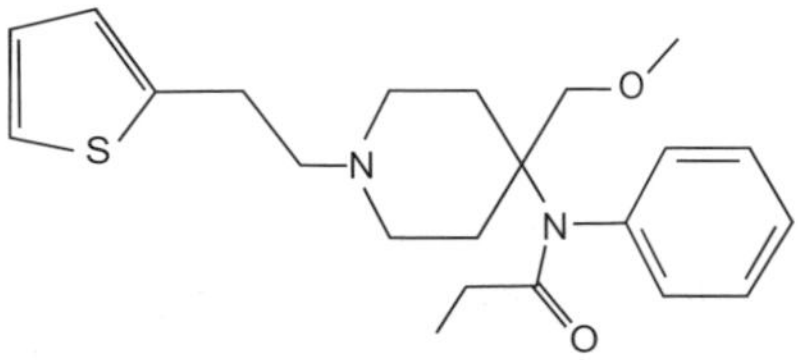

Figure 117.3.

analgesic effects. The key behind the OROS® technology is the tablet core, which is made up of a "drug" layer containing the drug (hydromorphone), a "push" layer made up of an osmo-polymer composition and a semi-permeable membrane that encapsulates these two layers [1]. This semi-permeable membrane is only pervious to water but not to hydromorphone or the osmotic layer [2]. A hole measuring 6.35 micrometers in diameter is made with laser precision within this semi-permeable membrane, allowing drug to be released [1,3].

The driving force behind this system is the absorption of water from the gastrointestinal tract. Water passes from the gastrointestinal tract into the "push" layer at a controlled rate determined by the semi-permeable membrane [1]. The absorbed water suspends hydromorphone and causes the osmotic layer to expand. This expansion of the osmotic layer pushes against the drug layer, which forces the hydrated hydromorphone out through the laser-drilled orifice (Figure 117.4) The rate of drug release is directly proportional to the rate that water enters the tablet core [1].

Studies have concluded that the OROS® system provides a constant stable level of release of hydro-

morphone over a 24 hour period [1,5]. Measurable release of hydromorphone begins after about 2 hours [1]. Thereafter the release is constant for up to 18 hours with peak plasma concentrations occurring around 13–16 hours [1]. Plasma concentrations reach a broad and flat plateau within 6 to 8 hours and remain at this plateau for 24 hours [1]. Steady state is achieved in 48 hours [1]. Pharmacokinetics are linear. Gastric pH, GI motility and the presence of food have a minimal effect on drug absorption or metabolism in healthy patients [4].

This OROS® hydromorphone technology is currently being marketed in Europe under the tradename Jurnista. It has not yet been approved for sale in the USA.

A search of current ongoing or pending clinical trials involving this medication at clinicaltrials.gov reveals the following: safety and efficacy of OROS® Hydromorphone compared with oral morphine, OROS® Hydromorphone in patients with chronic osteoarthritis, and the use of OROS® Hydromorphone in cancer patients.

A search of completed studies also reveals the following: effectiveness and tolerability of OROS® Hydromorphone and Hydromorphone IR in chronic pain, safety and tolerability of OROS® Hydromorphone in long-term use for cancer pain, effectiveness versus placebo for chronic low back pain, in chronic non-malignant pain, safety and impact on quality of life, randomized open-label for safety and effectiveness in short-term use for post-operative pain, dose proportionality studies, OROS® Hydromorphone versus morphine in cancer patients, and safety and effectiveness in patients with osteoarthritis.

It remains unclear whether or when OROS® Hydromorphone will be approved and available for prescription.

Common doses/uses: 8 mg, 16 mg, 32 mg, 64 mg.

Potential advantages

Patient compliance – facility of once a day dosing; steady and long duration of analgesia; stable plasma levels for 24 hours; reduced variability – GI pH, motility, and food have minimal effect on absorption and metabolism.

Potential disadvantages

Toxicity: a previous formulation of extended-release hydromorphone marketed under the name Palladone® utilized a distinct technology but was pulled from

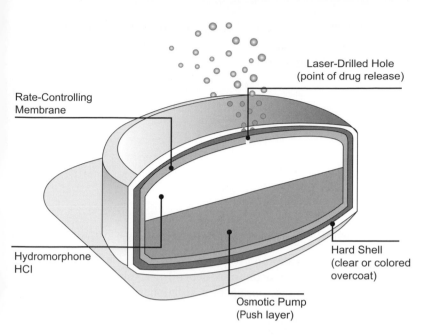

Figure 117.4. OROS® technology.

Laser-Drilled Hole
(point of drug release)

Rate-Controlling
Membrane

Hydromorphone
HCl

Hard Shell
(clear or colored
overcoat)

Osmotic Pump
(Push layer)

the US market secondary to drug dumping. This is a potential concern for all extended-release drug formulations.

Tamper-resistance: the capsule is not hardened and drug may be extruded and adulterated, and possibly abused.

Drug interactions: same as hydromorphone.

Decreased plasma concentrations may result from gastrointestinal hyper-motility syndromes due to excretion before absorption.

A "ghost" of the outer lining of the capsule will be passed in feces. This should be explained to patients.

Drug-related adverse events

Common/serious adverse events for hydromorphone: respiratory depression, dependence, tolerance, nausea/vomiting, constipation, sedation, pruritus.

Reported adverse events for trials involving OROS hydromorphone include: headache, asthenia, and nausea, occurring in 31%, 28%, and 28% of patients, respectively [5].

Subcutaneous extended-release sufentanil

Mode of activity

Sufentanil is a potent mu opioid receptor agonist. Like other opioids, its major and minor sites of action are at spinal and supraspinal opioid receptors. It is primarily metabolized by the liver with a small degree of intestinal metabolism. Although sufentanil is primarily used during induction and maintenance of general anaethesia, it can provide powerful analgesia in acute and chronic pain settings.

How it works

Chronogesic™ is a subcutaneously implantable drug dispensing osmotic pump that can provide benefits of continuous drug delivery for several months and possibly up to 1 year [1]. The DUROS® delivery system is the technology behind Chronogesic™ and was FDA-approved as a drug delivery technology in March 2000. The device is a 4 × 44 mm rod with a titanium housing which has a 155 microliter reservoir [6]. Similar to the OROS® technology, this system works by osmosis of water from the body. Water is slowly drawn through a semi-permeable polyurethane poly-membrane into the osmotic engine. Salt located in the "engine compartment" acts as the osmotic agent which draws water in from the body [6]. The osmosis of the water causes expansion of this compartment which then exerts pressure on a piston that displaces the sufentanil located in the drug reservoir [1]. Sufentanil is released in a continuous and highly controlled fashion (Figure 117.5). The system can be set up to deliver sufentanil at different concentrations from rates of 3.3 mg/day to 13.3 mg/day [1]. The titanium housing

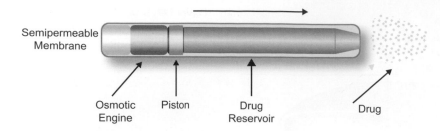

Figure 117.5. Sufentanil transdermal system.

Semipermeable Membrane

Osmotic Engine

Piston

Drug Reservoir

Drug

Actual Size: 4mm x 45mm

protects and stabilizes the drug inside thus allowing delivery of medication for months. Delivery is possible for up to 1 year.

The subcutaneous sufentanil system is placed by a physician, with recommended placement under the patient's arm. It can be done as a simple outpatient procedure in the office setting. The procedure is easy and only local anesthetic in the desired area is required prior to implantation. This can be done in as quickly as a few minutes. Removal or replacement is also simple and can be done in the office setting [6,7].

Development of the Chronogesic™ subcutaneous sufentanil system was halted during phase III clinical trials at the discretion of DURECT Corporation secondary to a design flaw that caused a small fraction of units to prematurely shut down delivery of the drug prior to the end of the intended delivery period. Clinical trials are on hold and will resume when redesign of the delivery system is complete [2]. Due to this development, trial information is not readily available.

Common doses/uses: subcutaneous 3.3 to 13.3 mg/day.

Potential advantages

Prolonged analgesic delivery system; steady and long duration of analgesia; 100% patient compliance; avoids therapeutic troughs and peaks in plasma concentration which may potentially diminish opioid tolerance.

Potential disadvantages

Premature shutdown in the delivery of drugs prior to end of the intended delivery time; possibility of drug dumping; small interventional procedure required for implantation, small risk of infection and subcutaneous reaction.

Drug-related adverse events

Common/serious adverse events (sufentanil): respiratory depression, dependence, tolerance, nausea/vomiting, constipation, sedation, pruritus.

Transdermal extended-release sufentanil

Mode of activity

Sufentanil is a potent mu opioid receptor agonist. Like other opioids, its major and minor sites of action are at spinal and supraspinal opioid receptors. It is currently being studied as an analgesic for use in chronic pain settings.

How it works

Sufentanil is approximately 7.5 times more potent than fentanyl, with greater opioid-receptor affinity. This potency allows a dramatic decrease in transdermal patch size. TRANSDUR™ sufentanil has been evaluated in phase II clinical trials by ENDO Pharmaceuticals [7]. Patients were converted from oral opioids and transdermal fentanyl to transdermal sufentanil. Dose potency relationships and dosing titration regimens were established; safety and tolerability have been demonstrated at these doses with documented effective analgesia provided. Proposals for phase III trials are undergoing FDA review. Two titration regimens are expected to be studied in phase III trials. A conversion factor between oral morphine and transdermal sufentanil has been established with plans for additional testing in upcoming phase III trials [7].

Common doses/uses:

Available in dose equivalents to fentanyl:

1. 100 μg/h
2. 25 μg/h.

Potential advantages

Longer duration of use – 7 days (versus 3 days for fentanyl patches); smaller patch size improves patient comfort/compliance (about 1/5 current fentanyl patch size); improved skin adhesion (versus fentanyl patches); improvement in skin irritation amongst other patch technology; prolonged analgesic delivery system; steady duration of analgesia.

Potential disadvantages

Allergy/pruritus to adhesive; lack of adhesiveness – similar to transdermal fentanyl patches, patients may have difficulty bathing, swimming, and showering.

Drug-related adverse events

Common/serious adverse events (sufentanil): respiratory depression, dependence, tolerance, nausea/vomiting, constipation, sedation, pruritus.

References

1. Gupta S, Sathyan G. Providing constant analgesia with OROS® hydromorphone. *J Pain Symptom Manage* 2007;**33**(2):S19–S24.

2. Palangio M, Northfelt D, Portenoy R, Brookoff D, Doyle R, Dornseif B, Damask M. Dose conversion and titration with a novel, once-daily, OROS® osmotic technology, extended-release hydromorphone formulation in the treatment of chronic malignant or nonmalignant pain. *J Pain Symptom Manage* 2002;**23**(5):355–368.

3. Rathbone M, Hadgraft J, Roberts M, Lane M. *Modified-Release Drug Delivery Technology*, 2nd ed. Vol. 1. New York: Informa Healthcare, 2008.

4. Sathyan G, Xu E, Thipphawong J, Gupta SK. Pharmacokinetic profile of the 24-hour controlled release OROS® formulation of hydromorphone in the presence and absence of food. *BMC Clin Pharmacol* 2007;7:2.

5. Sathyan G, Xu E, Thipphawong J, Gupta SK. Pharmacokinetic investigation of dose proportionality with a 24 hour controlled-release formulation of hydromorphone. *BMC Clin Pharmacol* 2007;7:3.

6. Wright J, Yum S, Johnson RM. DUROS® Osmotic Pharmaceutical Systems for Parenteral & Site-Directed Therapy. *Drug Deliv Technol* 2003; 3:64–73.

7. www.durtec.com

Section 12
Chapter

118

New and Emerging Analgesics

Extended-duration bupivacaine

Tiffany Denepitiya-Balicki and Mamatha Punjala

Generic Names: extended-duration bupivacaine, liposomal bupivacaine

Trade/Proprietary Names: Depobupivacaine, Exparel™

Drug Class: local anesthetic

Manufacturer: Pacira Pharmaceuticlals, 5 Sylvan Way, Parsippany, NJ 07054

Chemical Structure: see Figure 118.1

Chemical Name: 1-butyl-N-(2,6-dimethylphenyl) piperidine-2-carboxam

Chemical Formula: $C_{18}H_{28}N_2O$

Introduction

Currently available long-acting local anesthetics including bupivacaine and ropivacaine rarely last over 12 hours, thereby limiting their usefulness to

471

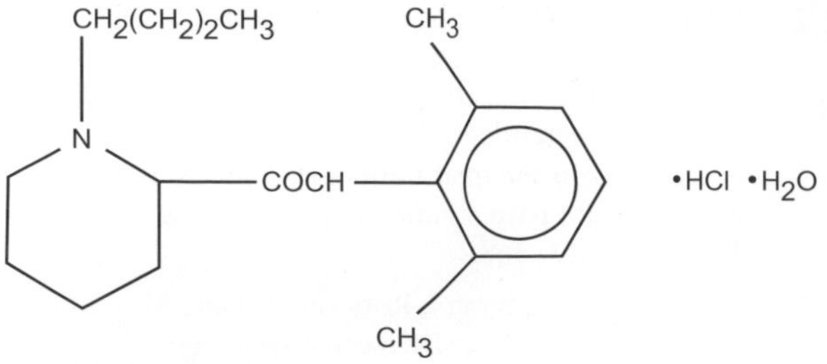

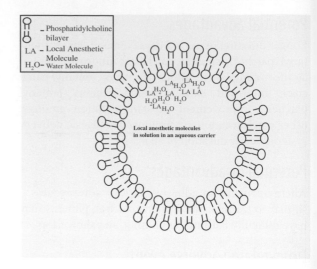

Figure 118.1.

Figure 118.2. Liposome structure. (With permission from Kuzma PJ, et al. Progress in the development of ultra-long-acting local anesthetics. *Regional Anesthesia* 1997; **22**:543–551.)

control moderate to severe post-operative pain unless repeated administration or continuous-infusion dosing are employed. An additional limitation of local anesthetics is the high drug plasma concentrations and systemic toxicity related to rapid absorption or intravascular injection. Development of controlled-release delivery systems which alter local anesthetic pharmacodynamics and pharmacokinetics offer the promise of improved extended post-operative pain management. Encapsulation of local anesthetic molecules into a liposomal carrier provides a safe and reliable method to extend duration of activity and improve post-operative pain management [1–3].

Mode of activity

Liposomes are bilayered lipid vesicles that are 1–3 μm in size. As a result of the bilayer structure, a separation of environments is created with resultant internal and external compartments (Figures 118.2 and 118.3) [3]. Lipid-soluble drugs are concentrated within the lipid bilayer, while water-soluble drugs can accumulate within the inner aqueous compartment [1]. Following depot injection, liposomes within the injectate suspension slowly dissolve over time and the entrapped medication diffuses into tissue [3]. In addition to being an excellent depot, liposomes possess the added benefits of being biocompatible, having the ability to be given by most routes, and decrease the exposure of toxin agents to susceptible tissues [1,2].

Because liposomes come in different shapes and sizes, the performance of each varies with their structure. The liposomes that will carry analgesics should fulfill certain criteria, including but not limited to: sterility, no neurotoxicity, no adverse effects, structural stability, and lengthened duration of action from the current standard [1]. While most liposomal local anesthetics are still being tested in humans, animal studies provide promising results. In rabbits, liposomal bupivacaine has been shown to provide a longer period of pain relief than plain bupivacaine, without motor block or side effects [1,2]. A second major advantage associated with liposomal delivery is that tissue and plasma levels of drug are maintained for prolonged periods while peak plasma concentrations observed with standard immediate-release preparations are avoided (Figure 118.4). This more favorable release kinetic profile would be expected to minimize neuro- and cardiotoxic adverse events associated with local anesthetics. One potential disadvantage of liposomal drug delivery is their unregulated or unpredictable dissolution rate and leakage of drug contents. Leakage, particularly in the case of local anesthetics, could lead to toxicity [1]. Other potential disadvantages include the low payload of analgesic and the moderate inherent stability of the molecule secondary to van der Waals forces among liposomes in a given solution [3]. A recently developed liposomal preparation (DepoFoam™) appears to have overcome problems associated with earlier products and offers several advantages for sustained and highly stable drug delivery [4]. The preparation has been approved for use as a delivery vehicle for epidural morphine (DepoDur™) and other pharmacological agents (Table 118.1). It is currently being evaluated as a carrier vehicle for extended-duration bupivacaine. Other liposomal carriers are being evaluated for extended-duration mepivacaine preparations [5].

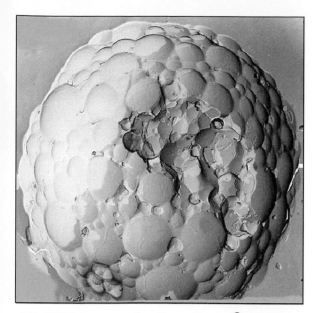

FF-SEM image of a DepoFoam® Particle

Figure 118.3. Scanning electron microscopic image of a drug-encapsulating liposome, DepoFoam™ I.

Table 118.1. DepoFoam™, multivesicular liposomes

1. Particles are suspended in isotonic saline
2. Liposomes are 1–3 μm in diameter
3. Liposomes are composed of phospholipids, triglycerides, and cholesterol
4. The solution can be injected with fine (20–24 gauge) needles
5. Drug is delivered over a period of 1–30 days
6. Shelf life is 2 years
7. Well tolerated, few adverse or allergic reactions noted

Microspheres

Microspheres are another modality for analgesics to be delivered over prolonged periods of time. Essentially, microspheres are synthetic biodegradable (similar to suture material) entities that are larger than liposomes. Like the liposomes, the physical characteristics of microspheres and their speed of degradation are key to release kinetics and duration of drug effect. While most microsphere pharmacokinetic information has been derived from animal studies, early human application has yielded promising results. Microspheres containing bupivacaine produce a prolonged nerve block (10 hours to 5.5 days duration). In the study, researchers found that adding varying amounts of dexamethasone prolonged the duration of the nerve block; however, the mechanism by which this occurs could not be accounted for [1]. One adverse event associated with microspheres that may limit their overall usefulness is inflammatory skin reactions that may or may not be allergic in nature.

Liposomal bupivacaine

A promising example of long-acting local anesthetics is liposomal bupivacaine (LB, DepoBupivicaine or ExpareL™). Liposomal bupivacaine (LB, Exparel™) is an extended-release liposomal injection of bupivacaine intended for single-dose administration which can provide several days of pain management following surgery. It is administered into the surgical wound prior to closure of facial and skin layers. Liposomal bupivacaine is currently in phase II and phase III trials. To date the preparation has been tested in ten wound infiltration clinical trials involving 350 volunteers and more than 1000 patients recovering from various types of surgery. In these trials LB had a low adverse event profile, no toxicology signals, and no QTc changes in doses ranging up to 750 mg [5].

In a randomized active-control phase II study the efficacy and safety of LB were evaluated in 103 patients recovering from total knee replacement surgery [6]. Following completion of surgery, patients received a single intra-operative dose of LB or immediate-release bupivacaine (Bup) via local infiltration. Liposomal bupivicaine effectively controlled moderate to severe pain for more than 72 hours in dose-dependent fashion, with significant reduction in opioid rescue. The pertinent clinical findings included the following. Patients receiving LB 450 mg reported average pain intensity scores of 5.0 cm vs. 7.0 cm for the Bup active control ($P < 0.05$). Pain intensity was also lower, with patients treated with LB 450 mg requiring significantly lower doses of opioid rescue throughout the entire evaluation period, and experiencing 30% less nausea and vomiting than patients treated with Bup. Of importance was the finding that 8% of patients treated with LB required no rescue opioid during the study period versus 0% in the active control group.

Two pivotal phase III placebo-controlled trials have been conducted in patients recovering from orthopedic and soft-tissue procedures [7]. In a recently completed hemorrhoidectomy trial, patients treated with 300 mg LB reported statistically signifi-

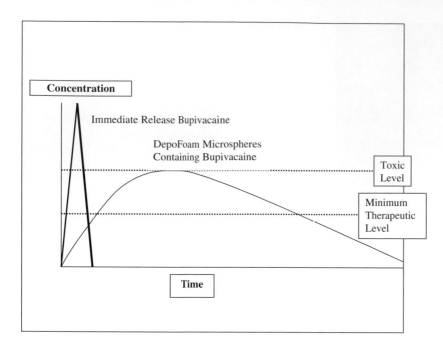

Figure 118.4. Bupivacaine plasma levels: immediate-release preparation versus a liposomal-release preparation (DepoFoam).

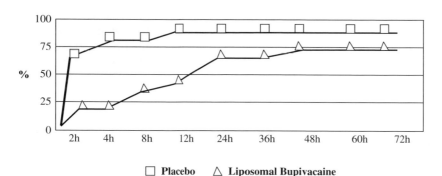

Figure 118.5. Phase III hemorrhoidectomy trial: time to first opioid rescue.

cant reductions in total pain intensity (NRS) in hours 0–72 ($P < 0.001$). Differences were statistically significant at 12, 24, 36, 48, 60, and 72 h following administration ($P < 0.001$). Opioid requirements over 72 h were significantly reduced in the LB-treated group ($P < 0.008$) (Figure 118.5). Similar analgesic benefits were observed in a double-blind placebo-controlled trial performed in patients recovering from bunionectomy [7]. Following completion of surgery performed under Mayo block, patients received either LB, 120 mg ($n = 93$) or placebo ($n = 93$). Pain intensity scores during the first 36 hours were significantly reduced in the LB-treated group when compared to placebo ($P < 0.005$) (Figure 118.5). Opioid dose requirements over 36 h were also reduced in the LB group.

Future

The future of long-acting analgesics looks promising. The ability to administer a single dose of local anesthetic post-operatively may render the need for continuously infusing catheters unnecessary. Liposomal bupivacaine overcomes the limitations of conventional bupivacaine formulations and may be particularly useful in procedures where post-operative pain management is especially problematic and where prolonged analgesia can provide a significant improvement in pain relief and functionality. For example 534 000 patients undergo extremely painful TKA in the USA each year and that number is expected to increase as our population continues to age. The use of LB and other prolonged-duration local anesthetics in this and other painful surgical procedures may be particularly efficacious. Liposomal bupivacaine may also be useful for palliative nerve blocks, and for control of non-surgical pain such as long bone and rib fractures and for intra-articular injection. While LB may be considerably more expensive than immediate-release preparations, single-dose local anesthetic administration offers greater patient safety and cost-effectiveness than continuous-infusion techniques. It must be recognized that catheters are associated with potential drug-related toxicity and infection risks and that placement and maintenance can be challenging, time-consuming, and expensive.

References

1. Grant SA. The Holy Grail: long acting local anesthetics and liposomes. *Best Pract Res Clin Anesthesiol* 2002;**16**:345–352.

2. Holt DV, Viscusi ER, Wordell CJ. Extended-duration agents for perioperative pain management. *Curr Pain Headache Rep* 2007;**11**:33–37.

3. Kuzma PJ, et al. Progress in the development of ultra-long-acting local anesthetics. *Reg Anesth* 1997;**22**:543–551.

4. Mantripragada S. A lipid based depot (DepoFoam™) for sustained release drug delivery. *Prog Lipid Res* 2002;**41**:392–404.

5. de Araujo DR, Cereda CM, Brunetto GB, et al. Encapsulation of mepivacaine prolongs the analgesia provided by sciatic nerve block in mice. *Can J Anesth* 2004;**51**:566–572.

6. Bramlett KW. A single administration of DepoBupivacaine intraoperatively provides analgesia and reduction in use of rescue opiates compared with bupivacaine HCL in patients undergoing total knee arthroplasty. Biennial World Congress of the International College of Surgeons in Vienna, Austria (Poster) December 6, 2008.

7. Pacira Pharmaceuticals, Inc., Parsipany NJ. http://www.pacira.com/news-events.aspx. Unpublished data on file, 2009.

**Section 12
Chapter**

119

New and Emerging Analgesics

Morphine-6-glucuronide

Stephen M. Eskaros

Generic Name: morphine-6-glucuronide

Trade/Proprietary Name: none

Drug Class: opioid analgesic

Chemical Structure: formed by glucuronidation of morphine at the C-6 position; see Figure 119.1

Chemical Formula: $C_{23}H_{27}NO_8$

Introduction

Morphine remains the most widely used opioid analgesic for acute post-operative and chronic pain. Like all opioids, morphine exhibits a number of undesirable and even life-threatening properties. As such, an opioid agonist highly selective for the analgesia-mediating receptors and devoid of morphine's numerous side effects has long been sought. One of morphine's metabolites, morphine-six-glucuronide (M6G), may prove to have such a profile. Several synthesis pathways for M6G exist and it is currently in phase III clinical trials as an opioid analgesic.

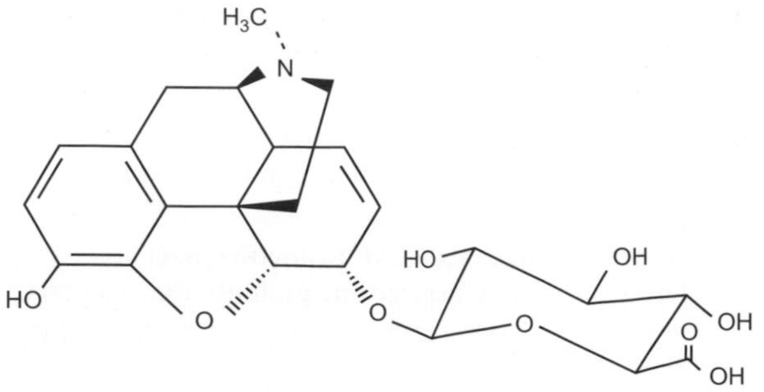

Figure 119.1.

Metabolism

Approximately 10–15% of an exogenous dose of morphine is converted to M6G by a specific glucuronosyl transferase found primarily in the liver and brain, though the kidneys may also play a role in its conversion. The same enzyme catalyzes the formation of morphine-3-glucuronide (M3G), which is pharmacologically inactive and morphine's most abundant metabolite (about 50%). M6G is excreted unchanged by the kidneys and its clearance has been shown to correlate with creatinine clearance.

Pharmacokinetics

It is estimated that the volume of distribution of M6G is 5–10 times smaller than that of morphine. Because it is considerably more polar than morphine and is not metabolized (only excreted), M6G has a slower onset and longer duration of action. Its plasma elimination half-time of 2–3 h is similar to that of morphine, but its blood-effect site equilibration half-time ($t_{1/2} \; K_{e0}$) is twice as long (6–8 h), mainly due to its slower passage across the blood–brain barrier. Studies suggest that subcutaneous M6G is completely bioavailable, but bioavailability of an oral dose is less than 15%. Significant enterohepatic cycling of M6G has been observed, and it appears that oral M6G is hydrolyzed to morphine in the gut followed by re-glucuronidation upon entering the plasma. Thus, an oral preparation of M6G would render little advantage over oral morphine for management of acute or chronic pain.

Pharmacodynamics

The relative potency of M6G to morphine is a topic of much debate. Animal data suggest M6G is equally or more potent than morphine, while it appears to be less potent in humans by a factor of 2–3. Early human studies suggested that small doses ≤ 0.1 mg/kg M6G provided no analgesia, but doses > 0.2 mg/kg were superior to placebo in relieving post-operative pain. Onset time varies between 15 and 30 min with doses ≥ 0.3 mg/kg.

Potential advantages and uses (Table 119.1)

M6G possesses many morphine-like properties, and several preliminary studies suggest it may provide analgesia comparable to morphine with similar onset and longer duration of action. It appears to induce less nausea and respiratory suppression, two of the most troublesome side effects of opioid analgesia, than

Table 119.1. Different opioid receptor types and subtypes

Receptors	Specific effects of each receptor subtype	Morphine affinity	M6G Affinity
M	Sedation, euphoria	+++	+
μ_1	Supraspinal analgesia, peripheral analgesia, euphoria, prolactin release		
μ_2	Spinal analgesia, respiratory depression, physical dependence, gastrointestinal effects, bradycardia, pruritus, dopamine, and growth hormone release		
Δ	Modulation of μ receptor function and dopaminergic neurons	+	++
δ_1	Spinal and supraspinal analgesia		
δ_2	Supraspinal analgesia		
K	Sedation, gastrointestinal effects	++	−
κ_1	Spinal analgesia, diuresis, miosis		
κ_2	Psychotomimesis, dysphoria		
κ_3	Supraspinal analgesia		

equipotent doses of morphine. This may be a result of lower affinity for the μ_2 receptor subtype, thought by many to be largely responsible for the respiratory and GI effects of opioids. In one study comparing morphine and M6G for post-operative pain following abdominal surgery, morphine induced PONV in more than twice as many subjects compared with M6G. Evidence also suggests that M6G causes less depression of respiration and of the ventilatory response to isocapnic hypoxia. These preliminary studies suggest M6G may prove to be equally efficacious as morphine in relieving pain with longer duration of action and superior safety and side-effect profiles.

Multiple routes of M6G administration have been studied. As mentioned, bioavailability of enteral M6G is minimal and probably precludes its use as an oral agent. Intrathecal doses of 100–125 µg produce analgesia comparable to that of morphine 500 µg. Nebulized M6G is poorly absorbed with bioavailability less than 10%. However, one placebo-controlled trial found nebulized M6G to be superior to morphine in improving exercise tolerance in COPD patients despite inferior plasma absorption. This may be related to recent data suggesting the presence of opioid receptors in the lung, and possibly a local rather than centrally mediated mechanism responsible for inducing cough and breathlessness. Nebulized M6G would be an ideal agent to relieve shortness of breath if opiates act locally in the lung, as systemic toxicity would be minimized while exposing pulmonary tissue to large amounts of drug. Another promising finding of these initial studies is that a subcutaneous dose of M6G displays very similar pharmacokinetics to an intravenous dose. It is absorbed into the circulation fairly rapidly despite its large polar structure, probably due to absence of a basement membrane in the endothelium. Presence of basement membrane in lung tissue probably explains the slower absorption of nebulized M6G despite a much larger surface area. Maximal plasma concentration occurs approximately 30 min after a SC dose and >60 min in nebulized form.

Disadvantages

The biggest drawback of M6G is its tendency to accumulate in patients with renal dysfunction. Plasma elimination half-time in non-dialyzed patients with end-stage renal disease can approach 30 hours. Another disadvantage is its slow passage across the blood–brain barrier, prolonging its onset of action relative to morphine.

Randomized controlled trials

Table 119.2 summarizes the findings of randomized, controlled clinical trials on the efficacy of M6G in

Table 119.2. Randomized, double-blind clinical trials on the efficacy of intravenous M6G for post-operative pain

Ref.	Population	Design	Placebo	Outcome
Motamed et al. [6]	37 patients after open knee surgery	M6G or morphine at skin closure followed by post-operative PCA	Yes	M6G 7 mg/70 kg was not better than placebo
Cann et al. [2]	144 patients after laparoscopic gynecological surgery	M6G or morphine bolus doses	No	M6G 8.4 mg/70 kg is as effective as morphine with respect to analgesia but with less nausea/vomiting and sedation
Binning et al. [1]	68 patients following hip replacement surgery	M6G bolus followed by morphine PCA	No	M6G 30 mg/70 kg equivalent to morphine 10 mg/70 kg
Hanna et al. [5]	100 patients during/after joint replacement surgery	M6G versus morphine bolus and PCA	No	M6G analgesia similar to morphine
Dahan et al. [4][a]	62 patients following open abdominal surgery	M6G versus morphine bolus and PCA	No	M6G and morphine analgesia similar with 50% less nausea and vomiting in the M6G group
Smith et al. [8]	170 patients after knee replacement surgery	M6G 10, 20, or 30 mg/70 kg bolus followed by morphine PCA	Yes	M6G 30 mg/70 kg superior to placebo

[a]Single-center sub-analysis (multi-center population size = 517).
PCA, patient-controlled analgesia.

humans. All but one reported M6G to be better than placebo and comparable to morphine in analgesic efficacy. M6G was generally found to produce less systemic toxicity compared with morphine, though no study to date has been adequately powered to compare side-effect profiles.

Conclusions

Many authors of clinical trials evaluating M6G believe it is reliably effective and possesses desirable properties distinct from commercially available pain medications, warranting its availability as an opioid analgesic. The development of a powerful opioid with minimal risk of nausea and respiratory suppression would undoubtedly be welcomed by physicians treating acute and chronic pain. While M6G is currently being evaluated in phase 3 trials, larger clinical studies are needed to further characterize its safety and efficacy.

References

1. Binning S, Coggins S, Davidson A, Millinga KR. *Comparison of Two Dosing Regimens of Morphine-6-glucuronide Versus Morphine for Analgesia following Total Hip Replacement.* Prague: 4th congress of EFIC, Abstract No. 587.T (2003).

2. Cann C, Curran J, Milner T, Ho B. Unwanted effects of morphine-6-glucoronide and morphine. *Anaesthesia* 2002;**57**:1200–1203.

3. Dahan A, van Dorp E, Sarton E. Postoperative morphine-6-glucuronide versus morphine: equal analgesia but reduced nausea/vomiting. *Anesthesiology* 2007;**107**:A1744.

4. Dahan A, van Dorp E, Smith T, Yassen A. Morphine-6-glucuronide (M6G) for postoperative pain relief. *Eur J Pain* 2008;**12**(4):403–411. Review.

5. Hanna MH, Elliott KM, Fung M. Randomized, double-blind study of the analgesic efficacy of morphine-6-glucuronide versus morphine sulphate for postoperative pain in major surgery. *Anesthesiology* 2005;**102**:815–821.

6. Motamed C, Mazoit X, Ghanouchi K, et al. Preemptive intravenous morphine-6-glucuronide is ineffective for postoperative pain relief. *Anesthesiology* 2000;**92**: 355–360.

7. Penson RT, Joel SP, Roberts M, Gloyne A, Beckwith S, Slevin ML. The bioavailability and pharmacokinetics of subcutaneous, nebulized and oral morphine-6-glucuronide. *Br J Clin Pharmacol* 2002;**53**(4):347–354.

8. Smith TW, Binning AR, Dahan A. Efficacy and safety of morphine-6-glucuronide (M6G) for postoperative pain relief: a randomized, double-blind study. *Eur J Pain* 2009;**13**(3):293–299.Epub 2008 Jun 11.

Neostigmine

120

Rongjie Jiang and Balazs Horvath

Generic Name: neostigmine, neostigmine methylsulfate

Trade Name: Neostigmine™

Drug Class: acetylcholinesterase inhibitor

Manufacturer: Baxter Healthcare Corporation, Deerfield, IL 60015

Chemical Structure: see Figure 120.1

Chemical Name: dimethylcarbamate (*m*-hydroxyphenyl)trimethylammonium methylsulfate

Chemical Formula: $C_{12}H_{19}N_2O_2$; molecular wt 223.294 g/mol

Introduction

Neostigmine methylsulfate is a cholinesterase inhibitor commonly used for reversal of non-depolarizing neuromuscular blockade. Neuraxial administration of neostigmine as an analgesic agent is still in an experimental stage. A severe nausea side effect limits its intrathecal application. Recent studies employing epidural neostigmine have reported effective analgesia, opioid, and local anesthetic sparing effects, and reduction in opioid-related side effects [2].

Major and minor sites of action

Neostigmine is approved for the reversal of non-depolarizing neuromuscular blockade. It directly inhibits acetylcholinesterase, the key enzyme responsible for deactivation of acetylcholine (Ach) in central and peripheral cholinergic synapses. Increased concentration of Ach and activation of spinal cholinergic receptors suppress pain transmission [2]. Following administration of neostigmine, the concentration of Ach expressed at spinal cholinergic neuronal endings is increased, resulting in measurable analgesic effects. Also, perfusion of rat spinal cord with Ach increases nitric oxide (NO) synthesis, which

may also provide analgesic effects [10]. Following epidural administration, neostigmine concentration in CSF is about 1/10 of that observed with intrathecal dosing, which may explain the reduced incidence of nausea and vomiting observed in multiple studies when using it epidurally [6].

Receptor interaction

Neostigmine offers additive analgesic effects when combined with opioids and alpha-2-adrenoceptor agonists such as clonidine. Opioids and NE receptors modulate pain via descending inhibitory fibers, whereas Ach receptors are suppressive at local interneurons. This addition of local modulation of noxious transmission may explain the opioid and local anesthetic sparing potential of neostigmine.

Metabolic pathways, drug clearance and elimination

Neostigmine is hydrolyzed by cholinesterase to 3-hydroxyphenyltrimethylammonia and 3-hydroxyphenyldimethylamine. It is also metabolized by microsomal enzymes in the liver to its glucuronide conjugate. Eighty percent of neostigmine is eliminated in the urine within 24 hours as either an unchanged form (50%) or its inactive metabolites (30%). Renal excretion accounts for 50% of neostigmine clearance [11].

How supplied

Neostigmine injection is supplied in 10 mL multiple-dose vials (1mg/mL), in packages of 10. This preparation contains 1 mg/mL neostigmine methylsulfate, 1.8 mg/mL methylparaben and 0.2 mg/mL propylparaben in sterile water.

Indications for analgesia

At present neostigmine has not been FDA-approved for analgesia. The FDA non-approved indications

479

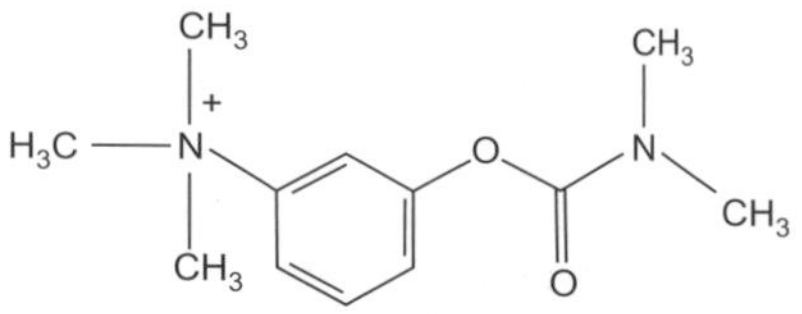

Figure 120.1.

include use as an adjunct to peripheral nerve block, and epidural and intrathecal administration as an adjunct in post-operative and labor analgesia.

Recent peer-reviewed trials suggest that neostigmine has measurable clinical efficacy; however, the studies were small and underpowered for safety determinations. When neostigmine given as a single bolus epidurally is combined with epidural bupivacaine at the end of the surgery, the analgesic effect lasts significantly longer than bupivacaine alone [12]. In early labor, a single bolus of 4 µg/kg neostigmine with 10 mg ropivacaine provided equivalent analgesia to 20 mg of ropivacaine [13]. When neostigmine is administered continuously in patient-controlled epidural analgesia during labor, it reduces hourly bupivacaine requirement by 19% to 25% [3].

Contraindications

Absolute [1]: neostigmine is contraindicated in patients with known hypersensitivity to neostigmine methylsulfate, intestinal or urinary tract obstruction, and mechanical peritonitis.

Relative [1]: neostigmine should be used cautiously in patients who have a history of asthma, bradycardia, cardiac arrhythmias, recent coronary occlusion, epilepsy, hyperthyroidism, peptic ulcer, or vagotonia.

Common doses

Intrathecally administered neostigmine produces dose-dependent side effects. At 150 µg, it causes mild nausea. At 500–750 µg, it causes severe nausea, vomiting, and sedation. At 750 µg, it causes anxiety [8]. The high incidence of nausea associated with neostigmine limits its use in spinal analgesia. Epidural neostigmine in combination with local anesthetics has a more acceptable side-effect profile. Neuraxial neostigmine doses evaluated in several clinical trials are presented in Tables 120.1 and 120.2.

Potential advantages

The recent studies employing epidural neostigmine have demonstrated significant analgesic efficacy, local

Table 120.1. Single bolus of epidural neostigmine [2]

Purpose	Dose (experimental)	Side effects	Duration
Post-operative pain for knee surgery	50–100 µg (1 µg/kg)	No changes from control group	~5 hours [7]
Post-operative pain for abdominal hysterectomy	10 µg/kg combined with bupivacaine 10 mg	No changes from control group	~223 min vs. control ~78 min [12]
Early labor pain	300 µg – 500 µg	To be determined (TBD)	TBD

Table 120.2. Continuous infusion of epidural neostigmine [3]

Purpose	Dose (experimental)	Side effects	Duration
Post-operative pain (adjunct)	PCEA: 0.125% bupivacaine plus neostigmine 4 µg/kg [4]	Epidural neostigmine 1–10 µg/kg is considered safe [5]	TBD
Labor analgesia (adjunct)	Bolus 80 µg then continuous with 4 µg/mL neostigmine in 1.25 mg/mL bupivacaine PCEA solution [3]	Moderate sedation [3]	Reduces bupivacaine usage by 19% to 25%

anesthetic sparing effects, and an acceptable side-effect profile. Unlike opioid analgesics, neostigmine does not produce respiratory depression, neonatal depression, or pruritus [1]. Theoretically, neostigmine has a potential to replace the lipophilic opioids such as fentanyl and sufentanyl as the primary analgesic adjunct to local anesthetic blockade. Epidural neostigmine administered in doses of 1–10 µg/kg is considered safe [5]. The exact safety profile has yet to be determined. Larger, direct comparison studies are needed.

Potential disadvantages

It is unclear whether epidural neostigmine or preservatives within the vial may be associated with neurotoxicity given the limited sample size within the existing studies. The antioxidants methyl- and propyl-paraben which are present in the commercially available neostigmine have not demonstrated neurotoxicity in animals [10]. Preservative-free neostigmine is not available in the USA. A much larger clinical trial is needed to assess the short- and long-term safety profile of neuraxial-administered neostigmine.

References

1. Neostigmine in Micromedex Healthcare Series and DrugDex Evaluations.

2. Eisenach J. Epidural neostigmine: will it replace lipid soluble opioids for postoperative and labor analgesia? *Anesth Analg* 2009;**109**(2):293–295.

3. Wong C. Neostigmine decreases bupivacaine use by patient-controlled epidural analgesia during labor: a randomized controlled study. *Anesth Analg* 2009;**109**(2):524–530.

4. Tekin, S. Comparison of analgesic activity of the addition to neostigmine and fentanyl to bupivacaine in postoperative epidural analgesia. *Saudi Med J* 2006;**27**(8):1199–1203.

5. Chia YY. The acotomy. *Anesth Analg* 2006;**102**(1):201–208.

6. Omais M. Epidural morphine and neostigmine for post-operative analgesia after orthopedic surgery. *Anesth Analg* 2002;**95**(6):1698–1701.

7. Lauretti GR. Postoperative analgesia by intraarticular and epidural neostigmine following knee surgery. *J Clin Anesth* 2000;**12**(6):444–448.

8. Hood DD, Eisenach JC. Phase I safety assessment of intrathecal neostigmine methylsulfate in humans. *Anesthesiology* 1995;**82**(2):331–343.

9. Cronnelly R, et al. Renal function and the pharmacokinetics of neostigmine in anesthetized man. *Anethesiology* 1979;**51**:222–226.

10. Eisenach JC, et al. Phase I human safety assessment of intrathecal neostigmine containing methyl- and propylparabens. *Anesth Analg* 1997;**85**:842–846.

11. Neostigmine package insert. Baxter, Deerfield, IL, June 2005.

12. Nakayama M, et al. Analgesic effect of epidural neostigmine after abdominal hysterectomy. *J Clin Anesth* 2001;**13**(2):86–89.

13. Roelants F, et al. The effect of epidural neostigmine combined with ropivacaine and sufentanil on neuraxial analgesia during labor. *Anesth Analg* 2003;**96**(4):1161–1166.

Section 12 Chapter 121

New and Emerging Analgesics

Buprenorphine transdermal

Martin Hale

Generic Name: buprenorphine transdermal delivery system

Proprietary Names: Transtec™ (transdermal 3-day delivery system), Norspan™, BuTrans™, ResTiva™ (transdermal 7-day delivery systems)

Class of Drug: opioid analgesic

Manufacturers: Napp Pharmaceuticals Limited, Cambridge Science Park, Milton Road, Cambridge, UK; Purdue Pharma LP, One Stamford Forum, Stamford, CT

Chemical Structure: see Figure 121.1

Chemical Name: (2S)-2-[(−)-(5R,6R,7R,14S)-9α-cyclopropylmethyl-4,5 epoxy-6,14-ethano-3-hydroxy-6-methoxymorphinan-7-yl]-3,3-dimethylbutan-2-ol

Chemical Formula: $C_{29}H_{41}NO_4$; molecular wt 467.6

481

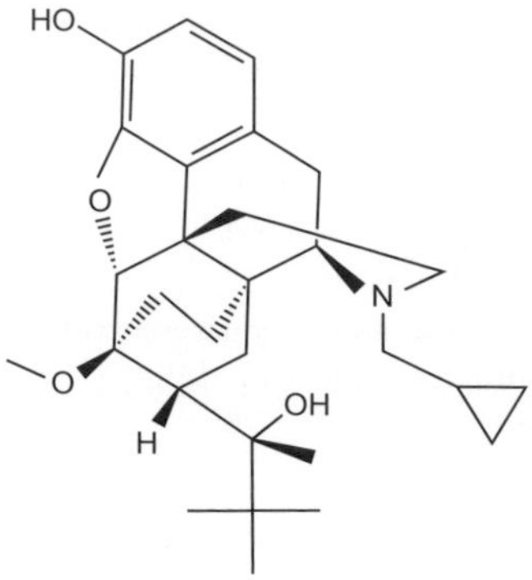

Figure 121.1.

Introduction

Buprenorphine is a semi-synthetic, highly lipophilic opioid analgesic derived from thebaine, approved for the management of moderate to severe acute and chronic pain [1,2]. Buprenorphine has poor oral bioavailability; however, it provides effective analgesia following parenteral, sublingual, or neuraxial administration [1,2]. Transdermal buprenorphine delivery systems have been developed to improve convenience compliance and analgesic uniformity. A 3-day delivery transdermal system, named Transtec™, was developed and subsequently marketed in Europe in 2002, followed in 2004 by a 7-day preparation named Norspan™. Norspan™ is approved for use in 26 countries worldwide, and an identical preparation named BuTrans™ is currently undergoing phase III FDA trials. At the present time neither Norspan™ nor BuTrans™ are approved or available for prescription in the USA.

Major and minor sites of action

Buprenorphine's precise mechanism of analgesic action is unknown. However, it is believed to bind and activate spinal and supraspinal opioid receptors. Buprenorphine has high affinity for mu opioid receptors, where it behaves as a partial agonist. At low to moderate doses buprenorphine is 25 to 50 times more potent than morphine; however, an analgesic ceiling effect is noted with increasing dose [1,2]. Buprenorphine also has agonist binding properties at delta and opioid-like receptors (ORL-1) and antagonistic effects at kappa subtypes [1].

Buprenorphine is metabolized in the liver by CYP3A4 and N-dealkylated to form norbuprenorphine. It is also conjugated with glucuronic acid to form buprenorphine-3β-O-glucuronide and norbuprenorphine-3β-O-glucuronide. Approximately 2/3 of buprenorphine is eliminated unchanged in feces [1–3].

Common doses/uses

Norspan/BuTrans is available in three strengths: the patches contain 5, 10 and 20 mg of buprenorphine and are designed to release buprenorphine at a controlled rate of 5, 10 and 20 µg/h.

Each patch provides a steady delivery of buprenorphine for up to 7 days. Steady state is achieved during the first application. After removal of the patch, buprenorphine concentrations decline approximately 50% in 12 hours.

Buprenorphine transdermal delivery system (BTDS) patches have been shown to successfully treat moderate to severe chronic pain. Double-blind studies have demonstrated its effectiveness in treating cancer pain as well as chronic lumbar pain [4] and chronic osteoarthritis pain of the hip and knee.

Contraindications

Absolute: contraindicated in patients with hypersensitivity to buprenorphine or the patch excipients (oleyl oleate, povidone, levulinic acid, adhesive matrix), opioid-dependent patients for narcotic withdrawal treatment, patients with severely impaired respiratory function, or in patients who have used MAO inhibitors in the past 2 weeks. BTDS has not been studied in patients under 18 years of age.

Relative: caution should be used in patients with convulsive disorders, head injury, shock, a reduced level of consciousness, intracranial lesions or increased intracranial pressure, or in patients with severe hepatic impairment.

Overdose deaths have been reported with buprenorphine in combination with ethanol and benzodiazepines.

Transdermal buprenorphine has a latency to onset and peak effect, and is not recommended for analgesia in the immediate post-operative period, or when analgesic requirements are varying rapidly.

Potential advantages

Seven-day transdermal delivery provides many benefits from the perspectives of pain management and public health. Opioids with full mu agonist activity are generally assumed to provide the strongest pain relief, but also carry a higher risk of respiratory depression and other side effects. Fentanyl is the only opioid in a transdermal dosage form currently marketed in the USA. The availability of a transdermal opioid with a potentially lower side-effect profile (e.g. respiratory depression) may offer advantages in patients with pulmonary disease. Buprenorphine appears to have a ceiling for cardiorespiratory and subjective effects and a high safety margin even when taken by the IV route [5]. Confirmed cases of overdose death in patients taking only buprenorphine are rare. Most cases of overdose death involve the use of buprenorphine in combination with sedatives and/or alcohol.

Transdermal buprenorphine may provide convenience and other benefits in certain populations (e.g. older adults who have difficulty swallowing pills and/or have trouble opening medication bottles, and individuals dependent on others for assistance with taking medication). The once per week, four patch changes per month dosing schedule should facilitate adherence with the prescribed regimen of medication administration for the control of pain [6]. No coordination is required with eating schedules because food consumption does not affect drug delivery by the transdermal route.

Abuse and diversion of any opioid product is of concern. However, buprenorphine appears to have a lower abuse liability than other morphine-like drugs, reflected in the FDA listing of buprenorphine as a C-III [7]. Furthermore, the transdermal system is not particularly attractive to opioid abusers, given their ready access to a broad range of opioids that produce stronger euphoria and require little or no tampering [7]. In addition, opioid abusers would be expected to find buprenorphine less desirable than morphine-like drugs due to its pharmacological ceiling limitation on euphoria and the possibility that its administration may precipitate opioid withdrawal symptoms.

Potential disadvantages

Abuse: all opioids have associated risk of misuse, abuse, addiction, and diversion. Evaluations prior to prescribing opioids should include: (a) proper assessment of the patient, (b) proper prescribing practices, and (c) periodic re-evaluation of therapy,

Toxicity: manifestations of acute opioid overdose include pinpoint pupils, sedation, hypotension, respiratory depression, and/or death. In cases of overdose, BTDS should be removed immediately. After BTDS removal mean buprenorphine concentrations decrease approximately 50% in 12 hours (range 10–24 h), with an apparent terminal half-life of ~26 hours. Naloxone may not be as effective in reversing respiratory depression produced by buprenorphine [1–3]. High doses of naloxone hydrochloride, 10–35 mg/70 kg, have been reported to be used in the management

of buprenorphine overdose. The risk of overdose and death is increased with concurrent abuse of BTDS with alcohol, benzodiazepines, sedatives, tranquilizers, antidepressants, and other substances.

Interactions: concomitant treatment with CYP3A4 inhibitors may lead to elevated plasma concentrations with intensified efficacy of buprenorphine. Co-administration of buprenorphine and CYP3A4 enzyme inducers could lead to increased clearance which might result in reduced efficacy.

Patients should avoid direct exposure of the BTDS application site to heating pads, electric blankets, heat lamps, saunas, hot tubs, and heated water beds, because an increase in absorption of buprenorphine may occur. Caution should be used when treating febrile patients as fever may increase absorption, resulting in increased plasma concentrations of buprenorphine.

Withdrawal: buprenorphine doses should be tapered gradually to prevent signs and symptoms of withdrawal in the physically dependent patient; introduction of appropriate immediate-release opioid medication should be considered.

Drug-related adverse events

In an efficacy and safety trial of BTDS in opioid-exposed subjects with moderate to severe low back pain, the most frequently reported adverse events were those typically associated with opioid therapy (e.g. nausea, headache, vomiting, constipation, somnolence, dizziness) and application-site pruritus, typical of a transdermal delivery system [4]. BTDS treatments were found to be generally well-tolerated and safe.

Conclusions

The advantages of transdermal buprenorphine are primarily related to the convenience and improved compliance associated with a 7-day analgesic delivery system. The preparation may be particularly useful in elderly patients with moderate pain that cannot be controlled with non-opioid analgesics and others who are at risk for respiratory depression with pure mu agonists.

References

1. Gutstein HB, Akil H. Chapter 23: Opioid analgesics. In Hardman JG, Limbird LE, Gilman AG, eds. *Goodman & Gilman's The Pharmacological Basis of Therapeutics*, 10th ed. New York: McGraw-Hill, 2005, pp. 569–619.

483

2. Way WL, Fields HL, Schumaker MA. Chapter 31: Opioid analgesics. In Katsung BG, ed. *Basic & Clinical Pharmacology*, 9th ed. Lange Medical Books/ McGraw-Hill, 2004.

3. http://emc.medicines.org.uk/ – BuTrans – summaries of product characteristics.

4. Steiner D, Munera, C, Hale, M, Ripa, S, Landau, C, The efficacy and safety of buprenorphine transdermal system (BTDS) in subjects with moderate to severe low back pain. APS 28th Annual Meeting, San Diego, CA. May 8, 2009.

5. Umbricht, A, Huestis, M, Cone, E, Preston, K, Effects of high-dose intravenous buprenorphine in experienced opioid abusers. *J Clin Psychopharmacol* 2004;24(5).

6. Bradley C. Compliance with drug therapy. *Prescriber's J* 1999;**39**(1).

7. http://www.fda.gov/ – FDA recommendation to reschedule buprenorphine – 11/23/01.

**Section 12
Chapter**

122

New and Emerging Analgesics

Nicotine (transdermal)

Dmitri Souzdalnitski, Imanuel Lerman and Keun Sam Chung

Generic Name: nicotine

Trade/Proprietary Names: Nicoderm, Habitrol, Nicorette, ProStep

Drug Class: acetylcholine receptor agonist

Manufacturer: Alza Pharmaceuticals, 1900 Charleston Road Mountain View, CA 94039; CIBA-Geigy, Summit, NJ; generic (multiple)

Chemical Structure: see Figure 122.1

Chemical Name: *S*-3-(1-methyl-2-pyrrolidinyl) pyridine

Molecular Formula: $C_{10}H_{14}N_2$; class: autonomic ganglia stimulant

Introduction

Nicotine is a tertiary amine composed of a pyridine and a pyrrolidine ring obtained, from the tobacco plant (*Nicotiana tabacum*). It was initially identified by Posselt and Reiman in 1828. Nicotine is a colorless to pale yellow, freely water-soluble, oily, hygroscopic volatile liquid, strong base with pKa = 8.5 with a characteristic pungent odor. It turns brown on exposure to air or light. Of its two stereoisomers, *S*(−) nicotine is the more active, and it is the prevalent form in tobacco [1].

Mechanism of action

Nicotine functions as an agonist at a subtype of acetylcholine receptors, termed "nicotinic receptors". Nicotinic acetylcholine receptors (nAChRs) are extremely variable in their molecular structure. They are composed of five subunits to form a ligand-binding site and an ionic pore. The variability of nAChRs subunit combinations and their location are responsible for diverse, sometimes paradoxical, physiological and pharmacological effects of nicotine, including pain relief [1,2].

1. Nicotine is a prominent central nervous system stimulant. Primary sites of action of nicotine in the brain are thought to be pre-junctional, causing the release of other neuro-transmitters. Nicotine rewarding properties are related to its ability to increase dopamine in the mesolimbic system, similarly to other drugs of abuse.

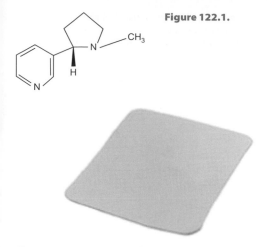

Figure 122.1.

Figure 122.2. Nicotine patch.

2. Nicotine is known to induce β-endorphin and enkephalins, which are thought to be fundamental for the manifestations of its rewarding properties.
3. Morphine and other opioids produce analgesia in part releasing acetylcholine and stimulating nAChRs. Nicotine stimulates the same nAChRs.
4. Nicotine is a potent stimulator of stretch or pressure mechanoreceptors of the skin, mesentery, tongue, lung, and stomach, which may contribute to its pain-relieving mechanisms.
5. Nicotine has anti-inflammatory properties.
6. Nicotine acts as an alpha-2 noradrenergic receptor agonist in a way similar to clonidine, another adjunct to pain management.
7. At the same time it promotes a discharge of epinephrine from the adrenal medulla, as well as discharge of catecholamines from sympathetic nerve endings, resulting in activation of spinal cord and brain descending inhibitory pain pathways.

Nicotine induces nausea, vomiting, and occasionally diarrhea by both central and peripheral actions.

Future research will clarify the role and relative contribution of specific actions of nicotine to alleviation of pain.

Pharmacokinetics

Absorption

Nicotine is easily absorbed from the respiratory tract, buccal membranes, skin, and intestines, but not from the stomach.

Distribution

Delivery via a transdermal patch provides a sustained plasma nicotine concentration, typically lower than venous blood concentrations after tobacco smoking (Figure 122.2). On the other hand, a nasal spray and a vapor inhaler provide immediate 10-fold higher arterial blood concentrations immediately following inhalation compared to venous concentrations after a nicotine patch application.

Metabolism

Nicotine is rapidly metabolized to cotinine, the major metabolite of nicotine, via the cytochrome P450 pathway by cytochrome P450 (CYP2A), mainly in the liver. Other metabolites included nicotine-1′-N-oxide and 3-hydroxycotinine and conjugated metabolites, also produced for the most part in the liver but also in the kidney and lung. Only about 10–20% of nicotine remains unchanged. The relationship of nicotine and CYP450 remains undiscovered. Nicotine has a half-life of about 2–4 hours, and cotinine has a half-life of approximately 16–20 hours. While cotinine is thought to be an inactive metabolite it may contribute to development of tolerance to nicotine by prolonged weak stimulation of cholinergic receptors. Nicotine and its metabolites are eliminated by the kidney. About 10% of nicotine is excreted with urine unaltered. Nicotine is also excreted in the milk of lactating women.

Indications (non-FDA-approved)

Acute surgical pain

Nicotine is not FDA-approved for any pain indications. Nevertheless, data obtained from recent clinical trials suggest it may provide limited analgesic benefits in post-surgical settings [3–5]. Transdermal nicotine, 5 mg, applied once immediately prior to induction of general anesthesia for pelvic or abdominal surgical procedures, reduced post-operative pain scores in non-smokers. There was no increased benefit of nicotine with doses larger than 5 mg [3]) (Table 122.1).

Another recent study revealed that the pre-operative application of a 7 mg nicotine patch resulted in a significant (31%) reduction in opioid consumption in non-smoking patients undergoing radical retropubic prostatectomy [4]. Peri-operative administration of a high-dose transdermal nicotine patch (21 mg/24 hours) for 3 days did not improve post-operative pain control or decrease the analgesic requirement after

Table 122.1. Nicotine transdermal patch as an adjunct for post-operative pain control: indications and techniques

Indications	Advantages	Transdermal nicotine patch application	Primary pain control program
Pelvic and abdominal open or laparoscopic surgeries [3]	Decreased pain scores by 25–40%, tendency to decrease opioid consumption	5 mg/16 h × 1 patch applied immediately before surgery to glabrous skin away from the surgery site. The patches to be removed at bedtime on the same night of surgery	Morphine PCA, NSAIDs
Radical retropubic prostatectomy [4]	Decreased opioid consumption by 1/3, tendency to decrease pain scores for the first 24 h after the surgery	7 mg/24 h × 1 patch applied behind the ear 30–60 min before surgery	Intravenous morphine patient-controlled analgesia (PCA) and nonsteroidal anti-inflammatory drugs (NSAIDs)
Abdominal hysterectomy [5]	Improves discharge eligibility	21 mg/24h patch applied before, and on post-operative days 1 and 2.	Morphine PCA

pelvic gynecological surgery. This study was different from others in the way that it included both smokers and non-smokers [5].

Chronic pain and cancer pain

There are no RCTs of nicotine for chronic non-malignancy pain or cancer pain. The existing data suggest that chronic nicotine users may actually be more sensitive to pain than non-smokers. Symptoms are more pronounced in smokers with more severe nicotine dependence [6]. The association between the intensity of pain in chronic pain states and smoking status was explained by higher levels of substance P (P for pain) in the cerebral spinal fluid and lower plasma beta-endorphin levels than in non-smokers. There are similarities between hypersensitivity to pain induced by chronic nicotine use and opioid-induced hyperalgesia and opioid-induced tolerance in chronic pain states. Further research is needed to explore and explain these effects.

Adverse reactions

Serious reactions: nicotine dependence, fetal harm risk.

Common reactions: nausea, local erythema, local edema, rash, withdrawal symptoms, headache, palpitations, tachycardia, HTN, hiccups, constipation, flatulence, diarrhea, paresthesias, arthralgias, chest discomfort, insomnia, abnormal dreams [7].

Less common adverse events: fever, hypothermia, thirst.

Contraindications

Hypersensitivity, severe arrhythmias, acute myocardial infarction within 2 weeks, worsening or severe angina [7].

Relative contraindications and cautions

Caution if asthma or reactive airway disease, cardiovascular, peripheral vascular diseases, hepatic impairment, renal impairment, hyperthyroidism, pheochromocytoma, insulin-dependent diabetes mellitus, peptic ulcer disease, or HTN are present [7].

Pregnancy: nicotine is a Pregnancy Category D medication and should not be used by pregnant women.

Drug abuse and dependence: there is a significant risk of addiction associated with the use of nicotine.

Drug interactions

Combination of nicotine and dofetilide, a class III antiarrhythmic drug, is contraindicated since it may increase levels of both drugs with QT prolongation and arrhythmias [7]. Combination with bupropion may increase risk of hypertension secondary to possible additive effects. Combination with insulin may increase insulin requirements. Combination with metformin may increase metformin levels and risk of lactic acidosis, and may decrease hypoglycemic agent efficacy. Blood sugar monitoring recommended for combinations of nicotine with some other diabetic medications, including acarbose, miglitol, pioglitazone, repaglinide, rosiglitazone, sitagliptin, sulfonylureas. Combination with ergot alkaloids or caffeine may increase risk of peripheral vasoconstriction, ischemia.

Common doses

Adult dosing: 7 mg, 14 mg, or 21 mg–24h patch [7]; renal dosing – caution advised if severe impairment; hepatic dosing – caution advised if hepatic impairment; pediatric dosing is currently unavailable and not applicable for nicotine.

Potential advantages

Potential advantages of nicotine include its opioid-sparing effect in multimodal post-operative analgesia, easy use and administration, and cost-effectiveness [1,3–5]. It has been shown recently that use of transdermal nicotine patch significantly improves discharge eligibility scores [7]. Discharge home earlier may allow considerable savings for each treated patient without compromising patient safety and patient satisfaction. If confirmed, this finding may attract a significant number of healthcare providers and payers to nicotine use for post-operative pain control.

Potential disadvantages

Addiction potential is the main disadvantage of use of nicotine for pain control. Public access to this drug makes its use even less attractive than opioids. The fact that nicotine induces nausea, vomiting, and sometimes diarrhea may limit its usefulness as an analgesic as well.

References

1. Benowitz NL. Nicotine and postoperative management of pain. *Anesth Analg* 2008;**107**(3): 739–741.

2. Trigo JM, Zimmer A, Maldonado R. Nicotine anxiogenic and rewarding effects are decreased in mice lacking beta-endorphin. *Neuropharmacology* 2009;**56**(8):1147–1153.

3. Hong D, Conell-Price J, Cheng S, Flood P. Transdermal nicotine patch for postoperative pain management: a pilot dose-ranging study. *Anesth Analg* 2008;**107**(3):1005–1010.

4. Habib AS, White WD, El Gasim MA, et al. Transdermal nicotine for analgesia after radical retropubic prostatectomy. *Anesth Analg* 2008;**107**(3):999–1004.

5. Turan A, White PF, Koyuncu O, Karamanliodlu B, Kaya G, Apfel CC. Transdermal nicotine patch failed to improve post-operative pain management. *Anesth Analg* 2008;**107**(3):1011–1017.

6. Weingarten TN, Moeschler SM, Ptaszynski AE, Hooten WM, Beebe TJ, Warner DO. An assessment of the association between smoking status, pain intensity, and functional interference in patients with chronic pain. *Pain Physician* 2008;**11**(5):643–653.

7. http://www.epocrates.com/.

123

Local anesthetic bone paste

Vadim Tokhner and Inderjeet Singh Julka

Generic Names: methyl methacrylate cement plus lidocaine, hemostatic putty plus lidocaine

Trade/Proprietary Names: (Simplex™ Bone cement), Osteobond™, Orthostat™, Sterilized lidocaine (Xylocaine™)

Drug Class: local anesthetic

Manufacturers: Howmedica Osteonics Corporation, 325 Corporate Drive, Mahwah, NJ; Zimmer Holdings, 345 Main Street, Warsaw, IN; Orthocon, Inc., North Brunswick, NJ; Astra Pharmaceuticals, Shrewsbury, MA; Astra Zeneca Pharmaceuticals, Westboro, MA

Chemical Formula of Lidocaine: 2-(diethylamino)-N-(2,6-dimethylphenyl) ethanamide

Chemical Structure of Lidocaine: see Figure 123.1

Poly(methyl methacrylate) is an acrylic resin. It is a clear and a rigid vinyl polymer, made by free radical vinyl polymerization from the monomer methyl methacrylate (Figure 123.2).

Description

Bone cement is used for fixation of artificial joints/implants to the skeleton. It acts as a filler between the bone and the implant. It consists of poly(methyl methacrylate) (PMMA), which is a transparent thermoplastic. It is a synthetic polymer of methyl methacrylate. Addition of crystals of barium sulfate gives it radiopacity. Incorporation of substances such as local anesthetics [1], antibiotics, anti-inflammatory drugs, immunomodulators, osteogenic promoters, and diagnostic substances such as radioactive tracers into bone cement has been attempted. The combination of a local anesthetic with methyl methacrylate cement offers the promise of selective analgesia following surgery or injury to bone. Analgesia from incorporated local anesthetic is thought to be due to the elution of the drug into the surgical site. However, much research into the efficacy, duration of analgesia, and side effects needs to be done. Some elution behavior of local anesthetics has been preliminarily studied. It was found that prilocaine eluted the fastest and bupivacaine the slowest, with lidocaine between them [2]. Local anesthetics have also been shown to have some anti-microbial activity [3–5].

Orthocon Inc. is developing a novel extended-release bone hemostat containing lidocaine which is designed to stop bleeding and to provide local pain relief. This preparation utilizes the company's proprietary Orthostat™ hemostatic bone putty. Orthostat™ is a sterile, moldable, wax-like mixture of calcium stearate and alkylene oxide copolymer intended to control bleeding from the cut surface of bone. When applied manually to surgically incised or traumatically broken bone, the putty achieves local control of bleeding by acting as a mechanical tamponade. The new preparation combines Orthostat™ putty with lidocaine. It allows the local anesthetic to be slowly eluted and may be employed for relief of osteogenic pain following orthopedic surgery. The company expects to initiate a pivotal clinical trial with this product in the near future.

Mode of activity

Local anesthetic agents released from bone paste or putty can reversibly block the fast sodium channels of the neural cell membrane and prevent axonal depolarization. This leads to failure of noxious transmission and neuronal signaling within injured bone.

Indications

Patients undergoing orthopedic surgeries where bone cement is utilized can be considered as potential candidates for this approach.

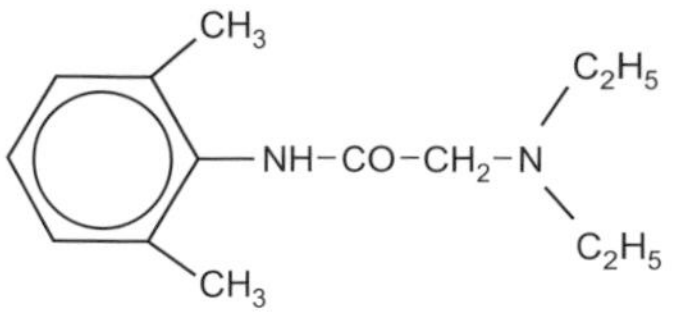

Figure 123.1.

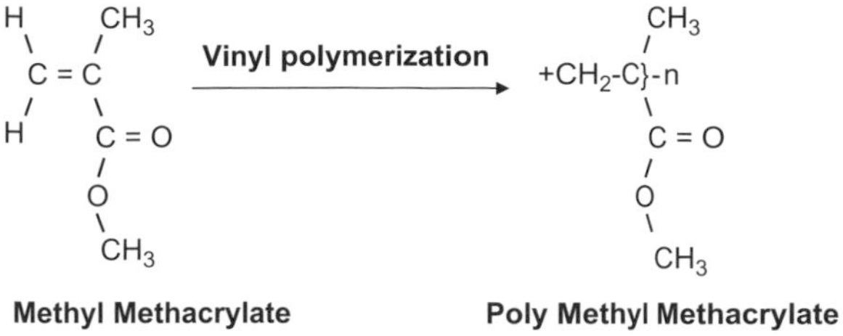

Methyl Methacrylate   Poly Methyl Methacrylate

Figure 123.2.

Common doses

An amount of 5% by weight of bone cement composition of a local anesthetic agent is thought to be effective [1].

Potential advantages

Various potential advantages may be present while providing analgesia by this method, including ease of use, tolerability, opioid-sparing effect, and possible reduction in opioid-related adverse events. Familiarity with the technique by the surgeons can be a potential advantage.

Elution profiles were studied and it was concluded that the amount of lidocaine released is proportional to the amount mixed with PMMA. It was found to peak at 6 hours and continued to elute up to 72 hours [1].

There was a 10% improvement in impact strength upon addition of lidocaine to CMW3 bone cement and it had little effect on compressive strength, flexural strength, or flexural modulus [1].

Potential disadvantages

Various potentially significant adverse reactions may occur due to hypersensitivity to any of the components (local anesthetics, bone cement and plastics).

Systemic reactions to local anesthetics including cardiac arrhythmia, bradycardia, cardiovascular collapse, increased defibrillator threshold, and heart block can occur.

Agitation, confusion, dizziness, euphoria, hallucinations, lightheadedness, seizure, slurred speech, somnolence, and coma can occur due to central nervous systemic effects. Dermatological manifestations such as angioedema and urticaria can be present. Patients may complain of metallic taste, nausea, and vomiting and present with bronchospasm, dyspnea, respiratory depression, and resultant respiratory arrest.

Disease-related concerns include liver dysfunction, which may lead to increased risk of local anesthetic toxicity.

Mixing lidocaine with bone cement is also found to increase the cement setting time [1].

References

1. US patent No 6,355,705 B1: date of patent 03/12/2002. Inventor David M Bond; John F. Rudan.

2. Bond DM, Rudan J, Kobus SM, Adams MA. Depot local anesthetic in polymethylmethacrylate bone cement: a preliminary study. *Clin Orthop Relat Res* 2004;**418**:242–245.

3. Ravin CE, et al. In vitro effects of lidocaine on anaerobic respiratory pathogens and strains of Hemophilus influenzae. *Chest* 1977;**72**:439–441.

4. Rosenburg PH, et al. Antimicrobial activity of bupivacaine and morphine. *Anesthesiology* 1985;**62**:178–179.

5. Schmidt RM, et al. Antimicrobial activity of local anesthetics: lidocaine and procaine. *J Infect Dis* 1970;**121**:597–607.

Peripheral kappa agonists

Derek Chalmers

Generic Name: peripheral kappa agonist

Trade/Proprietary Name: CR845

Drug Class: opioid analgesic

Manufacturer/Developer: Cara Therapeutics Parrot Drive, Trumbull, CT

Chemical Structure: see Figure 124.1

Chemical Name: D-Phe-D-Phe-D-Leu-D-Lys-[γ-(4-*N*-piperidinyl)amino carboxylic acid], acetate salt

Introduction

CR845 is a novel peripherally restricted, all-d-amino acid tetrapeptide kappa opioid selective agonist under development for the treatment of acute and chronic pain. It belongs to a novel class of opioid ligands which has a reduced ability to cross the blood–brain barrier and therefore acts without inducing central side effects [1]. It is currently available as an intravenous formulation in a sterile isotonic 0.04 M acetate buffer of pH 4.5 composed of acetic acid, sodium acetate trihydrate, sodium chloride, and water, with addition of hydrochloric acid for pH adjustments.

Mechanism of action

CR845 acts to reduce pain by selectively activating kappa opioid receptors located on peripheral nerve terminals, and kappa receptors on certain immune cells. CR845 has no activity at the mu or delta subtypes of opioid receptors, or other known receptors. Stimulation of kappa receptors by CR845 results in the initiation of an intracellular cascade that leads to the inhibition of ion channels necessary for peripheral nerve activity and culminates in reduced afferent nerve activity. Activation of kappa receptors on immune cells results in reduced release of nerve-sensitizing pro-inflammatory molecules.

Pharmacokinetics

Absorption: intravenous CR845 is completely absorbed after infusion with peak plasma levels at the end of infusion.

Distribution: CR845 exhibits a low volume of distribution in humans related to its high level of solubility. Highest concentrations are found in the plasma compartment with minimal to no exposure predicted in the central nervous system (CNS) based on preclinical distribution analysis. CR845 has a plasma half-life of approximately 2 hours

Metabolism: CR845 is not a substrate for hepatic drug-metabolizing enzymes and is eliminated as an unchanged parent compound via biliary and urinary excretion.

Indications (non-approved)

Acute surgical pain: CR845 may be effective in treating visceral, inflammatory, and neuropathic pain in the acute post-operative setting. CR845 is particularly indicated under conditions in which surgical procedures, such as abdominal laparoscopic approaches, are likely to induce post-operative pain with a prominent visceral pain component. In a recent randomized double-blind evaluation performed in women recovering from laparoscopic vaginal hysterectomy, patients treated with CR845 benefited from reductions in pain intensity and IV-PCA morphine requirements [2].

Contraindications

Hypersensitivity: at this stage of clinical development, CR845 is contraindicated in patients with a known hypersensitivity to any component of this product or opioids in general.

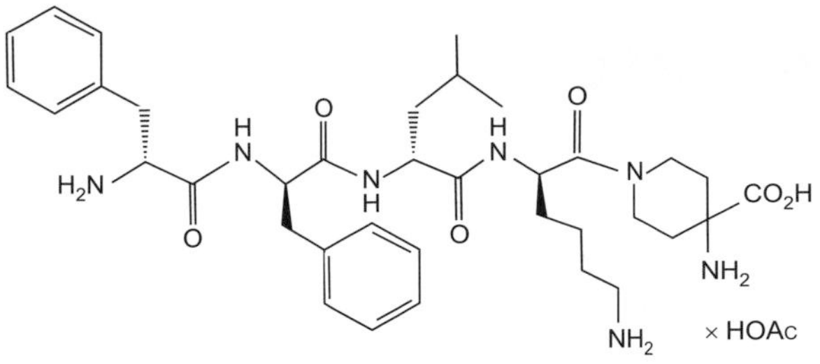

Figure 124.1.

Drug abuse and dependence

CR845 has not been systematically studied in humans for its potential in relation to abuse, tolerance, or physical dependence. However, it is likely that CR845's peripherally restricted distribution would limit its ability to induce CNS-related responses associated with dependence.

Potential advantages

CR845 offers the potential advantage of opioid-like analgesia in the absence of classical opioid side effects. Due to CR845's lack of central nervous system activity and pharmacological selectivity for the kappa opioid receptor, CR845 does not produce CNS-mediated respiratory depression, nausea or vomiting, sedation, or cognitive dysfunction. In addition, CR845's activation of peripheral kappa opioid receptors may act to treat visceral pain with a higher degree of efficacy than that available with traditional opioids, such as morphine. Moreover, the drug's lack of activity at peripheral mu opioid receptors may result in a lack of gastrointestinal and bladder-related side effects, such as post-operative ileus and urinary retention, and lead to improved patient recovery times. CR845 may be used in a multimodal approach with reduced doses of centrally acting opioids.

Potential disadvantages

The administration of IV CR845 results in an acute diuretic effect manifest as an increase in mean urine flow rate and a resultant negative fluid balance. Patients should be monitored for fluid balance on an ongoing basis.

Drug-related adverse events

The most frequently reported AE after CR845 administration is facial paresthesia. This usually manifests as mild "tingling" or numbness around the face and nose and subsides within minutes after drug administration. Mild to moderate orthostatic tachycardia has also been observed with CR845 use and is most probably secondary to negative fluid balance induced by increased urine flow rate.

References

1. Vanderah TW, Largent-Milnes T, Lai J, et al. Novel D-amino acid tetrapeptides produce potent antinociception by selectively acting at peripheral κ-opioid receptors. *Eur J Pharmacol* 2008;**583**:62–72.

2. Cara Therapeutics, 2010. Unpublished data on file.

Cannabinoid agonists

Yasser F. Shaheen and Aziz M. Razzuk

Generic Names: delta-9-tetrahydrocannabinol, dronabinol, nabilone

Proprietary Names: Marinol®, Cesamet®, Sativex®

Manufacturer: Solvay Pharmaceuticals, Inc., Marietta, GA; Valeant Pharmaceuticals International; GW Pharmaceuticals, London, UK

Drug Class: central-acting analgesic

Chemical Structures: Δ^9-THC (dronabinol; Marinol®), see Figure 125.1; nabilone (Cesamet®), see Figure 125.2; cannabidiol, see Figure 125.3

IUPAC Names: dronabinol, $(-)$-$(6aR,10aR)$-6,6,9-trimethyl-3-pentyl-6a,7,8,10a-tetrahydro-6H-benzo[c]chromen-1-ol; nabilone, $(6aR,10aR)$-1-hydroxy-6,6-dimethyl-3-(2-methyloctan-2-yl)-7,8,10,10a-tetrahydro-6aH-benzo[c]chromen-9-one; cannabidiol, 2-[(6S)-3-methyl-6-prop-1-en-2-ylcyclohex-2-en-1-yl]-5-pentyl-benzene-1,3-diol

Introduction

Cannabis sativa is the genus and species name of a flowering plant which has been used medicinally for thousands of years. Delta-9-tetrahydrocannabinol (Δ^9-THC) is responsible for almost all the psychoactive effects of cannabis, but is only one of more than 60 similar compounds found in cannabis which, together, are collectively known as cannabinoids. Cannabinoid agonists that share the basic chemical structure of delta-9-tetrahydrocannabinol have been increasingly studied in recent years for potential benefits in various types of pain and pain syndromes.

To gain FDA approval of a drug, the molecule must be relatively safe and the doses standardized, among other things. The inhalation of natural cannabis smoke or oral consumption of the plant parts is either unsafe, the dose cannot be standardized practically, or both. Cannabis smoke carries similar health risks to cigarette smoke and there are hundreds of different compounds beyond the cannabinoids that vary in concentration from plant to plant, making dose standardization infeasible. Current cannabinoid agonists are either synthesized Δ^9-THC or synthetic analogs of Δ^9-THC or are chemical extracts from pharmaceutically standardized cannabis plants.

To date, only two cannabinoid agonist drugs have been approved by the FDA for use in the USA. Dronabinol is a Schedule III synthetic form of Δ^9-THC and is marketed as Marinol® capsules. Nabilone is marketed as Cesamet® and is a Schedule II synthetic analog of Δ^9-THC. Neither of these drugs is approved for pain, however. Dronabinol is approved for nausea and vomiting associated with cancer chemotherapy in patients for whom standard antiemetics are inadequate and for AIDS patients with anorexia and weight loss. Nabilone is approved for treating cancer patients with chemotherapy-induced nausea and vomiting (CINV) for whom conventional therapy failed. However, there are a number of clinical trials and case reports demonstrating that dronabinol and nabilone provide moderate analgesic effects in humans.

One other drug, Sativex® (GW Pharmaceuticals, London, England) is currently undergoing phase IIb/III trials in the USA for the treatment of patients with advanced cancer whose pain is not controlled with opioid medications. The trials were expected to be completed by the end of 2009, after which FDA approval will be sought by the manufacturer to market Sativex in the USA with its partner, Otsuka Pharmaceutical Co. Ltd. Sativex is an oral mucosal spray which delivers a mixture of Δ^9-THC and cannabidiol. Cannabidiol is one of the phyto-cannabinoids found in cannabis which has no psychoactivity itself, but reduces the psychoactive side effects of Δ^9-THC when

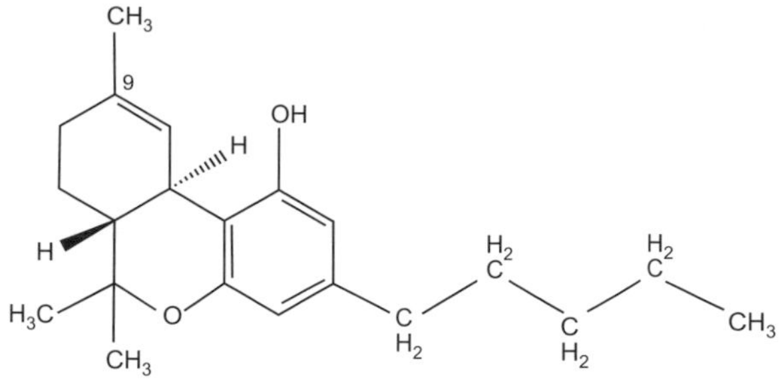

Figure 125.1.

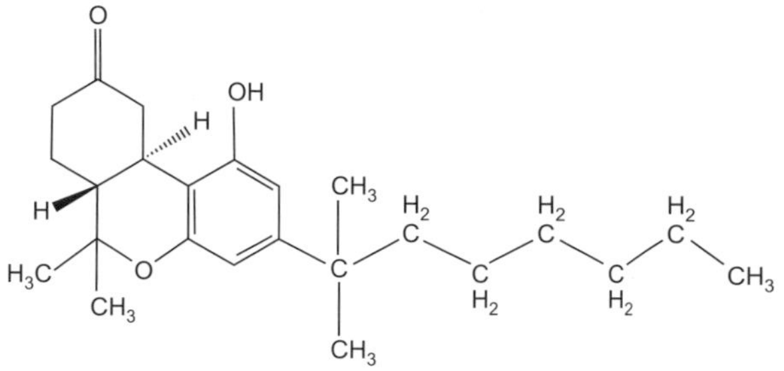

Figure 125.2.

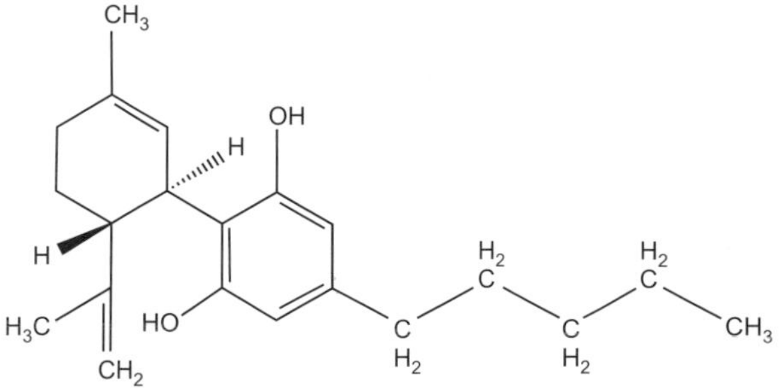

Figure 125.3.

administered in combination. Sativex is extracted from pharmaceutical-grade cannabis standardized to give a reproducible proportion of Δ⁹-THC and cannabidiol. This cannabis is grown in a secret location by the manufacturer in the UK.

Of the four stereoisomers of Δ⁹-THC, the *trans* (−) isomer occurs naturally in cannabis and is many times more potent than the other isomers. Dronabinol refers specifically to this isomer. Nabilone is more potent than dronabinol and differs in that the methyl group has been replaced by a carbonyl group on C-9 and the alkyl side chain is branched and longer. Cannabidiol differs from dronabinol in that the pyran ring is broken. This difference renders it essentially devoid of psychoactivity.

Mode of activity

The cannabinoid agonists act on cannabinoid receptors that have been found in high concentrations in areas of the brain dealing with pain control. These receptors are also found peripherally and are capable of modulating nociception as well. The receptors clearly identified thus far are designated CB_1 and CB_2 (for cannabinoid-1 and cannabinoid-2). CB_1 is primarily found in the central nervous system but can also be found in the peripheral nervous system. CB_2 is found in cells and tissues involved with immune function and in microglial cells, centrally. They are both G protein-coupled receptors located on the presynaptic terminals of neurons. Central CB_1 receptors are responsible for the psychoactive side effects of cannabinoid agonists, which are one of the primary difficulties in the use of cannabinoids for pain management.

CB_1 and CB_2 are part of the endogenous cannabinoid system known as the endocannabinoid system. This system also includes the naturally occurring ligands (endocannabinoids) of these receptors as well as associated metabolic enzymes. Two of these endocannabinoids are *N*-arachidonoyl ethanolamine or anandamide and 2-arachidonoyl glycerol or 2-AG. They are not stored in synaptic vesicles, but rather are synthesized on demand within the postsynaptic membrane. They are then released as retrograde messengers acting on CB_1 and CB_2 receptors on the presynaptic membrane resulting in an inhibitory effect on neurotransmitter release. Although Δ⁹-THC acts on the same receptors as anandamide and 2-AG, producing similar effects, its chemical structure is very different from these two endocannabinoids. The endocannabinoid system is found throughout the central and peripheral nervous systems as well as in many other tissues and performs a vast array of functions in a multitude of processes. Its involvement in nociception is still being elucidated and a variety of methods to manipulate it for control of pain are being studied intensively at institutions all over the world.

The absorption and metabolism of the cannabinoid agonists also impact their effectiveness in the management of pain symptoms. Greater than 90% of dronabinol is absorbed and then readily metabolized hepatically via microsomal hydroxylation to a mixture of metabolites, with 11-hydroxy-Δ⁹-THC being the main active metabolite. They begin exerting their effect within 1 hour and within 4 hours reach peak effect, with psychoactivity lasting up to 6 hours. Elimination is primarily biliary with more than half being excreted in the feces and less than a fifth in the urine. Complete clearance of the drug takes days to weeks due to its highly lipid-soluble nature. Nabilone is more potent than dronabinol, but otherwise has similar onset of action, metabolism, and clearance.

Sativex contains approximately equal proportions of dronabinol and cannabidiol delivered in an oral spray providing an onset of action of only 15–40 minutes with peak effect occurring similarly to the oral drugs. The cannabidiol may decrease psychotropic effects either by competitive inhibition for the CB_1 receptor site and/or by decreasing the metabolism of dronabinol to 11-hydroxy-Δ^9-THC, which may be more psychoactive than Δ^9-THC.

Indications

Dronabinol and nabilone have not been approved for the treatment of pain, but there is increasing evidence that they have a useful role and have been prescribed in some pain states. Sativex, on the other hand, is in late-stage clinical trials to approve its use specifically for patients with intractable cancer pain. The literature also contains many reports of its utility in various types of pain.

Studies of cannabinoid agonists in acute post-operative pain have been mixed, with nabilone found to actually worsen post-operative pain in one report. However, there is evidence for their use with opioid drugs, adjunctively, for possible synergistic effects or to delay the development of opioid tolerance.

Cannabinoid agonists have been found to be more generally useful in the management of chronic pain. The individual drugs have rarely been compared head to head for efficacy in any single study, so it is still not clear which drug would be more beneficial for any particular pain syndrome. Furthermore, reported efficacy of an individual drug can vary substantially from study to study, even of the same pain syndrome.

Dronabinol has been found to be helpful to patients with chronic non-malignancy pain on stable dosages of opioids with persistent pain. Ten mg of dronabinol was as effective as 20 mg of dronabinol and had fewer side effects. The same dosage was effective in moderately reducing pain related to multiple sclerosis (MS). Benefit to patients with cancer pain has also been reported.

Nabilone was successful in reducing non-malignancy pain as well as cancer pain, where it also decreased opioid usage. At 1 mg per day, it reduced spasticity-related pain in MS. Case reports describing its use in neuropathic pain have been positive.

Sativex has generally been found to be more effective than the currently approved cannabinoid drugs in the management of pain. It has been reported to be useful in chronic non-malignancy pain, intractable cancer pain, and peripheral and central neuropathic pain, including that related to MS. It has already been approved in Canada for the treatment of cancer pain refractory to opioid therapy and central neuropathic pain in MS. Studies have shown it to help patients with brachial plexus root avulsion and rheumatoid arthritis.

Contraindications

Since the cannabinoid agonists are not first-line drugs in the treatment of any of the various types of pain or pain syndromes, any potential risk of serious consequences from their use should be considered an absolute contraindication. Preexisting or genetic predisposition to serious psychiatric disorders such as schizophrenia or psychotic disorders, in general, would be an example. Precipitation or worsening of these and less serious psychiatric disorders has been reported. Caution and close monitoring of patients with less serious illnesses such as bipolar disorder, anxiety, or depression is necessary since the symptoms of these disorders could become manifest.

The cannabinoid agonists should be avoided in nursing mothers and have not been studied in pregnancy, pediatrics, or geriatrics, necessitating either avoidance in these groups, or, at least, careful consideration of risk versus benefit. In the elderly, evaluation of cardiovascular, hepatic, and renal disease should be undertaken. These drugs can cause tachycardia and orthostatic hypotension, especially initially, increasing the risk of myocardial infarction in patients with cardiovascular disease. Postural hypotension coupled with the common adverse effects of increased dizziness and drowsiness could lead to falls in the elderly.

These drugs can lower the seizure threshold in patients with a history of seizure disorder, which raises the concern for the potential of precipitation of seizures in this group of patients. Careful monitoring is advised in prescribing these drugs to patients already on other drugs that affect the CNS due to possible additive or synergistic effects. Although the potential risk of abuse of the cannabinoid agonists has been found to be low, care should be taken when prescribing these drugs to patients with a prior history of substance abuse, including alcohol. Of course, these drugs should be avoided in patients with known hypersensitivity to cannabinoids, the sesame oil in Marinol capsules, or the propylene glycol, ethanol, or peppermint oil in the Sativex spray.

Common doses/uses

The cannabinoid agonists suffer from a relatively increased adverse effect profile compared to other drugs used to treat pain. It is, therefore, generally recommended to titrate cannabinoid-based drugs for therapeutic effect, beginning with dosages at the lower end of the spectrum. Dronabinol dosages often range from 2.5 mg per day to 40 mg divided into four doses (QID). BID and TID dosing can be used for smaller total daily dosages. Early-morning dosing should be avoided due to a subsequent increase in adverse effects. Nabilone can be titrated beginning with 1 mg at bedtime or 0.5 mg for cannabinoid-naive patients and increased to BID dosing with a maximum daily dosage of 6 mg. Each actuation of the Sativex pump delivers 100 μL of an oro-mucosal spray containing 2.7 mg of Δ^9-THC and 2.5 mg of cannabidiol. The patient can self-titrate the number of sprays per day for symptomatic pain relief since the onset of action is fairly rapid. Patients usually reach a stable dosage range within 7–10 days and this often amounts to about 8–10 sprays per day.

Potential advantages

Cannabinoid agonists are especially advantageous in pain management due to a relative lack of toxicity, with reported deaths from overdose rare to nonexistent. This is attributable to their low potential for respiratory depression because of the lack of CB_1 receptors in the respiratory center of the brainstem. When used adjunctively, they are opioid-sparing and thereby reduce the risk of respiratory depression by opioids. In addition, Δ^9-THC stimulates beta endorphin production, delays development of tolerance to opioids, and limits withdrawal symptoms from opioids.

Although the cannabinoid agonists have a side-effect profile that is significant enough to limit widespread use among clinicians, they have few serious adverse effects. With continued usage, tolerance to the sedative effects develops while, at the same time, there is generally no loss of analgesic efficacy and even some increase in pain relief over a period of weeks to months. Dronabinol and nabilone assist with improved sleep, which helps increase pain tolerance. Nabilone is more potent than Δ^9-THC and has a longer half-life, requiring less frequent dosing. The abuse potential for these drugs is relatively low, presumably because of the slower rise in plasma levels due to oral intake as opposed to the rapid rise in plasma levels attained with smoked cannabis.

Long-term use of Sativex in a variety of pain syndromes has not demonstrated significant tolerance development to its analgesic effects. With normal usage, serum levels remain below the generally accepted minimum threshold for driving impairment, specifically, 5 ng/mL of Δ^9-THC. Few drug–drug interactions and virtually no withdrawal symptoms on abrupt cessation of therapy are further advantages to the use of Sativex.

Potential disadvantages

The main disadvantages of using cannabinoid agonists for the treatment of pain is their psychotropic side effects and potential for intoxication while generally providing only modest pain reduction. Patients need to be advised to abstain from driving, operating machinery, or engaging in other hazardous activities until the drug's effect on them is known. Caution and monitoring are required in the context of psychiatric disorders. It is possible to become psychologically or physiologically dependent on these drugs. Special care must also be taken with cardiac patients and the elderly.

Drug interactions include, among others, additive CNS depression when given to patients already on CNS depressants and additive tachycardia and/or hypertension when given to patients taking sympathomimetic drugs, anticholinergic drugs, and tricyclic antidepressants.

There may be issues of availability with nabilone since it is not generally considered a formulary drug. Also, since it is a Schedule II drug, restrictions on prescribing may complicate its use in chronic pain therapy. Sativex is a Schedule II drug in Canada, but it is uncertain whether it will be categorized as a Schedule II or Schedule III drug when ultimately approved in the USA.

The cost of cannabinoid agonist therapy for chronic pain is relatively high. Dronabinol and nabilone range in cost from several hundred dollars per month to even $1000–$2000 or more, depending on the dosage. It is not known what the cost of Sativex therapy will be once approved. In Canada, it is less expensive than the oral drugs, yet still costs up to several hundred dollars per month for the usual dosage regimen.

495

Table 125.1. Less common adverse events of individual cannabinoid agonists

Dronabinol	Nabilone	Sativex
Weakness	Weakness	Weakness
Depersonalization	Depersonalization	Depersonalization
Confusion	Confusion	Confusion
Palpitations	Headache	Headache
Anxiety	Sleep disturbance	Anxiety
Abdominal pain	Ataxia	Abdominal pain
Paranoia	Visual disturbance	Blurred vision
Abnormal thinking	Concentration difficulties	Memory problems
		Oral pain (due to spray)
		Oral irritation (due to spray)
		Abnormal taste (due to spray?)

Drug-related adverse events

Serious adverse events are uncommon with the cannabinoid agonists. Their interactions with the central nervous system are complex and not well understood, but include sympathomimetic effects that can lead to tachycardia and, occasionally, postural hypotension, which may lead to cardiac events in susceptible patients. Psychotic reactions and seizures can be precipitated in some patients with a history or genetic predisposition to these disorders.

The most common adverse events with cannabinoids are CNS-related, including dizziness, drowsiness, persistent appetite stimulation, conjunctival hyperemia, dry mouth, and the euphoria associated with the cannabinoid "high". Some of the less common adverse events associated with each individual cannabinoid agonist are listed in Table 125.1.

Treatment of minor adverse events may include reassurance, cessation of therapy, and supportive care. In cases of recent overdose, activated charcoal and a saline or sorbitol cathartic should be introduced into the stomach via nasogastric tube. Reassurance and/or benzodiazepines may be used if psychotic reactions, panic, or severe agitation are present. For hypotensive reactions, intravenous fluids and Trendelenburg positioning are usually adequate without the need for pressors or other drugs.

Summary

Currently, the analgesic potential of the cannabinoid agonists is generally modest, at best, and adverse effects can limit their potential benefit. However, for patients with intractable or chronic pain and chronic pain syndromes, there are often no effective treatments. The cannabinoid agonists should be considered as alternative or adjunctive analgesics in this subset of patients, since even modest alleviation of discomfort and opioid-sparing helps to lessen their total pain burden.

References

1. *American Hospital Formulary Service Drug Information 2008*. Bethesda, MD: American Society of Health-System Pharmacists, 2008, pp. 3007–3008.

2. Ashton JC, Milligan ED. Cannabinoids for the treatment of neuropathic pain: clinical evidence. *Curr Opin Investig Drugs* 2008;**9**:65–75.

3. A study of Sativex® for pain relief in patients with advanced malignancy. (SPRAY) ClinicalTrials.gov website. http://clinicaltrials.gov/ct2/show/NCT00530764?term=sativex&rank=68. Accessed July 20, 2009.

4. Canadian Agency for Drugs and Technologies in Health website. http://www.cadth.ca/media/pdf/310_sativex_cetap_e.pdf. September 2005. Accessed July 22, 2009.

5. Farquhar-Smith WP. Do cannabinoids have a role in cancer pain management? *Curr Opin Support Palliat Care* 2009;**3**:7–13.

6. Hosking RD, Zajicek JP. Therapeutic potential of cannabis in pain medicine. *Br J Anaesth* 2008;**101**:59–68.

7. Narang S, Gibson D, Wasan AD, Ross EL, Michna E, Nedelikovic SS, Jamison RN. Efficacy of dronabinol as

an adjuvant treatment for chronic pain patients on opioid therapy. *J Pain* 2008;**9**:254–264.

8. Pertwee RG. Cannabinoid pharmacology: the first 66 years. *Br J Pharmacol* 2006;**147**:S163–S171.

9. *Physicians' Desk Reference.* 63rd ed. Montvale, NJ: Physicians' Desk Reference, Inc., 2009, pp. 3163–3166.

10. Regence Rx Pharmacy Benefit Management website. http://www.regencerx.com/docs/physicianRx/cesamet0207.pdf. February 2007. Accessed July 22, 2009.

11. Russo EB. Cannabinoids in the management of difficult to treat pain. *Ther Clin Risk Manag* 2008;**4**:245–259.

12. Svendsen KB, Jensen TS, Bach FW. Does the cannabinoid dronabinol reduce central pain in multiple sclerosis? Randomised double blind placebo controlled crossover trial. *Br Med J* 2004;**329**:253–257.

Section 12
Chapter

126

New and Emerging Analgesics

Peripheral cannabinoid receptor agonists

Ho Dzung and Mark J. Lema

Generic Names: anandamide (endogenous ligand); tetrahydrocannabinol

Proprietary Names: CR701; WIN-55212–2; JWH-133; AM-1231

Drug Class: central- and peripheral-acting analgesic

Manufacturer: CR701: Cara Therapeutics, Shelton CT

Chemical Structures: see Figure 126.1

Introduction

Although cannabinoid drugs have been used recreationally and therapeutically for millennia little was known regarding their sites of activity and mechanisms of action. In recent years the pharmacological and behavioral properties of these molecules have been more thoroughly defined [1,2]. Development of ligands that preferentially bind to peripheral receptors may offer the promise of effective analgesia without the central nervous system effects of nonselective cannabinoids.

Description

Delta-9-tetrahydrocanabinol (THC), the active ligand in *Cannabis sativa* extract, was thought to exert its pharmacological effects by activating cannabinoid receptors in the central nervous system. These receptors were identified in 1988, and endogenous ligands termed endocannabinoids were isolated in 1992. Two major cannabinoid receptor subtypes termed CB_1 and CB_2 have been characterized [2–4]. Central CB_1 receptors are primarily localized in neocortex and the limbic system, and are responsible for many of the behavioral and analgesic effects of cannabinoid agonists. Peripheral CB_2 receptors and some CB_1 subtypes are primarily localized in immune cells such as leukocytes and mast cells, which have been shown to be involved in pain and inflammatory responses. CB_2 receptors are not present in the CNS; however, they are also found in peripheral nerve fibers and are particularly concentrated in injured neural endings.

The first endocannabinoid, anandamide, is an arachidonoyl ethanolamine, derived from fatty acids within the body. Its pharmacology is quite similar to THC although its chemical structure is different. Anandamide binds primarily to the central CB_1

497

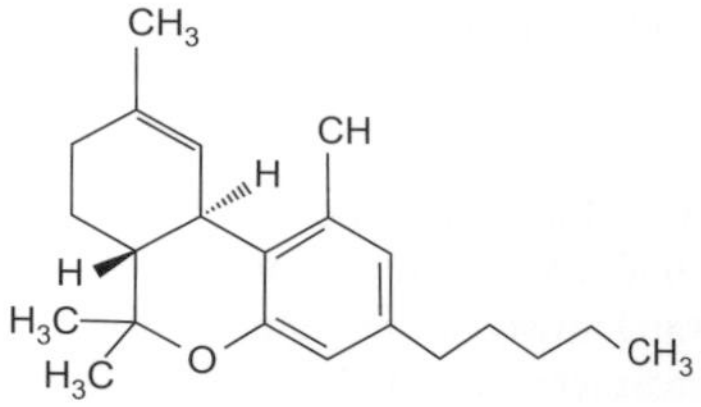

Figure 126.1.

THC

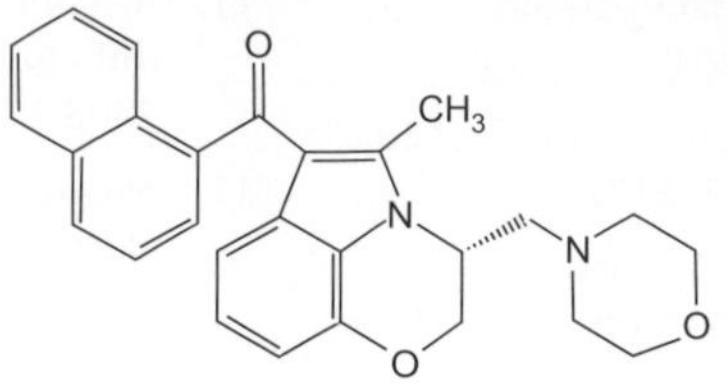

WIN-55212-2

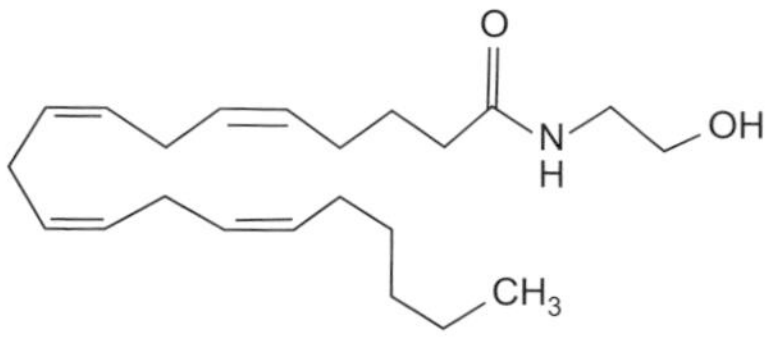

Anandamide

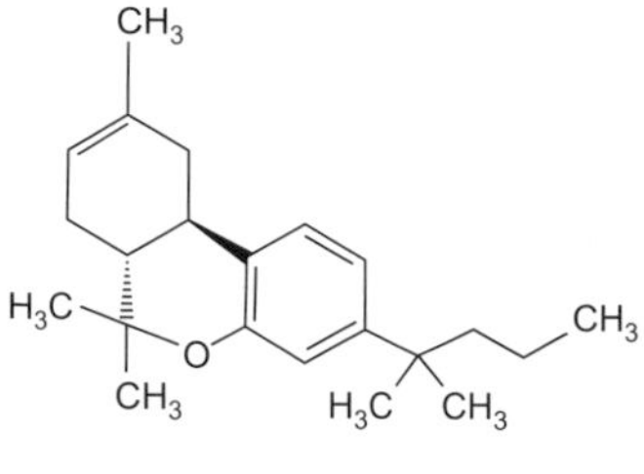

JWH-133

subtypes, and its potency is equivalent to THC. CB_1 agonists are associated with measurable analgesic effects; however, their behavioral effects, including suppression of locomotion, catalepsy, and hypothermia, are often problematic.

Recently a number of highly selective CB_2 receptor agonists have been developed [4–6]. These peripherally acting molecules have little to no activity in the central nervous system and minimal off-target activity on non-cannabinoid receptors, or various channels, transporters, and kinases [5,6]. Peripherally selective CB_2 agonists were synthesized by combining an active ligand with non-active chemical groups that either limit association with CB_1 receptors or decrease blood–brain barrier penetration and access to the CNS. Limitations in CNS access may provide important clinical advantages over nonselective cannabinoids, since the psychoactive effects of cannabinoids are caused by their interactions at central CB_1 receptors. Psychoactivity and other adverse effects including euphoria, ataxia, dizziness, and confusion have diminished patient tolerability. Unlike nonselective cannabinoids, peripherally selective agonists would also be expected to have lower psychological dependency, abuse, and diversion risks. Peripheral CB_2 receptors may be an appropriate target for eliciting relief of inflammatory pain without the CNS effect. CB_2 receptor agonists in development can inhibit inflammation and inflammatory hyperalgesia and offer the promise

of providing safe and effective analgesia [7]. Synthetic CB_2 ligands have also been found to attenuate neuropathic pain and mechanical and thermal hyperalgesia in animal nerve ligation models

A number of peripherally selective CB_2 agonists, including WIN-55212–2, JWH-133, HU-308, and CR701, have been developed and are being evaluated in early phase II safety and analgesic efficacy trials. The compound HU-308 is highly selective for the CB_2 receptor subtype, with a selectivity over 5000 times greater for CB_2 vs. CB_1. A second CB_2 agonist, CR701, that has high selectivity and minimal CNS access is being evaluated at Cara Therapeutics [6]. This compound has demonstrated efficacy in animal models of inflammatory and neuropathic pain. A similar compound, CB-13, is a potent agonist at both the CB_1 and CB_2 receptors, but has very poor blood–brain barrier penetration. It produces only peripheral effects at low doses, with symptoms of central effects such as catalepsy only appearing at much higher dose ranges. It has antihyperalgesic properties in animal studies and has progressed to preliminary human trials. A final compound, AM1241, appears to be particularly effective in controlling neuropathic pain. Ibrahim et al. [8] tested the hypothesis that CB_2 receptor activation would reverse the sensory hypersensitivity observed in neuropathic pain states. AM1241 dose-dependently reversed tactile and thermal hypersensitivity produced by ligation of the L5 and L6 spinal nerves in rats. These effects were not antagonized by a CB_1 receptor antagonist, suggesting that they were produced by actions of AM1241 at CB_2 receptors. AM1241 was also active in blocking spinal nerve ligation-induced tactile and thermal hypersensitivity in mice lacking CB1 receptors (CB1−/− mice), confirming that AM1241 reverses sensory hypersensitivity independent of actions at CB_1 receptors.

Mode of activity

Peripherally selective cannabinoid agonists exert their major and minor effects by selectively activating peripheral CB_2 receptors. Cannabinoid receptors are $G_{i/o}$-linked seven-transmembrane-domain G protein-coupled receptors. CB_2 agonists mediate analgesia by preventing the release of noxious and inflammatory mediators from a variety of cell types including neutrophils, macrophages, and mast cells. As mentioned above, CB_2 receptors also inhibit afferent conduction in inflamed or injured nerve fibers. Recent data indicate that CB_2 expression is up-regulated in injured peripheral neurons and may play a role in neuropathic pain, particularly painful neuromas. Other studies exhibit a possible spinal location of microglia and macrophages expressing CB_2 receptors. Activation of these receptors leads to improvement of central sensitization, hyperalgesia, and allodynia while also providing anti-inflammatory effects.

Metabolic pathways

Clearance and elimination pathways for peripherally selective cannabinoids have yet to be clearly defined. THC is metabolized to 11-OH-THC (11-hydroxy-THC) by the human body by almost exclusive first-pass hepatic metabolism. More than 50% of THC is excreted in the feces.

Indications (approved/non-approved)

There are no approved indications for peripheral cannabinoid agonists for the treatment of pain. Animal models and clinical trials display possible use for inflammatory, visceral, and neuropathic pain. Doses for pain management in humans have yet to be determined.

Contraindications (based on dronabinol usage)

Absolute: known sensitivity and allergic reactions to cannabinoids, marijuana, or sesame oil.

Relative: patients with coronary risk factors (tachycardia and orthostatic hypotension), dementia (fall precautions), mood disorders (anxiety, confusion, dizziness).

Potential advantages

When employed as analgesics, CB_2 agonists may offer improved safety by avoiding psychoactive effects commonly observed with nonselective agonists. This may also permit use of higher and potentially more efficacious doses with greater patient tolerability. This is a very important advantage, because despite clear analgesic effects in animal models, THC and other nonselective cannabinoids have not proven to be effective analgesics in humans. The major factor responsible for this lack of clinical efficacy has been a very high side-effect profile of these agents that severely limits dose. Proper utilization of CB_2 agonists may not only eliminate psychoactive effects, but, when employed in a multimodal regimen, may also limit opiate use and their associated side effects. Experimental cannabinoids such as JWH-133 and CR-701 exhibit fewer adverse reactions due to more selectivity for CB_2 receptors, but provide effective analgesia in animal studies. When used as a sole analgesic, CB_2 agonists are shown to alleviate neuropathic pain and mechanical hyperalgesia. They have not been studied as part of a multimodal regimen; however, CB2 receptor agonists enhance the effect of μ opioid receptor agonists in a variety of models of analgesia, and combinations of cannabinoids and opioids may produce synergistic effects [9]. There is also evidence that CB_2 agonists enhance the analgesic effect of nonsteroidal anti-inflammatory drugs (NSAIDs), raising the possibility that combination therapy could reduce NSAID dose and minimize the potential for gastrointestinal and cardiovascular disturbances [9].

Potential disadvantages

Toxicity: toxicity is extremely low with no reported cases. Absorption is limited by serum lipids, which can become saturated with THC, mitigating toxicity. LD_{50} of THC is 1270 mg/kg for male rats and 730 mg/kg for female rats from oral doses. Accumulation of metabolites is directly associated with increased incidence of adverse effects.

Drug interactions: no significant drug–drug interactions are noted. Treatment for any possible interactions should include the discontinuation of cannabinoid treatment.

Adverse events observed with nonselective agonists may not be as common or pronounced with peripherally selective CB_2 cannabinoids. They include potential for abuse, confusion, ataxia, memory loss, psychosis, dizziness, hypotension, sedation, euphoria, paranoia, and dry mouth. Less common adverse events include: orthostatic hypotension, abdominal pain, nausea, vomiting, anxiety, myalgias, increased appetite, nightmares, flushing, visual difficulties, and headache. No specific antagonists are currently in use, but adverse effects can be cared for individually.

Availability: due to the potential for abuse, there is legal debate about the therapeutic use of natural cannabinoids. It is to be noted that use of cannabinoids may be habit-forming and possibly lead to abuse of other substances. This may not be the case for peripherally selective agonists. Currently CB_2 receptor agonists are only available for experimental analgesic trials.

References

1. Hanus L, Breuer A, Mechoulam R, Fride E. HU-308: a specific agonist for CB(2), a peripheral cannabinoid receptor. *Proc Natl Acad Sci USA* 1999;**96**(25): 14228–14233.

2. Roxane Laboratories, Inc. Q & A about therapy with Marinol (dronabinol). Pamphlet. Columbus, OH, 1997.

3. Brownjohn PW, Ashton JC. Novel targets in pain research: the case for CB2 receptors as a biorational pain target. *Curr Anaesth Crit Care* 2009;**20**:198–203.

4. LaBuda CJ, Koblish M, Little PJ. Cannabinoid CB2 receptor agonist activity in the hindpaw incision model of postoperative pain. *Eur J Pharmacol* 2005;**527**:172–174.

5. Gardin A, Kucher K, Kiese B, Appel-Dingemanse S. Cannabinoid receptor agonist 13, a novel cannabinoid agonist: first in human pharmacokinetics and safety. *Drug Metab Dispos* 2009;**37**(4):827–833.

6. Chalmers D. Cara Therapeutics, personal communication. 2009

7. Quartilho A, Mata HP, Ibrahim MM, et al. Inhibition of inflammatory hyperalgesia by activation of peripheral CB2 cannabinoid receptors. *Anesthesiology* 2003;**99**:955–960.

8. Ibrahim MM, Deng H, Zvonok A, et al. Activation of CB2 cannabinoid receptors by AM1241 inhibits experimental neuropathic pain: pain inhibition by receptors not present in the CNS. *Proc Natl Acad Sci USA* 2003;**100**(18):10529–10533.

9. Philip Malan T Jr, Mohab M Ibrahim, Josephine Lai, et al. CB2 agonists, analgesia without psychoactive effects. *Curr Opin Pharmacol* 2003;**3**:62–67.

Section 12
Chapter

127

New and Emerging Analgesics

Injectable capsaicin

Muhammad K. Ghori

Generic Name: injectable capsaicin

Trade Name: Adlea™

Manufacturer: Anesiva Inc., San Francisco, CA; note: Anesiva merged with a second company on August 5, 2009, and is now called Arcion Therapeutics Inc.

Class: peripheral-acting TRPV-1 antagonist-type analgesic

Chemical Structure: see Figure 127.1

Chemical Name: 8-methyl-*N*-vanillyl-*trans*-6-nonenamide

Chemical Formula: $C_{18}H_{27}NO_3$; molecular wt 305.41

Introduction

The injectable analgesic Adlea™ is a concentrated and purified form of capsaicin (8-methyl-N-vanillyl-6-nonenamide). It is an unapproved preparation, currently in phase 3 trials for relief of post-surgical acute pain, nerve trauma-induced neuropathic pain, and for chronic musculoskeletal, tendon-related, and arthritic pain.

Description

Capsaicin is an alkaloid derived from plants and has been a common ingredient in food and spices for many centuries. It is concentrated in the seeds and inner stem of chili peppers and is the active ingredient responsible for making them taste hot. Low-concentration capsaicin is widely available and is a frequently used topical analgesic for patients with chronic arthritic joint and back pain. Topical gels and creams are often combined with NSAIDs and narcotic analgesics for severe pain due to sprains, strains, joint pains, and for other types of arthritis. A higher-concentration topical capsaicin has also been approved for postherpetic neuralgia-related neuropathic pain [1,2].

This new injectable preparation Adlea™ (formerly named ALRGX 4975 98% Pure) employs purified capsaicin in very high concentration. In October 2006 the FDA granted orphan drug status for Adlea™ for the treatment of pain related to interdigital neuroma (Morton's neuroma).

The manufacturer is currently evaluating Adlea™ for the management of acute pain following orthopedic surgery and for chronic joint pain. Currently, long-acting, site-specific Adlea™ is being evaluated in several clinical trials, including pain related to interdigital neuroma, post-traumatic neuropathic pain, knee joint osteoarthritis pain, and post-surgical pain following bunionectomy, total knee replacement, and arthroscopic shoulder surgery.

Mode of activity

Capsaican is a TRPV-1 agonist. TRPV1 (also termed the capsaican receptor) is a polymodal nociceptor exhibiting a dynamic threshold of activation that is markedly reduced in inflammatory conditions [3]. TRPV1 knock-out mice are devoid of post-inflammatory thermal hyperalgesia. TRPV receptors are in abundance on unmyelinated C fiber peripheral endings and respond to a variety of noxious mediators. Once activated these fibers transmit localized and

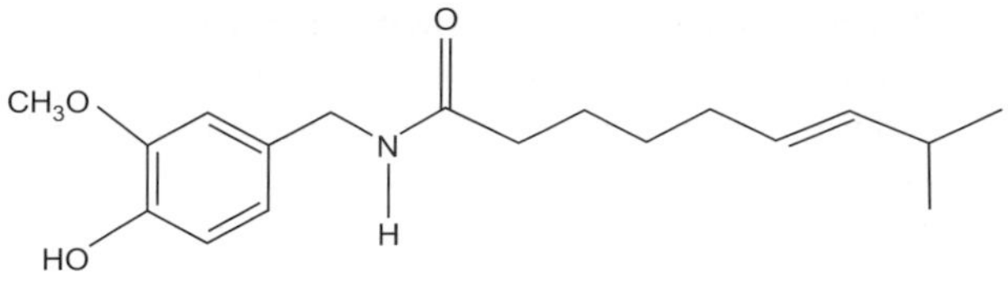

Figure 127.1.

highly intense pain impulses (gnawing pain, deep, aching pain) to the spinal cord and higher centers. Following local application, Adlea initially stimulates these receptors, releases additional substance P, and causes immediate complaints of severe burning pain. Continued exposure to capsaicin depletes stores of substance P, and eventually destroys the terminal nerve endings, thereby minimizing or preventing subsequent C fiber activation. Adlea's effects are highly selective at C fiber TRPV1 receptors. For this reason its application does not have any clinically measurable effects on A-delta and A-alpha fibers, and it does not block temperature or touch sensations [3].

Potential indications

1. Post-operative pain: total knee replacement, bunionectomy, total hip replacement, arthroscopic shoulder surgery, hernia repair.
2. Acute and chronic pain: pain due to tendinitis of the elbow, interdigital neuromas, moderate to severe osteoarthritis of the knee, neuropathic pain occurring secondary to trauma and nerve injury [4].
3. As adjuvant therapy: clinically significant opioid-sparing effect. It may be useful in elderly debilitated patients in whom respiratory and CNS depression due to narcotic overdose needs to be avoided.
4. Limited data indicate that capsaicin may be effective for relief of migraine headache, cancer-related pain and diabetic and HIV neuropathy [5].

Clinical trials and doses

1. Total knee arthroplasty: in a randomized, double-blind, phase 3 trial (ACTIVE 1) Adlea (15 mg in 60 mL of solution, 0.25 mg /mL) was compared with placebo in 217 patients undergoing total knee arthroplasty. Adlea was injected into the wound at the end of surgery. Post-operative pain

improvement from the 4–48 hours period was significantly improved in the active group ($P = 0.005$). In a similar but more extended trial (ACTIVE-2), reductions in post-operative pain and improved range of motion continued for 6 weeks following surgery. There was a significant reduction in opioid requirements during this time period ($P = 0.005$).

2. Bunionectomy: this phase 2 dose-ranging trial in 185 patients evaluated 100, 500 and 1000 μg doses of Adlea vs. placebo during the first 32 hours following bunionectomy. Pain relief was statistically improved and need for ketorolac rescue reduced in the higher-dose group vs. the two lower-dose groups and placebo during the first 32 hours post-op. All three doses were well tolerated with similar side effects to placebo. In a randomized double blind phase 3 study of 301 patients, Adlea 1 mg in 4 mL solution (0.25 mg/mL) injected into the surgical wound was compared with placebo for pain relief following bunionectomy [6]. Study results showed less pain in the Adlea group; however, the reduction was not significant during the first 2–32 hours when compared with placebo ($P = 0.07$). During this interval a secondary endpoint (opioid consumption) was significantly reduced in the Adlea group ($P = 0.012$). Another secondary end point, the numeric of post-operative pain rating score from 4 to 48 hours, also showed statistically significant reductions in the Adlea-treated group ($P = 0.004$). There was no difference in wound healing, safety profile or sensory testing around the wound, which demonstrated the selectivity of Adlea's effect on noxious C fibers.

3. Osteoarthritis of knee joint: a small phase 2 study ($n = 12$) found that patients with end-stage osteoarthritis reported significant pain relief for 6 weeks after receiving a single injection of Adlea in the knee joint. In an open label phase 2 study of 55 patients suffering from osteoarthritis of the knee joint, a statistically significant reduction of pain ($P = 0.001$) was noted in one of four groups treated with stepped doses of Adlea (100 μg first week, 300 μg second week and 1000 μg third week).

4. Tendinitis of the elbow joint: in a small phase 2 trial, tendinitis of the elbow was studied in 45 patients. Patients were treated with lidocaine followed by placebo or Adlea (100 μg) in painful tendinitis of the elbow joint. Reduced pain and increased functionality from baseline was noted by 60% of patients treated with Adlea.

5. Interdigital neuroma: in this double-blind, placebo-controlled phase 2 study of 58 patients with severe interdigital neuroma-related pain, those treated with a single injection of Adlea reported significant improvement in symptoms for up to 4 weeks. The Adlea group reported 59% less pain, which was significantly better than placebo (36% less pain) throughout the 4-week observation period.

Pharmacokinetics/pharmacodynamics

Subcutaneous injection of capsaicin in rats resulted in a rise in blood concentration, reaching a maximum at 5 hours. Highest concentration was found in kidney, and lowest in liver. Direct plasma levels of Adlea™ have yet to be reported in any of the clinical trials. Plasma levels were measured following application of the high dose (640 μg/cm^2) capsaican dermal patch Qutenza™ (NGX-4010). Plasma concentration from 173 patients with post-herpetic neuralgia, HIV-related neuropathy, and painful diabetic neuropathy showed a maximum plasma concentration of 17.8 ng/mL. The capsaicin levels declined very rapidly, with a mean population elimination half-life of 1.64 hours. Mean area under the curve and C_{max} values after a 60 minute application were 7.42 ng/mL and 1.86 ng/mL respectively. Application of NGX-4010 for 90 minutes resulted in capsaicin area under the curve and C_{max} values approximately 1.78- and 2.15-fold higher than observed in patients treated for 60 minutes. Low systemic exposure and very rapid elimination half-life of capsaicin after NGX-4010 administration are unlikely to result in systemic effects and support the overall safety profile of this investigational cutaneous patch. Mild transient increase in liver enzymes was seen more often in the capsaicin-treated group. Metabolism and elimination data for Adlea are expected to be similar to topical and transdermal capsaicin.

Contraindications

At this time, the only absolute contraindication for Adlea is patient hypersensitivity to capsaicin or capsinoid products. Relative contraindications would include patients with elevated liver enzymes, patients showing signs of septic arthritis, age less than 2 years, and patients on ACE inhibitors.

Common doses

Dosing will be based on clinical trial safety and efficacy data, and contingent upon FDA approval.

Potential advantages and disadvantages

Adlea is a selective peripheral-acting analgesic that can be used for acute and chronic pain management [5,6]. It may be employed in a multimodal analgesic regimen with opioids and NSAIDs. Its long-lasting analgesic and narcotic-sparing effect may reduce the incidence and severity of opioid-related sedation, nausea, vomiting, and constipation.

The NSAID-sparing effect of capsaicin can reduce the unwanted side effects of NSAIDs such as platelet-related aggregation abnormalities, peptic ulcer problems, or cardiovascular and renal complications. It may be particularly useful in the elderly, who are often intolerant to opioids and NSAIDs.

Potential disadvantages are burning stinging pain and hyperalgesia at the injection site; possible neurotoxicity if injected directly into a nerve. Persistent redness and erythema; occasional cough with ACE inhibitors

Pain and hyperthermia at the injection site can be reduced by pre-administration neural blockade, and administration during general anesthesia. Ideally, Adlea may be applied to patients receiving anesthesia and post-operative analgesia with epidural and peripheral neural blockade catheters. Residual pain may be controlled with local application of ice packs, local anesthetic infiltration, and oral acetaminophen.

In conclusion, Adlea appears to exhibit promise as a novel analgesic in the treatment of acute surgical pain, osteoarthritis, and conditions of chronic neuropathic pain. It remains unclear whether or when it will receive FDA approval. The merging of Anesevia into a larger company may improve the chances for funding and completion of outstanding clinical trials.

References

1. Wong GY, Gavva NR. Therapeutic potential of vanilloid receptor TRPV1 agonists and antagonists as analgesics: recent advances and setbacks. *Brain Res Rev* 2009;**60**(1)267–277, Epub 2008 Dec 25.

2. Aasvang EK, Hansen JB, Kehlet H. The effect of wound instillation of a novel purified capsaicin formulation on post herniotomy pain. *Anesth Analg* 2008;**107**(1):9–10.

3. Final report on capsaicin. *Int J Toxicol* 2007:**26**(suppl. 1):3–106.

4. Remadevi R, Szallisi A. Adlea(ALGRX-4975) an injectable capsaicin (TRPV1 Receptor agonist) formulation for longstanding pain relief. *IDrugs* 2008;**11**(2):120–132.

5. Babbar S, Marier JF, Bley K. Pharmacokinetic analysis of capsaicin after topical administration of a high-concentration capsaicin patch to patients with peripheral neuropathic pain. NeurogesX inc, San Mateo, California 94404, USA.

6. Stoker DG, Gottleib I, Comfort S. A single instillation of a highly purified capsaicin formulation decreases postoperative pain after bunionectomy. IASP annual meeting, 2008.

New and Emerging Analgesics

TRPV-1 ion channel blockers

Jeanette Derdemezi

Generic Names: transient receptor potential vanilloid (TRPV) channel antagonist, capsazepine, iodo-resiniferatoxin (I-RTX), MK-2295

Trade/Proprietary Name: none at present

Drug Class: ion channel blocker

Manufacturer/developer: Sandoz (Novartis), Novartis International AG, CH-4002 Basel, Switzerland; Merck Pharmaceuticals, P.O. Box 100, One Merck Drive, Whitehouse Station, NJ 08889

Chemical Structure: see Figure 128.1

Chemical Name: *N*-[2-(4-chlorophenyl)ethyl]-1,3,4,5-tetrahydro-7,8-dihydroxy-2*H*-2-benzazepine-2-carbothioamide

Chemical Formula: $C_{19}H_{21}ClN_2O_2S$

Introduction

Transient receptor potential vanilloid (TRPV) channel blockers (antagonists) are new drugs, which are not currently approved for clinical use, yet have great analgesic potential. An example of this class of drugs is capsazepine, a synthetic analog of capsaicin [1], which inactivates TRPV1 channels by competitively occupying TRPV1 binding sites in sensory neurons. Although capsazepine, the first TRPV antagonist, exhibited certain analgesic and anti-inflammatory properties, its effects were of low potency as well as variable within different species. As a result, capsazepine never reached the clinical arena. It is used now in the laboratory as an investigating tool for the study of other TRPV antagonists. The next compound studied was iodo-resiniferatoxin (I-RTX), an analog of resiniferatoxin (RTX). This drug was more potent than capsazepine and more specific for TRPV receptors but lacked consistent analgesic effects. The functional importance of the TRPV channels in pain was further elucidated with the cloning of the vanilloid

receptor [2]. The search for the perfect TRPV antagonist has been intensified and currently there are several drugs undergoing clinical trials. The new generation of TRPV antagonists has structures completely different from the agonists and therefore they are devoid of partial agonistic effect. Newer compounds that are in phase 2 clinical trials are: SB-705498 (for migraine, made by GSK), NGD-8243/MK-2295 (for acute pain, made by Neurogen/Merck), and GRC (for acute pain, made by Glenmark/Eli Lilly). Some other compounds useful for the treatment of chronic pain are in phase 1 clinical trials (AMG-517, AZD-1386,ABT-102) [3].

Mode of action

Ion channels are integral membrane proteins found in every cell. Transient receptor potential (TRP) channels are nonselective monovalent and divalent cation channels, first described in the visual system of *Drosophila*. TRP channels, which got their name because mutations in this gene cause a transient voltage response, are important structures for Ca^{2+} homeostasis and other regulatory and physiological functions. When intracellular Ca^{2+} stores are depleted, these channels open, allowing extracellular Ca^{2+} to enter the cell. TRP channels are classified into six families according to their amino acid sequence and homology: TRPC (canonical), TRPM (melastatin), TRPL (mucolilpins), TRPP (polycystins), TRPA (ankyrin), and TRPV (vanilloid receptors) [4].

TRPV channels are further classified into six subfamilies: TRPV1, TRPV2, TRPV3, TRPV4, TRPV5, and TRPV6. The subtypes TRPV 1, 2, 3, and 4 are called thermo TRPs [4] since all of them are activated by different degrees of temperature. In 1997 the TRPV1 (capsaicin, vanilloid) receptor was cloned from rodent posterior dorsal root ganglia [2] and since then has been studied extensively. Activation of TRPV1 receptors is associated with pain formation

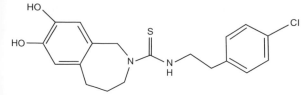

Figure 128.1.

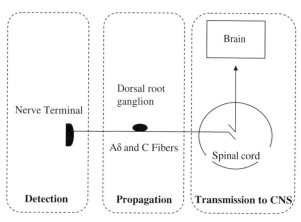

Figure 128.2. Schematic representation of signal detection propagation and transmission.

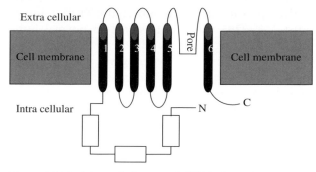

Figure 128.3. Schematic diagram of a TRPV1 channel.

and propagation via the afferent neurons into the posterior horn of the spinal cord and other CNS locations, where they release glutamate and other neuropeptides Meanwhile there is release of pro-inflammatory substances from the periphery (Figure 128.2). Due to their role in pain detection, transmission, amplification, and sensitization, TRPV channels have become the target for the development of new analgesics.

Structure of TRPV channels

The TRPV receptor contains six transmembrane domains designated S1–S6. These domains anchor the channel to the cellular membrane. Between S5 and S6 there is a pore. TRPV possess three ankyrin repeats. This transmembrane protein has an extracellular surface and an intracellular surface (Figure 128.3). Factors that activate and regulate this channel act in different domains. Antagonists of this channel may act in different areas of the complex molecule, the pore, the capsaicin site, the extracellular area, or the intracellular area, leading to its inactivation.

Location: TRPV1, a nonselective cation channel with a preference for calcium, is abundant in the peripheral sensory and central nervous system as well as other organ cells. TRPV channels are found in small

unmyelinated (C), less myelinated (Ad) fibers of primary afferent neurons as well as in the dorsal root and trigeminal and nodose ganglia. In addition they are located in the dorsal horn of the spinal cord (especially in lamina I and the inner surface of lamina II), the spinal nucleus of the trigeminal tract and in the fibers deriving from the nodose ganglia. The expression of these receptors (channels) in the pathway of the pain ties them closely to initiation and transduction of pain. TRPV channels have been located in areas other than the sensory system such as the urothelial cells, the gastroesophageal junction, in the mast cells, lymphocytes, and keratinocytes. The presence of TRPV channels in mast cells emphasizes their role in the inflammatory process.

TRPV1 channels are activated by many physical, mechanical and chemical stimuli and endogenous ligands, and therefore have been described as "polymodal receptors". TRPV1 is stimulated by:

1. temperatures above 42°C
2. pH less than 5.5 (protons)
3. capsaicin, piperine
4. spider venoms
5. jellyfish
6. lipids such as anandamide
7. pro-inflammatory neuropeptides, such as prostaglandins, ATP, NGF, bradykinin, CGRP (calcitonin gene-related peptide).

When TRPV channels are stimulated by the above factors, the proteins undergo a configurational change which allows Ca^{2+} followed by Na^+ to enter the cytoplasm causing depolarization. In addition, Ca^{2+} entering the cytoplasm causes the release of many neuropeptides (kinins, substance P, prostaglandins,) which further activate the TRPV channel. TRPV1 antagonists can interfere in all these levels, thereby decreasing inflammatory pain, acute pain, and chronic pain.

505

In a preliminary human trial, the TRPV1 antagonist MK-2295 was administered to normal individuals for 14 days. In addition to reductions in experimental pain and hyperalgesia, these subjects also displayed a marked increase in threshold to heat-related discomfort. Some patients did not report discomfort despite exposure to unpleasant temperatures around 48°C. While this finding may offer therapeutic benefits, it could result in thermal injury.

Ideal TRPV1 antagonist (drug profile)

For clinical use the TRPV1 antagonists should be able

1. to block activation of the channel (heat, proton, ligand)
2. to be potent
3. to have bioavailability
4. to be highly selective
5. to have minor, if any, side effects
6. to be soluble.

Potential indications of TRPV1 antagonists

The new TRPV agents will be useful alone or in combination with other agents in the following conditions:

1. Hyperalgesia (some types)
2. Post-operative pain
3. Inflammatory pain (osteoarthritis, rheumatoid arthritis)
4. Neuropathic pain (diabetic, AIDS neuropathy)
5. Bone cancer pain [5]
6. Visceral pain
7. Migraine pain.

Advantages of TRPV blockers

The advantage of these agents is that they act at the nociceptor level; therefore by blocking TRPV channels they can interfere with pain at the site of its formation rather its propagation.

Potential disadvantages

TRPV channels are expressed in cells outside the sensory system and therefore mediate many physiological functions. Blocking these channels can lead to untoward effects from other systems. The following are some well-documented and some potential side effects.

1. Hyperthermia which is not responding to antipyretics (TRPV channels are found in the hypothalamus, where they may play a role in temperature regulation).
2. Insensitivity to potentially damaging thermal stimulation.
3. Hypertension (this is a potential untoward effect that may occur with prolonged use).
4. Gastric ulcers.

Based on these potential risks, systemic administration of TRPV1 antagonists may be restricted; however, topical application may offer greater safety and analgesic effectiveness.

References

1. Bevan S, et al. Capsazepine: a competitive antagonist of the sensory neurone excitant capsaicin: *Br J Pharmacol* 1992;**107**:544–552.
2. Caterina MJ, Schumacher MA, Tominaga M, Rosen TA, Levine JD, Julius D. The capsaicin receptor: a heat-activated ion channel in the pain pathway. *Nature* 1997;**389**:816–824.
3. Pal M, Angaru S, Kodimuthali A, Dhingra N. Vanilloid receptor antagonists: emerging class of novel anti-inflammatory agents for pain management. *Curr Pharm Des* 2009;**15**:1008–1026.
4. Cortright DN, Szallasi A. TRP channels and pain. *Curr Pharm Des* 2009;**15**:1736–1749.
5. Nilius B, Owianik G, Voets T, Peters JA. Transient receptor potential cation channels in disease. *Physiol Rev* 2007;**87**:165–217.

129

Neramexane

Dajie Wang

Generic Name: neramexane

Trade/Proprietary Name: none at present

Class of Drug: uncompetitive NMDA antagonist

Manufacturer: Forest Laboratories, Inc., 909 Third Avenue, New York, NY 10022; Merz Pharmaceuticals, Frankfurt, Germany

Chemical Structure: see Figure 129.1

Chemical Name: 1-amino-1,3,3,5,5-pentamethyl-cyclohexane hydrochloride

Introduction

Neramexane is a central-acting N-methy-D-aspartate receptor antagonist which first underwent preclinal trials in Germany. In 1998, it was investigated for both neuroprotective and alcololholism effects. In 2001, it continued onto phase II trials for alcoholism and a phase I trial for pain. In 2001, Forest Laboratories Inc. entered into an agreement with Merz & Co. (Germany) and brought the drug to the USA [1,2]. Pre-clinical animal models have been trialed with neramexane, looking at its effects on various entities, including neuropathic pain [3]. A phase 1b trial revealed promising results for treatment of neuropathic pain; however, the subsequent phase II trial showed no superiority to existing treatments [4,5]. A phase III trial is currently under investigation for tinnitus [1,2].

Mode of activity

Neramexane is an open-channel blocker against the NMDA receptor. It has moderate affinity to the NMDA receptor, with strong voltage-dependency and fast-onset blocking kinetics.

Metabolic pathways, drug clearance and elimination: in the phase I study, an oral dose (5–40 mg) demonstrated a plasma half-life of approximately 29–42 hours. Metabolism has not been clearly elucidated yet. After administration of a single dose, 30–40% of the drug was excreted from the kidney unchanged [3].

Indications

Specific indications have not been approved by the FDA. Several clinical trials have used neramexane for Alzheimer's disease, tinnitus, alcohol substitution, and pain. A phase III trial for moderate to severe Alzheimer's disease failed to achieve significance in the end points tested. For tinnitus, a phase III trial is ongoing.

Preliminary analgesic trials

In a rat model of diabetic neuropathic pain, treatment with neramexane (12.3, 24.6, and 49.2 mg/kg per day) for 2 weeks via an osmotic minipump significantly reduced symptoms of mechanical hyperalgesia and allodynia. Administration of memantine (20 mg/kg per day) was comparable to gabapentin (50 mg/kg per day) [3].

In a phase Ib human investigation the analgesic and anti-hyperalgesic properties of neramexane were tested in 18 subjects following intradermal capsaicin [4]. The patients received either a single dose of neramexane (40 mg PO), flupirtine (100 mg), or placebo in a double-blind, randomized, cross-over study. Pain intensity following intradermal capsaicin injection as well as pain evoked by pinpricks was significantly reduced by neramexane (−22% to −30% vs. placebo). Dynamic mechanical allodynia (pain to light touch) was also significantly attenuated by neramexane (−28% vs. placebo). Flupirtine showed no analgesic or anti-hyperalgesic effect. The finding that a single low dose of neramexane had a marked analgesic effect in a human surrogate model of neurogenic hyperalgesia could not be duplicated in a subsequent phase II trial [5].

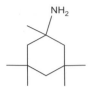

Figure 129.1.

Contraindications

Not available for clinical use.

Common doses/uses

Oral doses between 5–50 mg were used in the clinical trials [3].

Potential advantages/disadvantages

This drug is not available for clinical use, although it may be effective for neuropathic pain.

Drug-related adverse events

There were no serious adverse events in all the trials and no subjects were taken out of the trials for adverse

drug reactions. The most frequent adverse events were fatigue, daze, and dizziness [3].

References

1. Neramexane. *Drugs R D.* 2002;**3**(1):19–20.

2. Goldman-Sachs Global Healthcare. Goldman Sachs Global Healthcare Conference. Forest Laboratories Inc., Company Presentation, 2006.

3. Chen SR, Samoriski G, Pan HI. Antinociceptive effects of chronic administration of uncompetitive NMDA receptor antagonists in a rat model of diabetic neuropathic pain. *Neuropharmacology* 2009;**57**:121–126.

4. Klein T, Magerl A, Hanschmann M, et al. Antihyperalgesic and analgesic properties of the N-methyl-d-aspartate (NMDA) receptor antagonist neramexane in a human surrogate model of neurogenic hyperalgesia. *Eur J Pain* 2008;**12**:17–29.

5. Rammes G. Neramexane: a moderate-affinity NMDA receptor channel blocker: new prospects and indications. *Exp Rev Clin Pharmacol* 2009;**2**(3): 231–238.

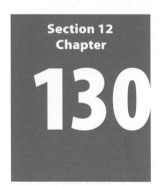

Section 12
Chapter

130

New and Emerging Analgesics

Nociceptin

Juan Jose Egas and Bijal Patel

Introduction

Nociceptin (orphanin FQ) is a novel neuropeptide whose actions have yet to be completely elucidated. However, stimulation of the nociceptin receptor has been implicated in the modulation of many neurobehavioral processes, including pain, substance dependence, sexual behavior, anxiety, locomotor activity, learning capacity, memory, and adaptation to stressful stimulus [1–6]. Continued research in this area has the potential to lead to a new class of drugs for pain medicine and beyond.

History

Detailed characterization of opioid receptors began in 1992 with the identification and cloning of the OP1 (delta) receptor, followed by subsequent identification and cloning of OP2 (kappa) and OP3 (mu) receptors. All of these receptors are G-coupled proteins that have seven transmembrane domains and share 60% of structural homology. In 1994, a new receptor subtype was identified and was originally given the name "opioid receptor like-1" (ORL-1). This subtype has typical opioid receptor characteristics, such as a G-coupled protein, seven transmembrane domains and also sharing up to 60% of structural homology with mu opioid receptors. This homology is particularly strong in the transmembrane domains and less in the extracellular domains (up to 80% in the second, third and seventh transmembrane domains) [1]. Its gene was localized to murine chromosome 2 and was named Oprl1 [2]. Despite this receptor's close homology to the traditional opioid receptors, investigators were initially unable to find an endogenous binding ligand, thus leading to its original classification as an orphan receptor [2]. However, 1 year after its discovery, an endogenous ligand neuropeptide was found simultaneously by two groups of investigators. A French group led by Meunier named the ligand nociceptin to denote its presumed pronociceptive activity, while a Swiss group led by Reinscheid named it orphanin FQ, referring to its affinity to the "orphan" opioid receptor [2].

The nociceptin/orphanin FQ neuropeptide

Like most neuropeptides, nociceptin/orphanin FQ (NC OF FQ) originates from a larger precursor peptide, in this case prepro-nociceptin, whose gene has been localized to chromosome 8 (8p21). Nociceptin/orphanin FQ is a heptadecapeptide, which also shares some structural homologies with the classic endogenous opioid neuropeptide dynorphin A. Both neuropeptides are composed of 17 amino acids, and contain the same last two amino acids at the carboxyl terminus [2]. Despite these structural similarities, both neuropeptides do not share cross affinity with their respective ligand receptors. NC OF FQ has no affinity to any of the traditional opioid receptors (does not bind or compete) and its actions cannot be antagonized by nonselective antagonists of opioid receptors, such as naloxone. NC OF FQ's affinity for traditional opioid receptors can be enhanced by replacing the alanine at position one by tyrosine. Although the tyrosine analog interacts with the traditional opioid receptors, it still preserves some affinity for OP4 receptors and can induce naloxone-resistant actions [2].

Stimulation of this receptor system by an agonist will elicit a pre-junctional inhibitory effect. It is believed that this inhibition occurs through the same cellular mechanisms and transduction pathways that occur with classic opioid receptor stimulation: (a) facilitating inward K^+ currents; (b) inhibition of Ca^{2+} entry to the cells through voltage-gated N-type calcium channels; (c) suppression of adenylate cyclase with a subsequent decrease of intracellular cAMP levels. All of these events will lead to an inhibition of neuronal excitability and a decrease of neurotransmitter release.

Nociceptin orphanin FQ CNS distribution

Research studies have identified the distribution of NC OF FQ and OLR-1 through mRNA detection techniques (which is the main determinant of active expression of the genes implicated in the synthesis of NC OF FQ). Through these techniques, this system was found to extend to many areas of the CNS, including the cortex, ventral forebrain, hypothalamus, amygdala, mammilary bodies, claustrum, anterior olfactory nucleus, hippocampus, mesolimbic pathways (nucleus accumbens), periaqueductal gray, pontine nuclei, interpeduncular nucleus, substantia nigra, raphe complex, locus coerulus, and ventral and dorsal horns of the spinal cord [2]. Receptors have also been found in the sympathetic, parasympathetic, and sensory nerves.

There have been conflicting data regarding the modulatory effects of nociceptin on pain. Both antinociception and pro-nociception effects have been noted by several authors. The route of administration and dose administered seem to be paramount as determinants of its predominant effect. A decrease in the nociceptive threshold is contradictory to the general belief that stimulation of opioid receptors produces analgesia and anti-hyperalgesia. In animal studies, intracerebroventricular (ICV) injections of NC OF FQ provided supraspinal analgesia including stress-induced-anti-nociception. Spinal administration of NC OF FQ produces a dose-dependent analgesia, giving a bell-shaped dose-response curve. Low doses of intrathecal NC OF FQ produce a spontaneous pain effect similar to that elicited by intrathecal administration of substance P and/or NMDA agonists. It is believed that this pro-nociceptive action of low-dose NC can be in part mediated by the activation of the substance P system [1]. The pro-nociceptive effect is reflected by caudally directed scratching, licking, and biting behaviors in test animals, all of which can be eliminated by pre-treatment with morphine, capsaicin, and neurokinin-1 receptor antagonists [1]. On the other hand, high doses of intrathecal NC produce analgesia similar to that evoked by classic opioid receptor agonists. Pre-treatment with high intrathecal doses of NC can block the scratching, bitting, and licking behaviors induced by intrathecal administration of substance P. Prolonged administration of NC will result in tolerance similar to that observed with opioid; however, there is no cross-tolerance noted between NC and morphine, indicating that the actions of the two compounds are mediated by different receptors [1].

Supraspinal effects of NC OF FQ can be pro-nociceptive and block analgesia provided by endogenous and exogenous opioid compounds. It can also counteract analgesia from alpha-2 receptor agonists (clonidine), GABA B receptor agonists (baclofen), and electroacupuncture [2]. It is believed its anti-analgesic effects are mediated through interactions at other sites of the neuronal circuit acting as a "functional antagonist" rather than a direct interaction with classic opioid receptors [2]. The pro-nociceptive action of NC OF FQ is completely absent in OP4 receptor knockout mice and, similar to the classic opioid receptors, prolonged stimulation of OP4 will produce tolerance to its anti-opioid effects [1]. At the same time, this pro-nociceptive, anti-analgesic effect of NC OF FQ has been questioned by several authors. An ICV injection may not be considered an ideal method for reproducing its true physiological role. Diffusion and spread of this compound will be dependent on a concentration gradient limiting its spread into deeper structures. There is also a question by using this route how it will affect populations of opioid-like receptors that would not be normally activated by endogenously released NC OF FQ [2].

Nociceptin/orphanin FQ in inflammatory pain models

It is well known that peripheral nerve injury or inflammatory states induce neuronal plastic changes in the spinal cord. These plasticity changes are responsible for the production and maintainance of persistent pain states, allodynia, and hyperalgesia occurring in both affected areas (primary sensitization) and non-affected areas (secondary sensitization). In inflammatory states, the NC OF FQ system is up-regulated [4]. This is reflected by increased NC levels and binding in the spinal cord, specifically at the level of the dorsal horns – mainly limited to the superficial laminae I and II. Inflammatory states also induce the expression of

the prepro-NC gene at the dorsal root ganglion, giving a short-lived burst of NC levels lasting for less than 6 hours [1].

Injection of CFA or formalin will induce tissue injury acompanied by an inflammatory state characterized by thermal hyperalgesia and mechanical allodynia [4,5]. Both effects are induced by an up-regulation of pro-inflammatory cytokines, nitric oxide synthase, and CGRP at the level of the dorsal root ganglion and spinal neurons [4]. It is widely accepted that pre-treatment with mu opioid agonists can prevent or reduce the formation of secondary hyperalgesia and allodynia after tissue injury [3]. This effect is a consequence of the inhibition of ascending excitatory nociceptive transmission pathways and activation of inhibitory systems with decreased propagation of action potentials in nociceptive neurons.

In animal studies using formalin for inducing inflammatory pain, morphine was compared to nociceptin efficacy in treating several stages of pain. It was shown that local, peripheral, and spinal morphine pre-treatment prevented both hyperalgesia and secondary allodynia from happening with a limited efficacy in treating pain once both phenomena are well established. Like morphine, local, peripheral, and spinal administration of nociceptin was also able to prevent or reduce both phenomena, but to a lesser extent. Post-treatment with NC was more effective than both morphine and pre-treatment with NC in reducing long-term effects of formalin in pain [3]. In another study, pre-treatment with NC produced a long-lasting attenuation of inflammatory pain after CFA injection by suppressing the up-regulation of inflammatory mediators and c-fos gene expression [4]. Through these data, we can conclude that NC OP FQ administration has the potential to both prevent the spinal cord sensitization induced by inflammatory states and suppress pain transmission in the spinal cord once the neuroplastic changes associated with sensitization are established.

Nociceptin/orphanin FQ agonists for substance abuse

In addition to pain modulation, nociceptin/orphanin FQ has been implicated in reducing, or even completely blocking, the rewarding effects and tolerance of substances that have abuse and dependency potential. NC and its receptor are located throughout the reward areas of the brain, including a high denisty of receptors in the central nucleus of the amygdala [7]. Several studies have shown that NC may block the rewarding properties of morphine. This action was demonstrated by blocking conditioned place preference (CPP – a possible indirect way to measure reward) through the ICV administration of NC in test animals that were given subcutaneous morphine [8]. The anti-tolerance and anti-addictive effects are limited not only to opioids, but potentially also extend to other substances such as cocaine, alcohol, and amphetamines [1,2,6]. This anti-addiction effect could give us the possibility of developing bifunctional opioids that will act on both mu opioid and NC receptors that could function as non-addictive analgesics, devoid of any abuse potential, or even lead to medications for treatment of drug addiction.

Theoretically, combination mu/NC agonists may be able to balance the therapeutic and side-effect profiles of opioid analgesics by reducing the reward effect and tolerance development. In a study using mice and bimodal opioids with both mu and NC activity, it was concluded that NC full agonist activity is required to attenuate morphine-induced rewarding effects. Between the compounds used with both NC partial and mu partial agonist activity, it was found that these compounds still have analgesic properties without the rewarding and addictive effects of pure mu opioid stimulation [6]. Likewise, kappa opioid receptor stimulation has also been implicated in reducing the rewarding effect of mu opioid stimulation and this is associated, as with NC receptor stimulation, to a decrease of dopamine release in the mesolimbic pathway (nucleus accumbens). Mixed kappa/mu opioid ligands, such as nalbuphine, have potent antinociceptive effects and are less addictive compared to morphine. It appears that a bifunctional compound with NC and mu agonist activity may be useful in decreasing opioid withdrawal and increasing compliance in addicts. Buprenorphine is a partial mu agonist that has been succesfully used to treat chronic pain and drug addiction, and this effect has been attributed in part to its ability to stimulate NC receptors [6].

Nociceptin/orphanin FQ as an anxiolytic

In animal studies, NC was shown to act as an anxiolytic by limiting the behavioral inhibition that would be associated with stressful/anxiety-provoking situations [1,7].

It was specifically found to play a role in the response to acute, extreme stress conditions, rather than affecting all aspects of the response to anxiety. The mechanism of action is not clearly understood; however, it is believed that its impact is focused on the inhibitory effects of NC on serotoninergic mechanisms primarily at two sites. The first site is the dorsal raphe nucleus neurons where NC increases K^+ conductance, thereby resulting in inhibition. NC is also believed to act on the cortical serotoninergic nerve terminals through the inhibition of 5-HT release. Additional studies have demonstrated that non-peptide OP4 agonists have anxiolytic effects, suggesting the possibility of a new class of anxiolytic medication without any abuse potential, such as is often seen with drugs such as benzodiazapenes [1].

Adverse effects

With the possibility of new drugs targeting NC and its receptor, one must consider the potential systemic effects with such administration. NC has the potential to effect systems such as the cardiovascular and renal systems. IV administration of NC resulted in species-based cardiovascular changes in test animals, showing transient hypotension and bradycardia in test rats, but an increase in both heart rate and blood pressure in sheep [1]. With regard to renal function, IV administration of NC resulted in increased water excretion and decreased urinary sodium excretion according to one study. This effect is probably due to the inhibition of oxytocin and vasopressin by NC. ICV injection of NC in test animals led to an increase in food consumption [1]. However, unlike other effects, this one was shown to be antagonized by naloxone.

Summary

The relatively recent discovery of the neuropeptide nociceptin/orphanin FQ, and its receptor system, offers the possibility of future treatment modalities in the field of pain medicine. As described, this system can play a role in pain relief, anxiolysis, and substance abuse associated with opioids, and other central-acting drugs. Although much research remains, these potential effects with regard to pain, anxiety, and substance abuse, as well as numerous other systemic effects, encourage further work in the area.

References

1. Calo G, et al. Pharmacology of the nociceptin receptor. *Br J Pharmacol* 2000;**129**:1261–1283.

2. Mogil J, et al. The molecular abd behavioral pharmacology of the orphanin FQ/nociceptin peptide and receptor family. *Pharmacol Rev* 2001;**53**:381–415.

3. Ambriz-Tututi M. Role of opioid receptor in formalin-induced secondary allodynia and hyperalgesia in rats. *Eur J Pharmacol* 2009;**619**:25–32.

4. Chen Y. Activation of the nociceptin opioid system in rat sensory neurons produces antinociceptive effects in inflammatory pain: involvement of inflammatory mediators. *J Neurosci Res* 2007;**85**:1478–1488.

5. Chen Y. Nociceptin and its receptor in rat dorsal root ganglion neurons in neuropathic and inflammatory

pain models: implications on pain processing. *J Peripher Nerv Syst* 2006;**11**:232–240.

6. Toll L. Comparison of the anti-nociceptive and anti-rewarding profiles of novel bifunction nociceptin/orphanin FQ receptor (NOPr)-mu opioid receptor (MOPr) ligands: implications for theurapeutic applications. *J Pharmacol Exp Ther* 2009;**331**(3):954–964.

7. Ciccocioppo R, et al. Nociceptin/orphanin FQ and drugs of abuse. *Peptides* 2000;**21**:1071–1080.

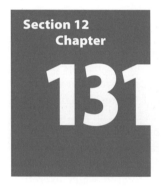

Section 12
Chapter

131

New and Emerging Analgesics

Anti-nerve growth factor

Allison Gandey and Roger Chou

Generic Names: nerve growth factor antibodies (anti-NGF)

Trade/Proprietary Names: Tanezumab™, Antibody PG110, JNJ-42160443

Drug Class: monoclonal antibody

Manufacturers: Pfizer Pharmaceuticals, 235 East 42nd Street, New York, NY 10017; PanGenetics BV, Heath House, Princes Mews, Royston, SG8 9RT, UK; Johnson and Johnson, One Johnson & Johnson Plaza, New Brunswick, NJ 08933

Description

Management of chronic pain is often challenging since commonly prescribed analgesics do not have direct effects on damaged nerves, but, rather, nonspecific effects on pain receptors and other mediators of pain. Neurotoxins are a new class of medications that are being evaluated as potential analgesics. Using these medications, researchers hope to achieve pain relief by suppressing the activity of injured nerve tissue and directly targeting the source of some types of chronic pain. A challenge in developing these medications is that in addition to affecting nerves causing pain, they could also damage other nerves, including those in the brain and spinal cord. Neurotoxins could therefore cause serious harm related to unintended nerve damage, and are undergoing careful testing to understand how well they selectively affect already damaged nerves.

Anti-nerve growth factor is the first highly selective neurotoxin to be investigated for use in humans. Discovered in the 1950s, investigators found that this immunotoxin stunts neural growth [1]. Researchers Rita Levi-Montalcini and Victor Hamburger observed that a substantial increase in the size of sympathetic ganglia coincided with the extensive branching of sympathetic axonal terminals in tumors. They reasoned that tumors were releasing a neurotrophin – a protein that promotes the growth and development of neurons.

The researchers named this sympathetic neurotrophin nerve growth factor and found that it could be administered to newborn mice to promote supernormal development of the sympathetic nervous system.

Rita Levi-Montalcini with biochemist Stanley Cohen went on to develop an immunotoxin to nerve growth factor and discovered that it severely suppressed growth and development of sympathetic noradrenergic neurons. For this and related findings, they were awarded the 1986 Nobel Prize in Medicine.

The use of anti-nerve growth factor antibodies for pain relief is experimental. Some studies have suggested that nerve growth factors can mediate injury-induced or inflammatory pain. Anti-nerve growth factor antibodies may prove to be effective in post-traumatic and post-surgical analgesia. Advocates suggest the agents will provide pain relief without impairing bone healing.

Tanezumab™

Pfizer's investigational drug Tanezumab is currently being studied for the treatment of a variety of painful conditions, such as osteoarthritis, pain associated with bone metastases, endometriosis, and low back pain [2].

Tanezumab is a monoclonal antibody that targets nerve growth factor. It is administered intravenously and has been linked to a number of adverse events, including abnormal peripheral sensation and neuropathy with hyperesthesia. This suggests that effects of Tanezumab are not completely selective for injured nerve tissue. More studies are needed to understand the frequency and severity of neuropathy, as well as how long such drug-induced symptoms persist.

A phase 3 trial evaluating the efficacy and safety of Tanezumab in osteoarthritis of the knee is currently recruiting patients. A similar trial evaluating three doses of tanezumab in osteoarthritis of the hip is also under way.

Results from a phase 2 trial of the investigational drug in chronic low back pain suggest it reduced pain and improved physical function more effectively than naproxen [3].

The 220 trial participants had chronic nonradiculopathic low back pain for at least 3 months that required regular analgesic medication. Investigators report a single intravenous infusion of Tanezumab 200 μg/kg provided durable efficacy over a 12-week period (Table 131.1).

Table 131.1. Patients achieving ≥50% treatment response

Treatment	Week 6 (%)	Week 12 (%)
Tanezumab	56.8	48.9
Naproxen	34.1	34.1
Placebo	19.5	29.3

The researchers report abnormal peripheral sensation in 12.5% of those taking Tanezumab, 3.4% of those taking naproxen, and 2.4% of those on placebo. There were two cases of severe hyperesthesia in the Tanezumab group. There was also a case of peripheral neuropathy with hyperesthesia.

The analgesic effect of Tanezumab appears promising, but more research is needed to understand how it would be used to manage chronic pain. Even if it is shown to be more effective than standard medications, peripheral neuropathy is a potentially serious adverse event that could limit its use as a first-line medication. Also, the cost of Tanezumab has not yet been determined. In addition to the price of Tanezumab itself, an additional cost consideration is that it is administered intravenously [4]. Compared to other medications for chronic pain, a potential advantage of Tanezumab is that it is dosed infrequently.

Antibody PG110

PanGenetics Limited is investigating another nerve growth factor inhibitor. The investigational agent known as PG110 is being studied for the treatment of osteoarthritis pain.

The humanized antibody is administered intravenously. A phase 1 study evaluating the safety and tolerability of PG110 is currently recruiting participants. The randomized, double-blind, placebo-controlled, single-ascending-dose trial will evaluate PG110 in patients with pain from osteoarthritis of the knee.

Potential adverse events remain unknown, but, like Tanezumab, this nerve growth factor inhibitor may be linked to abnormal peripheral sensation, neuropathy, and hyperesthesia. PG110 is also administered intravenously.

Many questions remain about the analgesic potential of anti-nerve growth factor antibodies. The new drugs could provide an exciting treatment alternative affording potent analgesia without impairing bone healing. Possible benefits will have to be weighed carefully against the risks of these powerful and potentially harmful neurotoxins.

References

1. Kostrzewa RM. Evolution of neurotoxins: from research modalities to clinical realities. *Curr Protoc Neurosci* 2009; Unit 1.18.

2. ClinicalTrials.gov.

3. American Pain Society 28th Annual Meeting: Poster 268 presented May 7, 2009.

4. Gandey A. Tanezumab investigated for low back pain. *Medscape Medical News*. http://www.medscape.com/viewarticle/703204.

Index

515

529